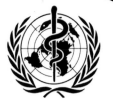

World Health Organization Classification of Tumours

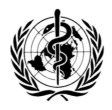

WHO   OMS

International Agency for Research on Cancer (IARC)

Pathology and Genetics of Tumours of Soft Tissue and Bone

Edited by

Christopher D.M. Fletcher
K. Krishnan Unni
Fredrik Mertens

IARCPress
Lyon, 2002

World Health Organization Classification of Tumours

Series Editors   Paul Kleihues, M.D.
Leslie H. Sobin, M.D.

Pathology and Genetics of Tumours of Soft Tissue and Bone

Editors   Christopher D.M. Fletcher, M.D.
K. Krishnan Unni, M.D.
Fredrik Mertens, M.D.

Coordinating Editor   Wojciech Biernat, M.D.

Layout   Lauren A. Hunter

Illustrations   Lauren A. Hunter
Georges Mollon

Printed by   LIPS
69009 Lyon, France

Publisher   IARCPress
International Agency for
Research on Cancer (IARC)
69008 Lyon, France

This volume was produced in collaboration with the

International Academy of Pathology (IAP)

The WHO Classification of Tumours of Soft Tissue and Bone
presented in this book reflects the views of a
Working Group that convened for an
Editorial and Consensus Conference in
Lyon, France, April 24-28, 2002.

Members of the Working Group are indicated
in the List of Contributors on page 369.

Published by IARC Press, International Agency for Research on Cancer,
150 cours Albert Thomas, F-69008 Lyon, France

Enquiries should be addressed to the
Communications Unit, International Agency for Research on Cancer, 69008 Lyon, France,
which will provide the latest information on any changes made to the text and plans for new editions.

Format for bibliographic citations:
Fletcher C.D.M., Unni K.K., Mertens F. (Eds.): World Health Organization
Classification of Tumours. Pathology and Genetics of Tumours of Soft Tissue
and Bone. IARC Press: Lyon 2002

IARC Library Cataloguing in Publication Data

Pathology and genetics of tumours of soft tissue and bone /
        editors, C.D.M. Fletcher ... [et al.]

        (World Health Organization classification of tumours ; 4)

        1. Bone Neoplasms 2. Genetics 3. Pathology
        4. Soft Tissue Neoplasms   I. Fletcher, C.D.M.
        II. Series

        ISBN 92 832 2413 2   (NLM Classification: W1)

Contents

WHO Classification of Soft Tissue Tumours

This new WHO classification of soft tissue tumours, in line with other volumes in this new series, incorporates detailed clinical, histological and genetic data. The explosion of cytogenetic and molecular genetic information in this field over the past 10-15 years has had significant impact on soft tissue tumour classification and also on our understanding of their biology.

The major changes which are reflected in the new classification include a revised categorization of biological behaviour which allows for two distinct types of intermediate malignancy, identified respectively as 'locally aggressive' and 'rarely metastasizing'. The new classification, most importantly, acknowledges the poorly defined nature of the categories known as malignant fibrous histiocytoma (MFH) (which in reality represents undifferentiated pleomorphic sarcoma) and haemangiopericytoma (most examples of which are closely related to solitary fibrous tumour). The uncertain line of differentiation in so-called angiomatoid MFH and extraskeletal myxoid chondrosarcoma has resulted in their reclassification into the chapter of Tumours of uncertain differentiation. However, the Working Group has avoided changes in nomenclature until these tumour types are better understood, for fear of causing confusion in routine clinical practice. Multiple newly recognized entities, which have become established since the 1994 classification, are now included and it seems likely that this trend of clinically relevant and carefully defined subclassification of soft tissue tumours will continue in the future.

WHO classification of soft tissue tumours

ADIPOCYTIC TUMOURS

Benign
Lipoma	8850/0*
Lipomatosis	8850/0
Lipomatosis of nerve	8850/0
Lipoblastoma / Lipoblastomatosis	8881/0
Angiolipoma	8861/0
Myolipoma	8890/0
Chondroid lipoma	8862/0
Extrarenal angiomyolipoma	8860/0
Extra-adrenal myelolipoma	8870/0
Spindle cell/	8857/0
Pleomorphic lipoma	8854/0
Hibernoma	8880/0

Intermediate (locally aggressive)
Atypical lipomatous tumour/	
Well differentiated liposarcoma	8851/3

Malignant
Dedifferentiated liposarcoma	8858/3
Myxoid liposarcoma	8852/3
Round cell liposarcoma	8853/3
Pleomorphic liposarcoma	8854/3
Mixed-type liposarcoma	8855/3
Liposarcoma, not otherwise specified	8850/3

FIBROBLASTIC / MYOFIBROBLASTIC TUMOURS

Benign
Nodular fasciitis	
Proliferative fasciitis	
Proliferative myositis	
Myositis ossificans	
fibro-osseous pseudotumour of digits	
Ischaemic fasciitis	
Elastofibroma	8820/0
Fibrous hamartoma of infancy	
Myofibroma / Myofibromatosis	8824/0
Fibromatosis colli	
Juvenile hyaline fibromatosis	
Inclusion body fibromatosis	
Fibroma of tendon sheath	8810/0
Desmoplastic fibroblastoma	8810/0
Mammary-type myofibroblastoma	8825/0

Calcifying aponeurotic fibroma	8810/0
Angiomyofibroblastoma	8826/0
Cellular angiofibroma	9160/0
Nuchal-type fibroma	8810/0
Gardner fibroma	8810/0
Calcifying fibrous tumour	
Giant cell angiofibroma	9160/0

Intermediate (locally aggressive)
Superficial fibromatoses (palmar / plantar)	
Desmoid-type fibromatoses	8821/1
Lipofibromatosis	

Intermediate (rarely metastasizing)
Solitary fibrous tumour	8815/1
and haemangiopericytoma	9150/1
(incl. lipomatous haemangiopericytoma)	
Inflammatory myofibroblastic tumour	8825/1
Low grade myofibroblastic sarcoma	8825/3
Myxoinflammatory	
fibroblastic sarcoma	8811/3
Infantile fibrosarcoma	8814/3

Malignant
Adult fibrosarcoma	8810/3
Myxofibrosarcoma	8811/3
Low grade fibromyxoid sarcoma	8811/3
hyalinizing spindle cell tumour	
Sclerosing epithelioid fibrosarcoma	8810/3

SO-CALLED FIBROHISTIOCYTIC TUMOURS

Benign
Giant cell tumour of tendon sheath	9252/0
Diffuse-type giant cell tumour	9251/0
Deep benign fibrous histiocytoma	8830/0

Intermediate (rarely metastasizing)
Plexiform fibrohistiocytic tumour	8835/1
Giant cell tumour of soft tissues	9251/1

Malignant
Pleomorphic 'MFH' / Undifferentiated	
pleomorphic sarcoma	8830/3
Giant cell 'MFH' / Undifferentiated	
pleomorphic sarcoma	
with giant cells	8830/3
Inflammatory 'MFH' / Undifferentiated	
pleomorphic sarcoma with	
prominent inflammation	8830/3

---

* Morphology code of the International Classification of Diseases for Oncology (ICD-O) {726} and the Systematize Nomenclature of Medicine (http://snomed.org).

SMOOTH MUSCLE TUMOURS
Angioleiomyoma	8894/0
Deep leiomyoma	8890/0
Genital leiomyoma	8890/0
Leiomyosarcoma (excluding skin)	8890/3

PERICYTIC (PERIVASCULAR) TUMOURS
Glomus tumour (and variants)	8711/0
malignant glomus tumour	8711/3
Myopericytoma	8713/1

SKELETAL MUSCLE TUMOURS

Benign
Rhabdomyoma	8900/0
adult type	8904/0
fetal type	8903/0
genital type	8905/0

Malignant
Embryonal rhabdomyosarcoma	8910/3
(incl. spindle cell,	8912/3
botryoid, anaplastic)	8910/3
Alveolar rhabdomyosarcoma	
(incl. solid, anaplastic)	8920/3
Pleomorphic rhabdomyosarcoma	8901/3

VASCULAR TUMOURS

Benign
Haemangiomas of	
subcut/deep soft tissue:	9120/0
capillary	9131/0
cavernous	9121/0
arteriovenous	9123/0
venous	9122/0
intramuscular	9132/0
synovial	9120/0
Epithelioid haemangioma	9125/0
Angiomatosis	
Lymphangioma	9170/0

Intermediate (locally aggressive)
Kaposiform haemangioendothelioma	9130/1

Intermediate (rarely metastasizing)
Retiform haemangioendothelioma	9135/1
Papillary intralymphatic angioendothelioma	9135/1
Composite haemangioendothelioma	9130/1
Kaposi sarcoma	9140/3

Malignant
Epithelioid haemangioendothelioma	9133/3
Angiosarcoma of soft tissue	9120/3

CHONDRO-OSSEOUS TUMOURS
Soft tissue chondroma	9220/0
Mesenchymal chondrosarcoma	9240/3
Extraskeletal osteosarcoma	9180/3

TUMOURS OF UNCERTAIN DIFFERENTIATION

Benign
Intramuscular myxoma	8840/0
(incl. cellular variant)	
Juxta-articular myxoma	8840/0
Deep ('aggressive') angiomyxoma	8841/0
Pleomorphic hyalinizing	
angiectatic tumour	
Ectopic hamartomatous thymoma	8587/0

Intermediate (rarely metastasizing)
Angiomatoid fibrous histiocytoma	8836/1
Ossifying fibromyxoid tumour	8842/0
(incl. atypical / malignant)	
Mixed tumour/	8940/1
Myoepithelioma/	8982/1
Parachordoma	9373/1

Malignant
Synovial sarcoma	9040/3
Epithelioid sarcoma	8804/3
Alveolar soft part sarcoma	9581/3
Clear cell sarcoma of soft tissue	9044/3
Extraskeletal myxoid chondrosarcoma	9231/3
("chordoid" type)	
PNET / Extraskeletal Ewing tumour	
pPNET	9364/3
extraskeletal Ewing tumour	9260/3
Desmoplastic small round cell tumour	8806/3
Extra-renal rhabdoid tumour	8963/3
Malignant mesenchymoma	8990/3
Neoplasms with perivascular epithelioid	
cell differentiation (PEComa)	
clear cell myomelanocytic tumour	
Intimal sarcoma	8800/3

Soft tissue tumours: Epidemiology, clinical features, histopathological typing and grading

C.D.M. Fletcher
A. Rydholm
S. Singer

M. Sundaram
J.M. Coindre

The large majority of soft tissue tumours are benign, with a very high cure rate after surgical excision. Malignant mesenchymal neoplasms amount to less than 1% of the overall human burden of malignant tumours but they are life-threatening and may pose a significant diagnostic and therapeutic challenge since there are more than 50 histological subtypes of STS, which are often associated with unique clinical, prognostic and therapeutic features. Over the past decade, our understanding of these neoplasms has increased significantly, both from a histopathological and genetic point of view. The close interaction of surgical pathologists, surgeons and oncologists has brought about a significant increase in disease-free survival for tumours which were previously almost invariably fatal {1960}, the overall 5-year survival rate for STS in the limbs now being in the order of 65-75% {1960}. Careful physical examination and radiographic evaluation to evaluate the size, depth and location of the mass, along with signs of neurovascular involvement are essential for designing the best therapeutic approach.approach.

Epidemiology

Benign mesenchymal tumours outnumber sarcomas by a factor of at least 100. The annual clinical incidence (number of new patients consulting a doctor) of benign soft tissue tumours has been estimated as up to 3000/million population {1830} whereas the annual incidence of soft tissue sarcoma is around 30/million {861,1663}, i.e. less than 1 percent of all malignant tumours. There are no data to indicate a change in the incidence of sarcoma nor are there significant geographic differences.

Age and site distribution

At least one-third of the *benign tumours* are lipomas, one-third fibrohistiocytic and fibrous tumours, 10 percent vascular tumours and 5 percent nerve sheath tumours. There is a relation between the type of tumour, symptoms, location and patient's age and gender. Lipomas are painless, rare in hand, lower leg and foot and very uncommon in children {1830}, multiple (angio)lipomas are sometimes painful and most common in young men, angioleiomyomas are often painful and common in lower leg of middle-aged women, whereas half of the vascular tumours occur in patients younger than 20 years {1524}. Of the benign soft tissue tumours 99% are superficial and 95% are less than 5 cm in diameter {1524}.

Soft tissue sarcomas may occur anywhere but three fourths are located in the extremities (most common in thigh) and 10 percent each in the trunk wall and retroperitoneum. There is a slight male predominance. Like almost all other malignancies, soft tissue sarcomas become more common with increasing age; the median age is 65 years. Of the extremity and trunk wall tumours one-third are superficial with a median diameter of 5 cm and two-thirds are deep-seated with a median diameter of 9 cm {861}. Retroperitoneal tumours are often much larger before they become symptomatic. One tenth of the patients have detectable metastases (most common in the lungs) at diagnosis of the primary tumour. Overall, at least one-third of the patients with soft tissue sarcoma die because of tumour, most of them because of lung metastases.

Three fourths of soft tissue sarcomas are histologically classified as high grade pleomorphic (malignant fibrous histiocytoma [MFH]-like) sarcoma, liposarcoma, leiomyosarcoma, synovial sarcoma, and malignant peripheral nerve sheath tumours and three fourths are highly malignant (histological malignancy-grades 2 and 3 in three-tiered grading systems, grades 3 and 4 in four-tiered systems) {861}. The distribution of histotypes varies over time and between researchers, probably because of changing definitions of histotypes (compare the evolution of the concept of MFH, page 120). The age-related incidences vary; embryonal rhabdomyosarcoma occurs almost exclusively in children, synovial sarcoma mostly in young adults, whereas pleomorphic high grade sarcoma, liposarcoma and leiomyosarcoma dominate in the elderly.

Aetiology

The aetiology of most benign and malignant soft tissue tumours is unknown. In rare cases, genetic and environmental factors, irradiation, viral infections and immune deficiency have been found associated with the development of usually malignant soft tissue tumours. There are also isolated reports of soft tissue sarcomas arising in scar tissue, at fracture sites and close to surgical implants {1125}. However, the large majority of soft tissue sarcomas seem to arise de novo, without an apparent causative factor. Some malignant mesenchymal neoplasms occur in the setting of familial cancer syndromes (see below and Chapter 21). Multistage tumourigenesis sequences with gradual accumulation of genetic alterations and increasing histological malignancy have not yet been clearly identified in soft tissue tumours.

Chemical carcinogens

Several studies, many of them from Sweden, have reported an increased incidence of soft tissue sarcoma after exposure to phenoxyacetic herbicides, chlorophenols, and their contaminants (dioxin) in agricultural or forestry work {607,608}. Other studies have not found this association. One explanation for different findings may be the use of herbicides with different dioxin contaminations {4,2333}.

Radiation

The reported incidence of post-irradiation sarcoma ranges from some few per thousand to nearly one percent. Most incidence estimates are based on breast cancer patients treated with radiation as adjuvant therapy {1070}. The risk increases with dose; most patients have received 50 Gy or more and the median time between exposure and tumour diagnosis is about 10 years, although there is some evidence that this latent interval is decreasing. More than half of the tumours have been classified as so-called malignant fibrous histiocytoma, most often highly malignant. Patients with a germline mutation in the retinoblastomas gene (*RB1*) have a significantly elevated risk of developing post-irradiation sarcomas, usually osteosarcomas.

Viral infection and immunodeficiency
Human herpes virus 8 plays a key role in the development of Kaposi sarcoma and the clinical course is dependent on the immune status of the patient {2232}. Epstein-Barr virus is associated with smooth muscle tumours in patients with immunodeficiency {1368}. Stewart-Treves syndrome, development of angiosarcoma in chronic lymphoedema, particularly after radical mastectomy, has by some authors been attributed to regional acquired immunodeficiency {1895}.

Genetic susceptibility
Several types of benign soft tissue tumour have been reported to occur on a familial or inherited basis (for review see Chapter 21 and reference {2242}). However these reports are rare and comprise an insignificant number of tumours. The most common example is probably hereditary multiple lipomas (often angiolipomas) {1062}. Desmoid tumours occur in patients with the familial Gardner syndrome (including adenomatous polyposis, osteomas and epidermal cysts) {859}. Neurofibromatosis (types 1 and 2) is associated with multiple benign nerve tumours (and sometimes also non-neural tumours). In around 2% of the patients with neurofibromatosis type1 malignant peripheral nerve sheath tumours develop in a benign nerve sheath tumour {1997}. The Li-Fraumeni syndrome {954} is a rare autosomal dominant disease caused by germline mutations in the *TP53* tumour suppressor gene, which seems to be of importance for sarcomagenesis. Half of the patients have already developed malignant tumours at age 30, among them, in more

than 30% of cases, soft tissue and bone sarcomas. The inherited, or bilateral form of retinoblastoma, with a germline mutation of the *RB1* locus, may also be associated with sarcoma development.

Clinical features
Benign soft tissue tumours outnumber sarcomas by at least 100 to 1, although it is almost impossible to derive accurate numbers in this regard. Most benign lesions are located in superficial (dermal or subcutaneous) soft tissue. By far the most frequent benign lesion is lipoma, which often goes untreated. Some benign lesions have distinct clinical features but most do not. Some non-metastasizing lesions, such as desmoid-type fibromatosis or intramuscular haemangioma, require wide excision comparable to a sarcoma, otherwise local recurrence is very frequent. Since excisional biopsy or 'shelling out' of a sarcoma is inappropriate and often may cause difficulties in further patient management, then it is generally advisable to obtain a diagnostic biopsy (prior to definitive treatment) for all soft tissue masses >5 cm (unless a very obvious subcutaneous lipoma) and for all subfascial or deep-seated masses, almost irrespective of size.
Most soft tissue sarcomas of the extremities and trunk wall present as painless, accidentally observed tumours, which do not influence function or general health despite the often large tumour volume. The seemingly innocent presentation and the rarity of soft tissue sarcomas often lead to misinterpretation as benign conditions. Epidemiological data regarding size and depth distribution for benign and malignant soft tissue tumours in Sweden have been used to formulate simple guidelines for the suspicion of a sarcoma: superficial soft tissue lesions that are larger than 5 cm and all deep-seated (irrespective of size) have such a high risk (around 10 percent) of being a sarcoma {1524,1830} that such patients should ideally be referred to a specialized tumour centre before surgery for optimal treatment {143,862,1831}.

Imaging of soft tissue tumours
Magnetic resonance imaging (MRI) is the modality of choice for detecting, characterizing, and staging soft tissue tumours due to its ability to distinguish tumour tissue from adjacent muscle and fat, as well

as to define relationships to key neurovascular bundles. Additionally, it aids in guiding biopsy, planning surgery, evaluating response to chemotherapy, restaging, and in the long-term follow-up for local recurrence. Although MR imaging may not always reliably predict the histological diagnosis of a mass or its potential biologic activity, several conditions can be reliably diagnosed based on their characteristic pathological and signal pattern, location of mass, relationship to adjacent structures, multiplicity, and clinical history. MR imaging accurately defines tumour size, relationship to muscle compartments, fascial planes, and bone and neurovascular structures in multiple planes; it provides information on haemorrhage, necrosis, oedema, cystic and myxoid degeneration, and fibrosis.
MR imaging provides better tissue discrimination between normal and abnormal tissues than any other imaging modality. Most masses show a long T1 and long T2. However, there are a group of lesions that show a short T1 and short T2. Masses with relatively high signal intensity on T1 are lipoma, well-differentiated liposarcoma, haemangioma, subacute haemorrhage, and some examples of Ewing sarcoma/peripheral PNET. Clumps or streaks of high signal within the low signal intensity mass on T1-weighted sequences might be encountered in haemangioma, myxoid liposarcoma, infiltrative intramuscular lipoma, and lipomatosis of nerve. Tumours that may have a low signal on T2 include diffuse-type giant cell tumour, clear-cell sarcoma and fibromatosis. Soft tissue masses that do not demonstrate tumour-specific features on MR imaging should be considered indeterminate and biopsy should always be obtained to exclude malignancy.

MRI-guided biopsy. Radiologists should be cautious when asked to perform biopsies of indeterminate soft tissue tumours. Caution has to be exercised in three respects: Selection of an appropriate pathway, coordination with the treating surgeon, and participation of a pathologist comfortable with interpreting percutaneous biopsies. The radiologist should undertake biopsies only at the request of the treating surgeon and not necessarily at the request of the patient's initial physician. In collaboration with the treating surgeon, the needle tract (which needs to be excised with the tumour) can be established and the patient well served.

Spiral CT is preferable for examining sarcomas of the chest and abdomen, since air / tissue interface and motion artefacts often degrade MRI quality. A baseline chest CT scan at the time of diagnosis for evidence of lung metastasis is important, particularly for sarcomas >5 cm, for accurate staging of patients. Early studies suggest that *positron emission tomography (PET)* has clinical potential by determining biological activity of soft tissue masses {522,565,700,1293}. The technique is selectively used for distinguishing benign tumours from high grade sarcomas, pretreatment grading of sarcomas, and evaluation of local recurrence. Its role, vis-à-vis, MR imaging which remains the mainstay, is yet to be defined.

Biopsy

Given the prognostic and therapeutic importance of accurate diagnosis, a biopsy is necessary (and appropriate) to establish malignancy, to assess histological grade, and to determine the specific histological type of sarcoma, if possible. A treatment plan can then be designed that is tailored to a lesion's predicted pattern of local growth, risk of metastasis, and likely sites of distant spread. A large enough sample from a viable area of sarcoma is usually required for definitive diagnosis and accurate grading. Most limb masses are generally best sampled through a longitudinally oriented incision, so that the entire biopsy tract can be completely excised at the time of definitive resection. An incisional biopsy with minimal extension into adjacent tissue planes is the ideal approach for most extremity masses. Excisional biopsy should be avoided, particularly for lesions greater than 2 cm in size, since such an approach will make definitive re-excision more extensive due to the contamination of surrounding tissue planes. For deep-seated lesions, a core biopsy approach may be used to establish a diagnosis, however, the limited tissue obtained with this technique may make definitive grading and prognostication difficult. Fine needle aspiration (FNA) cytology is generally best limited to those centres with a high case volume and with a well-integrated multidisciplinary team,

since careful clinicoradiologic correlation and considerable experience are required in order to make accurate diagnoses. A particular problem with needle biopsies and FNA is the inevitability of limited sampling, which impacts not only diagnostic accuracy but also the possibility of triaging tissue for ancillary diagnostic techniques such as cytogenetics and electron microscopy.

Terminology regarding biological potential

As part of this new WHO classification of Soft Tissue Tumours, the Working Group wished to address the problems which have existed regarding definition of a lesion's biological potential, particularly with regard to the current ambiguity of such terms as 'intermediate malignancy' or 'borderline malignant potential.' With this goal in mind, it is recommended to divide soft tissue tumours into the following four categories: benign, intermediate (locally aggressive), intermediate (rarely metastasizing) and malignant. Definitions of these categories are as follows:

Benign

Most benign soft tissue tumours do not recur locally. Those that do recur do so in a non-destructive fashion and are almost always readily cured by complete local excision. Exceedingly rarely (almost certainly <1/50,000 cases, and probably much less than that), a morphologically benign lesion may give rise to distant metastases. This is entirely unpredictable on the basis of conventional histological examination and, to date has been best documented in cutaneous benign fibrous histiocytoma.

Intermediate (locally aggressive)

Soft tissue tumours in this category often recur locally and are associated with an infiltrative and locally destructive growth pattern. Lesions in this category do not have any evident potential to metastasize but typically require wide excision with a margin of normal tissue in order to ensure local control. The prototypical lesion in this category is desmoid fibromatosis.

Intermediate (rarely metastasizing)

Soft tissue tumours in this category are often locally aggressive (see above) but, in addition, show the well-documented ability to give rise to distant metastases

FNCLCC grading system: definition of parameters

Tumour differentiation	
Score 1:	sarcomas closely resembling normal adult mesenchymal tissue (e.g., low grade leiomyosarcoma).
Score 2:	sarcomas for which histological typing is certain (e.g., myxoid liposarcoma).
Score 3:	embryonal and undifferentiated sarcomas, sarcomas of doubtful type, synovial sarcomas, osteosarcomas, PNET.

Mitotic count	
Score 1:	0-9 mitoses per 10 HPF*
Score 2:	10-19 mitoses per 10 HPF
Score 3:	≥20 mitoses per 10 HPF

Tumour necrosis	
Score 0:	no necrosis
Score 1:	<50% tumour necrosis
Score 2:	≥50% tumour necrosis

Histological grade	
Grade 1:	total score 2,3
Grade 2:	total score 4,5
Grade 3:	total score 6, 7, 8

Modified from Trojani et al. {2131}.
PNET: primitive neuroectodermal tumour
*A high power field (HPF) measures 0.1734 mm^2

in occasional cases. The risk of such metastases appears to be <2% and is not reliably predictable on the basis of histomorphology. Metastasis in such lesions is usually to lymph node or lung. Prototypical examples in this category include plexiform fibrohistiocytic tumour and so-called angiomatoid fibrous histiocytoma.

Malignant

In addition to the potential for locally destructive growth and recurrence, malignant soft tissue tumours (known as soft tissue sarcomas) have significant risk of distant metastasis, ranging in most instances from 20% to almost 100%, depending upon histological type and grade. Some (but not all) histologically low grade sarcomas have a metastatic risk of only 2-10%, but such lesions may advance in grade in a local recurrence, and thereby acquire a higher risk of distant spread (e.g., myxofibrosarcoma and leiomyosarcoma).

It is important to note, that in this new classification scheme, the intermediate categories do not correspond to histologically determined intermediate grade in a soft tissue sarcoma (see below), nor do they correspond to the ICD-O/1 category described as uncertain whether benign or malignant. The locally aggressive subset with no metastatic potential, as defined above, are generally given ICD-O/1 codes , while the rarely metastasizing lesions are given ICD-O/3 codes.

Histological grading of soft tissue sarcomas

The histological type of sarcomas does not always provide sufficient information for predicting the clinical course and therefore for planning therapy. Grading, based on histological parameters only, evaluates the degree of malignancy and mainly the probability of distant metastasis. Staging, based on both clinical and histological parameters, provides information on the extent of the tumour.

The concept of grading in STS was first properly introduced by Russell et al in 1977 {1826}, and was the most important factor of their clinico-pathological classification. Several grading systems, based on various histological parameters, have been published and proved to correlate with prognosis {401,1335,1525,2131, 2183}. The two most important parameters seem to be the mitotic index and the extent of tumour necrosis {401,2131, 2183}. A three-grade system is recommended, retaining an intermediate histological grade (grade 2) of malignancy. Grade particularly indicates the probability of distant metastasis and overall survival {50,155,385,773,930,1335,1711, 1833}, but is of poor value for predicting local recurrence which is mainly related to the quality of surgical margins. Moreover, the initial response to chemotherapy has been reported to be better in patients with a high grade tumour than in patients with a low grade one {385,672}.

The two most widely used systems are the NCI (United States National Cancer Institute) system {401,402} and the FNCLCC (French Fédération Nationale des Centres de Lutte Contre le Cancer) system {385,386,387,851,2131}.

According to the methodology defined in 1984 {401} and refined in 1999 {402}, the NCI system uses a combination of histological type, cellularity, pleomorphism

Comparison of the NCI and FNCLCC systems for the histological grading of soft tissue tumours

Histological type	NCI grading system	FNCLCC grading system
Well differentiated liposarcoma	1+(*)	1
Myxoid liposarcoma	1+	2
High grade myxoid liposarcoma (round cell liposarcoma)	2-(**) 3	3
Pleomorphic liposarcoma	2 3	3
Dedifferentiated liposarcoma		3
Fibrosarcoma		
Well differentiated	1+	1
Conventional	2	2
Poorly differentiated	3	3
Pleomorphic sarcoma (MFH, pleomorphic type)		
With storiform pattern	2	2
Patternless pleomorphic sarcoma	3	3
With giant cells		3
With prominent inflammation		3
Myxofibrosarcoma (MFH, myxoid-type)	1+ 2 3	2
Leiomyosarcoma		
Well differentiated	1+	1
Conventional	2	2
Poorly differentiated / pleomorphic / epithelioid	3	3
Pleomorphic rhabdomyosarcoma	2 3	3
Embryonal / alveolar rhabdomyosarcomas	3	3
Myxoid chondrosarcoma	1 2 3	
Mesenchymal chondrosarcoma	3	3
Osteosarcoma	3	3
Ewing sarcoma / PNET	3	3
Synovial sarcoma	2 3	3
Epithelioid sarcoma	2 3	
Clear cell sarcoma	2 3	
Angiosarcoma	2 3	

Modified from Costa et al {401}, Costa {402} and Guillou {851}. The original diagnostic terms are shown in parentheses.
MFH: malignant fibrous histiocytoma; PNET: primitive neuroectodermal tumour.
(*) + grade is attributed by a combination of histological type, cellularity, pleomorphism and mitotic rate.
(**) - grade is attributed according to the extent of tumour necrosis (< or > 15%).

and mitotic rate for attributing grade 1 or 3. All the other types of sarcomas were classified as either grade 2 or grade 3 depending on the amount of tumour necrosis, with 15% necrosis as the threshold for separation of grade 2 and grade 3 lesions.

The FNCLCC system is based on a score obtained by evaluating three parameters selected after multivariate analysis of several histological features: tumour differentiation, mitotic rate and amount of tumour necrosis {2131}. A score is attributed independently to each parameter and the grade is obtained by adding the three attributed scores. Tumour differentiation is highly dependent on histological type and subtype {851}. The reproducibility of this system was tested by 15 pathologists: the crude proportion in agreement was 75% for tumour grade but only 61% for histological type {387}. Guillou et al. {851} performed a comparative study of the NCI and FNCLCC sys-

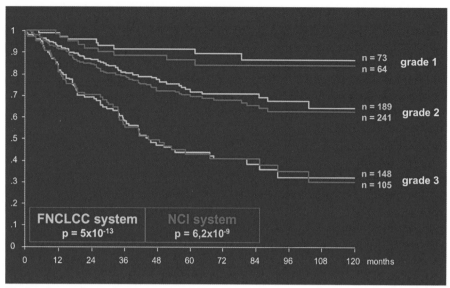

Fig. A.1 Comparison of overall survival curves for a cohort of 410 patients with soft tissue sarcomas graded according to the NCI and FNCLCC systems. Reproduced from Guillou et al {851}.

tems on a subgroup of 410 patients. In univariate analysis both systems were of good prognostic value, although grade discrepancies were observed in 34% of the cases. In the NCI system, there were more grade 2 tumours, and use of the FNCLCC resulted in a better correlation with overall and metastasis-free survival. Because of some limitations and pitfalls of grading, some rules must be respected in order to get the highest performance and reproducibility of the system:
>Grading should be used only for untreated primary soft tissue sarcomas.
>Grading should be performed on representative and well processed material.
>Grading is not a substitute for a histological diagnosis and does not differentiate benign and malignant lesions, and, before grading a soft tissue lesion, one must be sure that one is dealing with a true sarcoma and not a pseudosarcoma.
>Grading is not applicable to all types of soft tissue sarcoma. Because of the over- all rarity of STS, grade is used on the whole group of sarcomas considered as a single entity, but the significance of the histological parameters used in grading systems differs for various sarcomas. Therefore, grade is of no prognostic value for some histological types, such as MPNST {386,902} and its use is not recommended for angiosarcoma, extraskeletal myxoid chondrosarcoma, alveolar soft part sarcoma, clear cell sarcoma and epithelioid sarcoma {5,851,1102} . In a recent study {386}, it was shown that the FNCLCC grading was the most important predictive factor for metastasis for pleomorphic sarcomas, unclassified sarcomas and synovial sarcomas and the second and third independent factor for leiomyosarcomas and liposarcomas.

Parameters of grading must be carefully evaluated and, particularly, mitosis counting should be done rigorously.

Staging

Staging of soft tissue sarcomas is based on both histological and clinical information. The major staging system used for STS was developed by the International Union against Cancer (UICC) and the American Joint Committee on Cancer (AJCC) and appears to be clinically useful and of prognostic value. This TNM system incorporates histological grade as well as tumour size and depth, regional lymph node involvement and distant metastasis. It accommodates 2, 3, 4-tiered grading systems.

Therapy

Once the histological diagnosis and grade is established and the work-up for distant metastasis performed, a multidisciplinary team of surgeons, radiation oncologists and medical oncologists can design the most effective treatment plan for the patient.

Surgery

Although surgery remains the principal therapeutic modality in soft tissue sarcoma, the extent of surgery required, along with the optimum combination of radiotherapy and chemotherapy, remains controversial. In designing a treatment plan, the multidisciplinary team must balance the goal of minimizing local and distant recurrence with the aim of preserving function and quality of life. A properly executed surgical resection remains the most important part of the overall treatment. In general, the scope of the excision is dictated by the size of the tumour, its anatomical relation to normal structures (e.g. major neurovascular bundles) and the degree of function that would be lost after operation. If severe loss of function is likely, the key question is whether this can be minimized by use of adjuvant /neoadjuvant radiotherapy or chemotherapy. For subcutaneous or intramuscular high grade soft tissue sarcoma smaller than 5 cm, or any size low grade sarcoma, surgery alone should be considered if a wide excision with a good 1-2 cm cuff of surrounding fat and muscle can be achieved. If the excision margin is close, or if there is extramuscular involvement, adjuvant radiotherapy should be added to the surgical resection to reduce the probability of local failure. However, irrespective of grade, post-operative radiotherapy is probably used more often than strictly necessary. In fact, Rydholm et al. {1832} and Baldini et al. {115} have shown that a significant subset of subcutaneous and intramuscular sarcomas can be treated by wide margin excision alone, with a local recurrence rate of only 5-10%.

Adjuvant and neoadjuvant chemotherapy

For high grade sarcomas, greater than 5 cm, there are several possible approaches to treatment that are based on not only achieving good local control but also reducing the risk of developing subsequent systemic metastasis. The value of systemic chemotherapy depends on the specific histological subset of the sarcoma. Chemotherapy is usually indicated as primary "neoadjuvant" therapy in the treatment of Ewing sarcoma and rhabdomyosarcoma. Adjuvant chemotherapy is indicated for these specific tumour types, even if the primary site has been resected, because of the very high risk of metastasis. For other histological types of soft tissue sarcoma the value of systemic chemotherapy remains controversial. The histological type and location of disease are important predictors of sensitivity to chemotherapy and thus may help in decisions on the potential benefit of chemotherapy. The majority of the randomized chemotherapy trials have shown no significant impact on overall survival; however they have found that chemotherapy does improve disease-free survival, with improved local and loco-regional control {3,51,64,245,612}. The majority of these trial data came from the era before the standard use of ifosfamide. A single randomized trial of adjuvant chemotherapy involving an anthracycline (epirubicin) plus ifosfamide has been performed in Italy. Although designed to detect only differences in disease-free survival (and with only relatively short follow-up), this trial is reported to show relapse-free and overall survival differences associated with systemic chemotherapy administration {3}. These results require confirmation before adjuvant chemotherapy for all sarcomas is accepted as standard practice. Given the limitations of the randomized trial data cited above and that the benefit in systemic disease control may be relatively small, the preoperative use of neo-adjuvant chemotherapy with an anthracycline and ifosfamide can be justified in carefully selected patients with large, high grade tumours and in certain histological types most likely to respond to such chemotherapy (e.g. synovial sarcoma and myxoid/round cell liposarcoma).

Multimodal protocols
For the treatment of large, high grade extremity sarcomas several sequencing schedules of chemotherapy, radiation and surgery have been developed. There are three general approaches {1960}:
  1. Neoadjuvant chemotherapy
     > surgery > adjuvant chemotherapy
     + post-operative radiotherapy.
  2. Neoadjuvant chemotherapy
     interdigitated with preoperative
     radiotherapy > surgery > adjuvant
     chemotherapy
  3. Neoadjuvant chemotherapy >
     preoperative radiotherapy > surgery
     > adjuvant chemotherapy

One major advantage to giving the chemotherapy alone and directly prior to

TNM Classification of soft tissue sarcomas

Primary tumour (T)	TX:	primary tumour cannot be assessed
	T0:	no evidence of primary tumour
	T1:	tumour ≤ 5cm in greatest dimension
		T1a: superficial tumour*
		T1b: deep tumour
	T2:	tumour > 5cm in greatest dimension
		T2a: superficial tumour
		T2b: deep tumour
Regional lymph nodes (N)	NX:	regional lymph nodes cannot be assessed
	N0:	no regional lymph node metastasis
	N1:	regional lymph node metastasis

Note: Regional node involvement is rare and cases in which nodal status is not assessed either clinically or pathologically could be considered N0 instead of NX or pNX.

| Distant metastasis (M) | M0: | no distant metastasis |
| | M1: | distant metastasis |

G Histopathological Grading
Translation table for three and four grade to two grade (low vs. high grade) system

TNM two grade system	Three grade systems	Four grade systems
Low grade	Grade 1	Grade 1
		Grade 2
High grade	Grade 2	Grade 3
	Grade 3	Grade 4

Stage IA	T1a	N0,NX	M0	Low grade
	T1b	N0,NX	M0	Low grade
Stage IB	T2a	N0,NX	M0	Low grade
	T2b	N0,NX	M0	Low grade
Stage IIA	T1a	N0,NX	M0	High grade
	T1b	N0,NX	M0	High grade
Stage IIB	T2a	N0,NX	M0	High grade
Stage III	T2b	N0,NX	M0	High grade
Stage IV	Any T	N1	M0	Any grade
	Any T	Any N	M1	Any grade

From references {831,1979}.
Superficial tumour is located exclusively above the superficial fascia without invasion of the fascia; deep tumour is located either exclusively beneath the superficial fascia, or superficial to the fascia with invasion of or through the fascia. Retroperitoneal, mediastinal and pelvic sarcomas are classified as deep tumours.

surgery (approach 1) is the ability to determine if the sarcoma is progressing on therapy and thus avoid potential toxicity of additional adjuvant chemotherapy in those patients who have measurable disease that appears to be resistant to such therapy.

The retroperitoneal and visceral sarcomas represent a particularly complex challenge for the treating physician. Because of their large size, their tendency to invade adjacent organs, and the difficulty in achieving a clean margin surgical resection, the survival rate for retroperitoneal sarcomas is 20-40% of that for extremity soft tissue sarcoma. The most important prognostic factors for survival in retroperitoneal sarcoma are the completeness of the surgical resection and the histological grade {1247, 1959}. Despite an aggressive surgical approach to eradicate tumour, local control is still a significant problem that ultimately leads to unresectable local disease and death in many cases. Well differentiated and dedifferentiated liposarcoma account for the majority of retroperitoneal sarcomas and they frequently recur locally and multi-focally within the retroperitoneum, with distant metastasis to lung only occurring in 20% of those patients who have dedifferentiated high grade liposarcoma {578,937}. In contrast, patients with retroperitoneal high grade leiomyosarcoma often (in greater than 50% of patients) develop distant metastasis to liver or lung, which is usually the limiting factor for outcome.

CHAPTER 1

Adipocytic Tumours

Adipocytic tumours represent the largest single group of mesenchymal tumours, due to the high prevalence of lipomas and angiolipomas. Liposarcomas represent the single most common type of soft tissue sarcoma. Its principal histological subtypes (well differentiated, myxoid, and pleomorphic) are entirely separate diseases with different morphology, genetics, and natural history. Most types of adipocytic neoplasm have distinctive karyotypic aberrations which can be of considerable help in diagnosis.

Principal changes and advances since the 1994 WHO classification have been
> the recognition that atypical lipomatous tumour and well differentiated liposarcoma are essentially synonymous and that site-specific variations in behaviour relate only to surgical resectability,
> the inclusion of two newly characterized entities, myolipoma and chondroid lipoma, and
> the renaming of fibrolipomatous hamartoma of nerve as lipomatosis of nerve.

Descriptions of angiomyolipoma and myelolipoma are provided in the Urogenital and Endocrine volumes, respectively.

Lipoma

G.P. Nielsen
N. Mandahl

Definition
Lipoma is a benign tumour composed of mature white adipocytes and is the most common soft tissue mesenchymal neoplasm in adults.

ICD-O code   8850/0

Epidemiology
Conventional lipoma occurs over a wide age range but is most common between the ages of 40 and 60 years and is more frequent in obese individuals {601}. Lipomas are rare in children. Approximately 5% of patients have multiple lipomas.

Sites of involvement
Conventional lipoma can arise within subcutaneous tissue (superficial lipoma) or within deep soft tissues (deep lipoma) or even on the surfaces of bone (parosteal lipoma) {1079,1800}. Deep seated lipomas that arise within or between skeletal muscle fibres are called *intramuscular* or *intermuscular lipomas*, respectively {685,1113}. Intramuscular lipoma arises during mid to late adulthood and involves skeletal muscle in a variety of locations including the trunk, head and neck region, upper and lower extremities {685,1113}. Intermuscular lipoma arises between muscles most frequently in the anterior abdominal wall, and involves a similar age group as the intramuscular lipoma. So-called *lipoma arborescens* (villous lipomatous proliferation of synovial membrane) is characterized by fatty infiltration of the subsynovial connective tissue and may represent a reactive process.

Clinical features
Lipomas usually present as a painless soft tissue mass, except for larger ones that can be painful when they compress peripheral nerves. Superficial lipomas are generally smaller (<5cm) than the deep seated ones (>5cm). Patients with lipoma arborescens are usually adult men that complain of gradual swelling of the affected joint {324,837,875,1343,

1982}. Imaging studies show a homogeneous soft tissue mass that is isodense to the subcutaneous tissue and demonstrates fat saturation. Attenuated fibrous strands can be seen but they are not as prominent as seen in the atypical lipomas. Intramuscular lipomas are more variably circumscribed, and lipoma arborescens shows diffuse fatty infiltration of the synovium.

Aetiology
Unknown. Lipomas are more common in obese individuals.

Macroscopy
Grossly, lipomas are well circumscribed and have a yellow, greasy cut surface. Different types are basically similar in appearance, however bone formation can be seen in osteolipoma and grey glistening nodules may be seen in chondrolipoma. Intramuscular and intermuscular lipoma do not show any specific gross features except that a portion of skeletal muscle is often attached to the periphery of the tumour. In lipoma arborescens the entire synovium assumes a nodular and papillary appearance and has a bright yellow cut surface.

Histopathology
Conventional lipoma is composed of lobules of mature adipocytes. The cells are identical to the surrounding adipose tissue except for slight variation in the size and shape of the cells in lipomas. Lipomas can occasionally have areas of bone formation (osteolipoma), cartilage (chondrolipoma), abundant fibrous tissue (fibrolipoma), or extensive myxoid change (myxolipoma). Intramuscular lipoma may be either well demarcated from the surrounding skeletal muscle or, more often, shows an infiltrative growth pattern with mature adipocytes infiltrating and encasing skeletal muscle fibres that often show evidence of atrophy. In lipoma arbor-escens the subsynovial connective tissue is infiltrated by mature adipocytes; scattered inflammatory cells are also usually present.

Immunophenotype
Mature adipocytes stain for vimentin, S100 protein and leptin {1610}.

Ultrastructure
Lipoma is composed of cells that have a large, single lipid droplet compressing a peripherally situated nucleus.

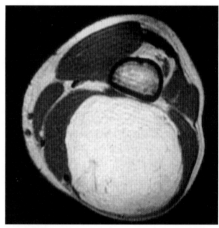

Fig. 1.01 Image of a deep seated conventional lipoma showing a well circumscribed, homogenous tumour with the same characteristics as the adjacent subcutaneous fat.

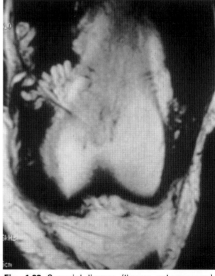

Fig. 1.02 Synovial lipoma (lipoma arborescens) demonstrating a fatty infiltration of the synovium that assumes papillary appearance.

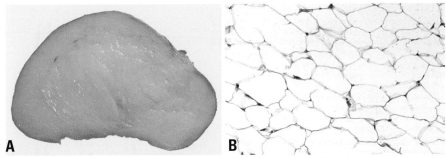

Fig. 1.03 Conventional lipoma. **A** Grossly, the tumour is well circumscribed and has a homogenous yellow cut surface. **B** The mature adipocytes vary only slightly in size and shape and have small eccentric nuclei.

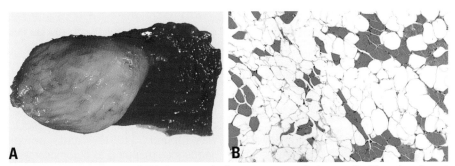

Fig. 1.04 Intramuscular lipoma. **A** This intramuscular lipoma appears well circumscribed from the adjacent skeletal muscle (right). **B** Mature adipocytes infiltrate and encase skeletal muscle fibres.

Pinocytotic vesicles are present and external lamina is seen surrounding the cells {1110}.

Genetics
Cytogenetics
Lipomas have been analysed extensively by chromosome banding. In larger cytogenetically investigated series, chromosome aberrations have been found in 55-75% of the cases {1320,2020,2271}. Among the abnormal tumours, about 75% show seemingly balanced karyotypes and in more than 50% there is a single abnormality in at least one clone {1477}. On average, signs of clonal evolution is found in every sixth tumour. Numerical chromosome changes are rare and randomly distributed, and chromosome numbers deviating from 46 are exceedingly rare. The pattern of cytogenetic aberrations is quite heterogeneous, but three cytogenetically defined subgroups have been distinguished: 1) the major subgroup consisting of tumours with aberrations involving 12q13-15, 2) tumours with aberrations involving 6p21-23, and 3) tumours with loss of material from 13q. Patients with and without aberrations of 12q13-15 show no differences with respect to age distribution and gender. The frequency of abnormal karyotypes seems to be higher among older patients {2020,2271}. Otherwise, no clear, consistent correlations between clinical and cytogenetic data have been identified.

Tumours with 12q13-15 aberrations
About two-thirds of tumours with abnormal karyotypes show aberrations of 12q13-15, which has been found to recombine with a large number of bands in all chromosomes except 16 and Y. The preferred rearrangement, seen in more than 20% of tumours with 12q13-15 aberrations, is t(3;12)(q27-28;q13-15). Other recurrent recombination partner regions, present in 3-7% of these tumours, are 1p36, 1p32-34, 2p22-24, 2q35-37, 5q33, 11q13, 12p11-12, 12q24, 13q12-14, 17q23-25, and 21q21-22. The majority of these aberrations originate through translocations or insertions. One in six of these tumours show more or less complex intrachromosomal rearrangements - including primarily inversions, but also deletions and duplications - leading to recombination between 12q13-15 and other segments of chromosome 12, primarily 12p11-12 and 12q24.

Tumours without 12q13-15 aberrations
Among these tumours, constituting one-third of lipomas with acquired chromosome aberrations, all chromosomes except 20 have been involved, but the only distinct clustering of breakpoints seen is to 6p21-23, 13q11-22, and, less often, 12q22-24, together constituting about half of this group of tumours. Involvement of 6p21-23, mostly in the form of seemingly balanced translocations, has been found in more than 20% of these tumours. The only recurrent translocation partner has been 3q27-28 in two cases. Aberrations affecting the long arm of chromosome 13 are dominated by deletions, which have been found in slightly less than 20% of the cases. Most aberrations are interstitial deletions with breakpoints in 13q12-14 and 13q22, respectively. There is an overlap between 6p21-23 rearrangements and 13q deletions, with some tumours showing both aberrations, but more often these aberrations occur as sole anomalies.

Simultaneous involvement of 6p21-23 and 12q13-15 is uncommon, in contrast to the coexistence of 12q13-15 aberrations and 13q losses. In tumours with combinations of 6p, 12q, and 13q aberrations, 13q is mostly involved in bal-

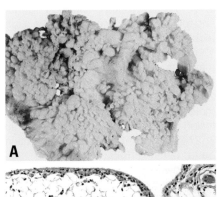

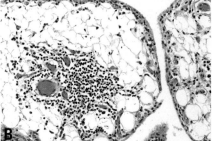

Fig. 1.05 A Synovial lipoma (lipoma arborescens). The entire synovium is bright yellow and has a nodular or papillary appearance. **B** Synovial lipoma (lipoma arborescens). The subsynovial connective tissue has been replaced by mature adipocytes. Note also scattered chronic inflammatory cells.

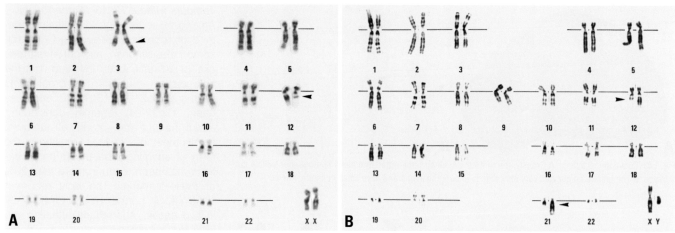

Fig. 1.06 A Karyotype from a lipoma showing the most common structural rearrangement, a translocation t(3;12)(q27;q15). **B** Lipoma with t(12;21)(q15;q22) as the sole chromosomal aberration. Arrowheads indicate breakpoints.

anced translocations when recombining with 6p21-23 or 12q13-15, whereas deletions in 13q are predominating when aberrations of 6p21-23 or 12q13-15 are present but recombine with other chromosome segments.

Among tumours without rearrangements of 12q13-15 or 6p21-23 or loss of 13q sequences, one-fifth of the breakpoints coincide with those recurrently recombining with 12q13-15.

Molecular genetics

The *HMGIC* (a.k.a. *HMGA2*) gene, encoding a family member of the high mobility group of proteins, located in 12q15 is affected in at least some lipomas with rearrangements of 12q13-15 {90,1890}. In tumours with t(3;12)(q27-28;q13-15), the consequence at the molecular level is the formation of a fusion gene involving *HMGIC* and *LPP* in 3q27-28, a member of the LIM protein gene family {1696}. In addition, this fusion gene has been observed in a few cases with complex karyotypic changes including 12q13-15 but not 3q27-28 and in cases with normal karyotypes, indicating that cytogenetic analysis underesti-

mates the frequency of tumours with recombination between these two chromosome segments {1696}. In all cases, the chimeric *HMGIC/LPP* transcript is expressed, whereas the reciprocal *LPP/HMGIC* transcript is expressed only occasionally. Alternative fusion transcripts, encoding the three DNA binding AT-hook domains of HMGIC and two or three LIM domains of LPP have been reported, thus excluding the 3´ acidic, protein-binding domain and the N-terminal leucine-zipper motif, respectively. The preferred breakpoints are in the large intron 3 of *HMGIC* and *LPP* intron 8. The chimeric transcript is not unique for lipomas of the soft tissues but has also been detected in parosteal lipoma and pulmonary chondroid hamartoma {1698,1803}.

Rearrangement of *HMGIC* has been detected also in tumours with changes involving 12q13-15 and other chromosome segments. In a single case of lipoma with t(12;13)(q13-15;q12), an *HMGIC/LHFP* fusion transcript has been reported {1697}. Also in this case, the breakpoint was in *HMGIC* intron 3. In lipomas with recombination between

12q13-15 and 12p11, due to inversion, fusion of putative but yet unidentified gene sequences in 12p11 with *HMGIC* was found {1081}, and ectopic sequences mapping to chromosome 15 have been implicated {90}. Possibly, the related *HMGIY* (*HMGA1B*) gene is the target, directly or indirectly, in lipomas with 6p21-23 aberrations; split FISH signals, using probes covering *HMGIY*, have been reported in cases with translocations involving 6p {1082,2083}. Transcriptional activation of *HMGIC* or *HMGIY* is indicated by immunohistochemical studies, and correlates well with cytogenetic findings of breakpoints in the regions where these two gene loci are located {2083}.

Prognostic factors

The subclassification of conventional lipoma does not have any prognostic significance except for the infiltrating intramuscular lipoma that has a higher local recurrence rate, therefore total removal of the involved muscle or a compartmental resection has been suggested for these infiltrating tumours in order to minimize local recurrence {206}.

Lipomatosis

G.P Nielsen
A.E. Rosenberg

Definition
Lipomatosis is a diffuse overgrowth of mature adipose tissue. It occurs in a variety of clinical settings and can affect different anatomic regions of the body.

ICD-O code   8850/0

Synonyms
Madelung disease, Launois-Bensaude syndrome.

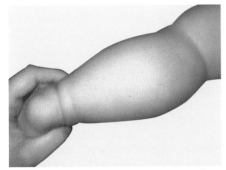

Fig. 1.07 Lipomatosis presenting as diffuse enlargement of the lower leg in an infant

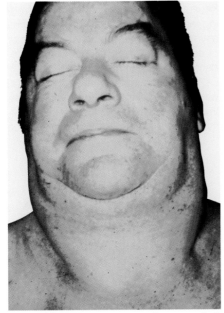

Fig. 1.08 Patient showing typically symmetrical, massive expansion of the neck.

Epidemiology
Diffuse lipomatosis usually occurs in individuals under 2 years of age but it may also arise in adults {1574}. Pelvic lipomatosis most frequently affects black males who range in age from 9 to 80 {839,944,1135}. Symmetric lipomatosis develops in middle aged men of Mediterranean origin. Many patients have a history of liver disease or excessive alcohol consumption. Steroid lipomatosis manifests in patients on hormonal therapy or have increased endogenous production of adrenocortical steroids. HIV lipodystrophy is frequently seen in AIDS patients treated with protease inhibitors but is also seen in patients receiving other forms of anti-retroviral therapy {234,1175}.

Sites of involvement
Diffuse lipomatosis involves the trunk, large portion of an extremity, head and neck, abdomen, pelvis or intestinal tract. It may be associated with macrodactyly or gigantism of a digit {836,1365,1616}. Symmetric lipomatosis manifests as symmetric deposition of fat in the upper part of the body particularly the neck. In pelvic lipomatosis there is diffuse overgrowth of fat in the perivesical and perirectal areas. Steroid lipomatosis is characterized by the accumulation of fat in the face, sternal region or the upper middle back (buffalo hump). HIV-lipodystrophy typically shows the accumulation of visceral fat, breast adiposity, cervical fat pads, hyperlipidemia, insulin resistance as well as fat wasting in the face and limbs {400,1461}.

Clinical features
In most forms of lipomatosis the patients present with massive accumulation of fat in the affected areas that may mimic a neoplasm. Additionally patients with symmetric lipomatosis can have neuropathy and central nervous system involvement {1541,1712}. Accumulation of fat in the lower neck areas in these patients can also cause laryngeal obstruction, and compression of the

vena cava. Patients with pelvic lipomatosis frequently complain of urinary frequency, perineal pain, constipation, and abdominal and back pain. Bowel obstruction and hydronephrosis may eventually develop. Imaging studies in all forms of lipomatosis show accumulation of fat and are only helpful in determining the extent of its accumulation and excluding other processes.

Aetiology
The basic mechanism underlying lipomatosis is not well understood. In symmetric lipomatosis point mutations in mitochondrial genes have been implicated in its pathogenesis {1140}. The similarity between HIV lipodystrophy and benign symmetric lipomatosis suggests a similar pathogenesis in that mitochondrial DNA damage may be induced by the drugs being used to treat HIV {153,400}.

Macroscopy
The gross appearance of lipomatosis is the same for all of the different subtypes. The lesions consist of poorly circumscribed aggregates of soft yellow fat that is identical in appearance to normal fat. The only differences are the site of involvement and the distribution of the fat.

Histopathology
All of the different types of lipomatosis have identical morphologic features, consisting of lobules and sheets of mature adipocytes that may infiltrate

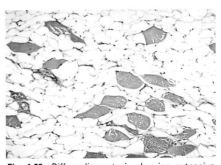

Fig. 1.09 Diffuse lipomatosis showing extensive skeletal muscle infiltration of mature adipocytes.

other structures such as skeletal muscle.

Immunophenotype
The adipose tissue stains for vimentin and S-100, similar to normal fat.

Ultrastructure
The adipocytes have the features of white fat.

Genetics
An association with several genetic disorders has been reported, and an autosomal dominant inheritance is suggested {1377}.

Prognostic factors
All idiopathic forms of lipomatoses have a tendency to recur locally after surgery.

The treatment is palliative surgical removal of excess fat. Massive accumulation of fat in the neck region may cause death due to laryngeal obstruction. The fat in steroid lipomatosis regresses after steroid levels have been lowered. Experimental drugs such as recombinant growth hormones have been used to treat HIV-lipodystrophy.

Lipomatosis of nerve

G.P. Nielsen

Definition
Lipomatosis of nerve is characterized by infiltration of the epineurium by adipose and fibrous tissue. The tissue grows between and around nerve bundles thereby causing enlargment of the affected nerve.

ICD-O code   8850/0

Synonyms and historical annotations
Fibrolipomatous hamartoma, lipofibroma, fibrolipomatosis, intraneural lipoma of the median nerve, perineural lipoma, median nerve lipoma, macrodystrophia lipomatosa, neural fibrolipoma.

Epidemiology
Lipomatosis of nerve is frequently first noted at birth or in early childhood, but

patients may not present for treatment until early or mid adulthood. In the largest reported series the patients ranged in age from 11 to 39 years. Because the constituent tissues are normal components of the epineurium, some have considered this lesion to be a hamartoma of the nerve sheath {445, 2103}. In some cases it is associated with macrodactyly of the digits inervated by the affected nerve.
Associated macrodactyly was present in approximately 1/3 of patients, including 5 females and 2 males {1952}. Females predominate when lipofibroma is accompanied by macrodactyly, whereas males are more commonly affected when macrodactyly is absent.

Sites of involvement
The median nerve and its digital branches are most commonly affected followed by the ulnar nerve {189,1952}. The process has also been reported to involve unusual sites such as the cranial nerves and the brachial plexus {176,1726}.

Clinical features
Patients present with a gradually enlarging mass in the affected area that may be asymptomatic or associated with motor or sensory deficits. Patients with macrodactyly have symmetrical or asymmetrical enlargement of the affected finger(s) with enlargement of the involved bones. Imaging studies show fusiform enlargement of the nerve with fatty infiltration

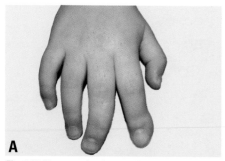 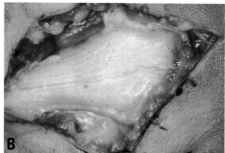 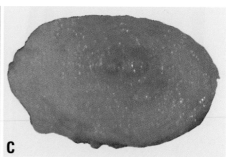

Fig. 1.10 Lipomatosis of nerve. **A** A clinical picture showing macrodactyly of the second and third fingers. **B** An intraoperative view of lipomatosis of nerve showing a transition between the normal nerve (left) and the affected area (right). **C** Cross section reveals nerve bundles entrapped within fibroadipose tissue.

{474} and MRI findings are virtually pathognomonic {1336}.

Aetiology
The aetiology is unknown. Lipomatosis of nerve is not associated with any syndrome nor is there any known hereditary predisposition.

Macroscopy
Grossly there is fusiform enlargement of the nerve by yellow fibrofatty tissue, which is generally confined within the epineurial sheath.

Histopathology
The epineurial and perineurial compartments of the enlarged nerve are infiltrated by mature adipose tissue admixed with fibrous tissue which dissects between and separates individual nerve bundles {1952}. Concentric perineurial fibrous tissue is a prominent feature. The affected nerve may also show other changes such as perineural septation, microfascicle formation and pseudoonion bulb formation mimicking an intraneural perineurioma {1882}. Metaplastic bone formation is rarely present {551}.

Immunophenotype
Immunohistochemical studies are not helpful in diagnosing this lesion as all of its components are seen in normal nerves.

Ultrastructure
There are no characteristic ultrastructural findings. The nerve bundles demonstrate onion bulblike formations with one or two nerve fibres and peripheral perineural cells {99}.

Prognostic factors
Lipomatosis of nerve is a benign lesion with no effective therapy. Surgical excision usually causes severe damage of the involved nerve. Division of the transverse carpal ligament may relieve neurological symptoms.

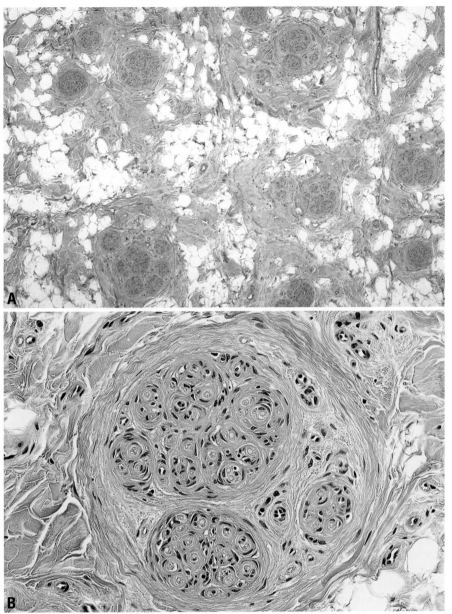

Fig. 1.11 A Epineural infiltration of fibroadipose tissue separating nerve bundles. **B** The nerves show pseudoonion bulb formation and perineural fibrosis.

Lipoblastoma / Lipoblastomatosis

R. Sciot
N. Mandahl

Definition
A lobulated, localized (lipoblastoma) or diffuse (lipoblastomatosis) tumour, resembling fetal adipose tissue.

ICD-O code
8881/0

Synonyms
Foetal lipoma, embryonic lipoma, infantile lipoma.

Epidemiology
Both tumours are most commonly found in the first three years of life. They may occasionally be present at birth or in older children. There is a male predilection {348,391,1410,2196}.

Sites of involvement
The extremities are most commonly involved, but locations in the mediastinum, retroperitoneum, trunk, head & neck, and various organs (lung, heart, parotid gland) have been described {273,500,525,1002,1010,1177,1192, 1352,1654,1713,1720,1762,2134,2149}.

Clinical features
Most patients present with a slowly growing soft tissue nodule/mass, well circumscribed and confined to the subcutis in case of lipoblastoma, infiltrating the deeper muscle in case of lipoblastomatosis. Depending on the location, the tumour may compress adjacent structures, such as the trachea. Imaging reveals a mass with adipose tissue density, but does not allow distinction from lipoma and liposarcoma {1777}.

Macroscopy
Notwithstanding exceptions, lipoblastomas are relatively small lesions (2-5 cm), showing fatty looking tissue with gelatinous areas.

Histopathology
Lipoblastoma shows a lobulated appearance with an admixture of mature and immature adipocytes, the latter corresponding to lipoblasts in various stages of development. Depending on the age of the patient, lipoblasts may be very scarce. Connective tissue septa separate the lobules. The lobulation is less prominent in lipoblastomatosis, in which entrapped muscle fibres frequently occur. The matrix can be quite myxoid, with a plexiform vascular pattern, thus mimicking myxoid liposarcoma. The latter tumour, which is exceptionally rare under the age of 10, usually shows nuclear atypia and does not show the pronounced lobulated pattern of lipoblastoma {223}. However, in rare cases molecular genetic analysis may be required for definitive distinction. Occasionally, lipoblastoma(tosis) may show extramedullary haematopoiesis or cells resembling brown fat. Cellular maturation has been described, leading to a lipoma-like picture. When fascicles of primitive mesenchymal cells are present in the septa, lipoblastoma resembles infantile lipofibromatosis or infantile fibromatosis {658}. The lobulated aspect, the at least focal myxoid stroma and plexiform capillaries, as well as the over-

whelming fat component with lipoblasts, help to separate lipoblatoma(tosis) from these lesions.

Ultrastructure
Lipoblastoma(tosis) strongly resembles normal developing fat, with a spectrum ranging from primitive mesenchymal cells to multivacuolated lipoblasts and mature lipocytes {223}.

Genetics
Typically, lipoblastomas have simple, pseudodiploid karyotypes with structural chromosome aberrations. The characteristic cytogenetic feature is rearrangement of 8q11-13, which has been found in the vast majority of cases. The only chromosome segments that, so far, have been found to be involved in recurrent recombinations with 8q11-13 are 3q12-13, 7p22, and 8q24, but several other chromosome segments have been the translocation partners in single cases. Numerical changes are rare, but gain of chromosome 8 has been found in cases with or without simultaneous rearrangement of 8q11-13.

To date, two different fusion genes have been reported to result from the chromosomal rearrangements, *HAS2/PLAG1* in three cases and *COL1A2/PLAG1* in a single case {945}. The *PLAG1* gene is located in 8q12, *HAS2* in 8q24 and *COL1A2* in 7q22. The genomic breakpoint of *PLAG1* seems to be in intron1, resulting in loss of exon 1. The entire *HAS2* 5′ untranslated region is involved in the fusion gene, which is probably under control of the *HAS2* promoter, leading to transcriptional up-regulation of *PLAG1* and production of a full-length PLAG1 protein. The *COL1A2-PLAG1* fusion gene encodes a chimeric protein containing the first amino acids of COL1A2 and full-length PLAG1. These fusion genes seem to act through a promoter-swapping mechanism {105,945}. An alternative mechanism associated with lipoblastoma tumourigenesis may act through excess copies of chromosome 8 {792}. Since +8 may be present

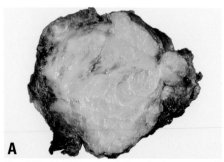
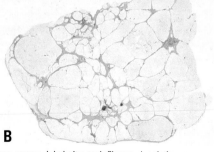

Fig. 1.12 Lipoblastoma. **A** Grossly, the tumour shows vague lobularity and fibrous / gelatinous areas. **B** Low power view. Note the prominent lobulation.

26 Adipocytic tumours

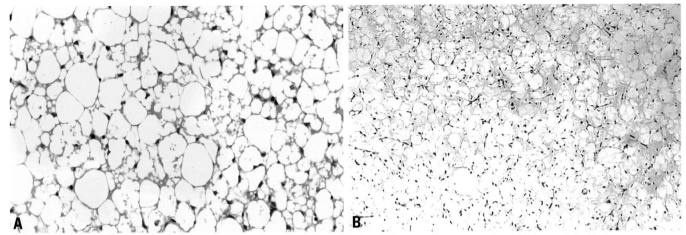

Fig. 1.13 A Admixture of multivacuolated lipoblasts and mature adipocytes. **B** 315 Delicate plexiform vascular pattern and myxoid changes in lipoblastoma.

in tumours both with and without changes of 8q12, the effect of *PLAG1* rearrangement might be reinforced by gain of chromosome 8 in some cases. Whether the extra copies of the *PLAG1* gene are normal or have point mutations is not known. By in situ hybridization it has been shown that split *PLAG1* signals are present in both classical, myxoid, and lipoma-like lipoblastomas as well as in a variety of mesenchymal cell components, indicating the mutation to occur in a progenitor cell that then differentiates {792}.

Prognostic factors

Lipoblastoma(tosis) is fully benign and malignant transformation or metastasis does not occur. Recurrences are described in 9% to 22% of cases, mainly in lipoblastomatosis. Therefore wide total excision of diffuse lesions is advised {348,391,1410,2196}.

Angiolipoma

R. Sciot
N. Mandahl

Definition

A subcutaneous nodule consisting of mature fat cells, intermingled with small and thin-walled vessels, a number of which contain fibrin thrombi.

ICD-O code   8861/0

Epidemiology

Angiolipomas are relatively common and usually appear in the late teens or early twenties. Children and patients older than 50 years are rarely involved. There is a male predominance and an increased familial incidence has been described (5% of all cases) {230,357, 942,977,1062,1232}. The mode of inheritance is not clear.

Sites of involvement

The forearm is the most common site, followed by the trunk and upper arm. Spinal angiolipomas and intramuscular haemangiomas, previously also called 'infiltrating angiolipomas', are different lesions {878,2148}.

Clinical features

Angiolipomas most frequently present as multiple subcutaneous small nodules, usually tender to painful. There is no correlation between the intensity/occurrence of pain and the degree of vascularity {527}.

Macroscopy

Angiolipomas appear as encapsulated yellowish to reddish nodules, most often less than 2 cm in diameter.

Histopathology

Angiolipomas typically consist of two mesenchymal elements: mature adipocytes and branching capillary sized vessels, which usually contain fibrin thrombi. The vascularity is more prominent in the subcapsular area {527}. The relative proportion of adipocytes and vessels varies and some lesions are almost completely composed of vascular channels. These 'cellular' angiolipomas should be distinguished from angiosar-

coma and Kaposi sarcoma {983}. Interstitial mast cells may be prominent and in older lesions, increased fibrosis is present.

Genetics

With a single exception, all cytogeneti-

cally investigated tumours have had a normal karyotype {1905}.

Prognostic factors

Angiolipomas are always benign and show no tendency to recur. Malignant transformation does not occur.

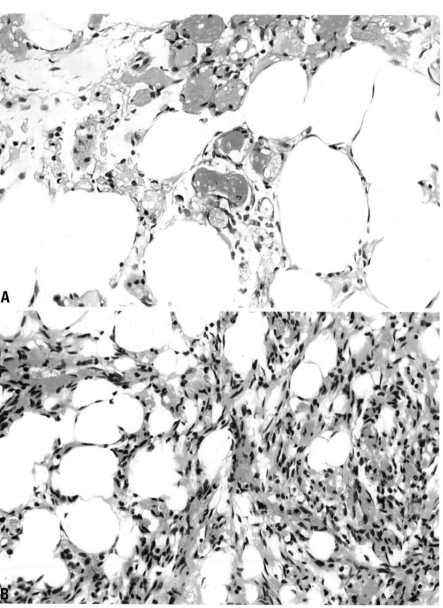

Fig. 1.14 Angiolipoma. **A** The tumour consists of mature adipocytes and capillaries, some of which contain microthrombi. **B** Cellular angiolipoma, in which the vessels predominate.

Myolipoma of soft tissue

J.M. Meis-Kindblom
L.G. Kindblom

Definition
Myolipoma of soft tissue is a benign tumour exhibiting features of mature smooth muscle and mature adipose tissue.

ICD-O code   8890/0

Synonym
Extrauterine lipoleiomyoma.

Epidemiology
Myolipoma of soft tissue is an extremely rare lesion occurring in adults, with a male to female ratio of 1:2 {1393}.

Sites of involvement
The majority of cases are deeply located and involve the abdominal cavity, retroperitoneum, and inguinal areas. The trunk wall and extremities may also be involved; such cases are subcutaneous and may grow deeply to involve the superficial muscular fascia {1393}.

Clinical features
Most lesions present as a palpable mass; the remainder are incidental findings.

Macroscopy
Deep-seated myolipomas of soft tissue range between 10 and 25 cm in size; the average size is 15 cm. Smaller lesions are seen in the subcutis. A completely or partially encapsulated lipomatous tumour intermingles with strands and nodules of firm white-tan, fibrillary to whorled areas corresponding to smooth muscle.

Histopathology
The smooth muscle component usually dominates with a muscle to fat ratio of 2:1. Smooth muscle tends to be evenly distributed and arranged in short fascicles, resulting in a sieve-like pattern as it traverses the fat. Individual smooth muscle fibres have deeply acidophilic fibrillary cytoplasm that becomes fuchsinophilic with the Masson trichrome stain. Nuclear chromatin is evenly dispersed, nucleoli are inconspicuous and no appreciable mitotic activity is seen. Equally important is the absence of any atypia in the mature lipomatous component of myolipoma. Floret cells and lipoblasts are not seen, nor are medium calibre thick-walled blood vessels as

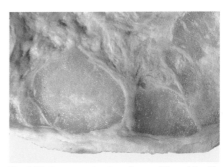

Fig. 1.15 An encapsulated myolipoma of the pelvis with clear fatty and smooth muscle components.

seen in angiomyolipoma. Sclerosis and focal inflammation may be present in the fat.

Immunophenotype
Diffusely and strongly positive smooth muscle actin and desmin immunostaining confirm the presence of smooth muscle in myolipoma.

Prognostic factors
Myolipoma does not recur. Complete surgical resection is curative.

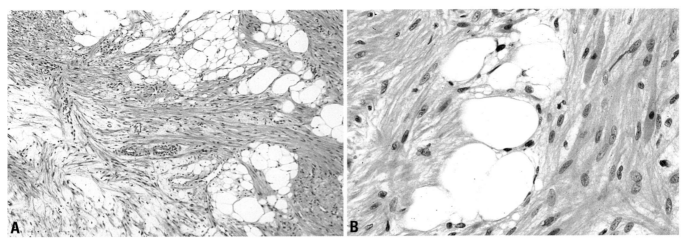

Fig. 1.16 A,B Mature adipose tissue and mature smooth muscle arranged in short fascicles are seen in a myolipoma of the distal extremity.

Chondroid lipoma

L.G. Kindblom
J.M. Meis-Kindblom
N. Mandahl

Definition

Chondroid lipoma is a unique and recently recognized benign adipose tissue tumour containing lipoblasts, mature fat, and a chondroid matrix. It bears a strikingly close resemblance to myxoid liposarcoma and extraskeletal myxoid chondrosarcoma.

ICD-O code   8862/0

Epidemiology

Chondroid lipoma is rare and affects primarily adults with a male:female ratio of 1:4 {1396} without racial predilection.

Sites of involvement

This tumour occurs most commonly in the proximal extremities and limb girdles. However, the trunk and head and neck areas may also be affected. Chondroid lipoma is often deep-seated, involving skeletal muscle or deep fibrous connective tissues. Those cases involving the subcutis tend to impinge on the superficial muscular fascia.

Clinical features

The majority of patients present with a painless mass of variable duration. There is a recent history of enlargement in roughly one-half of cases.
Reports of imaging studies of this lesion are exceedingly sparse {1277,2320}.

Macroscopy

Most chondroid lipomas are 2–7 cm in size, although cases with haemorrhage may be significantly larger {1396}. Tumours are typically well circumscribed and yellowish, suggesting fatty differentiation.

Histopathology

Chondroid lipoma is often encapsulated and occasionally multilobular. Its histologic hallmarks are nests and cords of abundant uni- and multivacuolated lipoblasts embedded in a prominent myxoid to hyalinized chondroid matrix admixed with a variable amount of mature adipose tissue. The lipoblast nuclei are small and uniform, ranging from oval, reniform to multilobated in shape, with evenly dispersed chromatin and small nucleoli. The cytoplasm is finely vacuolated, containing small lipid droplets and PAS positive glycogen. Cells may have granular eosinophilic cytoplasm. Chondroid lipoma is highly vascular and not infrequently contains haemorrhage and fibrosis.
Toluidine blue and alcian blue stains at controlled pHs confirm the typical presence of chondroitin sulfates in the matrix {1116}.

Immunophenotype

Lipoblasts are weakly S100 protein positive whereas stronger staining is seen with increasing adipocytic maturation {1116}. Vimentin is uniformly positive in all cells; cytokeratins are detected in rare cases, corresponding ultrastructurally to tonofilaments. EMA is uniformly negative. Proliferative index with MIB1 is <1%.

Ultrastructure

Primitive cells sharing features of embryonal fat and embryonal cartilage are seen, as well as lipoblasts, preadipocytes and mature fat. Cytoplasmic knobby protrusions are often seen. The matrix has features resembling cartilage, including thin filaments, thin collagen fibres and numerous proteoglycan particles {1116,1559}.

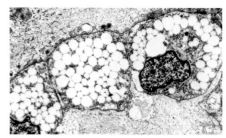

Fig. 1.18 EM of lipoblasts arranged in cords and a prominent chondroid matrix.

Cytogenetics

Two chondroid lipomas reported have displayed a seemingly balanced translocation, t(11;16)(q13;p12-13), in one case as the sole anomaly {1477}. Recurrent involvement of 11q13 has been found also in ordinary lipoma and hibernoma. However, in these tumour entities, 11q13 has never been found to recombine with 16p12-13 {1477}.

Prognostic factors

Chondroid lipoma does not recur locally or metastasize. Surgical excision is curative.

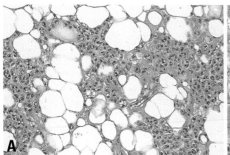
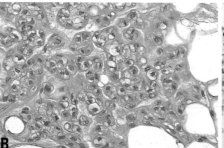
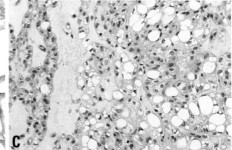

Fig. 1.17 Chondroid lipoma. **A** Mature fat and nests of small lipoblasts. **B** High magnification shows cellular details. **C** Mature fat and nests of small lipoblasts in chondroid lipoma showing a more prominent myxoid matrix.

Spindle cell lipoma / Pleomorphic lipoma

M.M. Miettinen
N. Mandahl

Definition
Spindle cell and pleomorphic lipoma, ends of a common histological spectrum, are circumscribed subcutaneous lesions occurring typically on the neck and back usually of males and composed of a variable admixture of bland spindled cells, hyperchromatic rounded cells, and multinucleate giant cells associated with ropey collagen.

ICD-O codes
Spindle cell lipoma   8857/0
Pleomorphic lipoma   8854/0

Sites of involvement
Spindle cell / pleomorphic lipomas occur predominantly in the posterior neck and shoulder area. Face, forehead, scalp, buccal-perioral area and upper arm are less common sites, and occurrence in the lower extremity is distinctly rare.

Clinical features
Spindle cell / pleomorphic lipomas typically present in older men with a median age of over 55 years, and only 10% of patients are women {60,102,595,684, 1944}. The tumour forms an asymptomatic, mobile dermal or subcutaneous mass, and there is often a long history. Rare patients have multiple lesions, and familial occurrence has been reported, mostly in men {633}. Spindle cell / pleomorphic lipomas have benign behaviour and conservative local excision is considered sufficient.

Macroscopy
Grossly spindle cell lipoma / pleomorphic lipoma forms an oval or discoid yellowish to greyish-white mass depending on the relative extent of the fatty and spindle cell components. The tumour often has a firmer texture than ordinary lipoma, but some examples have a gelatinous texture.

Histopathology
Histologically, at one end at the histological spectrum, spindle cell lipoma is composed of bland mitotically inactive

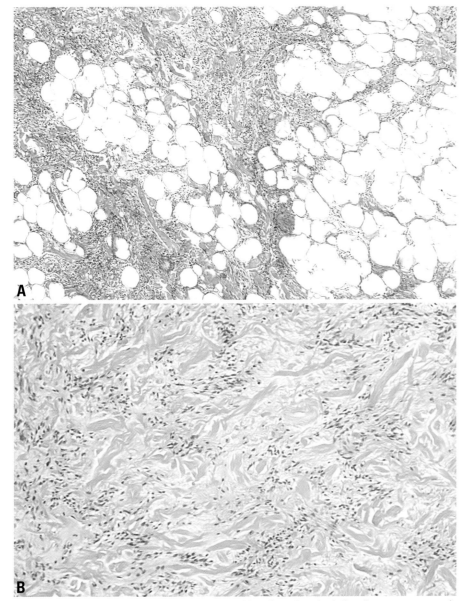

A

B

Fig. 1.19 Spindle cell lipoma. **A** The relative proportions of the adipocytic and spindle cell components are variable. **B** Some lesions are almost devoid of adipocytes and show vague nuclear palisading. Note the typically ropey collagen bundles.

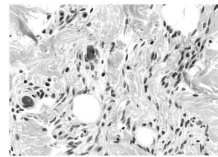

Fig. 1.20 Spindle cell lipoma. Typical case with bland spindle cells in a background with thick collagen fibres and a small number of adipocytes.

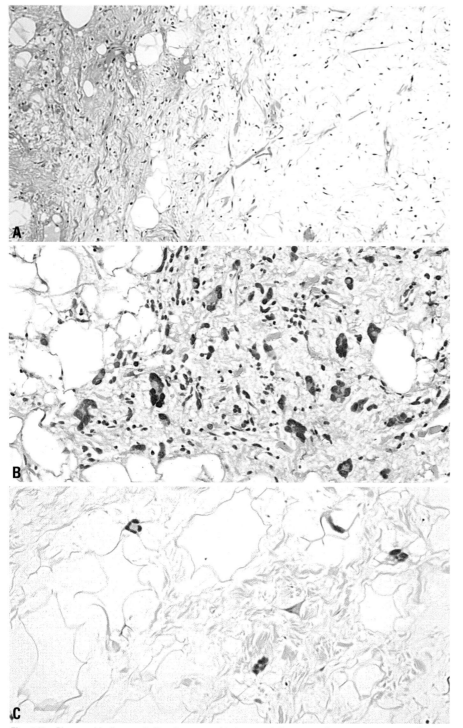

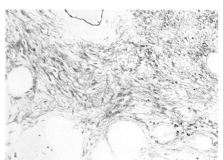

Fig. 1.22 Immunopositivity for CD34 is a consistent feature of the spindle cell component.

vascular slits ("pseudoangiomatoid variant") {911}.

At the opposite end of the spectrum, pleomorphic lipoma is characterized by small spindled and rounded hyperchromatic cells and multinucleated giant cells with radially arranged nuclei in a "floret-like" pattern, like petals of flowers. Cases with features intermediate between classic spindle cell lipoma and pleomorphic lipoma quite often occur.

Immunophenotype
The spindle cells in both spindle cell and pleomorphic lipomas are strongly positive for CD34 and may rarely be positive for S100 protein {626,2059,2102}.

Cytogenetics
Spindle cell lipomas and pleomorphic lipomas show similar cytogenetic aberrations. The karyotypes are, on average, more complex than those found in ordinary lipomas and are frequently hypodiploid, often with multiple partial losses, no gain of sequences, and few balanced rearrangements. Monosomy or partial loss of chromosomes 13 and/or 16 have been found in seven to eight out of ten cases. Half of the tumours with involvement of chromosome 16 have had a breakpoint in 16q13, and all of them have had loss of 16q13-qter. The most frequently lost segments of chromosome 13 include 13q12 and 13q14-q22. Other chromosome segments lost in two to three of the ten cases are 6pter-p23, 6q15-q21, 10pter-p15, 10q23-qter, and 17pter-p13 {442}.

Prognostic factors
These are benign lesions which only rarely recur locally.

Fig. 1.21 Pleomorphic lipoma. **A** Prominent myxoid change of the stroma is not an uncommon feature. **B** Classical example showing numerous floret-like multinucleate cells. **C** Some pleomorphic lipomas consist almost entirely of mature adipocytes with admixed multinucleated stroma cells, often having floret-like nuclei.

spindled cells arranged in parallel registers between the fat cells and associated with thick rope-like collagen bundles. {60,595,684,1944}. Large numbers of mast cells are often seen in between the spindle cells, and lymphocytes and plasma cells may occur, especially in pleomorphic lipoma. Some spindle cell lipomas show myxoid stromal change or display slit-like cleavage spaces resembling

Hibernoma

M.M. Miettinen
J.C. Fanburg-Smith
N. Mandahl

Definition
Hibernoma is a rare benign adipose tumour composed at least in part of brown fat cells with granular, multivacuolated cytoplasm. This brown fat component is admixed in variable proportion with white adipose tissue. Residual brown fat, mostly seen around cervical and axillary lymph nodes, should not be classified as hibernoma.

ICD-O codes   8880/0

Epidemiology
Recognized since around the turn of the century {1424}, hibernoma comprises 1.6% of benign lipomatous tumours and approximately 1.1% of all adipocytic tumours in AFIP files. Based on AFIP data on 170 cases {747}, hibernoma occurs predominantly in young adults, with a mean age of 38 years. 60% occur in the third and fourth decades, only 5% occur in children 2-18 years, and 7% in patients over 60 years. There is a slight male predominance {747}.

Sites of involvement
Hibernoma occurs in a wide variety of locations. The most common site is the thigh, followed by the trunk, upper extremity, and head and neck. The myxoid and spindle cell variants tend to be located in the posterior neck and shoulders, similar to spindle cell lipoma {747}. Less than 10% occur in the intra-abdominal or thoracic cavities {19}.

Clinical features
Hibernoma is a relatively slow growing tumour of the subcutis. At least 10% of cases are intramuscular. Hibernomas are usually painless. MRI reveals non-fat septations in hibernoma, not found in lipoma. By CT scan, hibernoma has a tissue attenuation intermediate between fat and skeletal muscle and enhances with contrast {1172}.

Aetiology
The aetiology of hibernoma is unknown, although many lesions arise at the sites where brown fat is normally found in hibernating animals and human fetuses/newborns {754}.

Macroscopy
The median size for hibernoma is 9.3 centimeters, range 1-24 centimeters {747}. Hibernomas are lobular, well-demarcated, and vary in colour from yellow to brown. They have a greasy, soft, and spongy cut surface {747,1113}.

Histopathology
Histologically, hibernomas vary in the content and appearance of the polygonal brown fat cells, the associated small capillary proliferation, and the stromal background, resulting in six variants. Most tumours contain large numbers of multivacuolated brown fat cells with abundant, granular cytoplasm and a

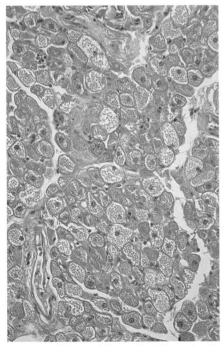

Fig. 1.23 Hibernoma. The eosinophilic variant is composed mostly of granular-appearing, multivacuolated brown fat cells with prominent nucleoli.

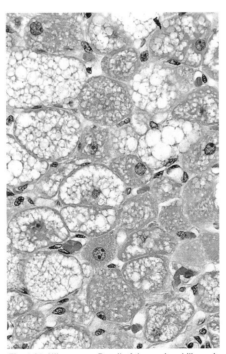

Fig. 1.24 Hibernoma. Detail of the eosinophilic variant with granular, multivacuolated brown fat cells and prominent nucleoli.

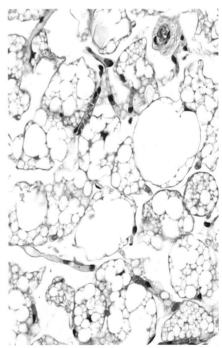

Fig. 1.25 Hibernoma. The pale cell variant has a pale tinctorial quality of the multivacuolated brown fat cells.

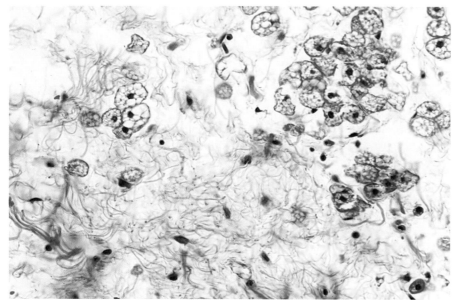

Fig. 1.26 Hibernoma. The myxoid variant has a myxoid background with floating brown fat cells.

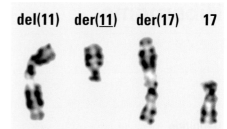

Fig. 1.28 Hibernoma. Partial G-banded karyotype showing a translocation t(11;17)(q13;p13).

Immunophenotype

Hibernoma cells are variably, sometimes strongly, positive for S100 protein. The spindle cell variant has a CD34 positive spindle cell component, similar to spindle cell lipoma, whereas the other hibernoma variants are negative for CD34 {747}.

Genetics

Although hibernomas frequently show somewhat more complex chromosome changes than ordinary lipomas and lipoblastomas, the karyotypes are near- or pseudodiploid. The only recurrent aberration is the involvement of 11q13-21, most often 11q13, in structural rearrangements, which in the majority of cases affect three or more chromosomes. No chromosome band has been involved more than once as a translocation partner.

Metaphase FISH analyses have demonstrated that the chromosomal rearrangements are more complex than can be detected by chromosome banding analysis {793}. The aberrations not only affect the obviously rearranged chromosome 11, but also the seemingly normal homologue. Both heterozygous and homozygous deletions have been detected, with deletions comprising segments up to 4 Mb. Homozygous deletion of the multiple endocrine neoplasia type I tumour suppressor gene *MEN1* has been found in four of five tumours, whereas all five hibernomas investigated showed heterozygous loss of *PPP1A* {793}. Yet, no conclusive evidence of the pathogenetically important event is available.

Prognostic factors

Hibernoma is a benign tumour that does not recur with complete local excision {747}. All morphologic variants have the same good prognosis.

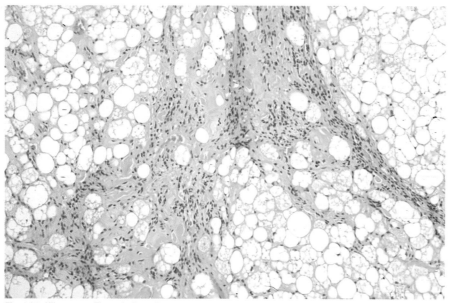

Fig. 1.27 Hibernoma. The spindle cell variant, a hybrid tumour between hibernoma and spindle cell lipoma, shows brown fat cells, mature white fat cells, scattered mast cells, bland spindled cells.

small, central nucleus, the granular or eosinophilic variant. The brown fat cells vary from pale staining to variably eosinophilic, and some cases have a mixture of pale and eosinophilic cells, the mixed variant, while other cases have pure pale brown fat cells, the pale variant. Some hibernomas contain small clusters of brown fat amidst ordinary white fat, the "lipoma-like" variant. Multivacuolated lipoblast-like cells are often seen. Rare variants with myxoid stroma (myxoid variant), or a spindle cell component, with thick bundles of collagen fibres, scattered mast cells, and mature adipose tissue (spindle cell variant), a hybrid between hibernoma and spindle cell lipoma, have been described. Mitoses are exceptional and cytological atypia is unusual. Such features should not be equated with malignancy as the biologic behaviour of hibernoma is invariably benign. However, scattered normal brown fat cells may be found in an otherwise classic myxoid or well differentiated liposarcoma.

Atypical lipomatous tumour / Well differentiated liposarcoma

A.P. Dei Tos
F. Pedeutour

Definition

Atypical lipomatous tumour (ALT) / well-differentiated (WD) liposarcoma is an intermediate (locally aggressive) malignant mesenchymal neoplasm composed either entirely or in part of a mature adipocytic proliferation showing significant variation in cell size and at least focal nuclear atypia in both adipocytes and stromal cells. The presence of scattered hyperchromatic, often multinucleate stromal cells and a varying number of monovacuolated or multivacuolated lipoblasts (defined by the presence of single or multiple sharply marginated cytoplasmic vacuoles scalloping an enlarged hyperchromatic nucleus) may contribute to the morphologic diagnosis. Use of the term 'atypical lipomatous tumour' is determined principally by tumour location and resectability.

ICD-O code   8851/3

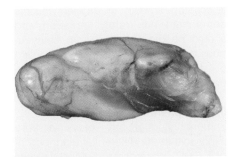

Fig. 1.29 Atypical lipomatous tumour / Well differentiated liposarcoma. Surgical specimen showing a well circumscribed, lobulated mass.

Terminology in clinical practice

The fact that WD liposarcoma shows no potential for metastasis unless it undergoes dedifferentiation led, in the late 1970s, to the introduction of terms such as atypical lipoma or atypical lipomatous tumour {626}, particularly for lesions arising at surgically amenable locations in the limbs and on the trunk since, at these sites, wide excision should usually be curative and hence the designation 'sarcoma' is not warranted. However, the variable, sometimes controversial application of this new terminology has represented a source of potential diagnostic confusion {620, 1112, 2246}. Atypical lipomatous tumour and WD liposarcoma are synonyms describing lesions which are identical both morphologically and karyotypically (see below) and in terms of biologic potential. The choice of terminology is therefore best determined by the degree of reciprocal comprehension between the surgeon and the pathologist to prevent either inadequate or excessive treatment {486}. However, in sites such as the retroperitoneum and mediastinum it is commonly impossible to obtain a wide surgical excision margin and, in such cases, local recurrence (often repeated and ultimately uncontrolled) is almost inevitable and often leads to death, even in the absence of dedifferentiation and metastasis – hence, at these sites, retention of the term WD liposarcoma can readily be justified. Spindle cell/pleomorphic lipoma must be kept separated from the atypical lipoma category as it is morphologically as well as cytogenetically distinct, rarely recurs and has no potential to dedifferentiate (see page 31).

Synonyms

Atypical lipoma, adipocytic liposarcoma, lipoma-like liposarcoma, sclerosing liposarcoma, spindle cell liposarcoma, inflammatory liposarcoma.

Epidemiology

ALT/WD liposarcoma accounts for about 40-45% of all liposarcomas and therefore represents the largest subgroup of aggressive adipocytic neoplasms. These lesions mostly occur in middle aged adults with a peak incidence in the 6th decade. Convincing examples in childhood are extremely rare. Males and females are equally affected with the obvious exception of those lesions affecting the spermatic cord {588,678, 2242}.

Sites of involvement

ALT/WD liposarcoma occurs most frequently in deep soft tissue of the limbs, especially the thigh, followed by the retroperitoneum, the paratesticular area and the mediastinum {588, 678, 2242}. These lesions may also arise in subcutaneous tissue and, very rarely, in skin.

Clinical features

ALT/WD liposarcoma usually presents as a deep-seated, painless enlarging mass

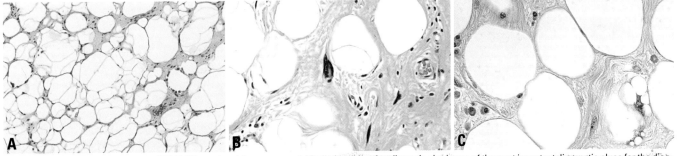

Fig. 1.30 Atypical lipomatous tumour / Well differentiated liposarcoma. **A** Marked variation in adipocytic size is one of the most important diagnostic clues for the diagnosis. **B** The presence of atypical, hyperchromatic stromal cells represents a common finding. **C** A varying number of lipoblasts can be seen in well-differentiated liposarcoma but their presence does not make (nor is required for) a diagnosis of liposarcoma.

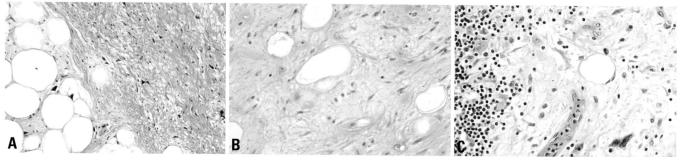

Fig. 1.31 Atypical lipomatous tumour / Well differentiated liposarcoma. **A** The presence of scattered bizarre stromal cells, exhibiting marked nuclear hyperchromasia set in a fibrillary collagenous background represent the most important diagnostic feature of sclerosing variant. **B** Neural-like spindle cell proliferation in a fibrous and / or myxoid background, associated with an atypical lipomatous component that usually includes lipoblasts, characterize the spindle cell variant. **C** Bizarre, often multinucleate cells in the stroma are an important diagnostic clue in the inflammatory variant. Note the accompanying inflammatory component.

that can slowly attain a very large size, particularly when arising in the retroperitoneum. Retroperitoneal lesions are often asymptomatic until the tumour has exceeded 20 cm in diameter and may be found by chance.

Macroscopy
ALT/WD liposarcoma consists usually of a large, usually well-circumscribed, lobulated mass. In the retroperitoneum there may be muliple discontiguous masses. Rarely an infiltrative growth pattern may be encountered. Colour varies from yellow to white (and firm) depending on the proportion of adipocytic, fibrous and/or myxoid areas. Areas of fat necrosis are common in larger lesions.

Histopathology
ALT/WD liposarcoma can be subdivided morphologically into four main subtypes: adipocytic (lipoma-like), sclerosing, inflammatory {2234} and spindle cell {490}. The presence of more than one morphological pattern in the same lesion is common, particularly in retroperitoneal tumors.
Microscopically, ALT/WD liposarcoma is composed of a relatively mature adipocytic proliferation in which, in contrast to benign lipoma, significant variation in cell size is easily appreciable. Focal adipocytic nuclear atypia as well as hyperchromasia also contributes to the usual morphologic picture and scattered hyperchromatic as well as multinucleate stromal cells are often identified. Hyperchromatic stromal cells tend to be more numerous within fibrous septa. A varying number (from many to none) of monovacuolated or multivacuolated lipoblasts may be found. It is commonly believed that lipoblasts represent the

hallmark of any liposarcoma subtype; however, it is important to emphasise that the mere presence of lipoblasts does not make (nor is required for) a diagnosis of liposarcoma.
Sclerosing liposarcoma ranks second in frequency among the group of ALT/WD liposarcoma. This pattern is most often seen in retroperitoneal or paratesticular lesions. Microscopically, the main histological finding is the presence of scattered bizarre stromal cells, exhibiting marked nuclear hyperchromasia and associated with rare multivacuolated lipoblasts set in an extensive fibrillary collagenous stroma. As occasionally the fibrous component may represent the majority of the neoplasm, lipogenic areas (which are often limited in extent) can be easily overlooked or even missed in a small tissue sample. Extensive sampling of the surgical specimen is therefore mandatory, and blocks should be taken from any area showing variation in gross appearance.
Inflammatory liposarcoma represents a rare variant of ALT/WD liposarcoma, occurring most often in the retroperitoneum, in which a chronic inflammatory infiltrate predominates to the extent that the adipocytic nature of the neoplasm can be obscured. In such instances, the differential diagnosis is mainly with non adipocytic lesions such as inflammatory myofibroblastic tumour, Castleman disease and Hodgkin as well as non-Hodgkin lymphomas {78, 1174}. The inflammatory infiltrate is usually composed of polyphenotypic lymphoplasmacytic aggregates in which a B-cell phenotype tends to predominate. Cases exist in which a polyclonal T-cell population represents the main inflammatory component. When dealing with cases in

which the adipocytic component is scarce the presence of bizarre multinucleate stromal cells represents a useful diagnostic clue and should raise the suspicion of inflammatory liposarcoma.
The spindle cell variant of ALT/WD liposarcoma {490} is composed morphologically of a fairly bland neural-like spindle cell proliferation set in a fibrous and/or myxoid background and is associated with an atypical lipomatous component which usually includes lipoblasts. An interesting albeit rare finding in ALT/WD liposarcoma, is the presence of heterologous differentiation. In addition to metaplastic bone formation, a well differentiated smooth or striated muscle component can rarely be seen and should be distinguished from heterologous differentiation arising in the context of dedifferentiated liposarcoma (see page 38) {2063}.

Immunophenotype
Immunohistochemistry plays a very minor role in the differential diagnosis of ALT / WD liposarcoma. Adipocytic cells usually exhibit S-100 protein immunoreactivity that may be helpful in highlighting the presence of lipoblasts {493}. HMB-45 immunonegativity has proved useful in the differential diagnosis with angiomyolipoma that occasionally may mimic liposarcoma.

Genetics
The defining genetic features of ALT/WD liposarcoma cells are supernumerary circular ("ring") and giant rod chromosomes. These rings and giant markers contain amplification of the 12q14-15 region, including the *MDM2* gene, associated with co-amplification of various other chromosomal regions; they most

often lack alpha-satellite centromeric sequences.

Cytogenetics

The supernumerary ring and giant marker chromosomes have been observed as the sole change or concomitant with a few other numerical or structural abnormalities {1477}. Metaphase cells are usually near-diploid but often near-tetraploid. Random and non-random telomeric associations are frequently observed and may give a false impression of complexity to ALT/WD liposarcoma karyotypes {1322}. Cells containing either rings or giant markers or both can be observed in the same tumour sample. Varying stages of complexity are observed, from the simple, classical picture of a supernumerary ring or giant marker in addition to 46 apparently normal chromosomes up to more complex patterns showing several copies of rings and giant markers, telomeric associations, and other structural alterations.

Molecular cytogenetics and genetics

The combination of fluorescence in-situ hybridisation (FISH) using whole chromosome painting probes and comparative genomic hybridisation indicates that both supernumerary rings and giant markers are composed of interspersed amplified sequences consistently originating from the 12q14-15 region. A variety of other chromosomal regions, the most frequent of which are 12q21-22 and 1q21-25, have been shown to be co-amplified with 12q14-15 {434, 1678, 1680, 2053, 2072}. Investigations using FISH with unique probes and Southern blotting showed that *MDM2*, located in 12q14-15, was consistently amplified, usually accompanied by amplification of neighbouring genes, such as *SAS*, *CDK4*, and *HMGIC*. This 12q14-15 amplification is not observed in lipomas and its detection may therefore serve to distinguish ALT/WD liposarcoma from benign adipose tumours. More centromeric genes, located in 12q13, such as *GLI* or *DDIT3* (*CHOP*), have not been shown to be amplified. Nuclear blebs, anaphase bridges, and strings or micronuclei containing the amplified regions are frequently observed. The *TP53* gene is usually not subject to mutations in ALT/WD liposarcoma {1706,

1889}. Another striking feature of ALT/WDLPS supernumerary chromosomes is that they have a functional centromere, as indicated by positive labeling with anti-CENPC antibodies that bind to the kinetochore, but they do not contain alpha-satellite sequences, and C-banding is often negative {1962}.

Prognostic factors

The most important prognostic factor for ALT/WD liposarcoma is anatomic location. Lesions located in surgically amenable soft tissue do not recur following complete (preferably wide) excision with a clear margin. Tumours occurring in deep anatomic sites such as retroperitoneum, spermatic cord or mediastinum tend to recur repeatedly to the extent that they may cause the patient's death as a result of uncontrolled local effects or they may dedifferentiate and metastasise. The ultimate risk of dedifferentiation varies according to site and lesional duration and is probably >20% in the retroperitoneum but < 2% in the limbs. Overall mortality ranges from essentially 0% for ALT of the extremities to more than 80% for WD liposarcomas occurring in the retroperitoneum if the patients are followed up for 10-20 years. Median time to death ranges between 6 and 11 years {1290, 2246}.

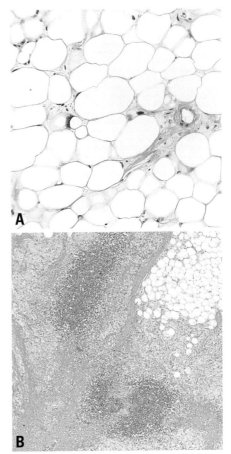

Fig. 1.32 Atypical lipomatous tumour / Well differentiated liposarcoma. **A** Lipoma-like subtype. **B** In the inflammatory subtype, the inflammatory infiltrate often predominates and may obscure the adipocytic nature of the neoplasm.

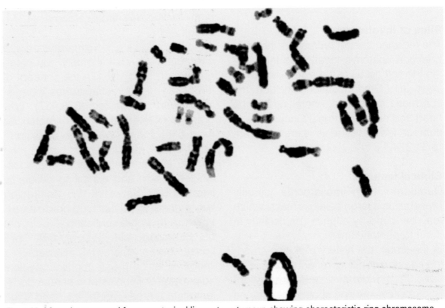

Fig. 1.33 Metaphase spread from an atypical lipomatous tumour, showing characteristic ring chromosome.

Dedifferentiated liposarcoma

A.P. Dei Tos
F. Pedeutour

Definition
Malignant adipocytic neoplasm showing transition, either in the primary or in a recurrence, from atypical lipomatous tumour/well differentiated liposarcoma to non-lipogenic sarcoma of variable histological grade, usually at least several milimeters in diameter.

ICD-O code   8858/3

Epidemiology
Dedifferentiation occurs in up to 10% of well differentiated (WD) liposarcomas of any subtype, although the risk of dedifferentiation appears to be higher when dealing with deep seated (particularly retroperitoneal) lesions and is significantly less in the limbs.
This most probably represents a time-dependent more than a site-dependent phenomenon. Dedifferentiated liposarcoma affects basically the same patient population as WD liposarcoma (see page 35).
No sex predilection is observed. About 90% of dedifferentiated liposarcomas arise "de novo" while 10% occur in recurrences {678, 2242}.

Sites of involvement
The retroperitoneum represents the most common anatomic location, outnumbering the soft tissue of the extremities by at least 3:1. Other locations include the spermatic cord and, more rarely, the head and neck and trunk. Occurrence in subcutaneous tissue is extremely rare {678, 2242}.

Clinical features
Dedifferentiated liposarcoma usually presents as a large painless mass, which may be found by chance (particularly in the retroperitoneum).
In the limbs, the history of a long-standing mass exhibiting recent increase in size often indicates dedifferentiation. Radiological imaging shows coexistence of both fatty and non-fatty solid components which, in the retroperitoneum, may be discontiguous.

Macroscopy
Dedifferentiated liposarcoma usually consists of large multinodular yellow masses containing discrete, solid, often tan-grey non-lipomatous (dedifferentiated) areas. Dedifferentiated areas often show necrosis. The transition between the lipomatous and the dedifferentiated areas sometimes may be gradual.

Histopathology
The histological hallmark of dedifferentiated liposarcoma is represented by the transition from ALT/WD liposarcoma of any type to non-lipogenic sarcoma which, in most cases, is high grade. The extent of dedifferentiation is variable but most often this component is evident to the naked eye. The prognostic significance of microscopic foci of dedifferentation is uncertain. The transition usually occurs abruptly. However in some cases this can be more gradual and, exceptionally, low grade and high grade areas appear to be intermingled. Dedifferentiated areas exhibit a variable histological picture but most frequently they resemble unclassified 'MFH'-like pleomorphic sarcoma or intermediate to high grade myxofibrosarcoma {1374, 2246}.
Although, originally, dedifferentiation was characterized definitionally by high grade morphology {617}, the concept of low grade dedifferentiation has increasingly been recognized {578,937}. Low grade dedifferentiation is characterized most often by the presence of uniform fibroblastic spindle cells with mild nuclear atypia, often organized in a fascicular pattern and exhibiting cellularity intermediate between WD sclerosing liposarcoma and usual high grade areas. Low grade dedifferentiation should not be confused with WD spindle cell liposarcoma which is invariably a lipogenic lesion (i.e. it contains atypical adipocytes or lipoblasts), whereas dedifferentiated areas, both low and high grade are generally non lipogenic.
Dedifferentiated liposarcoma may exhibit heterologous differentiation in about 5-

10% of cases which apparently does not affect the clinical outcome. Most often the line of heterologous differentiation is myogenic or osteo/chondrosarcomatous but angiosarcomatous elements have also been reported. A peculiar "neural-like" or "meningothelial-like" whorling pattern of dedifferentiation has recently been described {636, 1538}. This pattern is often associated with ossification.
Dedifferentiated liposarcoma appears to exhibit less aggressive clinical behaviour when compared with other high grade pleomorphic sarcomas. Careful and extensive sampling is therefore mandatory, particularly in large retroperitoneal lesions, as the well differentiated component may be overlooked. Additionally, it should be noted that local recurrences of dedifferentiated liposarcoma may be entirely well differentiated {1374, 2246}.

Immunophenotype
Immunohistochemistry plays its main role in permitting the recognition of divergent differentiation and in excluding other tumour types.

Genetics
Cytogenetics
Similar to ALT/WD liposarcoma, dedifferentiated liposarcoma most often has ring or giant marker chromosomes {680,794, 1389,1425,1706,1962}. However, the number of karyotyped cases is presently too small to establish whether significant

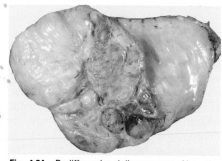

Fig. 1.34 Dedifferentiated liposarcoma. Note the solid, fleshy areas with haemorrhage, indicating the presence of a high grade component in this otherwise well differentiated retroperitoneal liposarcoma.

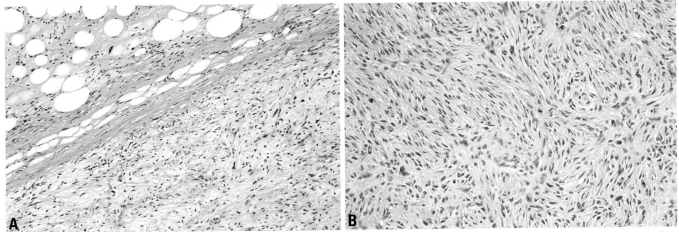

Fig. 1.35 Dedifferentiated liposarcoma. **A** Abrupt transition between well differentiated liposarcoma and high grade non lipogenic area is seen. **B** The morphology of the dedifferentiated component usually overlaps with so called storiform and pleomorphic MFH.

differences between the well differentiated and dedifferentiated types exist. A peculiarity of dedifferentiated liposarcoma might be the presence of multiple abnormal clones, with one or more containing supernumerary rings or large markers {1389,1425}.

Molecular cytogenetics and genetics
Comparative genomic hybridization and fluorescence in situ hybridisation analyses revealed amplification of the 12q13-21 region associated with the co-amplification of other regions, as also observed in WD liposarcomas {794, 1389, 1706, 1962, 2072}. Southern blot studies showed *MDM2* amplification in 5/5 retroperitoneal, but not in 4/4 non-retroperitoneal dedifferentiated liposarcoma cases {1706,1889}. These 4 non-retroperitoneal cases negative for *MDM2*

amplification were found to have *TP53* mutations, whereas in another series of 14 dedifferentiated liposarcoma, a majority of which expressed *MDM2*, *TP53* mutation was detected only in the dedifferentiated component of a single case {487}.

Prognostic factors
Dedifferentiated liposarcoma is characterized by a tendency to recur locally in at least 40% of cases. However, almost all retroperitoneal examples seem to recur locally if the patients are followed for 10-20 years. Distant metastases are observed in 15-20% of cases with an overall mortality ranging between 28 and 30% at 5 years follow-up {937, 1374, 2246}, although this figure is undoubtedly much higher at 10-20 years. The most important prognostic factor is represent-

ed by anatomic location, with retroperitoneal lesions exhibiting the worst clinical behaviour. The extent of dedifferentiated areas does not seem to predict the outcome. Interestingly, dedifferentiated liposarcoma, despite its high grade morphology, exhibits a less aggressive clinical course than other types of high grade pleomorphic sarcoma, although the basis for this difference is unknown {937, 1374, 2246}. Relative absence of complex karyotypic aberrations as well as integrity of the *TP53* gene in most cases (at variance with what is observed in high grade pleomorphic sarcomas) may at least in part explain the discrepancy between morphology and clinical outcome {399,487}.

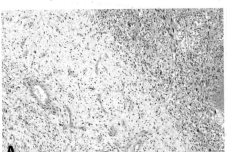
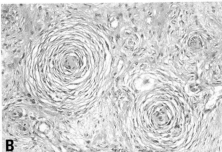
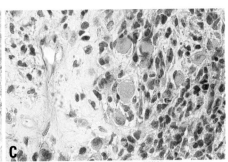

Fig. 1.36 Dedifferentiated liposarcoma. **A** Often the dedifferentiated component exhibits morphologic features indistinguishable from myxofibrosarcoma. **B** Rarely, dedifferentiated liposarcoma features a peculiar whorling growth pattern reminiscent of neural or meningothelial structures. **C** Approximately 5% of cases exhibit heterologous differentiation, most often myogenic. This example shows rhabdomyosarcomatous differentiation.

Myxoid liposarcoma

C. Antonescu
M. Ladanyi

Definition
A malignant tumour composed of uniform round to oval shaped primitive non-lipogenic mesenchymal cells and a variable number of small signet-ring lipoblasts in a prominent myxoid stroma with a characteristic branching vascular pattern. Included in this category are lesions formerly known as round cell liposarcoma.

ICD-O codes
Myxoid liposarcoma   8852/3
Round cell liposarcoma   8853/3

Synonyms
Myxoid / round cell (RC) liposarcoma, round cell liposarcoma.

Epidemiology
Myxoid liposarcoma (MLS) is the second most common subtype of liposarcoma, accounting for more than one third of liposarcomas and representing about 10% of all adult soft tissue sarcomas.

Sites of involvement
MLS occurs with predilection in the deep soft tissues of the extremities, and in more than two-thirds of cases arises within the musculature of the thigh. MLS rarely arises primarily in the retroperitoneum or in subcutaneous tissue.

Clinical features
MLS typically occurs as a large painless mass within the deep soft tissues of the limbs. MLS is a disease of young adults, with the age at presentation on average a decade younger than with other histological subtypes of liposarcoma. It has a peak incidence in the 4th and 5th decades of life and, although very rare, it is the commonest form of liposarcoma in patients younger than 20 years old. There is no gender predilection. MLS is prone to recur locally and one-third of patients develop distant metastases, but this is dependent on the histological grade. In contrast to other types of liposarcoma or other myxoid sarcomas of the extremities, MLS tends to metasta-

sise to unusual soft tissue (such as retroperitoneum, opposite extremity, axilla, etc) or bone (with predilection to spine) locations, even before spread to lung. In a significant number of cases, MLS patients present clinically with synchronous or metachronous multifocal disease {73}. This unusual clinical phenomenon most likely represents a pattern of haematogenous metastases to other sites by tumour cells seemingly incompetent to seed the lungs.

Macroscopy
Grossly, MLS are well-circumscribed, multinodular intramuscular tumours, showing a tan, gelatinous cut surface in predominantly low-grade tumours. In contrast, areas of RC component, representing high-grade sarcoma, have a white fleshy appearance. Gross evidence of tumour necrosis is uncommon.

Histopathology
At low-power MLS has a nodular growth pattern, with enhanced cellularity at the

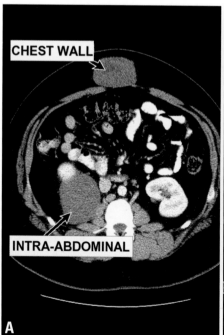

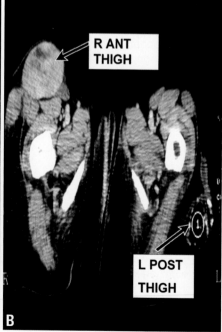

Fig. 1.37 A,B Myxoid liposarcoma. CT images of multifocal myxoid liposarcoma, showing synchronous soft tissue masses, likely representing multiple soft tissue metastases.

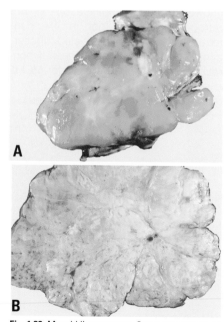

Fig. 1.38 Myxoid liposarcoma. Gross appearance of MLS with **(A)** a gelatinous cut surface in low grade myxoid areas and **(B)** a yellow-white appearance in the high grade round cell component.

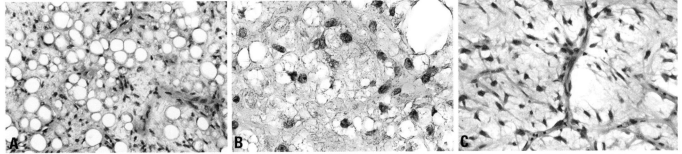

Fig. 1.39 Histological spectrum of myxoid liposarcoma (MLS). **A** Uniform round to oval shaped primitive nonlipogenic mesenchymal cells and a variable number of small lipoblasts in a prominent myxoid stroma. **B** Signet-ring lipoblasts with multivacuolated cytoplasm. **C** Delicate arborizing vasculature.

periphery of the lobules. There is a mixture of uniform round to oval shaped primitive nonlipogenic mesenchymal cells and small signet-ring lipoblasts in a prominent myxoid stroma, rich in a delicate, arborising, "chicken-wire" capillary vasculature. Frequently the extracellular mucin forms large confluent pools, creating a microcystic lymphangioma-like or

so-called "pulmonary oedema" growth pattern. Interstitial haemorrhage is common. Typically, MLS lacks nuclear pleomorphism, giant tumour cells, prominent areas of spindling, or significant mitotic activity. A subset of MLS shows histological progression to hypercellular or RC morphology, which is associated with a significantly poorer prognosis. The RC

areas are characterized by solid sheets of back-to-back primitive round cells with a high nuclear/cytoplasmic ratio and conspicuous nucleoli, with no intervening myxoid stroma {677}. The RC (hypercellular) areas may be composed of close-packed relatively small cells similar to those in the myxoid areas or may less often consist of larger rounded cells

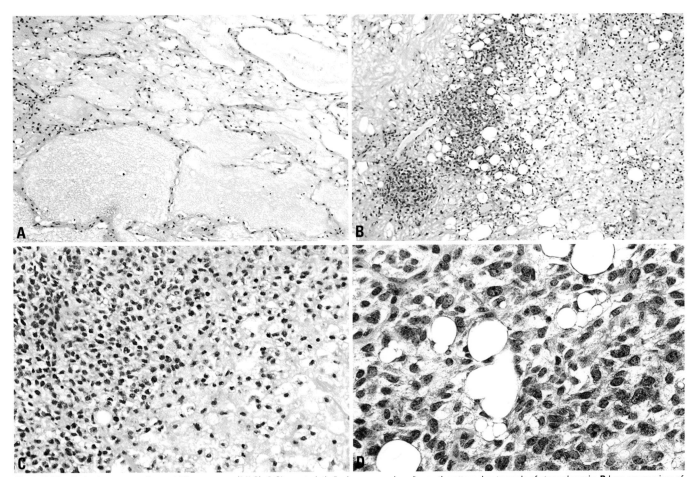

Fig. 1.40 Histological spectrum of myxoid liposarcoma (MLS). **A** Characteristic "pulmonary oedema" growth pattern due to pools of stromal mucin. **B** Low power view of a low grade MLS showing focal areas of increased cellularity. **C** High power view of a "transitional area", showing increased cellularity. Tumour cells are not closely packed, retaining a small amount of intercellular myxoid stroma. **D** Round cell MLS characterized by solid sheets of back-to-back primitive round cells with a high nuclear / cytoplasmic ratio and conspicuous nucleoli, with no intervening myxoid stroma.

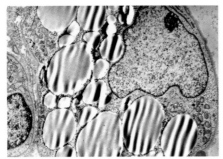

Fig. 1.41 Myxoid liposarcoma. Ultrastructural appearance of signet ring lipoblast, with microvesicular fat droplets.

with variable amounts of eosinophilic cytoplasm. These two morphologic patterns show no clear difference in prognosis but have been responsible for some of the confusion regarding definition of the round cell variant. The presence of gradual transition from myxoid to hypercellular/ RC areas, commonly observed in MLS, provides strong evidence that myxoid and RC liposarcoma represent a histological continuum of MLS. The so-called areas of transition are defined as areas of increased cellularity, not reaching the level of RC component and still retaining small amount of intercellular myxoid stroma. The existence of a morphologic spectrum, in which purely myxoid and RC liposarcoma represent the well and poorly differentiated components is supported by the same recurrent genetic alteration in both.

Immunophenotype

Although, for most MLS cases, immuno-histochemical studies are not needed for establishing a correct diagnosis, it can be useful in cases showing predominantly round cell morphology. In the majority of cases this shows a diffuse staining for S100 protein.

Ultrastructure

Ultrastructurally the proportion of undifferentiated cells, devoid of lipid droplets and rich in clusters of vimentin-type intermediate filaments, and signet-ring lipoblasts vary from case to case. Lipoblasts in variable stages of adipocytic maturation can be identified, containing either relatively few small lipid droplets, or large confluent lipid droplets that displace the nucleus to the periphery. Flocculent mucoid stromal material coating the cells and extracellular spaces is common.

Genetics

The karyotypic hallmark of myxoid and round cell liposarcoma is the t(12;16)(q13;p11) present cytogenetically in more than 90% of cases {2018, 2145}. The translocation leads to the fusion of the *DDIT3* (a.k.a. *CHOP*) and *FUS* (a.k.a. *TLS*) genes at 12q13 and 16p11, respectively, and the generation of FUS/DDIT3 hybrid protein {104, 410, 1687, 1741}. In rare cases of MLS a variant chromosomal translocation

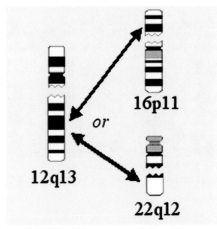

Fig. 1.42 Myxoid liposarcoma. Schematic illustration of the breakpoints involved in the specific translocations of myxoid/round cell liposarcoma, t(12;16)(q13;p11) and t(12;22)(q13;q12).

t(12;22)(q13;q12) has been described, in which *DDIT3* fuses instead with *EWS*, a gene highly related to *FUS* {1641}. *FUS/DDIT3* fusion transcripts occur as different recurrent structural variants based on the presence or absence of *FUS* exons 6 to 8 in the fusion product. Of the possible *FUS* genomic breakpoints, only breaks in *FUS* introns 5, 7, and 8 give rise to in-frame fusion transcripts joining *FUS* exons 5, 7, and 8, respectively, to exon 2 of *DDIT3* {1061, 1642}. Thus, three major recurrent fusion transcript types have been reported: type 7-2 (a.k.a. type I), seen in about 20% of cases, type 5-2 (a.k.a. type II), seen in approximately two-thirds of cases, and type 8-2 (a.k.a. type III), seen in about 10% {73, 1143, 1642}. Sequence analysis of the genomic t(12;16) breakpoints in *FUS* and *DDIT3* and associated functional studies suggest the involvement of translin and topoisomerase II in the process of translocation {971,1061}.

The monoclonal origin of the synchronous and/or metachronous multifocal MLS has been confirmed by comparing FUS/DDIT3 or EWS/DDIT3 genomic rearrangement structure in tumours from different sites {66}.

The presence of the *FUS/DDIT3* fusion is highly sensitive and specific for the MLS entity, and is absent in other morphologic mimics, such as the predominantly myxoid well differentiated liposarcomas of the retroperitoneum and myxofibrosarcomas {67}. No convincing genetic evidence has been provided to date to

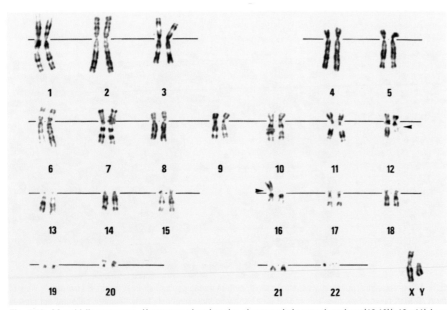

Fig. 1.43 Myxoid liposarcoma. Karyotype showing the characteristic translocation t(12;16)(q13;p11) in a myxoid liposarcoma. Arrowheads indicate breakpoints.

support the concept of mixed type liposarcoma composed of MLS and dedifferentiated liposarcoma.

Prognostic factors

High histological grade, often defined as ≥5%RC areas, presence of necrosis, and TP53 overexpression are predictors of unfavourable outcome in localized MLS {73, 1103, 1976}. The prognostic significance of more limited hypercellularity (transitional areas) is less certain. The clinical outcome of multifocal MLS is poor, regardless of its often bland or "low grade" histological appearance. In contrast with some other translocation-associated sarcomas, the molecular variability of fusion transcripts in MLS does not appear to have a significant impact on histological grade or clinical outcome {73}.

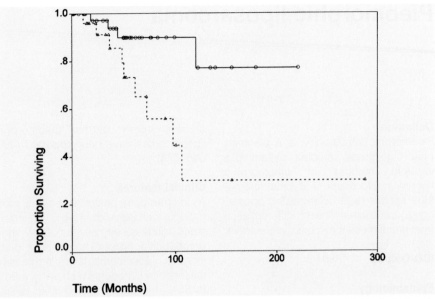

Fig. 1.44 Myxoid liposarcoma. Kaplan-Meier curve showing a correlation between high histological grade (≥5%RC) and disease specific survival in patients with localized MLS (From C.R. Antonescu et al. {73}).

Pleomorphic liposarcoma

T. Mentzel
F. Pedeutour

Definition
Pleomorphic liposarcoma is a pleomorphic, high grade sarcoma containing a variable number of pleomorphic lipoblasts. No areas of atypical lipomatous tumour (well differentiated liposarcoma) or another line of differentiation (malignant mesenchymoma) are evident.

ICD-O code   8854/3

Epidemiology
Pleomorphic liposarcoma represents the rarest subtype of liposarcoma, accounting for approximately 5% of all liposarcomas {101} and 20% of pleomorphic sarcomas {675}. The majority of neoplasms arise in elderly patients (>50 years) with an equal sex distribution.

Sites of involvement
Pleomorphic liposarcoma tends to occur on the extremities (lower>upper limbs), whereas the trunk and the retroperitoneum are less frequently affected; rare sites of involvement include the mediastinum, the paratesticular region, the scalp, the abdominal/pelvic cavities, and the orbit {290, 489, 548, 1139, 1445, 1609}. Although most cases arise in deep soft tissues, examples in subcutis or rare purely dermal pleomorphic liposarcomas have been reported {489, 548, 774}.

Clinical features
As in other deep seated sarcomas, most patients complain of a firm, enlarging mass; many cases have a notably short preoperative history. In general, pleomorphic liposarcoma is an aggressive mesenchymal neoplasm showing a 30% to 50% metastasis rate and an overall tumour associated mortality of 40% to 50% {548, 1445, 2332}. Many patients die within a short period of time {1445}, and the lung represents the preferred site of metastases {548}. In contrast, dedifferentiated liposarcomas and high-grade myxofibrosarcomas have a prolonged clinical course, whereas pleomorphic myogenic sarcomas of deep soft tissues show an even more aggressive clinical course emphasising the need for subclassification of pleomorphic sarcomas.

Macroscopy
Grossly, the neoplasms are typically described as firm, often multinodular lesions with white to yellow cut surfaces. In many cases myxoid areas and areas of necrosis are noted. The majority of neoplasms are large with a median greatest diameter of more than 10 cm.

Histopathology
Histologically, well circumscribed, non-encapsulated cases as well as ill defined and infiltrative neoplasms composed of a varying number of pleomorphic lipoblasts in a background of a high grade, pleomorphic sarcoma are seen. The majority of neoplasms consist of pleomorphic spindle shaped tumour cells and fascicles of spindled and smaller, round cells admixed with multinucleated giant cells (similar to so called malignant fibrous histiocytoma), as well as pleomorphic, multivacuolated lipoblasts, with bizarre, hyperchromatic and scalloped nuclei. In some cases only scattered pleomorphic lipoblasts are found, whereas sheets of pleomorphic lipoblasts are evident in other examples. Frequently, intra- and extracellular eosinophilic hyaline droplets or globules are noted, that most likely represent lysosomal structures. Rarely a prominent inflammatory infiltrate is evident. In a number of cases, areas with morphological features of pleomorphic sarcoma resembling intermediate to high

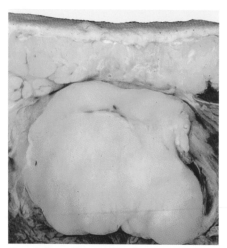

Fig. 1.45 Pleomorphic liposarcoma. Deep seated tumour with grey-white cut surface.

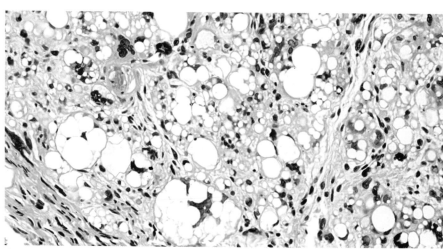

Fig. 1.46 Pleomorphic liposarcoma. Pleomorphic spindle and giant cells as well as pleomorphic lipoblasts which contain enlarged and hyperchromatic nuclei scalloped by cytoplasmic vacuoles.

grade myxofibrosarcoma associated with pleomorphic lipoblasts are noted. The recently described epithelioid variant of pleomorphic liposarcoma {1445} is composed predominantly of solid, cohesive sheets of epithelioid tumour cells with distinct cell borders, eosinophilic cytoplasm and round to oval nuclei with prominent nucleoli separated by narrow fibrous septa with thin-walled capillaries; at least focally, lipogenic differentiation with pleomorphic lipoblasts is noted also in these neoplasms. The mitotic rate is higher in the epithelioid variant, but areas of tumour necrosis are seen in the majority of cases irrespective of the morphological subtype. Most recently a small round cell variant containing pleomorphic lipoblasts and small round cells virtually indistinguishable from round cell liposarcoma has been proposed {1389}.

Immunophenotype
The tumour cells stain positively for vimentin, but despite unequivocal lipogenic differentiation S-100 protein is seen in less than half of the cases. Some cases of the epithelioid variant of pleomorphic liposarcoma show focal expression of epithelial markers, an important finding in the differential diagnosis of these lesions {774, 1445}.

Ultrastructure
Neoplastic cells of pleomorphic liposarcoma contain abundant and coalescing lipid droplets, numerous cytoplasmic organelles and surrounding plasma membranes {2231}.

Genetics
Cytogenetics
All 11 pleomorphic liposarcomas from which karyotypic data exist have shown high chromosome counts and complex structural rearrangements {1425,2018}. This complexity, represented by numerous unidentifiable marker chromosomes, non-clonal alterations, polyploidy and intercellular heterogeneity has made the detection of specific rearrangements difficult. The presence of ring, large marker, or double minute chromosomes has

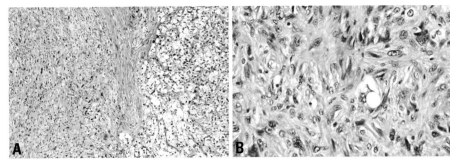

Fig. 1.47 Pleomorphic liposarcoma. In some neoplasms sheets of pleomorphic lipoblasts are seen (right part, **A**), whereas only scattered lipoblasts are present in other cases **(B)**.

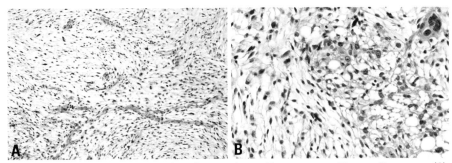

Fig. 1.48 This retroperitoneal neoplasm shows features of a myxoid sarcoma resembling myxofibrosarcoma **(A)**, however, focally, lipoblasts with hyperchromatic and scalloped nuclei were noted **(B)**

been reported in 6 of the 11 cases. The cytogenetic profile of pleomorphic liposarcoma appears therefore to be closer to other pleomorphic sarcomas than to well differentiated liposarcoma.

Molecular genetics
In contrast to well differentiated liposarcomas, amplification of the 12q14-15 region and the *MDM2* gene does not occur consistently in pleomorphic liposarcomas. A number of varied chromosomal gains and losses but no amplification of the 12q14-15 region were found in two cases studied by comparative genomic hybridisation {2072}. The amplification of *MDM2* was observed in approximately one third of the cases, and could be associated with the presence of ring chromosomes {1568, 1889}. *TP53* alterations, such as mutations in exons 7 or 8 or loss of heterozygosity, have been observed in 4/9 studied cases; all these 4 cases were negative for *MDM2* amplification {1889}.

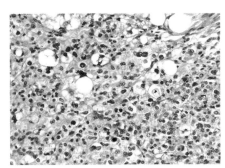

Fig. 1.49 Epithelioid variant of pleomorphic liposarcoma, characterized by sheets and clusters of atypical epithelioid tumour cells associated with pleomorphic lipoblasts (upper part).

Prognostic factors
Although no single morphological factor predicts the clinical prognosis reliably, tumour depth and size, more than 20 mitoses in 10 HPFs, and areas of tumour necrosis are associated with a worse clinical prognosis {548,1408,1445}.

Mixed-type liposarcoma

T. Mentzel
F. Pedeutour

Definition
Liposarcomas showing features of combined myxoid/round cell liposarcoma and atypical lipomatous tumour (well differentiated liposarcoma)/dedifferentiated liposarcoma or of myxoid/round cell liposarcoma and pleomorphic liposarcoma.

ICO-O codes
Mixed type liposarcoma   8855/3
Liposarcoma, NOS   8850/3

Epidemiology
True mixed-type liposarcomas are exteremely rare and occur predominantly in elderly patients {1416}.

Sites of involvement
Most cases of mixed-type liposarcoma appear to arise in retroperitoneal or intraabdominal locations. More rarely, examples in the mediastinum and in deep soft tissue of the extremities have been reported {1114, 1139, 1389, 1416}.

Clinical features
The patients usually present with a large painless tumour mass, that is noted sometimes incidentally.

Macroscopy
Given the location, most cases of mixed-type liposarcoma are large, and often present as multinodular masses with cystic and solid areas and grey-yellow cut surfaces.

Histopathology
The occurrence of myxoid areas in the group of atypical lipomatous tumour (well differentiated liposarcoma)/dedifferentiated liposarcoma is well recognized and especially in retroperitoneal and intraabdominal location quite common. However, in most cases, this reflects either myxoid degeneration or dedifferentiation with myxofibrosarcoma-like features in atypical lipomatous tumour (well differentiated liposarcoma) instead of a true mixed-type liposarcoma {67, 955, 1389}. Rare mixed-type liposarcomas show a combination of morphological features of myxoid/round cell liposarcoma (small undifferentiated mesenchymal cells, often univacuolated lipoblasts, and round cells set in a myxoid matrix with mucin pooling and a prominent plexiform capillary pattern), pleomorphic liposarcoma (features of pleomorphic sarcoma with a variable number of pleomorphic lipoblasts), and/or atypical lipomatous tumour (well differentiated liposarcoma) (adipocytes with marked variation in size and shape, nuclear atypia). Cases of so called dedifferentiated myxoid liposarcoma may represent mixed-type liposarcomas showing a combination of myxoid/round cell liposarcoma and dedifferentiated liposarcoma.

Genetics
In the three karyotyped cases of mixed-type liposarcoma, the presence of ring or giant marker chromosomes was observed either as the sole abnormality {680} or in association with complex rearrangements {794, 1389}. Amplification of the 12q14-15 region and, more specifically, of the *MDM2* gene has been found, but not *TP53* mutations {794, 1389, 1889}.

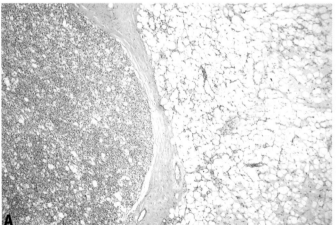 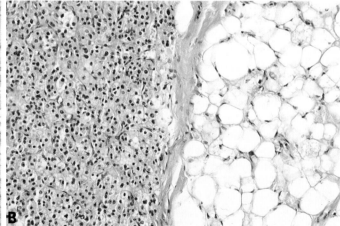

Fig. 1.50 This case of a mixed type liposarcoma shows morphological features of lipoma-like atypical lipomatous tumour (well differentiated liposarcoma) (right) and myxoid liposarcoma (left) **(A)**. High power view reveals small undifferentiated mesenchymal cells and lipoblasts set in a myxoid matrix with a plexiform vascular pattern in the myxoid liposarcoma areas **(B)**.

CHAPTER 2

Fibroblastic / Myofibroblastic Tumours

Fibroblastic / myofibroblastic tumours represent a very large subset of mesenchymal tumours. Many lesions in this category contain cells with both fibroblastic and myofibroblastic features, which may in fact represent functional variants of a single cell type. The relative proportions of these cell types vary not only between individual cases but also within a single lesion over time (often in proportion to cellularity). A significant subset of spindle cell and pleomorphic sarcomas are probably myofibroblastic in type but, to date, only low grade forms have been reproducibly characterized. Among lesions formerly known as malignant fibrous histiocytoma (MFH – see Chapter 3), at least some represent pleomorphic myofibrosarcomas.

Principal changes and advances since the 1994 WHO classification have been the characterization of numerous previously undefined lesions, including ischaemic fasciitis, desmoplastic fibroblastoma, mammary-type myofibroblastoma, angiomyofibroblastoma, cellular angiofibroma, Gardner fibroma, low grade fibromyxoid sarcoma, acral myxoinflammatory fibroblastic sarcoma, sclerosing epithelioid fibrosarcoma and low grade myofibroblastic sarcoma.

Conceptual changes have included the clearer recognition of solitary fibrous tumour in soft tissue and the realization that most cases of so-called haemangiopericytoma belong in this category, as well as the reclassification of lesions formerly labelled myxoid MFH as myxofibrosarcoma and the definitive allocation of these tumours to the fibroblastic category.

Nodular fasciitis

H.L. Evans
J.A. Bridge

Definition
Nodular fasciitis is a mass-forming fibrous proliferation that usually occurs in the subcutaneous tissue. It is composed of plump but uniform fibroblastic / myofibroblastic cells and typically displays a loose or tissue culture-like growth pattern. Intravascular fasciitis and cranial fasciitis are histologically similar lesions that extend into vessel lumens and involve the skull and overlying soft tissue, respectively.

Synonym
Pseudosarcomatous fasciitis.

Epidemiology
Nodular fasciitis is comparatively common among soft tissue mass lesions {39, 173,985,1136,1156,1399,1727,1940, 2000}. It occurs in all age groups but more often in young adults. Intravascular fasciitis {1727} and cranial fasciitis {1225} are rare. Intravascular fasciitis is found mostly in persons under 30 years of age, whereas cranial fasciitis develops predominantly in infants under 2 years of age. There is no sex predilection for nodular fasciitis or intravascular fasciitis, but cranial fasciitis is more frequent in boys.

Sites of involvement
Nodular fasciitis is usually subcutaneous, although occasional cases are intramuscular. Dermal localization is very rare {812} (see volume on skin tumours). Any part of the body can be involved, but the upper extremity, trunk, and head and neck are most frequently affected. Intravascular fasciitis is also chiefly subcutaneous. It occurs in small to medium-sized vessels, predominantly veins but occasionally arteries (or both). Cranial fasciitis typically involves the outer table of the skull and contiguous soft tissue of the scalp, and may extend downward through the inner table into the meninges.

Clinical features
Nodular fasciitis typically grows rapidly and has a preoperative duration in most, but not all, cases of not more than 1-2 months. Soreness or tenderness may be present. It usually measures 2 cm or less and almost always less than 5 cm. Intravascular fasciitis may enlarge more slowly but is also normally not more than 2 cm in size. Cranial fasciitis expands quickly, like nodular fascitis, and may become somewhat larger than the usual example of the latter. When the skull is involved, X-ray shows a lytic defect, often with a sclerotic rim. By contrast, nodular fasciitis presents as a nondistinctive soft-tissue mass on imaging studies, and there is little information on imaging of intravascular fasciitis.

Aetiology
Some patients with nodular fasciitis report trauma to the site of the lesion, but the majority do not. Birth trauma may be a factor in the genesis of cranial fasciitis.

Macroscopy
Grossly, nodular fasciitis may appear circumscribed or infiltrative but is not encapsulated. The cut surface varies from myxoid to fibrous, and occasionally there is central cystic change. Intravascular fasciitis ranges from nodular to plexiform, the latter contour resulting when there is extensive intravascular growth. Cranial fasciitis is typically cir-

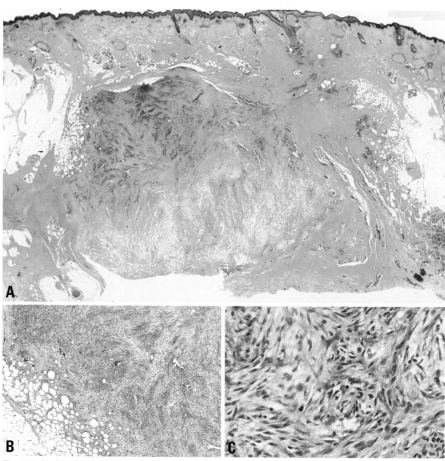

Fig. 2.01 Nodular fasciitis. **A** This low power view illustrates the typical subcutaneous location. **B** Detail from the same lesion showing infiltration of adjacent fat. **C** This high power view shows the typical plump but regular fibroblasts / myofibroblasts (From R. Kempson et al. {1086}).

cumscribed and rubbery to firm, and may be focally myxoid or cystic in its centre.

Histopathology

Nodular fasciitis is composed of plump but regular spindle-shaped fibroblasts (or myofibroblasts) lacking nuclear hyperchromasia and pleomorphism. Mitotic figures may be plentiful, but atypical mitoses would not be expected. The lesion may be highly cellular, but typically it is at least partly loose appearing and myxoid, with a torn, feathery, or tissue culture-like character. In more cellular areas, there is often growth in S- or C-shaped fascicles, and sometimes a storiform pattern. There is normally little collagen, but this may be increased focally, and keloidlike collagen bundles may be present and even occasionally prominent. Isolated cases may show extensive stromal hyalinization. Extravasated red cells, chronic inflammatory cells, and multinucleated osteoclastlike giant cells are other frequently identified features. The lesional border is typically, at least focally, infiltrative, although it may be well delineated; peripheral extension is often seen between fat cells in the subcutis and between muscle cells in intramuscular locations. Small vessels are numerous in some examples, resulting in a resemblance to granulation tissue, sometimes with poorly delimited margins. Intravascular fasciitis and cranial fasciitis are basically similar to nodular fasciitis histologically, although the former often displays a greater number of osteoclastlike giant cells. Intravascular fasciitis ranges from predominantly extravascular, with only a minor intravascular component, to predominantly intravascular. Osseous metaplasia is occasionally seen in nodular fasciitis (fasciitis ossificans) {450,1193} and cranial fasciitis.

Immunophenotype

Stains for SMA and MSA are usually positive, but desmin positivity is rare {1497}. These results are consistent with myofibroblastic differentiation but do not distinguish nodular fasciitis from many other

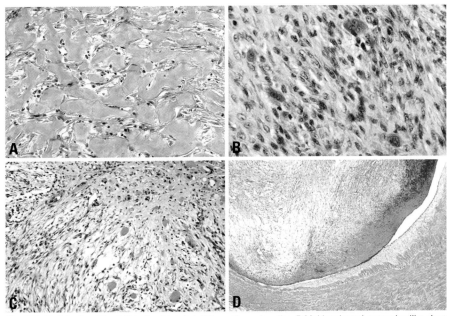

Fig. 2.02 Nodular fasciitis. **A** Note the thick, keloidlike collagen bundles. **B** Multinucleated, osteoclastlike giant cells are sometimes present. **C** Nodular fasciitis, intramuscular variant. There is a loose and "torn" appearance, but greater fibrosis than usual in one area (upper right). **D** Intravascular fasciitis. The intravascular location is demonstrated at scanning magnification (From R. Kempson et al. {1086}).

mesenchymal proliferations. CD68 staining is present in the osteoclast-like giant cells and occasionally in spindle cells. Keratin and S100 protein are typically negative.

Ultrastructure

By electron microscopy, nodular fasciitis demonstrates fibroblastic/myofibroblastic features; the cells are elongated, have abundant, often dilated rough endoplasmic reticulum, and sometimes demonstrate cytoplasmic filaments with dense bodies, pinocytotic vesicles, and cell junctions. Like the immunohistochemical profile, these findings are common to numerous mesenchymal entities.

Genetics

Assessment of DNA ploidy in nodular fasciitis using flow cytometry has shown these lesions to be diploid {575,1621}. In contrast, clonal chromosomal abnormalities have been detected by cytogenetic analysis in three cases of nodular fasciitis including a rearrangement of 3q21 with a group D acrocentric chromosome

in two {1869,2229}. The remaining case, a case of nodular fasciitis arising in the breast, exhibited a 2;15 translocation, loss of chromosomes 2 and 13, and several marker chromosomes {199}. Although the observation of clonality in these limited cases of nodular fasciitis would appear to support true neoplastic rather than reactive origin, it is possible that the culturing conditions used may favour growth of a particular clone or type of cell.

Prognostic factors

Recurrence of nodular fasciitis after excision is very rare. It has been observed occasionally (<2% of cases) after incomplete excision of *bona fide* examples, but in general recurrence should prompt reevaluation of the diagnosis. Metastasis does not occur. Intravascular fasciitis has the same innocent behaviour as nodular fasciitis, despite its sometimes prominent intravascular growth, as does cranial fasciitis.

Proliferative fasciitis and proliferative myositis

H.L.. Evans
J.A. Bridge

Definition

Proliferative fasciitis is a mass-forming subcutaneous proliferation characterized by large ganglion-like cells in addition to plump fibroblastic / myofibroblastic cells similar to those seen in nodular fasciitis. Proliferative myositis has the same cellular composition but occurs within skeletal muscle.

Epidemiology

Proliferative fasciitis and myositis are much less common than nodular fasciitis. Both occur predominantly in middle-aged or older adults {349,594,1093}, i.e., an older age group than for nodular fasciitis. A rare variant of proliferative fasciitis is described in children {1395}.

Site of involvement

Proliferative fasciitis develops most frequently in the upper extremity, particularly the forearm, followed by the lower extremity and trunk. Proliferative myositis arises predominantly in the trunk, shoulder girdle, and upper arm and less often in the thigh. By definition, proliferative fasciitis is subcutaneous and proliferative myositis is intramuscular.

Clinical features

Both proliferative fasciitis and proliferative myositis characteristically grow rapidly and are usually excised within 2 months of the time they are first noted. Proliferative fasciitis almost always measures less than 5 cm and is most often less than 3 cm. Proliferative myositis may be slightly larger but not greatly so. Either lesion may be painful or tender, but this is more common with proliferative fasciitis. There is not much experience with imaging of these conditions.

Aetiology

There is sometimes a history of trauma to the site of proliferative fasciitis and myositis, but more often there is not.

Macroscopy

Proliferative fasciitis typically forms a poorly circumscribed mass in the subcutaneous tissue and may extend horizontally along fascia. The rare childhood variant is often better circumscribed. Proliferative myositis is also poorly marginated and replaces a variable proportion of the involved muscle.

Histopathology

Both proliferative fasciitis and myositis contain plump fibroblastic/myofibroblastic spindle cells similar to those seen in nodular fasciitis but also demonstrate large cells with rounded nuclei, prominent nucleoli, and abundant amphophilic to basophilic cytoplasm. These features result in a resemblance to ganglion cells, and the cells are often described as ganglion-like. They usually have one nucleus but may have two or three. They vary in number in different examples and may be evenly or patchily distributed. Mitotic figures are found in both the spindle cells and ganglion-like cells and may be relatively numerous, but are not atypical. The stroma varies from myxoid to collagenous, and the lesional borders are typically infiltrative or even ill defined. Proliferative fasciitis may grow laterally along fascial planes, whereas proliferative myositis extends between individual muscle fibres and small groups, creating the characteristic "checkerboard" pattern. The childhood variant of proliferative fasciitis normally has better delineated borders than the adult form, greater cellularity, dominance of ganglion-like cells and more mitoses. Focal necrosis and acute inflammation may be present, in addition. Proliferative myositis may contain metaplastic bone, thus demonstrating kinship to myositis ossificans.

Immunophenotype

The immunohistochemical profile of proliferative fasciitis and myositis is similar to that of nodular fasciitis, with usual positivity for SMA and MSA and negativity for

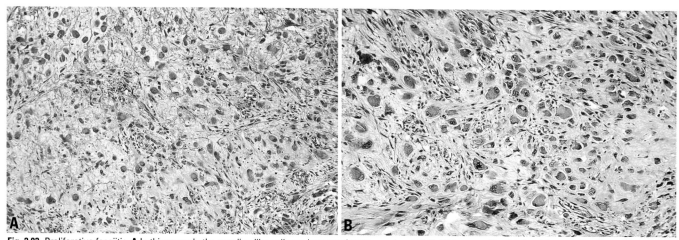

Fig. 2.03 Proliferative fasciitis. **A** In this example the ganglion-like cells are larger and more prominent. **B** On high power the details of the ganglion-like cells are better seen. (From R. Kempson et al. {1086}).

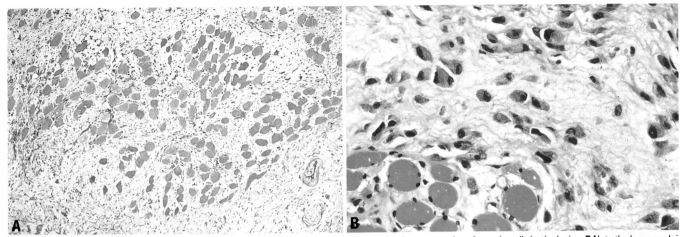

Fig. 2.04 Proliferative myositis. **A** Low power demonstrates the "checkerboard" pattern resulting from separation of muscle cells by the lesion. **B** Note the large nuclei and abundant amphophilic cytoplasm of the ganglion-like cells (From R. Kempson et al. {1086}).

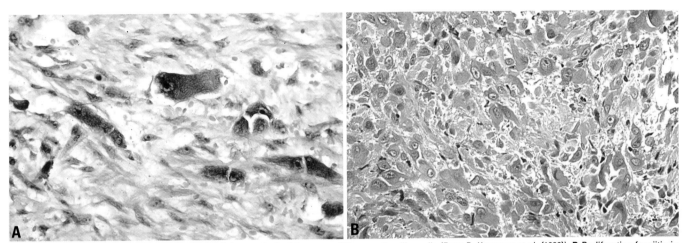

Fig. 2.05 A Proliferative myositis, showing in detail the cytological features of the ganglion-like cells (From R. Kempson et al. {1086}). **B** Proliferative fasciitis in childhood. Such lesions may readily be mistaken for rhabdomyosarcoma.

desmin {574,1295}.The ganglion-like cells, however, may stain only focally or weakly for actins. CD68 may stain some cells, but keratin and S100 protein are typically negative.

Ultrastructure
As with nodular fasciitis, the ultrastructural features of proliferative fasciitis and myositis are those of fibroblasts and myofibroblasts {574,1295}. The ganglion-like cells demonstrate abundant and dilated rough endoplasmic reticulum and lack neuronal characteristics.

Genetics
DNA flow cytometric analyses of proliferative fasciitis have revealed a uniformly diploid pattern {574,1295}. Trisomy 2 has been detected in a single case of proliferative fasciitis by standard cytogenetic evaluation {499}.
Cytogenetic studies of two cases of proliferative myositis have revealed distinct abnormalities {1371,1597}. An extra copy of chromosome 2 or trisomy 2 was detected in one case arising in the axilla of a 62-year-old male {1597}. The second case, arising in the rectus muscle of a 60-year-old female, showed the following translocation: t(6;14)(q23;q32) {1371}. Fluorescence in situ hybridization studies performed on uncultured cells of this latter case excluded the presence of trisomy 2.

Prognostic factors
Both proliferative fasciitis and myositis recur only rarely after local excision and do not metastasize.

Myositis ossificans and fibroosseous pseudotumour of digits

A.E. Rosenberg

Definition

Myositis ossificans (MO) and fibroosseous pseudotumour of digits (FP) are localized, self-limiting, reparative lesions that are composed of reactive hypercellular fibrous tissue and bone. Morphologically similar lesions may also occur in the subcutis, tendons or fascia and have been termed panniculitis ossificans and fasciitis ossificans, respectively. The rapid growth of these lesions that frequently arouses clinical suspicion in conjunction with their hypercellularity, cytological atypia, and mitotic activity makes them classic pseudosarcomas of soft tissues.

Synonyms

Pseudomalignant osseous tumour of soft tissue, extraosseous localized, nonneoplastic bone and cartilage formation, myositis ossificans circumscripta, myositis ossificans traumatica.

Epidemiology

MO and FP have a broad age distribution ranging from infancy to late adulthood (14 mos-95 years), however, they are characteristically encountered during young adulthood (mean age 32 years), and rarely occur in infants or the elderly {2,13,358,1588,2054}. Males are affected more frequently than females (3:2), however, females are more commonly involved in FP {559}. Patients with MO are typically physically active.

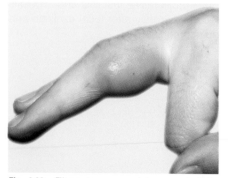

Fig. 2.06 Fibroosseous pseudotumour of digits presenting as a red and swollen mass.

Sites of involvement

MO may develop anywhere in the body including the extremities, trunk, and head and neck {2,805,1580,2054}. The most common locations are those most susceptible to trauma such as the elbow, thigh, buttock, and shoulder. MO-like lesions have also been reported in the mesentery {2277}. FP usually affects the subcutaneous tissues of the proximal phalanx of the fingers and less frequently the toes {559}.

Clinical features

The clinical and radiographic findings of MO parallel the stage of development of the lesion. In the early phase (1-2 weeks), the involved area is swollen and painful. Similarly, in FP the digit hurts and there is a localized fusiform swelling of the affected area.

Plain X-rays and CT scans of MO may demonstrate soft tissue fullness and oedema, whereas MRI reveals signal heterogeneity and high signal intensity on T2 weighted images {805,1169, 1580,1949,2277}. Two to six weeks after the onset of symptoms, flocculent dense calcifications become evident in the periphery of the mass and eventually produce a lacy pattern of bone deposition that sharply demarcates the periphery of the lesion in an eggshell-like fashion. In FP the lesional calcification has a more random distribution. In MO this correlates with the clinical progression for the affected site becomes more circumscribed and firm and eventually evolves into a painless, hard, well-demarcated mass. After a prolonged period of time the mass may remain stable or undergo partial or complete resorption. In older stable lesions MRI exhibits a well defined mass that possesses a rim of low signal intensity (mineralized bone) and contains intralesional regions of higher intensity representing marrow fat.

Aetiology

Soft tissue injury produced by a variety of mechanisms is believed to be the initiating event in most instances and a clear history of trauma is documented in 60-75% of cases {1580,1667}. In patients without a history of trauma, repetitive small mechanical injuries, ischaemia or inflammation have been implicated as possible causative factors. Initiation of the process is followed by proliferation of mesenchymal stem cells that produce activated fibroblasts and osteoblasts that grow in a centripetal fashion. The mechanisms underlying the characteristic pattern of zonation have not been clearly elucidated.

Macroscopy

Myositis ossificans manifests as a well delineated ovoid tan mass with a soft

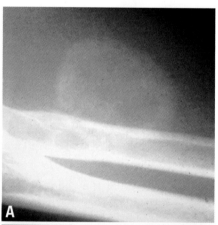

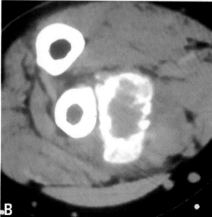

Fig. 2.07 Myositis ossificans. **A** Plain X-ray and **(B)** cross sectional CT of a forearm lesion of approximately 6 weeks duration with a well circumscribed, ossified periphery and a more lucent centre.

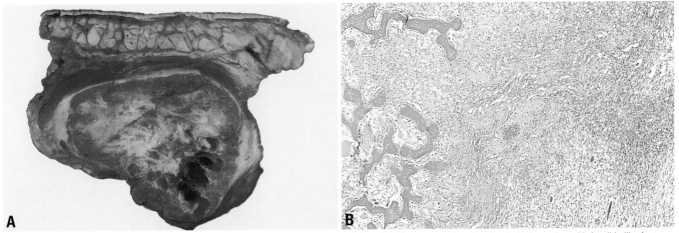

Fig. 2.08 Myositis ossificans. **A** Gross appearance of myositis ossificans in a young adult male. **B** Low power view showing typical zonation with fasciitis-like features (centre right), immature osteoid (centre) and bone formation at the periphery (left).

glistening centre and a firm, grey-white gritty periphery. The lesion ranges in size from 2-12 cm but most are approximately 5 cm in greatest dimension.

Histopathology

Myositis ossificans is characterized by a zonal proliferation of fibroblasts and bone-forming osteoblastic elements that progresses through various stages over time {1210}. In the early stages of development MO is most cellular, bearing a resemblance to nodular fasciitis, and is composed of numerous proliferating fibroblasts that are oriented randomly or in short intersecting fascicles. The fibroblasts have ill defined, tapering cell processes that consist of faintly eosinophilic cytoplasm and contain vesicular or finely granular nuclei with smooth nuclear membranes and nucleoli of variable size. Numerous mitoses may be present but atypical mitotic figures are uniformly absent. The stroma is richly vascular, oedematous or myxoid and contains fibrin, clusters of extravasated red blood cells, scattered chronic inflammatory cells, osteoclast-like giant cells and injured or atrophic myocytes. Peripherally, the fibroblastic component merges with ill defined trabeculae and sheets of unmineralized woven bone that harbour large osteocytes and demonstrate prominent osteoblastic rimming. In FP the bone is randomly distributed throughout the lesion. In some cases of MO, nodules of cellular hyaline cartilage with foci of enchondral ossification are present. Some late stage lesions of FP fuse with underlying periosteum and form an ostechondroma-like lesion. The most peripheral portions of MO are composed of well formed bony trabeculae and cortical-appearing bone which initially has a woven architecture but eventually is remodelled into lamellar bone. In most instances, the lesion is surrounded by a fibrous capsule that is typically oedematous in the early phases of development, but becomes progressively more collagenous over time. This histological pattern of zonation is most evident in cases of MO that are of at least three weeks duration. Eventually, the central cellular areas become progressively quiescent such that over a period of years, the lush, richly cellular and proliferative fibroblastic centre is transformed into a paucicellular, collagenous zone that ultimately undergoes ossification. Some cases appear to regress completely. In the end, the residual ovoid mass is composed merely of cortical and cancellous bone with fatty or haematopoietic marrow. In some cases of MO, especially those occurring in more superficial soft tissues, the zonal pattern is not well developed and the reactive bone may be located throughout the lesion.

Immunophenotype

The immunohistochemical staining pattern reflects the bidirectional differentiation characteristic of MO and FP. The

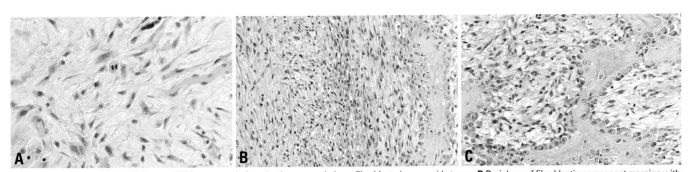

Fig. 2.09 Myositis ossificans. **A** Centre of MO composed of randomly arranged plump fibroblasts in a myxoid stroma. **B** Periphery of fibroblastic component merging with region containing trabeculae of woven bone. **C** Woven bone is prominently rimmed by osteoblasts.

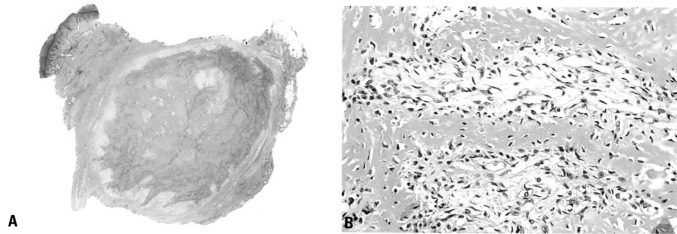

Fig. 2.10 A Fibroosseous pseudotumour of digits presenting as well circumscribed mass in subcutis. **B** Reactive woven bone lined by osteoblasts is present throughout the lesion.

centrally located fibroblasts and myofibroblasts express vimentin but may also stain with antibodies for actin, smooth muscle actin and desmin. The osteoblasts and osteocytes located in the periphery of the tumour typically express vimentin and osteocalcin.

Ultrastructure

The spindle cells have the characteristic ultrastructural features of fibroblasts and myofibroblasts including dilated rough endoplasmic reticulum and aggregates of cytoplasmic filaments occasionally associated with dense bodies {2,1722}. The bone forming cells demonstrate evidence of osteoblastic differentiation and contain many mitochondria and abundant dilated rough endoplasmic reticulum.

Prognostic factors

MO and FP have an excellent prognosis and rarely recur; however, lesions removed marginally or incompletely in the early stage of development have been known to regrow. There are rare examples of MO transforming into osteosarcoma but most of these reports are not well documented. Therefore, although the possibility of malignant transformation exists, this should be regarded as an extremely rare event and patients should be treated conservatively.

Ischaemic fasciitis

M. Michal

Definition
Ischaemic fasciitis (IF) is a distinctive pseudosarcomatous fibroblastic proliferation typically occurring over bony prominences, usually in immobilized patients.

Synonym
Atypical decubital fibroplasia.

Epidemiology
Ischaemic fasciitis most often occurs in immobilized patients as a result of prolonged pressure and impaired circulation {114,1498,1691}.

Sites of involvement
IF is usually localized over bony prominences subjected to intermittent pressure (e.g. greater trochanter or shoulder), where it forms a poorly circumscribed, painless soft tissue mass usually less than 10 cm in diameter {1498}. It is located in the subcutis, sometimes extending into the muscle tissue and dermis.

Clinical features
Most of the patients are elderly, with a peak incidence between the seventh and ninth decades of life. Patients are usually chronically immobilized. Females are affected slightly more commonly than males.

Histopathology
Histologically, IF is composed of multi-nodular zones of fibrinoid (coagulative) necrosis, fibrosis, myxoid changes involving adipose tissue and areas of vascular proliferation. Necrosis has a characteristic appearance consisting of central zone of liquefactive, fibrinoid necrosis having sharp uneven borders, staining deeply red to violet by H&E staining {233,2338}. Foci of necrosis are frequently surrounded by a fringe or pal-

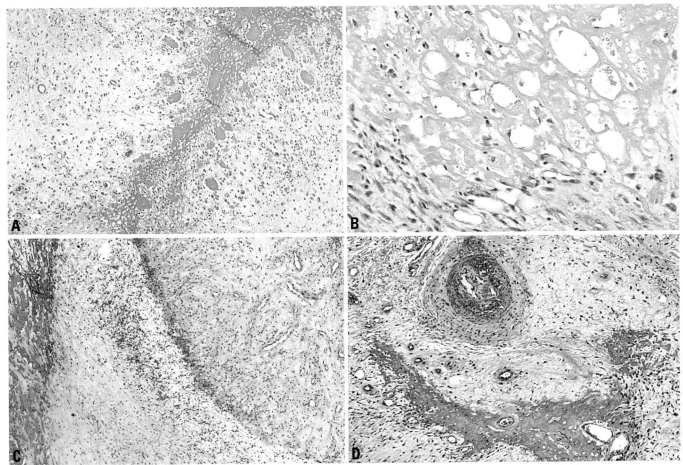

Fig. 2.11 Ischaemic fasciitis. **A** Medium power view showing fibrinoid necrosis and plump fibroblastic cells. **B** Note the prominent interstitial deposition of fibrin, associated with haemorrhage and reactive fibroblastic proliferation. **C** Foci of necrosis are frequently surrounded by a fringe or palisade of capillary proliferation and fibroblasts. **D** Necrosis has a characteristic appearance consisting of central zone of liquefactive and coagulative necrosis having sharp uneven borders, staining deeply red to violet by H&E. Muscular vessels reveal often a fibrinoid change within the wall with fibrin thrombi in various stage of recanalization.

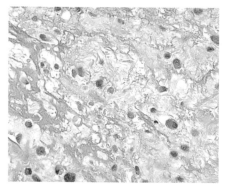

Fig. 2.12 Ischaemic fasciitis. High power view of the ganglion-like fibroblastic cells.

isade of capillary proliferation and fibroblasts. Muscular vessels reveal often fibrinoid change within the walls with fibrin thrombi in various stage of recanalization, and a small amount of secondary acute inflammation and extravasated RBC. Evidence of primary vasculitis or myositis is, however, never seen. Some of the fibroblasts are enlarged and even bizarre with abundant deep staining cytoplasm, large eccentric nuclei and smudged, hyperchromatic nucleus with prominent nucleoli. These cells resemble the fibroblasts in proliferative fasciitis.

Immunophenotype

Immunohistochemically the cells are vimentin positive and occasional fibroblastic cells are smooth muscle actin and CD68 positive. All cells are S100 protein and desmin negative. Enlarged, bizarre fibroblastic cells are CD34 positive {1498}.

Prognostic factors

These lesions may recur, due to persistence of the underlying cause rather than to intrinsic biological aggression. Most patients are cured by local excision.

Elastofibroma

H. Hashimoto
J.A. Bridge

Definition

An ill defined fibroelastic tumour-like lesion that occurs primarily in the soft tissue between the lower portion of the scapula and the chest wall of elderly persons and is characterized by a large number of coarse, enlarged elastic fibres.

ICD-O code   8820/0

Synonym

Elastofibroma dorsi.

Epidemiology

Although elastofibroma was originally considered as a rare lesion, there are geographically different distributions of this lesion, for example, many cases of elastofibroma have been detected in Okinawa, Japan {1526}. Elastofibroma or pre-elastofibroma-like changes have been found at autopsy in 13 to 17 % of elderly individuals {786,1030}.

Sites of involvement

Elastofibroma is almost always located in the connective tissue between the lower scapula and the chest wall, and lies deep to the latissimus dorsi and rhom-

boid major muscles, often with attachment to the periosteum of the ribs. Although it is unilateral in most cases, bilateral elastofibromas may be more common than previously recognized. Naylor et al. radiologically detected subclinical bilateral elastofibromas in many cases {1545}. Rare lesions have been reported in extrascapular locations, such as other parts of the chest wall, the upper arm, the hip region, and the gastrointestinal tract or other viscera.

Clinical features

Elastofibroma occurs almost exclusively in elderly individuals over the age of 50, with a peak between the seventh and eighth decades of life {1526}. There is a striking predominance in women. Elastofibroma is a slowly growing mass that only rarely causes pain or tenderness. Computed tomography (CT) and magnetic resonance imaging (MRI) allow a presumptive diagnosis of elastofibroma {1170}.

Aetiology

Although some have suggested that elastofibroma may be a response to repeated trauma or friction between the

lower scapula and the underlying chest wall {1031}, this has never been confirmed, particularly for examples located in extrascapular sites. Nagamine et al. described that approximately one-third of 170 patients with this lesion in Okinawa occurred within the same family lines, supporting a genetic predisposition in at least some patients {1526}. Enjoji et al. reported an elastofibromatous lesion of the stomach at the base of a peptic ulcer in a patient with bilateral subscapular elastofibromas, suggesting the possibility of an underlying systemic enzymatic defect {585}. The accumulation of large irregular elastic fibres in this lesion may be the result of abnormal elastogenesis rather than degeneration of preexisting elastic fibers.

Macroscopy

Elastofibroma is usually ill defined and rubbery, and exhibits grey-white fibrous tissue with interposing small areas of yellow fat. The mass varies from 2 cm up to 15 cm in diameter.

Histopathology

The lesion is composed of a mixture of paucicellular collagenous tissue and

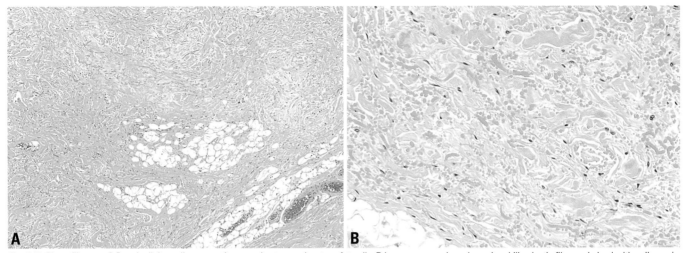

Fig. 2.13 Elastofibroma. **A** Paucicellular collagenous tissue and entrapped mature fat cells. **B** Large, coarse, densely eosinophilic elastic fibres admixed with collagen in an elastofibroma.

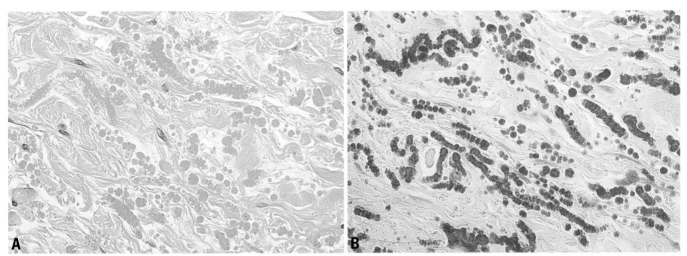

Fig. 2.14 Elastofibroma. **A** Elastic fibres arranged like beads or globules with serrated edges on a string in an elastofibroma. **B** Weigert's elastic stain highlights the bead-like arrangement of the abnormal elastic fibres in an elastofibroma.

large numbers of elastic fibers, associated with small amounts of mucoid stroma and entrapped mature fat cells. The elastic fibres are large, coarse, deeply eosinophilic, and fragmented into small, linearly arranged globules or serrated disks simulating beads on a string. Elastic stains reveal the large branched or unbranched fibres to have a dense core and irregular serrated margins. Although the elastin-like material is removed by prior treatment of the sections with pancreatic elastase, it is more resistant to the digestion than that of control skin {1531}.

Immunohistochemistry

The elastic fibres in elastofibroma are reactive with a specific antibody to elastin {733,1182}.

Ultrastructure

Elongated or globular masses with a central core of more electron-lucent material like mature elastic tissue surrounded by a fibrillary electron-dense substance like immature elastin are seen in a collageous stroma {159,733,1118, 1182,1753}. The constituent cells in close proximity to the elastic fibres have ultrastructural features of fibroblasts and myofibroblasts, some of which contain non-membrane-bounded dense granular bodies with an intensity similar to that of extracellular elastin in the cytoplasm, suggesting that these cells produce the extracellular elastin.

Genetics

Cytogenetic investigations of elastofibroma reveal that this lesion exhibits signifi-

cant chromosomal instability manifested as both clonal and non-clonal structural changes {141,1370,2188}. Aberrations of the short arm of chromosome 1 are particularly prominent. Additional studies are needed to define the potential biological significance of these chromosomal abnormalities in elastofibroma. The observation of familial occurrences of elastofibroma supports a genetic predisposition to this lesion of controversial aetiology {1526,1884}.

Prognostic factors

Elastofibroma is cured by simple excision. Local recurrence is very rare.

Fibrous hamartoma of infancy

H. Hashimoto

Definition

A paediatric, benign, poorly circumscribed, superficial soft tissue mass characterized by an organoid mixture of three components: well defined intersecting trabeculae of dense fibrocollagenous tissue, loosely textured areas of immature-appearing, small, rounded, primitive mesenchymal cells, and mature fat.

Epidemiology

Although in overall terms fibrous hamartoma of infancy is rare, accounting for approximately 0.02 % of all benign soft tissue tumours {1016}, this lesion is one of the relatively more common tumours of fibrous tissue in early childhood.

Sites of involvement

Fibrous hamartoma of infancy occurs most frequently in the anterior or posteri-or axillary fold, followed by the upper arm and shoulder, thigh, groin, back, and forearm {590,1476,1638,1998}. This lesion arises only exceptionally in the hands and feet {1029,1034,1794}. The feature helps distinguish fibrous hamartoma of infancy from calcifying aponeurotic fibroma, which occurs almost exclusively in the hands or feet.

Clinical features

The majority of fibrous hamartomas of infancy present in the first 2 years of life and up to 25 % are discovered at birth {519,570,590,1638}. They do not occur after puberty, although rare lesions have been reported in older infants. There is a striking predominance in boys {1638, 1998}, but there is no evidence of familial tendency or of association with any other congenital disorder. Fibrous hamartoma of infancy is almost always a solitary lesion, and usually a rapidly growing, freely movable mass in the subcutis or dermis, occasionally being attached to the underlying fascia and only rarely involving the skeletal muscle.

Macroscopy

Fibrous hamartoma of infancy is usually poorly circumscribed and exhibits grey-white tissue alternating with yellow fat. The amount of the fatty component varies from case to case. Most lesions are less than 5 cm in diameter, but tumours rarely reach larger than 10 cm {519}.

Histopathology

Fibrous hamartoma of infancy is characterized by three distinct components forming organoid structures. The well defined intersecting trabeculae of dense fibrocollagenous tissue are composed of fibroblastic and myofibroblastic spindle cells with bland, straight or wavy nuclei separated by varying amounts of collagen. The loosely textured islands interspersed among the fibrous trabeculae are made up of immature-appearing, small, rounded or stellate, primitive mesenchymal cells with scant cytoplasm embedded in a myxoid matrix containing abundant hyaluronidase-sensitive acid mucopolysaccharides. The primitive myxoid areas are frequently oriented around small veins. Mitotic figures are absent or few in either the fibroblastic or myxoid areas. The mature fat component is interspersed among the other two components. The relative proportions of these three components vary considerably between cases. Fat may be recognized only at the periphery or may be the major component. In some cases, especially in older children, a pronounced sclerosing process, that is somewhat reminiscent of disorderly fibrosis or neurofibroma, replaces the majority of the lesion {590}.

Immunohistochemistry

Both the fibroblastic and primitive cells are positive for vimentin. There are

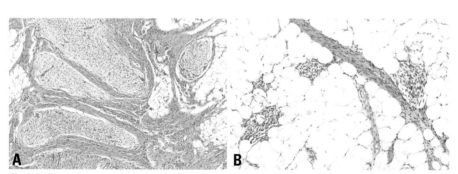

Fig. 2.15 Fibrous hamartoma of infancy. **A** Organoid pattern composed of trabeculae of dense fibrocollagenous tissue, with typical islands of loosely arranged spindle cells, and mature fat cells. **B** This case shows three distinct components, with mature fat predominating.

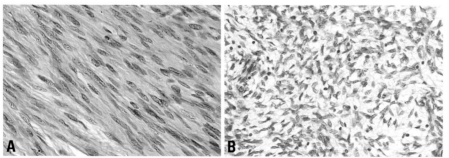

Fig. 2.16 Fibrous hamartoma of infancy. **A** Spindle cells in fibrous trabeculae are composed of bland fibroblastic or myofibroblastic cells with straight or wavy nuclei. **B** In the myxoid islands, note bland primitive spindle cells with scant cytoplasm.

actin-positive spindle cells only in the trabeculae, probably indicating myofibroblastic differentiation {686,845, 1440}. Desmin is usually negative, although some have described positive immunoreactivity to desmin in the trabecular component {845}.

Ultrastructure
A mixture of fibroblastic and myofibroblastic cells are seen in the trabecular component {830,845,1440}, whereas primitive mesenchymal cells with slender cytoplasmic processes and few intracytoplasmic organelles are found in the loosely textured myxoid areas.

Prognostic factors
Fibrous hamartoma of infancy is benign and usually cured by local excision. Rare recurrences are cured by reexcision {519,590,1998}.

Myofibroma / Myofibromatosis

B.P. Rubin
J.A. Bridge

Definition
Myofibroma and myofibromatosis are terms used to denote the solitary (myofibroma) or multicentric (myofibromatosis) occurrence of benign neoplasms composed of contractile myoid cells arranged around thin-walled blood vessels. Myofibroma(tosis) forms a morphological continuum with myopericytoma and so-called infantile haemangiopericytoma.

ICD-O codes
Myofibroma   8824/0
Myofibromatosis 8824/0

Synonyms
Infantile myofibromatosis, congenital generalized fibromatosis.

Epidemiology
Solitary and multicentric lesions can occur over an extremely wide age range that extends from newborns to the elderly {151,353,431,1970}. However, many cases are detected at birth or within the first two years of life. Myofibroma(tosis) is more common in males {353}. There are rare familial cases (see discussion of genetics). The relative frequency of solitary versus multicentric forms is unclear from the literature {353,2284}. This may be due to methodological differences in the types and completeness of radiological studies that were performed, as many lesions, even deep lesions and those affecting bone, may not be clinically apparent. In adults, solitary lesions are more common than multicentric tumours and this is probably also the case in children.

Sites of involvement
Approximately half of solitary myofibromas occur in the cutaneous/subcutaneous tissues of the head and neck region, followed by trunk, lower, and upper extremities {353}. The other half occur in skeletal muscle or aponeuroses, with a small number involving bone, predominantly the skull {353,894,1007, 1111}. Myofibromatosis (i.e., multicentric disease) involves both soft tissue and bone and frequently (from 15-20% of the time) occurs in the deep soft tissues and at visceral locations, including the lungs, heart, gastrointestinal tract, liver, kidney, pancreas, and rarely, the central nervous system {17,48,1828,1846}. Any bone can be involved but most often, the long bones are affected.

Clinical features
Lesions can be of short or of longstanding duration {431,679}. Cutaneous lesions have the appearance of purplish macules, simulating a vascular neoplasm. Subcutaneous lesions occur most often as painless, freely mobile masses while more deeply seated lesions may be fixed. Visceral lesions may cause symptoms referable to the organs that are involved. The radiological appearance of soft tissue lesions varies greatly, and can be well-circumscribed or infiltrative, often with calcification, either within or surrounding the lesions. Bony lesions characteristically occur as multiple elongated radiolucent lesions within the metaphyseal regions, sparing the region immediately adjacent to the epiphysis {1992}. A sclerotic margin forms invariably in more mature lesions, which also have central mineralization.

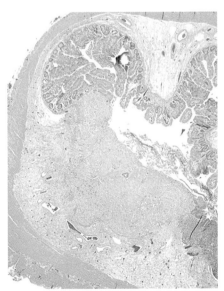

Fig. 2.17 580 Myofibroma / Myofibromatosis. Small bowel lesion in a newborn.

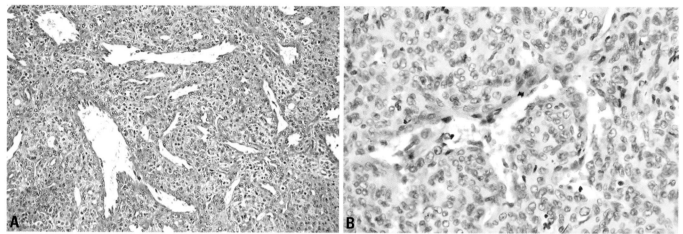

Fig. 2.18 Myofibroma / Myofibromatosis. **A** Primitive spindle cells with haemangiopericytoma-like blood vessels. **B** Note the perivascular growth pattern, underlying the close relationship with myopericytoma.

Aetiology

The aetiology of myofibroma(tosis) is unclear. There are rare familial cases, indicating a genetic component (see discussion of genetics).

Macroscopy

Nodules vary greatly in size, from 0.5 to 7 cm, with a median size of 2.5 cm {353}. Lesions within the dermis and subcutaneous tissue are better defined than those in the deep soft tissues and viscera. On cut surface, myofibromas have a firm, fibrous cut surface and are greyish white, light tan to brown, or purplish in colour. They often have central yellow / necrotic areas and / or cystic spaces filled with caseous-like material or haemorrhage.

Histopathology

At low power, there is a nodular or multinodular proliferation with a zoned appearance, due to regional variation of cell types. Usually within the periphery of the nodules, there are plump myofibroblasts arranged in short fascicles or whorls. These myofibroblasts are spindle shaped with pale pink cytoplasm and have elongated, tapering nuclei with a vesicular chromatin pattern and one or two small nucleoli. There is no significant atypia or pleomorphism. These myoid whorls or nodules often hyalinize, with a pseudochondroid appearance. Within the centre of the nodules, are less well differentiated, rounded, polygonal, or spindle-shaped cells, with slightly larger, hyperchromatic nuclei. These cells have relatively scant cytoplasm, and are arranged around thin-walled, irregularly

branching, haemangiopericytoma-like blood vessels {2037}. Occasional cases have a more random distribution of the two cell types and in some cases, the arrangement can be completely reversed (haemangiopericytoma-like appearance at the periphery and myofibroblastic cells in the middle) {151,353}. The haemangiopericytomatous component can predominate and this has led to the suggestion that most cases of so-

called infantile haemangiopericytoma, are actually cases of myofibroma(tosis) {353,1412}. Calcification, necrosis and stromal hyalinization are identified frequently. Mitotic activity is usually minimal although exceptional cases can have up to 10 per 10 high power fields. Another histological feature which merits attention, is the frequent presence of intravascular growth, which can lead to the mistaken diagnosis of malignancy {151,

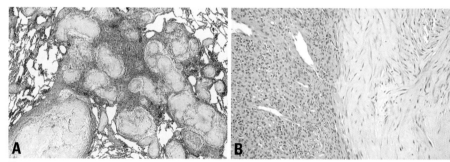

Fig. 2.19 Infantile myofibromatosis. **A** Lung is one of the more common visceral locations to be affected. Note the typically multinodular growth pattern. **B** High power view showing the typical cytologic features. On the left are the rounded, less well differentiated cells arranged around haemangiopericytoma-like blood vessels and on the right are the spindle-shaped myoid cells.

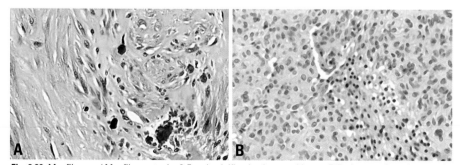

Fig. 2.20 Myofibroma / Myofibromatosis. **A** Focal calcification in a myoid area. **B** Both necrosis and apoptosis are often identified.

353}. This intravascular growth is in fact subendothelial and is not associated with true metastatic potential.

Immunophenotype
Both the myofibroblastic and more primitive component are positive for vimentin and smooth muscle actin, while the myofibroblastic component is more strongly positive for pan-actin HHF-35. Both components are negative for S100 protein, epithelial membrane antigen, and keratin {431,1412}.

Ultrastructure
Typical are prominent dilated rough endoplasmic reticulum, longitudinal filament bundles with dense bodies, and focal basal lamina {151,161,224,523,894}.

Genetics
Familial occurrence is too rare to allow any firm conclusions regarding the genetics of myofibromatosis. However, the documentation of affected cousins, half-siblings, and parent-offspring pairs suggests an autosomal dominant inheritance pattern {244,1037,2070}. The true incidence of myofibromatosis occurring in a familial setting may be higher than it appears as the lesions are frequently small and asymptomatic and tend to disappear spontaneously and thus, milder expressions of the disease in relatives could easily be overlooked {244}.

Prognostic factors
Some myofibromas regress spontaneously {146,161,353}. A small number of solitary lesions (<10%) recur, but there do not appear to be any factors that are predictive of recurrence and these recurrences are cured by local re-excision {353}. The extent and location of the visceral lesions determines the prognosis, with involvement of vital organs, leading to cardiopulmonary or gastrointestinal complications, causing death in rare cases {40,353,2284}. Pulmonary involvement appears to be an especially bad prognostic factor.

Fibromatosis colli

J. O'Connell

Definition
A benign, site-specific lesion that occurs in the distal sternocleidomastoid muscle of infants. The mass results in fusiform thickening of the muscle and cervicofacial asymmetry due to its shortening (torticollis).

Synonyms
Congenital muscular torticollis, sternocleidomastoid tumour of infancy, pseudotumour of infancy.

Epidemiology
Fibromatosis colli is uncommon. It occurs in approximately 0.4% of live births {1187}. There is no sex predilection. The majority of affected infants are diagnosed before 6 months of age {1187}. There is a high incidence of abnormal intrauterine positioning or difficult delivery in the affected infants {198,

1187,1863}. Additionally, there is a clear association with other musculoskeletal developmental abnormalities that are associated with abnormal intrauterine positioning, including forefoot anomalies and congenital hip dislocation {198, 1187,1863}.

Site of involvement
Fibromatosis colli typically affects the lower one-third of the sternocleidomastoid muscle. There is no predilection as to side.

Clinical features
The affected infants present with a smooth fusiform swelling of the distal sternocleidomastoid muscle {198,1187, 1863}. This usually measures less than 5.0 cm in length. The muscle typically is expanded although it rarely measures greater than 2.0 cm in width. Typically

the infants exhibit cervico-facial asymmetry with facial tilt due to the shortening

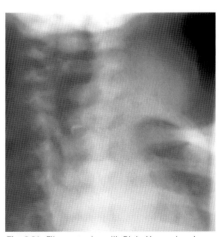

Fig. 2.21 Fibromatosis colli. Plain X-ray showing a soft tissue mass in the region of sternocleidomastoid muscle.

of the affected muscle {198,1187,1228, 1863}. Ultrasound investigation is useful and non-invasive. It demonstrates a uniform isoechoic mass confined to the muscle {407}. In real time this can be shown to move with the action of the muscle.

Aetiology
It is most likely that fibromatosis colli represents a cellular scar-like reaction to injury of the sternocleidomastoid muscle acquired in the last trimester of intrauterine growth, or at the time of delivery {198, 1187,1863}.

Macroscopy
The lesion appears as a tan gritty mass confined to the muscle. Regions of haemorrhage or necrosis are not present.

Histopathology
Like many presumed reactive proliferations, the microscopic appearance of fibromatosis colli varies depending on the time at which it is examined. Currently the favoured investigation of these masses is by fine needle aspiration cytology {1187}. This demonstrates cellular specimens with aggregates of uniform plump spindle cells embedded in myxoid to collagenous ground substance {1187}. Multinucleated skeletal myocytes may be admixed. These aspiration specimens correspond to the cellular proliferative phase of the process. Surgical specimens, which are obtained only from a minority of the patients at the time of tenotomy for persistent torticollis, usually demonstrate less cellular collagen-rich tissue that resembles scar or conventional fibromatosis. In these the lesion is composed of uniform plump fibroblastic and myofibroblastic cells embedded in a collagenous background {198,1228,1863}. Infiltration and entrapment of skeletal myocytes is evident.

Immunophenotype
The lesional cells exhibit positive staining for vimentin and muscle actins.

Prognostic factors
When diagnosed early, fibromatosis colli is managed in a non-surgical manner.

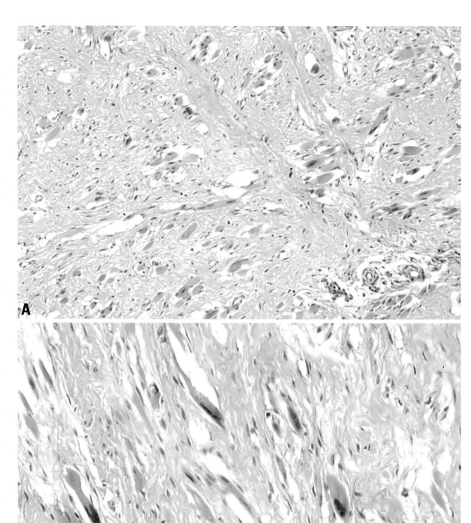

Fig. 2.22 Fibromatosis colli. **A** Note the diffuse pattern of scar-like fibroblastic proliferation within sterno-clei-domastoid muscle. **B** The entrapped skeletal muscle fibres commonly show both degenerative and reactive sarcolemmal nuclei.

The treatment involves passive stretching and physiotherapy {198}. Seventy percent of children will have complete resolution of the mass and demonstrate normal cervico-facial posture and movement with this approach {198}. Surgical intervention, principally tenotomy, is required in between 10 to 15% of patients {198}. Overall, 90% of patients achieve normal function and appearance following timely intervention {198}. The prognosis is worse in those infants who are diagnosed and treated when older than 1 year.

Juvenile hyaline fibromatosis

J. O'Connell

Definition

An apparently non-neoplastic disorder that typically presents in infancy, characterized by the accumulation of extracellular "hyaline material" within skin, somatic soft tissues and the skeleton, resulting in tumour-like masses. The hyaline material is produced by an aberrant population of fibroblasts. The clinical manifestations vary depending on the number, location and growth rate of the masses.

Synonyms

Molluscum fibrosum, mesenchymal dysplasia.

Epidemiology

Juvenile hyaline fibromatosis is an extremely rare disorder {1057,1094, 1313}. As of 1998 less than 50 cases had been reported in the literature {2279}. It typically presents in infancy {1057,1094, 1313,2279}. There is no sex predilection and affected infants are often the progeny of consanguineous parents {1057, 1094,1313,2279}. The clinical phenotype of affected children varies {1313}. Most of the time there is progressive increase in the number and size of superficial and deep nodules with resulting deformity and dysfunction. Survival into adulthood may occur {1078,1094}.

Sites of involvement

The tumour-like masses of hyaline material develop in the skin (particularly the face and neck resulting in papules and nodules), gums (producing "gingival hyperplasia"), periarticular soft tissues (resulting in joint contractures) and bones (especially the skull, long bones and phalanges) {1057,1078,1094,1313, 2279}.

Clinical features

Patients present with skin papules affecting the face and neck, in particular, around the ears. Perianal skin papules may resemble genital warts. Periarticular deposits of the hyaline material result in joint contractures, particularly involving the knees and elbows {1057,1078,1094,

1313,2279}. Imaging studies reveal generalized osteoporosis and discrete lytic lesions in the affected bones {1057, 1094,1480}.

Aetiology

The aetiology of juvenile hyaline fibromatosis is unknown. It appears to be transmitted in an autosomal recessive manner {1057,1094,1313}. Biochemical investigation of the hyaline material suggests increased extracellular chondroitin sulphate, and types I and VI collagen {250,1073}. Recently it has been suggested the fundamental defect may be a reduction in type III collagen production {250}.

Macroscopy

The nodules have a uniformly solid, white or waxy appearance.

Histopathology

The individual nodules obliterate the normal tissues in which they are found. They are composed of an admixture of plump fibroblastic cells associated with extracellular uniform hyaline material that is non-fibrillar and eosinophilic in haematoxylin and eosin stains. In younger patients or "newer lesions" the nodules are relatively more cellular {1362,1480}. The constituent fibroblasts have clear cytoplasm and may exhibit a vague fascicular arrangement. Nuclear atypia or necrosis is not seen. Older lesions are less cellular and the fibroblasts may appear compressed by the extracellular material. PAS stain is strongly positive and diastase resistant.

Immunophenotype

The fibroblastic cells label positively for vimentin. Stains for muscle actin and S100 protein are negative {14,1920}.

Ultrastructure

The lesional cells are fibroblasts and demonstrate numerous cystically dilated membrane-bound vesicles. These contain granular and filamentous material similar to the extracellular ground sub-

stance. Continuity between the vesicles and the extracellular space may be evident {1057,1313,1480,2279}.

Prognostic factors

The lesions are treated by surgical excision depending on their location. Local recurrence rates are high {1057}. The

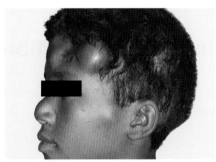

Fig. 2.23 Juvenile hyaline fibromatosis. Multiple subcutaneous nodules on the scalp and face are the most consistent finding.

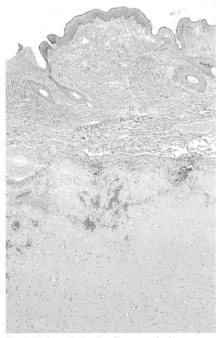

Fig. 2.24 Juvenile hyaline fibromatosis. Low power view of a typically well circumscribed hypocellular nodule in deep dermis / subcutis.

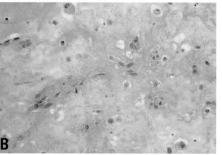
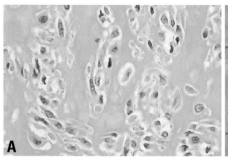

Fig. 2.25 Juvenile hyaline fibromatosis. **A** Cellular focus of a nodule. Note the clustered arrangement of the fibroblasts and the extracellular amorphous material. **B** An older nodule that is less cellular and dominated by the hyaline material.

prognosis is determined by the number, size and location of the nodules and the degree of the patient's functional impairment. A single case of oral squamous carcinoma arising in association with juvenile hyaline fibromatosis has been reported {1078}.

Inclusion body fibromatosis

J. O'Connell

Definition
A benign proliferation of fibroblastic and myofibroblastic cells that typically occurs on the digits of young children. It is named for the intracytoplasmic inclusions that are detected in a minority of the lesional cells.

Synonyms
Infantile digital fibromatosis, digital fibrous tumour of childhood, infantile digital fibroma.

Epidemiology
Inclusion body fibromatosis is rare.

Site of involvement
Typically, lesions develop on the dorsal aspect of digits of the hands or feet {148, 344,913,1791}. In a minority, more than one digit may be affected synchronously or asynchronously. Involvement of the thumb or big toe is extremely unusual. Rarely inclusion body fibromatosis occurs in extra-digital sites such as the soft tissues of the arm and breast {1702, 1738}.

Clinical features
Patients typically present in the first year of life {148,344,913,1791}. There is no

sex predilection. Occasionally clinically typical lesions present in older patients and conversely pathologically characteristic tumours occasionally develop in sites other than the digits {1702,1738}. Treatment is by local excision, with an effort to preserve function. Digital examples present as dome shaped swellings overlying the phalanges or interphalangeal joints. The nodules usually measure less than 2.0 cm and the overlying skin is typically taught and stretched. Occasional examples may erode bone. The extra-digital nodules present as nonspecific soft tissue masses.

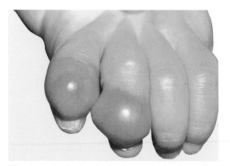
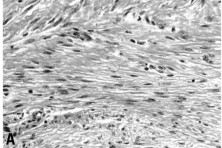
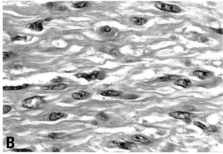

Fig. 2.26 Inclusion body fibromatosis. Two phalangeal nodules overlying the distal interphalangeal joints. Note the stretched overlying skin.

Fig. 2.27 Inclusion body fibromatosis. **A** Low power view demonstrating intersecting fascicles of spindle cells associated with extracellular collagen. **B** High power view shows the plump spindle cells, uniform nuclei and scattered intracytoplasmic eosinophilic round inclusions.

Macrosocopy

The lesions have a uniform white / tan appearance. They lack regions of haemorrhage or necrosis. They are typically ill defined.

Histopathology

The nodules are composed of intradermal sheets and fascicles of uniform spindle cells associated with varying amounts of extracellular collagen {344, 913,1702,1738}. They are non-encapsulated and fascicles of cells extend into adjacent tissues. Individual cells have central elongated nuclei and vaguely fibrillar cytoplasm. The diagnostic feature is the presence of intracytoplasmic, eosinophilic spherical "inclusions" {344, 913,1702,1738}. Inclusions are brightly trichrome positive and PAS negative. These are present in a minority of the cells and are not always uniformly distributed. The lesional cells lack nuclear atypia and mitoses are not prominent.

Immunophenotype

The lesional cells demonstrate positive staining for vimentin, and muscle actins {344,1515,1516,1702}. The latter stains often exhibit a parallel linear pattern beneath the cell membrane, in a so-called "tram-track" pattern. The eosinophilic globules demonstrate variable staining for actins in formalin fixed material {1515,1516,1702}. These vari-

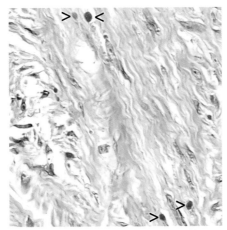

Fig. 2.28 Inclusion body fibromatosis. Masson trichrome stain shows the typical purple-red juxtanuclear rounded inclusions.

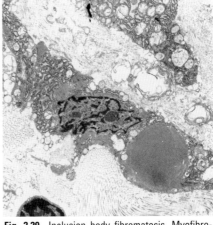

Fig. 2.29 Inclusion body fibromatosis. Myofibroblastic cell with a typical intracytoplasmic granular filamentous inclusion.

able results appear to be dependent upon the method of tissue preparation prior to immunohistochemical staining. Pretreatment with KOH has been reported to aid in demonstrating a positive staining result for actins within the inclusions {1515}.

Ultrastructure

The lesional spindle cells demonstrate ultrastructural features of myofibroblasts {344,913,1020,1516,1702}. They exhibit well formed rough endoplasmic reticulum and intracytoplasmic aggregates of filaments. These are concentrated beneath the cell membrane and focally show dense bodies. The inclusions lie free in the cytoplasm and have a granular / filamentous appearance {344,913, 1020,1516,1702}. Cytoplasmic actin filaments extend into the granular inclusions and may be demonstrated to be continuous with them {913}.

Prognostic factors

Local recurrence occurs in about 50% of cases {148,1791}. The main prognostic indicator is the adequacy of the primary excision. Metastasis does not occur.

Fibroma of tendon sheath

G. Farshid
J.A. Bridge

Definition
Fibroma of tendon sheath (FTS) is an uncommon, small, benign fibrous nodule that arises near tendinous structures, mostly in the hands of adult males.

ICD-O code   8810/0

Synonym
Tenosynovial fibroma.

Epidemiology
Most patients are in the fourth decade but FTS can occur at any age. Approximately 60% of lesions affect males. In the hands the right side is favoured. Multiplicity of lesions is rare. Familial or racial clustering is not reported.

Site of involvement
The thumb, index and middle fingers are the favoured sites of origin. Together with lesions of the volar aspect of hand and wrist, they account for 80% of cases. The anterior knee and plantar aspect of the foot are less commonly involved. Arms, elbows, toes, temporomandibular joint, trunk and neck are rarely affected.

Clinical features
FTS typically presents as a small, firm, slowly enlarging, painless mass. Impingement on nerves, carpal tunnel syndrome, pain, finger triggering and ulceration may occur.

A heterogeneous and lobulated mass with low signal intensity both in T1- and T2-weighted images may be seen on MRI. Smooth erosion into bone has been reported {2002}.

Aetiology
The predilection for specific digits of the right hand and the finding of fasciitis-like areas in some cases suggest a possible reactive origin. Injury is reported in 10% of cases. Clonal chromosome abnormalities have been demonstrated in one case.

Macroscopy
FTS forms a sharply-demarcated, multilobated and sometimes multinodular, fibrous mass, almost always <3 cm in diameter. The cut surface is homogenous, pale and solid.

Histopathology
FTS is composed of well-circumscribed nodules separated by deep, narrow clefts. The nodules are typically paucicellular, containing spindled fibroblasts embedded in a collagenous stroma. Scattered slit-like vascular channels are frequent {103,352,905,981,1736}. Some lesions may show hypercellularity, but the cellular areas usually merge with more typical paucicellular zones. These hypercellular examples resemble nodular fasciitis and often display typical mitotic figures, but coagulative necrosis

and nuclear hyperchromasia are not seen. Other less common histological features may include presence of stellate cells, pleomorphic bizarre cells, myxoid change, cyst formation, dense hyalinization and chondroid or osseous metaplasia.

Immunophenotype
The cells of FTS express SMA and vimentin.

Ultrastructure
Features of fibroblasts and myofibroblasts are identified.

Genetics
A clonal chromosomal abnormality, t(2;11)(q31-32;q12), has been described in one case {440}. Notably, an identical translocation has also been observed in desmoplastic fibroblastoma {1911}.

Prognostic factors
Up to 24% of lesions in the hands recur months to years after the diagnosis, sometimes repeatedly but non-destructively {352}. Because of adherence to tendinous structures local excision may be difficult. In view of their non-aggressive course, excision should aim to relieve symptoms but preserve function. Metastasis has never been reported in FTS.

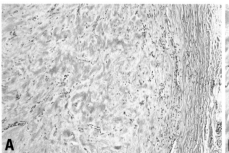 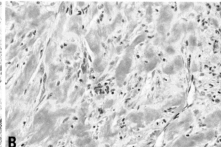 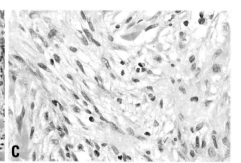

Fig. 2.30 Fibroma of tendon sheath. **A** Border of a well circumscribed nodule, showing **(B)** paucicellular spindle fibroblasts in a collagenous stroma. **C** Detail of a more cellular lesion.

Desmoplastic fibroblastoma

M.M. Miettinen
J.A. Bridge

Definition
A rare, benign, paucicellular tumour affecting mainly adult males, characterized by densely collagenous, predominantly stellate-shaped fibroblasts exhibiting bland cytological features. Myxoid stroma may be present.

ICD-O code
8810/0

Synonym
Collagenous fibroma.

Clinical features
This relatively uncommon tumour is usually diagnosed in men between the 5th and 7th decades (70%), and rarely in adolescents; only 25% of cases have been diagnosed in women. The tumour typically presents as an asymptomatic mass involving the subcutis, but fascial involvement is common and up to 25% of

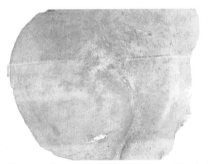

Fig. 2.31 Desmoplastic fibroblastoma. The lesion has a smooth, rounded contour.

cases involve skeletal muscle. It occurs in a variety of peripheral sites with the most common locations being the arm, shoulder, lower limb, back, forearm, hands and feet. The behaviour is benign, and none of the published clinicopathologic series had recurrences {622,900, 1447,1560}.

Macroscopy
The tumour is usually relatively small, measuring 1-4 cm in greatest dimension, but examples over 10 cm and as large as 20 cm have occurred. Grossly it appears as a well-circumscribed oval, fusiform-elongated, or disc-shaped mass, which may be lobulated. On sectioning the tissue is firm and homogeneous with cartilage-like consistency and pearl-grey colour.

Histopathology
Microscopically, desmoplastic fibroblastoma is relatively paucicellular with a prominent collagenous background. The tumour involves the subcutaneous fat in 70% of cases and extends into the skeletal muscle in 25% of cases. The margins are variably circumscribed. It is composed of scattered spindled or stellate-shaped fibroblasts and myofibroblasts. A minority of cases have variably, usually focally myxoid stromal change. The lesional blood vessels are usually inconspicuous with thin walls. Lower cellularity, lack of fascicular pattern, predomi-

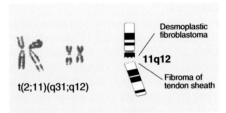

Fig. 2.34 Desmoplastic fibroblastoma showing a 2;11 translocation with a breakpoint at 11q12.

nance of amorphous collagenous stroma and inconspicuous vasculature separate it from desmoid tumour.

Immunophenotype
The tumour cells are positive for vimentin and are variably positive for alpha-smooth muscle actin and occasionally for keratins AE1/AE3. They are negative for desmin, EMA, S100 protein and CD34 {1447}.

Genetics
Clonal chromosomal abnormalities have been observed in two cases {1911}. Both exhibited abnormalities involving band 11q12. Notably, an identical 2;11 translocation has also been observed in a case of fibroma of tendon sheath {440}.

Prognostic factors
These lesions do not recur and do not metastasize.

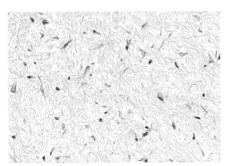

Fig. 2.32 Desmoplastic fibroblastoma. The tumour is paucicellular and composed of uniform, often stellate-shaped fibroblasts.

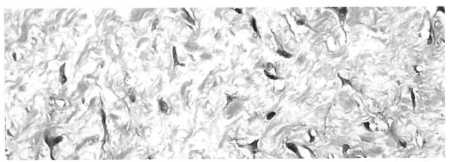

Fig. 2.33 Desmoplastic fibroblastoma. The tumour is paucicellular and composed of uniform, often stellate-shaped fibroblasts.

Mammary-type myofibroblastoma

M.E. McMenamin
J.A. Bridge

Definition

A benign mesenchymal neoplasm composed of spindle-shaped cells with features of myofibroblasts, embedded in a stroma that contains coarse bands of hyalinized collagen and conspicuous mast cells, and admixed with a variable amount of adipose tissue. The tumour is histologically identical to myofibroblastoma of breast.

ICD-O code   8825/0

Epidemiology

Lesions have arisen in adults with an age range of 35 to 67 years (median 55.5 years) and a male predilection (8 males, 2 females). The extramammary location of some myofibroblastomas has only recently been defined when 10 cases were reported {1382}. Therefore, conclusions related to epidemiology could alter with increased tumour recognition.

Sites of involvement

The most common location of mammary-type myofibroblastoma is the inguinal / groin area. Other reported sites include abdominal wall, buttock, back and vaginal wall. Lesions arise most commonly in subcutaneous tissue; however, cases have arisen deep to abdominal wall muscle, in the posterior vaginal wall and in a paratesticular location. There is an apparent predilection for myofibroblastomas to arise along the putative anatomic "milk-line" that extends from axilla to medial groin.

Clinical features

The tumours generally present as either painless masses or incidental lesions that are detected during surgical procedures such as inguinal hernia repair. Occasional lesions are tender or painful. Tumours have been described to be present for up to a year before clinical presentation. There are no imaging data.

Aetiology

Unknown. It has been postulated that myofibroblastomas arising in the breast may be related to a patient's hormonal status, in that lesions are relatively common in older men, e.g. in the setting of gynaecomastia and anti-androgen therapy {1381,2217}. Mammary-type myofibroblastoma of soft tissue arises most commonly in older adult males. The apparent predilection for origin of myofibroblastomas along a putative milk-line suggests the possible existence of hormonally-responsive mesenchymal tissue.

Macroscopy

Reported lesions ranged in size from 2 to 13 cm (median 5.8 cm). The tumours are well circumscribed and firm. The colour can be variable (white, pink, tan or brown). The cut surface may be whorled or nodular. Soft "mucoid"-appearing areas reflecting myxoid change were present in one case.

Histopathology

Tumours are unencapsulated but well circumscribed. They are composed of an admixture of spindle cells and adipose tissue and are morphologically identical to mammary myofibroblastoma {2217}. The spindle cells histologically resemble myofibroblasts and are characterized by oval to tapered nuclei with finely dispersed chromatin, small nucleoli, eosinophilic to amphophilic cytoplasm and poorly defined cytoplasmic borders. The spindle cells are frequently wavy in contour and generally are arranged in variably sized fascicles. The stroma is collagenous with broad bands of coarse hyalinized collagen that often adopt a zig-zag pattern. Stromal mast cells are usually numerous. Epithelioid change of the lesional cells and focal nuclear atypia with enlarged nuclei and multinucleation have been described {1382}. Such morphologic variation is well recognized in myofibroblastoma of breast {1381,2217}. The blood vessels in myofibroblastoma are generally not conspicuous, being small, often focally hyalinized and commonly having a perivascular lymphocytic infiltrate in contrast to the prominent medium to large vessels with markedly hyalinized walls

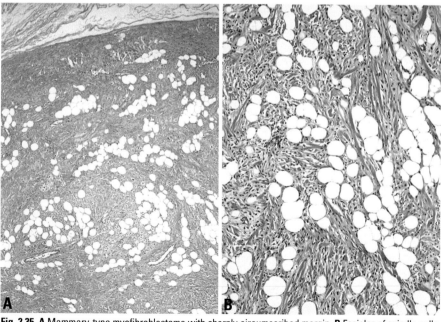

Fig. 2.35 A Mammary-type myofibroblastoma with sharply circumscribed margin. **B** Fasicles of spindle cells separated by coarse bands of intersecting hyalinized collagen. Note scattered adipose tissue.

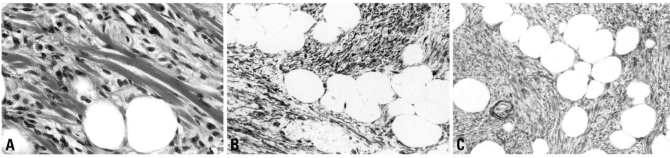

Fig. 2.36 Mammary-type myofibroblastoma. **A** Note the bland spindle cells with tapering nuclei, collagenous stroma and conspicuous mast cells. **B** The spindle cells are consistently immunopositive for desmin. **C** In most cases, the spindle cells are also positive for CD34.

that are characteristic in cellular angiofibroma or the large branching "haemangiopericytomatous" blood vessels that are seen in lipomatous haemangiopericytoma, two potential morphologic mimics. Mitotic figures range from 0-6 per 10 HPF.

Immunophenotype
As is characteristic of the breast counterpart, the typical immunophenotype of extramammary myofibroblastoma is diffuse co-expression by the spindle cells of desmin and CD34. Expression of smooth muscle actin is seen in a third of cases.

Genetics
Partial monosomy 13q has been detected in two cases, as well as partial monosomy 16q in one of these two cases {1670}. Similar rearrangements of 13q and 16q are characteristic of spindle cell lipoma {442}.

Prognostic factors
All tumours have followed a benign course following marginal local excision. However, the reported follow-up time is limited (up to 26 months).

Calcifying aponeurotic fibroma

G. Farshid

Definition
Calcifying aponeurotic fibroma (CAF) is a small tumour of the palms and soles of children with a propensity for local recurrence. Foci of calcification, palisaded round cells and radiating arms of fibroblasts characterise this lesion.

ICD-O code   8810/0

Synonym
Juvenile aponeurotic fibroma.

Epidemiology
CAF is very rare. The age range spans 0-64 with a median of 12 years. A slight male predisposition is found without familial or racial clustering. A case with multiple lesions has been reported {907}.

Sites of involvement
Palms, soles, wrists and ankles are typical sites of involvement. Back, arms, legs, neck and abdominal wall are rarely affected {657}. CAF arises near tendons, fascia and aponeuroses.

Clinical features
CAF presents as a solitary, small, slowly growing, poorly circumscribed non-tender mass. Plain X-rays show a soft tissue mass, possibly with stippled calcifications.

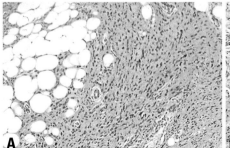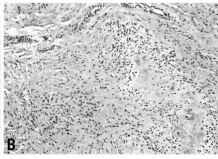

Fig. 2.37 Calcifying aponeurotic fibroma. **A** 1478 The spindle cell component resembles fibromatosis. **B** 1336 Paucicellular lesion with focal hyalinization.

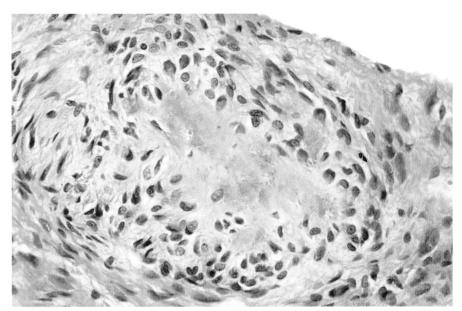

Fig. 2.38 Calcifying aponeurotic fibroma. Typical nodule with central hyalinization and incipient calcification.

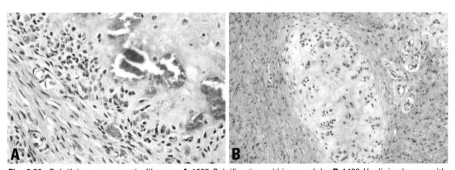

Fig. 2.39 Calcifying aponeurotic fibroma. **A** 1335 Calcification within a nodule. **B** 1489 Hyalinized area with chondroid features.

Macroscopy

CAF forms a firm, pale, infiltrative mass, usually <3 cm, with a gritty cut surface.

Histopathology

The typical lesion has two components: (1) nodular deposits of calcification, each surrounded by a palisade of round-ed, chondrocyte-like cells, arranged in short, parallel arrays, (2) a less cellular, spindled, fibroblastic component between the coalescent calcified nod-ules and emanating into the surrounding soft tissues.

The stroma of nodules is usually hyalin-ized but may have chondroid features.

Osteoclastic giant cells may border the calcium. The lesion may engulf nerves and blood vessels. Degenerate nuclei may be present in the calcified areas but coagulative necrosis or numerous mitoses are not features of CAF {43, 657}.

An uncommon variant seen in very young children has a more diffuse growth pattern. Greater cellularity and a paucity of the mineralised matrix also charac-terise CAF in the very young.

Immunophenotype

The limited number of cases examined have variably expressed vimentin, smooth muscle actin, muscle specific actin, CD99 and S100 protein {657}.

Ultrastructure

Cells with features of chondrocytes, fibroblastic cells and occasional myofi-broblastic cells are found on electron microscopy {1019}.

Prognostic factors

Up to 50% of patients experience local recurrence, usually within 3 years of diagnosis (range <1-9 yrs). This may be repeated but is not destructive or aggressive. Local recurrence is more likely in individuals <5 years of age but the likelihood of recurrence is not pre-dictable on the basis of morphology, location or the completeness of the pri-mary excision. The natural history of the lesion is one of reduced growth with age. Because local recurrence is not destruc-tive, re-excision should be considered only for symptomatic relief and should conserve functionally important struc-tures even if they are involved by tumour.

Angiomyofibroblastoma

Definition
A benign, well-circumscribed myofibroblastic neoplasm, usually arising in the pelviperineal region, especially the vulva, and apparently composed of stromal cells distinctive to this anatomic region. There may be morphologic overlap with cellular angiofibroma.

ICD-O code   8826/0

Epidemiology
Angiomyofibroblastoma is uncommon, having an incidence comparable to aggressive angiomyxoma.

These tumours arise predominantly in females, principally in adults between menarche and menopause {687,738, 1223,1564,1593}. Around 10% of patients are postmenopausal. Convincing examples have not been described before puberty. Rare cases occur in males {687,1593}.

Sites of involvement
Virtually all cases arise in pelviperineal subcutaneous tissue, with the majority arising in the vulva. Around 10-15% of cases are located in the vagina. Lesions in men occur in the scrotum or paratesticular soft tissue.

Clinical features
Most cases present as a slowly enlarging, painless, circumscribed mass. The most frequent preoperative diagnosis is Bartholin's gland 'cyst'. The aetiology is unknown.

Macroscopy
These lesions are well circumscribed but not encapsulated, with a tan/pink cut surface and a soft consistency. Necrosis is not seen. Most cases measure less than 5 cm in maximum diameter, although rare examples measuring up to 10 cm have been recognized.

Histopathology
Tumours are generally well demarcated by a thin fibrous pseudocapsule and, at low power, show varying cellularity with prominent vessels throughout. Vessels are mostly small, thin-walled and ectatic and are set in an abundant loose, oedematous stroma. The tumour cells are round-to-spindle shaped with eosinophilic cytoplasm and typically are concentrated around vessels. Mitoses are rare. Binucleate and multinucleate tumour cells are common. Some cases show very plasmacytoid or epithelioid cytomorphology and rare examples show degenerative ('ancient') nuclear hyperchromasia and atypia. Around 10% of cases have a variably prominent well differentiated adipocytic component. In post-menopausal patients the stroma is

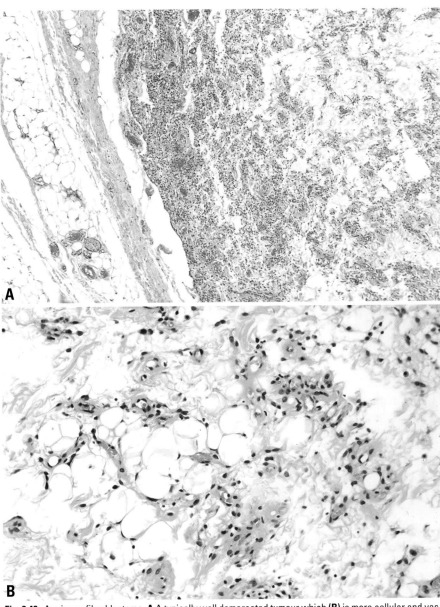

Fig. 2.40 Angiomyofibroblastoma. **A** A typically well demarcated tumour which **(B)** is more cellular and vascular than aggressive angiomyxoma. Note the adipocytic component.

Angiomyofibroblastoma   71

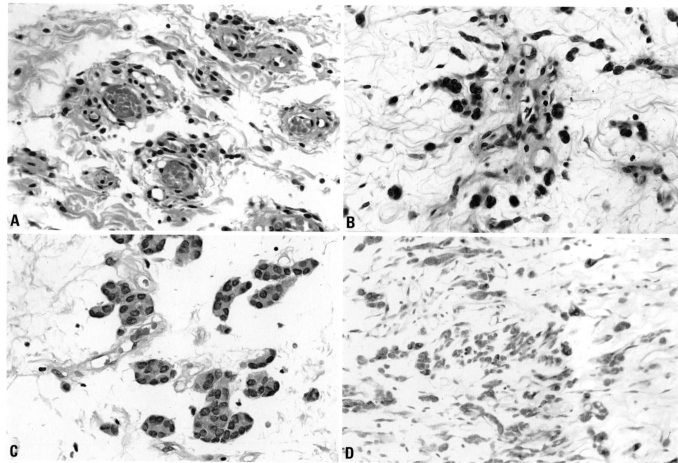

Fig. 2.41 Angiomyofibroblastoma. **A** Tumour cells and vessels are set in a loose oedematous stroma. **B** Binucleate and multinucleate cells are frequent and may have a plasmacytoid appearance. **C** In this example, the tumour cells are focally clustered with an epithelioid appearance. **D** Immunopositivity for desmin is a typical feature in most cases.

often less oedematous and more fibrous and there may be hyalinization of vessel walls. Some cases show morphologic overlap with cellular angiofibroma (see page 73) and rare cases show morphologic overlap with aggressive angiomyxoma {826}.

Immunohistochemistry

The majority of cases show strong and diffuse desmin positivity, while, at most, there is usually only focal positivity for smooth muscle actin or pan-muscle actin

{687,1564,1593}. Desmin staining may be reduced or absent in post-menopausal cases. Tumour cells are consistently positive for oestrogen receptor and progesterone receptor {1223, 1593}, occasionally positive for CD34 and negative for S100 protein, keratin and fast myosin.

Ultrastructure

Tumour cells show fibroblastic or myofibroblastic features by electron microscopy {687,1564}.

Prognostic factors

Angiomyofibroblastoma is entirely benign and has never been reported to recur locally, even after marginal local excision. There is one reported case of a clinically malignant counterpart of angiomyofibroblastoma {1566}.

Cellular angiofibroma

W.B. Laskin

Definition
Cellular angiofibroma (CA) is a benign, highly cellular and richly vascularised mesenchymal neoplasm that usually arises in the superficial soft tissues of the vulva and in the inguinoscrotal region of men. The tumour may be related to angiomyofibroblastoma, with which it shares certain morphological features.

ICD-O code   9160/0

Synonym
Male angiomyofibroblastoma-like tumour {1222}.

Epidemiology
Cellular angiofibroma is a rare neoplasm that has been described in small series {1222,1585} and in case reports {393, 413,1216}. Cellular angiofibroma has a peak incidence in the fifth through seventh decades of life.

Sites of involvement
Although the vulva and inguinoscrotal region are classic locations for cellular angiofibroma, rare examples of tumours microscopically resembling cellular angiofibroma have been described in the retroperitoneum {1584}, perineum {1585}, and subcutaneous tissue of the chest {770}.

Clinical features
Patients usually present with a painless mass. In males, the mass may be associated with hernia or hydrocoele {1222}.

Aetiology
The aetiology is unclear. However, the immunohistochemical expression of estrogen and progesterone receptor proteins in a small number of cases {1216, 1222} suggests that these hormones may have a role in the pathogenesis of the neoplasm.

Macroscopy
Cellular angiofibroma of the vulva is generally small (less than 3 cm) {1585}, whereas cases in males tends to be larger in size (range, 2.5 to 14 cm) {1222}. The tumours appear as round, oval, or lobulated well-circumscribed nodules. The consistency of the lesion varies from soft to rubbery and the cut surface is solid with a grey-pink to yellow-brown colour.

Histopathology
The tumours are typically well circumscribed and may or may not possess a fibrous pseudocapsule. Cellularity is variable. The main proliferating element is a spindle cell with a cytologically-bland, oval to fusiform nucleus and a

scanty amount of lightly eosinophilic cytoplasm with ill defined borders. Epithelioid-appearing neoplastic cells are focally present in some examples . Cytological atypia has been reported in a few cases {1222,1585}. The tumour cells grow in vague fascicles or in a random fashion. Although mitotic rate can be brisk in cellular angiofibroma {1585}, mitotic activity in male cases is typically negligible {1222}. Atypical mitotic figures and necrosis are absent. The vascular component consists of numerous small

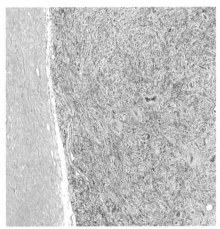

Fig. 2.42 Cellular angiofibroma is usually a well circumscribed neoplasm. A thick, fibrous pseudocapsule surrounds this example.

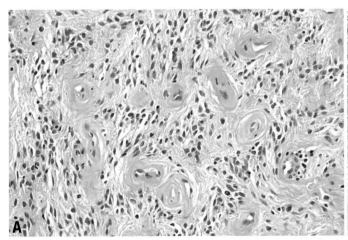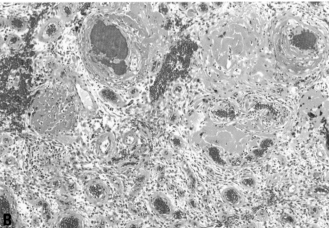

Fig. 2.43 Cellular angiofibroma. **A** The vascular component consists primarily of numerous small to medium-sized open vessels with hyaline walls. **B** Regressive and degenerative changes include organizing intraluminal thrombi, intramural inflammation, extravasated red blood cells, and haemosiderin deposits.

to medium-sized vessels distributed rather uniformly throughout the process. Perivascular hyaline fibrosis is present to some degree in all tumours. Intralesional fat in the form of small aggregates or individual adipocytes has been described in close to one-half of reported tumours {393,770,1222,1585} where it generally comprises less than 5% of the tumour area and is usually located near the periphery of the lesion. The stroma consists primarily of fine collagenous fibres. Additional stromal elements may include scattered thick bundles of eosinophilic collagen, a myxoid and oedematous stromal matrix, and hypocellular collagenous bands partitioning lesional tissue {1222}. Regressive or degenerative changes, including intravascular thrombi, extravasation of red blood cells and haemosiderin deposition, and cystic (pseudoangiomatous) stromal alteration are more common in males. Scattered mast cells are present in almost all tumours, whereas interstitial and perivascular chronic inflammation is more often noted in males.

Immunophenotype
The tumour cells show strong, diffuse expression of vimentin. CD34 expression has been documented in close to one-third of tumours tested {1216,1222, 1585}. Although cellular angiofibroma in females has consistently been shown not to express actin(s) or desmin {393,413, 770,1216,1585}, cases in males demonstrate more variable expression of muscle-specific and smooth muscle actin and desmin {1222}.

Prognostic factors
Although clinical follow-up data for CA is limited, only one case has been reported to recur {413,1216,1222,1585}. A complete (local) excision with uninvolved margins is adequate therapy for these benign neoplasms.

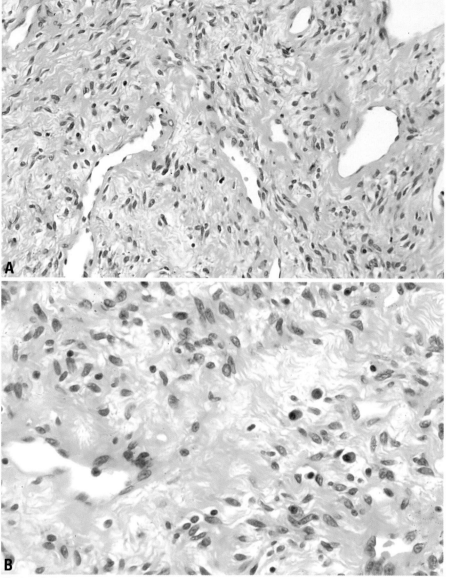

Fig. 2.44 Cellular angiofibroma. **A** Note the prominent dilated vessels with variably hyalinized walls and the short spindle cell fascicles. **B** The spindle cell cytomorphology is reminiscent of spindle cell lipoma. Note also the stromal mast cells.

Nuchal-type fibroma

M. Michal

Definition
Nuchal-type fibroma (NTF) is a rare benign hyalinized fibroblastic proliferation involving dermis and subcutis.

ICD-O code   8810/0

Synonym
Nuchal fibroma.

Epidemiology
NTF is significantly more common in men with a peak incidence during the third through fifth decades.

Sites of involvement
NTF typically affects the posterior neck region but can also occur in a number of other sites. Most of the extranuchal tumours are usually located in the upper back region, but other locations such as the face, extremities, and others can be encountered {600}. Because these extranuchal lesions are histologically indistinguishable from the nuchal examples, the designation nuchal-type fibroma was proposed to encompass all histologically similar lesions irrespective of their site of origin {1438}.

Clinical features
The mean greatest tumour dimension is slightly over 3 cm {1438}. It has hard consistency and white colour. The patients are usually asymptomatic. Interesting is the relationship between the patients with NTF and diabetes mellitus {11}. Up to 44% of patients with NTF in one series had diabetes mellitus {1438}.

Histopathology
NTF is an unencapsulated, poorly circumscribed, paucicellular lesion composed of thick, haphazardly arranged collagen fibres. In the central parts of the lesion, the collagen bundles intersect and form a vaguely lobular architecture. Compared with normal tissue from the nuchal area, NTFs show similarly thick collagen fibres. However, in NTF there is an expansion of collagenized dermis with encasement of adnexa, effacement of the subcutis with entrapment of adipocytes, and, in many cases, extension into the underlying skeletal muscle. A delicate network of elastic fibres is observed between the collagen fibres. Thus, NTFs appear to represent a local-ized accentuation of the poorly cellular, collagenous connective tissue that normally resides in these sites. Scant numbers of lymphocytes are present in a minority of cases, but inflammatory features are never prominent. Many NTFs contain a localized proliferation of nerve twigs, similar to that seen in traumatic neuromas {113}, and in rare cases, there can be also perineurial fibrosis, as seen in Morton neuroma. These changes are probably the result of repetitive minor trauma or a response by small nerves to the local accumulation of collagen. NTF is histologically indistinguishable from Gardner fibroma (see below).

Immunophenotype
Immunohistochemically the lesions are vimentin, CD34 and CD99 positive and negative with antibodies to actins and desmin {526,1438,2337}.

Prognostic factors
NTF often recurs but does not metastasize.

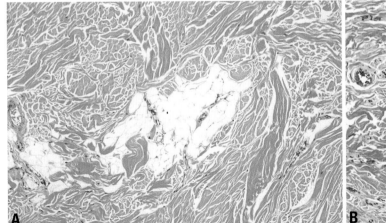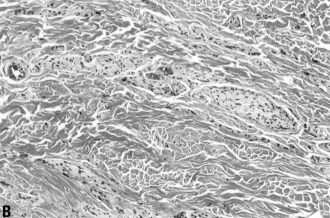

Fig. 2.45 Nuchal-type fibroma. **A** Entrapment of the adipose tissue by hypocellular collagenous tissue is a typical histological feature. **B** Note the tightly encased twigs of peripheral nerve.

Gardner fibroma

C.M. Coffin

Definition
Gardner fibroma is a benign soft tissue lesion consisting of thick, haphazardly arranged collagen bundles with interspersed bland fibroblasts, a plaque-like growth pattern with infiltration and entrapment of surrounding structures, and an association with desmoid-type fibromatosis and familial adenomatous polyposis / Gardner syndrome.

ICD-O code   8810/0

Epidemiology
Gardner fibroma is an uncommon soft tissue lesion. It affects predominantly infants, children, and adolescents. There is no sex predilection. Diagnosis of Gardner fibroma in early childhood can serve as the sentinel event for identifying Gardner syndrome kindreds and children with de novo *APC* germline mutations.

Sites of involvement
Gardner fibroma involves superficial and deep soft tissues of the paraspinal region, back, chest wall, flank, head and neck, and extremities {2227}. A similar mesenteric lesion has been reported as "desmoid precursor lesion" in patients with familial adenomatous polyposis {363}.

Clinical features
Patients with Gardner fibroma develop ill defined, plaque-like masses in superficial or deep soft tissue {2227}. The mass is usually asymptomatic, but may become painful with growth. Desmoid-type fibromatoses have arisen in the sites of Gardner fibromas {42,2227}. With imaging studies, Gardner fibroma appears as a dense plaque-like mass.

Macroscopy
Gardner fibroma ranges in size from 1 to 10 cm and involves superficial and deep soft tissues. The poorly circumscribed mass is firm, rubbery, and has a plaque-like appearance. The cut surface is white to tan-pink with scattered yellow areas representing entrapped adipose tissue {2227}.

Histopathology
The hypocellular proliferation of haphazardly arranged, coarse collagen bands contains scattered bland spindle cells and small blood vessels {2227}. The central portion of the lesion is uniform and displays a cracking artefact between the dense collagen bundles. Peripherally, the collagen extends into adjacent tissues and entraps fat, muscle, and nerves. A sparse mast cell infiltrate is present {2227}.

Immunophenotype
The spindle cells in Gardner fibroma are positive for vimentin and CD34 and negative for smooth muscle actin, muscle specific actin, desmin, oestrogen receptor, and progesterone receptor proteins {526,2226, 2227}.

Genetic susceptibility
Among the reported cases of Gardner fibroma, more than 90% were associated with Gardner syndrome, familial adenomatous polyposis, and/or *APC* mutation.

Prognostic factors
45% of patients developed subsequent desmoid-type fibromatoses {42,2227}. Accurate identification of Gardner fibroma, especially in childhood, is critical for recognizing underlying Gardner syndrome, addressing the high risk of development of classic desmoid-type fibromatosis, and instituting early and close monitoring of the patient and other relatives for manifestations of adenomatous polyposis coli {2227}. Consideration should also be given to the diagnosis of Gardner fibroma in paediatric lesions resembling nuchal-type fibroma {42,2226,2227}.

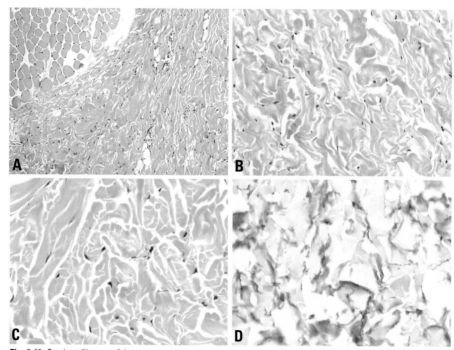

Fig. 2.46 Gardner fibroma. **A** Low power view of a paraspinal example in a young child showing a hypocellular fibrous lesion with entrapment of skeletal muscle and clusters of adipocytes. **B** Central areas of Gardner fibroma display hypocellular sheets of haphazardly arranged thick and thin collagen bands with sparse spindle cells. **C** Small bland spindle cells dispersed in cracks between collagen fibres. **D** CD34 staining identifies spindle cells between coarse collagen fibres.

Calcifying fibrous tumour

E. Montgomery

Definition
Calcifying fibrous tumour is a rare, benign fibrous lesion usually affecting children and young adults. It is paucicellular, with fibroblasts, dense collagenization, psammomatous and dystrophic calcification, and patchy lymphoplasmacytic infiltrates.

ICD-O code   8810/0

Synonyms
Childhood fibrous tumour with psammoma bodies {1809}, calcifying fibrous pseudotumour.

Epidemiology
Most soft tissue examples affect children and young adults without gender predilection {448,659,948,1306,1539}. Visceral examples usually occur in adults {157,337,868,1707}.

Sites of involvement
Tumours were originally described in the subcutaneous and deep soft tissues (extremities, trunk, neck, and scrotum) {659,1809} but have subsequently been reported all over the body, notably in the mesentery and peritoneum {157,337, 1148,1539,1951,2256}, pleura (sometimes multiple) {606,868,1707}, mediastinum {557}, and adrenal gland {571}.

Clinical features
Soft tissue examples present as painless masses. Visceral examples may produce site-specific symptoms {157,868,1707}. Radiographs show well marginated, non-calcified tumours. Calcifications are apparent on CT and may be thick and band-like or punctate {606}. On MRI, masses appear similar to fibromatoses, with a mottled appearance and a signal closer to that of muscle than fat {659}.

Aetiology
Although examples have followed trauma {1707,2336} and have occurred in association with Castleman disease {448} and inflammatory myofibroblastic tumours {1714,2176}, the pathogenesis remains unknown.

Macroscopy
Tumours are well marginated but unencapsulated, ranging in size from <1 to 15 cm. Some show indistinct boundaries with infiltration into surrounding tissues. On occasion, a gritty texture is noted on sectioning, which reveals a firm whitish lesion.

Histopathology
Tumours consist of well circumscribed, unencapsulated, paucicellular, hyalinized fibrosclerotic tissue with a variable inflammatory infiltrate consisting of lymphocytes and plasma cells. Lymphoid aggregates may be present. Calcifications, both psammomatous and dystrophic, are scattered throughout.

Immunophenotype
Lesional cells express vimentin and factor XIIIa, but usually lack actins, desmin, factor VIII, S100 protein, neurofilament protein, cytokeratins, CD34, and CD31. The immunophenotype differs from that of inflammatory myofibroblastic tumours in that most calcifying fibrous tumours

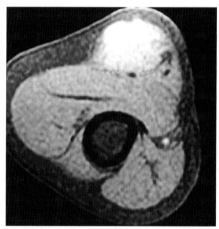

Fig. 2.47 Fat suppressed, gadolinium-enhanced T1 MRI of a calcifying fibrous tumour.

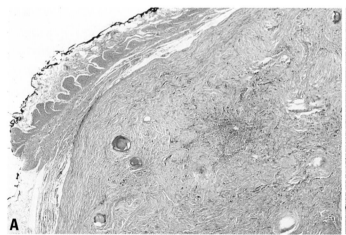
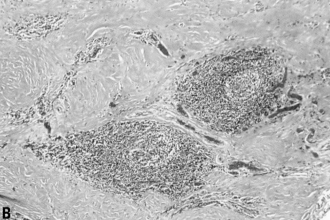

Fig. 2.48 A Calcifying fibrous tumour. The lesion is well marginated but not encapsulated. Note the psammomatous calcifications. **B** 530 Lymphoid follicles in this calcifying fibrous tumour.

lack actin and anaplastic lymphoma kinase (ALK) {948,1951}. Occasional lesions have expressed CD34 {948, 2256}.

Ultrastructure

On electron microscopy, fibroblasts are accompanied by collagen fibrils. The dystrophic and psammomatous calcifications are observed as electron-dense amorphous masses and laminated bodies, respectively, within the cytoplasm of fibroblasts and in the collagenous stroma. Cytoplasmic degeneration may be an initial event in intracytoplasmic calcification; extracellular calcified material often abuts fibroblasts {1306,1707}.

Prognostic factors

These lesions are benign; occasional recurrences are recorded and may be repeated {659,948}.

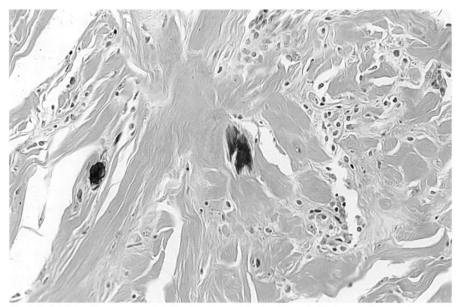

Fig. 2.49 Calcifying fibrous tumour. Calcifications are seen in a background with dense collagen and scattered plasma cells.

Giant cell angiofibroma

L. Guillou
J.A. Bridge

Definition
A non-recurring, benign neoplasm containing multinucleated giant stromal cells and angiectoid spaces. Giant cell angiofibroma may belong to the solitary fibrous tumour group.

ICD-O code
9160/0

Epidemiology
Described in 1995 {491}, giant cell angiofibroma (GCA) is a distinctive benign neoplasm which most often involves the orbital region and eyelids of middle-aged adults (median age : 45 years). Orbital GCA predominates in males {491,912}, whereas extraorbital lesions predominate in female patients {853,2109}.

Sites of involvement
GCA is usually observed in the orbital region, including the eyelids, the naso-lacrimal duct and the lacrimal sac region {491,912}. It has also been observed in the head and neck region outside the orbit (scalp, retroauricular region, parotid gland, cheek, submandibular region, buccal mucosa), as well as in the posterior mediastinum {740}, back, axillary and inguinal regions, retroperitoneum, and vulva {491,853,1454,2109}. Most extraorbital lesions are located subcutaneously.

Clinical features
GCA usually presents clinically as a slowly growing, sometimes painful {2109} mass.

Macroscopy
Grossly, GCAs are well circumscribed, variably encapsulated, small (median : 3 cm) lesions. Upon section, haemorrhagic and/or cystic changes may be observed. Soft tissue lesions tend to be larger than orbital-region tumours, sometimes measuring up to 10 cm {1950,2109}.

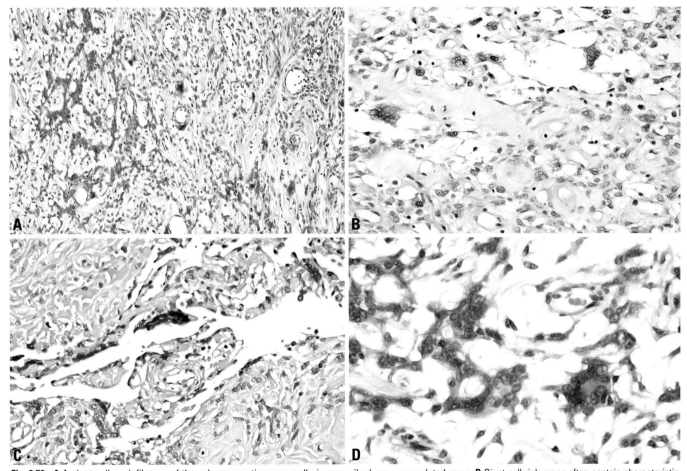

Fig. 2.50 **A** A giant cell angiofibroma of the vulva presenting as a well-circumscribed nonencapsulated mass. **B** Giant cell rich areas often contain characteristic medium-sized to small thick-walled vessels. **C** Multinucleated giant cells lining pseudovascular spaces in giant cell angiofibroma. **D** Morphological appearance of multinucleated giant stromal cells in giant cell angiofibroma.

Histopathology

The tumour displays a varying combination of cellular areas composed of bland round to spindle cells, collagenous or myxoid stroma with focal sclerotic areas, medium-sized to small thick-walled vessels, and multinucleated giant stromal cells, often lining angiectoid spaces {491,853,912,2109}. The number of giant cells may vary from one tumour to another, and pseudovascular spaces may occasionally be absent.

Immunophenotype

Mononuclear and multinucleated stromal cells are characteristically positive for CD34, CD99 and, less frequently, BCL2 {853,2109}.

Genetics

Cytogenetic analysis of one case arising in the orbit revealed abnormalities of chromosome band 6q13 {1988}.

Prognostic factors

Nearly all GCA show benign behaviour; recurrences after complete excision are exceptional {491,853,2109}.

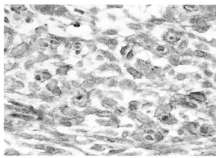

Fig. 2.51 Strong immunoreactivity of mono- and multinucleated stromal cells for CD34.

Superficial fibromatoses

J.R. Goldblum
J.A. Fletcher

Definition
Superficial fibromatoses are fibroblastic proliferations that arise in the palmar or plantar soft tissues and are characterized by infiltrative growth. They have a tendency toward local recurrence but do not metastasize.

ICD-O code
Palmar / plantar fibromatosis   8821/1

Synonyms
Palmar fibromatosis: Dupuytren disease, Dupuytren contracture.
Plantar fibromatosis: Ledderhose disease.

Epidemiology
Palmar fibromatosis tends to affect adults with a rapid increase in incidence with advancing age. Rarely, patients younger than 30 years of age are affected. The condition is three to four times more common in men and is most common in Northern Europe and in those parts of the world now settled by Northern Europeans {1455}. These lesions are quite rare in non-Caucasian populations {1478}. In contrast, plantar lesions have a much greater incidence in children and adolescents {45}. Although plantar lesions arise more commonly in men, the gender difference is not as great as that found in palmar lesions. Both forms of

fibromatosis have been linked with numerous other disease processes including other forms of fibromatosis. Approximately 5% to 20% of palmar fibromatoses are associated with plantar lesions, and up to 4% of patients also have penile fibromatosis (Peyronie disease) {195}.

Sites of involvement
Palmar lesions occur on the volar surface of the hand with a slight predilection for the right palmar surface. Almost 50% of cases are bilateral. Plantar lesions arise within the plantar aponeurosis, usually in non-weight-bearing areas. Cases arising in children tend to occur in the antero-medial portion of the heel pad {799}.

Clinical features
For palmar lesions, the initial manifestation is typically that of an isolated firm palmar nodule that is usually asymptomatic and which ultimately results in cord-like indurations or bands between multiple nodules and adjacent fingers. This often leads to puckering of the overlying skin, and flexion contractures principally affecting the 4th and 5th digits. Plantar lesions present as a firm subcutaneous nodule or thickening that adheres to the skin and is frequently associated with mild pain after long

standing or walking. Plantar lesions only exceptionally result in contraction of the toes {366}.

Aetiology
The pathogenesis is multifactorial and includes a genetic component, as many patients have a significant family history of this disease {1271}. Trauma likely also has a central role. The coexistence of these diseases with epilepsy, diabetes and alcohol-induced liver disease suggests that factors other than trauma are also important.

Macroscopy
Both lesions consist of small nodules or an ill defined conglomerate of several nodular masses intimately associated with the aponeurosis and subcutaneous fat. On cut section, both have a grey-yellow or white surface, although the colour depends on the collagen content of the lesion.

Histopathology
The proliferative phase is characterized by a cellular proliferation of plump, immature-appearing spindled cells that vary little in size and shape, have nor-mochromatic nuclei and small pinpoint nucleoli. Plantar lesions are often notably hypercellular. Mitotic figures are usually

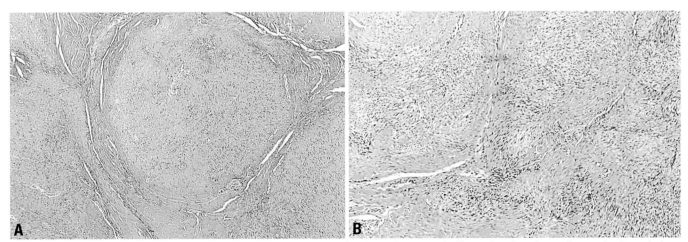

Fig. 2.52 A Low power view showing typically multinodular growth pattern (within tendoaponeurotic fibrous tissue), as is usually seen in plantar lesions. **B** In the early (proliferative) phase, palmar fascial or aponeurotic tissue is expanded by hypercellular spindle cell nodules.

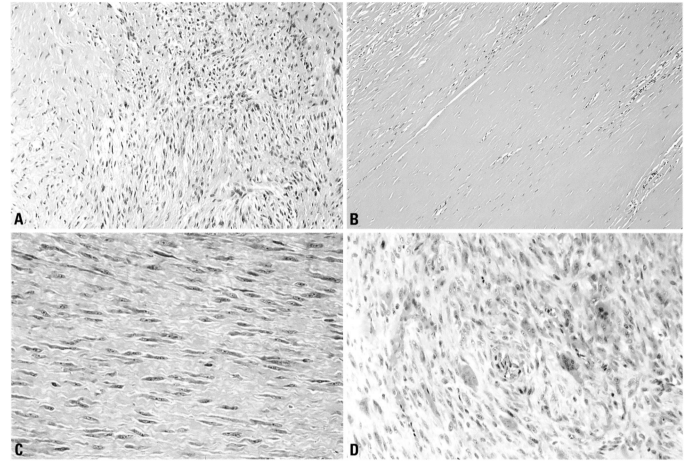

Fig. 2.53 A Early (proliferative) lesion of palmar fibromatosis showing bland fibroblastic / myofibroblastic cells. **B** Palmar fibromatosis. Late lesions associated with contracture consist largely of densely hyalinized hypocellular collageneous tissue. **C** High magnification view of cytologically bland cells in a palmar fibromatosis. In this example, the cells are widely separated by collagen. **D** Plantar fibromatosis may contain scattered osteoclastic giant cells.

infrequent but may be focally prominent, but the latter is not indicative of malignancy (e.g. fibrosarcoma). Cells are intimately associated with moderate amounts of collagen and elongated vessels. Older lesions are considerably less cellular and contain increased amounts of dense collagen. Occasional cases of plantar fibromatosis contain notable multinucleate giant cells {623}.

Immunophenotype
The cells strongly express vimentin and variably stain for muscle-specific and smooth muscle actin, depending upon the stage and degree of myofibroblastic differentiation.

Ultrastructure
Most cells have the features of fibroblasts, although a proportion of the cells has myofibroblastic features.

Genetics
Chromosome aberrations have been described in more than 50 cases, all showing near-diplod karyotypes. Simple numerical changes are typical, particularly gain of chromosomes 7 or 8 {1477}.

Prognostic factors
Risk of local recurrence is most closely related to the extent of surgical excision. Dermofasciectomy followed by skin grafting is associated with the lowest rate of local recurrence {275,873}. For plantar lesions, there appears to be an increased risk of local recurrence in those cases with multiple nodules, in patients with bilateral lesions, those with a positive family history and those who develop a postoperative neuroma {49,2216}.

Desmoid-type fibromatoses

J.R. Goldblum
J.A. Fletcher

Definition
Desmoid-type fibromatoses are clonal fibroblastic proliferations that arise in the deep soft tissues and are characterized by infiltrative growth and a tendency toward local recurrence but an inability to metastasize.

ICD-O codes
Aggressive fibromatosis   8821/1
Abdominal (mesenteric) fibromatosis
8822/1

Synonyms
Aggressive fibromatosis, musculoaponeurotic fibromatosis, desmoid tumour.

Epidemiology
Deep fibromatoses are rarer than their superficial counterparts and are encountered in two to four individuals per million population per year {1779}. In the paediatric population, these lesions have an equal sex incidence and most are extra-abdominal. Patients between puberty and 40 years of age tend to be female, and the abdominal wall is the favoured site in this group. Later in adulthood, these tumours are equally distributed between abdominal and extra-abdominal locations and occur equally in both genders {914}.

Sites of involvement
Extra-abdominal fibromatoses may be located in a variety of anatomic locations, although the principal sites of involvement are the shoulder, chest wall and back, thigh and head and neck. Abdominal tumours arise from musculoaponeurotic structures of the abdominal wall, especially the rectus and internal oblique muscles and their fascial coverings. Intra-abdominal fibromatoses arise in the pelvis or mesentery.

Clinical features
Extra-abdominal fibromatoses typically arise as a deep-seated, firm, poorly circumscribed mass that has grown insidiously and causes little or no pain. Some cases are multifocal. Although rare, some lesions cause decreased joint mobility or neurological symptoms. Abdominal wall lesions typically arise in young, gravid or parous women during gestation or, more frequently, during the first year following childbirth. Pelvic fibromatoses arise as a slowly growing palpable mass that is usually asymptomatic and is often mistaken for an ovarian neoplasm. Mesenteric lesions may be sporadic or arise in patients with Gardner syndrome. Most patients present with an asymptomatic abdominal mass, but some have mild abdominal pain. Less commonly, patients with mesenteric lesions present with gastrointestinal bleeding or an acute abdomen secondary to bowel perforation.

Aetiology
The pathogenesis is multifactorial and includes genetic, endocrine and physical factors. Features suggesting an underlying genetic basis include the existence of familial cases and the presence of these lesions, particularly mesenteric fibromatoses, in patients with Gardner syndrome {859}. Endocrine factors are implicated by the frequent occurrence of abdominal lesions during or after pregnancy. Trauma likely also serves as a contributory cause.

Macroscopy
These lesions are firm and cut with a gritty sensation. On cross section, the cut surface reveals a glistening white, coarsely trabeculated surface resembling scar tissue. Lesions in the abdomen may appear well circumscribed. Most tumours measure between 5 and 10 cm.

Histopathology
These lesions are typically poorly circumscribed with infiltration of the surrounding soft tissue structures. All are characterized by a proliferation of elongated, slender, spindle-shaped cells of uniform appearance, set in a collage-

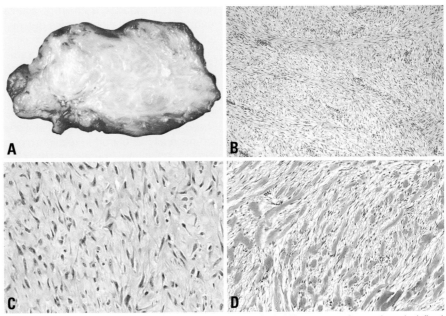

Fig. 2.54 Extra-abdominal desmoid fibromatosis. **A** Note the whorled fibrous cut surface and poorly defined margins to surrounding skeletal muscle. **B** Cellular proliferation of bland spindled cells arranged into ill defined long fascicles. Regularly distributed blood vessels are evident. **C** Cells are spindled or stellate in shape and have bland nuclear features. **D** Extensive keloid-like collagen deposition.

nous stroma containing variably prominent vessels, sometimes with perivascular oedema. The cells lack hyperchromasia or atypia and have small, pale-staining nuclei with 1 to 3 minute nucleoli. Cells are usually arranged in sweeping bundles. As with superficial fibromatoses, the mitotic rate is variable. Keloid-like collagen or extensive hyalinization may be present. Some lesions, particularly those arising in the mesentery and pelvis, have extensive stromal myxoid change and may show more fasciitis-like cytomorphology.

Immunophenotype
The cells strongly express vimentin and variably stain for muscle-specific and smooth muscle actin. Rare cells may also express desmin and S100 protein.

Ultrastructure
Most cells have the features of fibroblasts, although a proportion of the cells have myofibroblastic features.

Genetics
Desmoid-type fibromatoses may contain cell subpopulations with trisomies for chromosomes 8 and/or 20 {251,267,433, 476,689,1986}. These numerical chromosomal aberrations are typically found in no more than 30% of the fibromatosis cells, and it is unlikely that they play a crucial role at the inception of the tumours {267,476,689}. Some clinical series suggest a relationship between the trisomies and more advanced disease, but there is no consensus that any of these aberrations are prognostic in patients with newly-diagnosed fibromatoses {438,444,476,689, 1161,1431}. Inactivation of the *APC* tumour suppressor on chromosome arm 5q, occurring typically by point mutation or allelic deletion, is a potential initiating event in

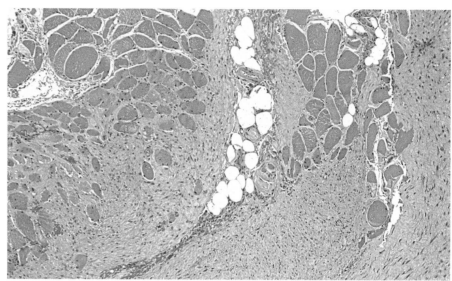
Fig. 2.55 Desmoid fibromatosis. Note the irregular infiltration into adjacent skeletal muscle and adipose tissue.

desmoid tumours. However, *APC* inactivation is found primarily in desmoid tumours from patients with familial polyposis, and is less common in patients with sporadic desmoid tumours {261, 447,785,1481,1640,1919,2327}. Germline *APC* mutations can result in familial desmoid tumour syndromes in which the polyposis component is either inconspicuous or even absent.

The APC protein binds to beta-catenin, which is an important cell signalling protein in the Wnt pathway. APC binding to beta-catenin induces a chain of events leading to degradation of beta-catenin, and inhibition of Wnt pathway signalling {1649,1819,1820}. Many sporadic desmoid tumours contain activating beta-catenin mutations, which render beta-catenin resistant to the normal inhibitory influence of APC {46,1249}. These beta-catenin activating mutations are generally "either/or" in relationship to *APC* inactivating mutations {9,1483,

1841,2101}. Because both types of mutation are manifested by stabilization of the beta-catenin protein, these molecular mechanisms can be addressed at a screening level by immunohistochemical staining for beta-catenin. Beta-catenin is strongly expressed in most desmoid tumours {9,1483}. Other distinctive genetic features, that distinguish desmoid tumours from most fibrosarcomas, include a paucity of *BCL2*, *RB1*, and *TP53* aberrations {966}.

Prognostic factors
Local recurrence is frequent and most closely related to the adequacy of surgical excision. However, attempts to achieve tumour-free resection margins may result in significant morbidity {1246, 1420}. Some cases may recur as a consequence of multicentricity. Despite the lack of metastatic potential, some desmoids prove fatal due to local effects, especially in the head and neck region.

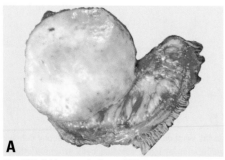
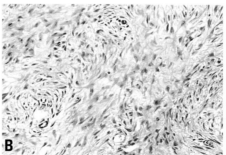
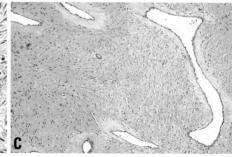

Fig. 2.56 A Mesenteric desmoid fibromatosis, presenting as a typically large, macroscopically circumscribed mass. The cut surface of mesenteric examples is often myxoid. **B** Mesenteric fibromatosis with extensive myxoid change. **C** Ectatic blood vessels with perivascular hyalinization in a mesenteric fibromatosis.

Lipofibromatosis

M.M. Miettinen
J.F. Fetsch

Definition

A histologically distinctive fibrofatty tumour of childhood, previously designated as infantile fibromatosis of non-desmoid type, with predilection for distal extremities.

Synonyms

Infantile fibromatosis, non-desmoid type.

Clinical features

This rare paediatric tumour was recently reported by Fetsch et al. {658}. It typically forms an ill defined slowly growing, painless mass in hands and feet and rarely occurs in the thigh, trunk and head. The tumour has been described exclusively in children from infancy to the early second decade and in some cases has been congenital; the median age for first surgery is 1 year. There is an over 2:1 male predominance.

Macroscopy

Grossly the lesion is yellowish or whitish tan, with a fatty component typically evident. It usually measures 1-3 cm and rarely exceeds 5 cm, with a median size of 2 cm.

Histopathology

Microscopically the tumour is composed of alternating streaks of mature adipose tissue and a fibrous spindle cell component mainly involving the septa of adipose tissue. This constellation resembles that of fibrous hamartoma of infancy, except that there is no primitive oval cell

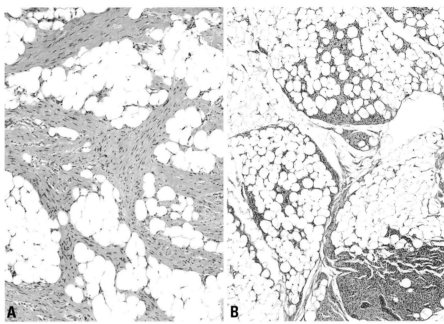

Fig. 2.57 Lipofibromatosis. **A** Even admixture of fibroblastic and adipocytic components. **B** The relative proportion of the two components is variable and the spindle cell areas may form delicate trabeculae.

component with myxoid stroma. The lesion differs from other forms of fibromatosis by the architectural preservation of fat and lack of solid fibrous growth. Mitotic activity is low and nuclear atypia is absent. Many cases contain minute collections of small vacuolated cells near the interface between the fibroblastic element and the mature adipocytes.

Immunophenotype

The spindle cells are often focally positive for CD34, BCL2, S100 protein, actins and EMA and may also be positive for CD99. No reactivity has been detected for desmin and keratins.

Prognostic factors

The tumour has a high rate of non-destructive local recurrence, but there is no metastatic potential. Congenital onset, male sex, mitotic activity in the fibroblastic component and incomplete excision may be risk factors for recurrence.

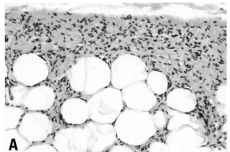
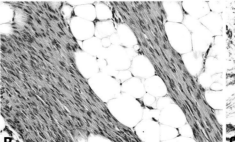
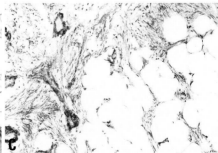

Fig. 2.58 Lipofibromatosis. **A** The spindle cell component is bland and may have a rather primitive fibroblastic appearance. **B** Fascicular growth of the fibroblastic element. **C** Focally positive immunostaining for smooth muscle actin, consistent with fibroblastic / myofibroblastic differentiation.

Extrapleural solitary fibrous tumour and haemangiopericytoma

L. Guillou
J.A. Fletcher
C.D.M. Fletcher
N. Mandahl

This section combines two neoplastic entities, the border between which has become increasingly blurred. In particular, the delineation of haemangiopericytoma as a separate entity may become obsolete since its histopathological features, as generally understood at the present time, are shared by a variety of soft tissue tumours.

Solitary fibrous tumour

Definition
A ubiquitous mesenchymal tumour of probable fibroblastic type which shows a prominent haemangiopericytoma-like branching vascular pattern. Morphologically, extrapleural solitary fibrous tumours (SFT) resemble pleural SFTs; most were termed haemangiopericytomas in the past.

ICD-O code
Solitary fibrous tumour   8815/1

Epidemiology
Extrapleural SFTs are uncommon mesenchymal neoplasms of ubiquitous location, observed in middle-aged adults between 20 and 70 years (median: 50 years), with no sex predilection. Occasional cases occur in children and adolescents.

Sites of involvement
SFTs may be found at any location. 40% of tumours are found in the subcutaneous tissue, others are found in the deep soft tissues of extremities or extra-compartmentally in the head and neck region (especially the orbit), thoracic wall, mediastinum, pericardium, retroperitoneum, and abdominal cavity. Other described locations include the meninges, spinal cord, periosteum as well as organs such as the salivary glands, lungs, thyroid, liver, gastro-intestinal tract, adrenals, urinary bladder, prostate, spermatic cord, testes, etc. {27,283,895,896,1406,1561,2062,2073, 2254}.

Clinical features
Most tumours present as well delineated, slowly growing, painless masses. Large tumours may give rise to compression symptoms, especially in the nasal cavity, the orbit and the meninges. Malignant tumours are often locally infiltrative {736, 737,896,2167}. Rarely, large tumours may be the source of paraneoplastic syndromes such as hypoglycaemia due to the production of an insulin-like growth factor {545}.

Macroscopy
Most SFTs present as well circumscribed, often partially encapsulated masses, measuring between 1 and 25 cm (median: 5 to 8 cm). On section, they frequently have a multinodular, whitish and firm appearance; myxoid and haemorrhagic changes are occasionally

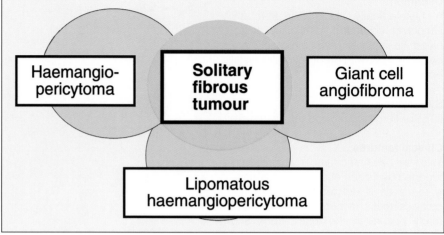

Fig. 2.59 Extrapleural solitary fibrous tumour and related lesions.

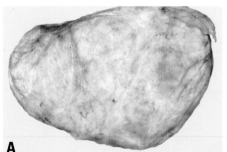

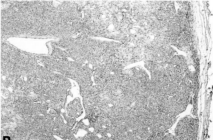

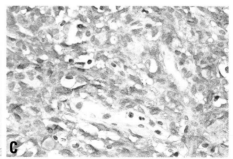

Fig. 2.60 A Gross appearance of an extrapleural solitary fibrous tumour. The lesion is well delineated and shows a multinodular and whitish appearance on cut section. **B** An extrapleural solitary fibrous tumour presenting as a well circumscribed but nonencapsulated mass. **C** Strong immunoreactivity of the tumour cells for CD99 in an extrapleural solitary fibrous tumour.

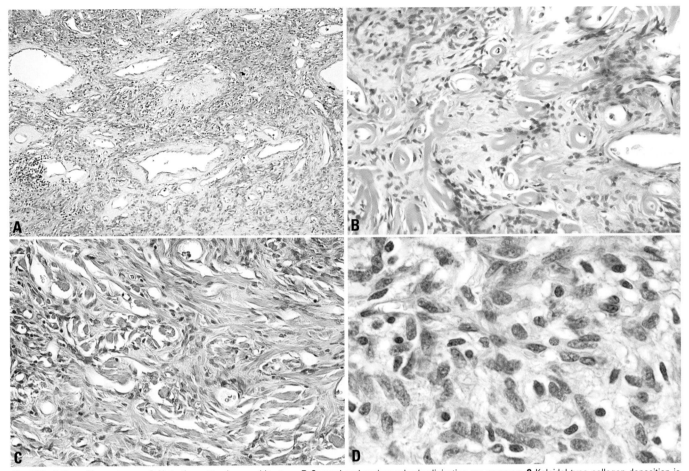

Fig. 2.61 Solitary fibrous tumour **A** Note the patternless architecture. **B** Stromal and perivascular hyalinization are common. **C** Keloidal-type collagen deposition is frequent. **D** Typically bland spindle cells with rather vesicular nuclei.

observed {736, 896, 1406, 1561, 2062, 2167}. Tumour necrosis and infiltrative margins (about 10% of cases) are mostly observed in locally aggressive or malignant tumours {737, 896, 2167}.

Histopathology

Typical SFTs show a patternless architecture characterized by a combination of alternating hypocellular and hypercellular areas separated from each other by thick bands of hyalinized, somewhat keloidal, collagen and branching haemangiopericytoma-like vessels. The non-atypical, round to spindle-shaped tumour cells have little cytoplasm with indistinct borders and dispersed chromatin within vesicular nuclei. Myxoid change, areas of fibrosis and interstitial mast cells are commonly observed. Mitoses are generally scarce, rarely exceeding 3 mitoses per 10 high-power fields. Some SFTs may contain mature adipocytes {1406, 2073} and/or giant multinucleated stromal cells {896}, overlapping morphologi-

cally with the so-called lipomatous haemangiopericytoma (see below) and giant cell angiofibroma (see above).

Malignant SFT are usually hypercellular lesions, showing at least focally moderate to marked cytological atypia, tumour necrosis, numerous mitoses (≥ 4 mitoses per ten high-power fields) and/or infiltrative margins {737, 896, 2167}. Rare cases show abrupt transition from conventional benign-appearing SFT to high grade sarcoma, likely representing a form of dedifferentiation.

Immunophenotype

Tumours cells in SFT are characteristically immunoreactive for CD34 (90 to 95% of cases) {283, 896, 1406, 1561, 2062, 2167, 2254}, and CD99 (70%) {1783}. 20 to 35% of them are also variably positive for epithelial membrane antigen, BCL2 {343, 2060}, and smooth muscle actin. Focal and limited reactivity for S100 protein, cytokeratins and/or desmin has also occasionally been reported {736, 2167}.

Ultrastructure

Ultrastructural features are nonspecific in SFT. Tumour cells often demonstrate features of fibroblastic, myofibroblastic and/or (arguably) pericytic differentiation {1406, 1556, 2073}.

Genetics

SFTs are cytogenetically heterogeneous {441, 682}. Demonstrable cytogenetic aberrations are particularly uncommon in smaller SFTs, but are found in most SFTs larger than 10 cm in diameter {1452}.

Prognostic factors

Although most cases are benign, the behaviour of SFT is unpredictable. Roughly, 10 to 15% behave aggressively, thus long-term follow-up is mandatory {736, 896, 2167}. There is no strict correlation between morphology and behaviour. However, most (but not all) histologically benign SFTs prove to be non-recurring and non-metastasizing lesions, and most histologically malignant tumours behave

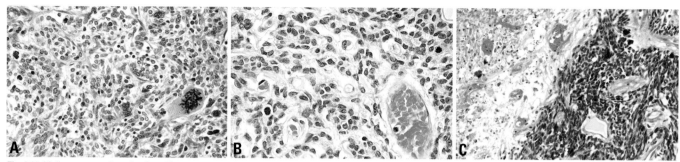

Fig. 2.62 Malignant extrapleural solitary fibrous tumours. **A** Hypercellularity and marked cytological atypia. Note the atypical mitosis. **B** Moderately cellular area with brisk mitotic activity. **C** Hypercellularity, marked cytological atypia, and areas of tumour necrosis (left).

aggressively. Lesions located in the mediastinum, abdomen, pelvis, and/or retroperitoneum also tend to behave more aggressively than those in the limbs {736,737,896,2167}. Metastases are most frequently observed in lungs, bone and liver {2167}.

Haemangiopericytoma

Definition
The residual group of lesions, previously combined under the term haemangiopericytoma, which closely resemble cellular areas of solitary fibrous tumour (SFT) and which appear fibroblastic in type. It has a range of clinical behaviour and is closely related to, if not synonymous with, SFT.

Historical annotation
Haemangiopericytoma (HPC), similar to malignant fibrous histiocytoma, is a term which has been used loosely to encompass a wide variety of neoplasms which have in common the presence of a thin-walled branching vascular pattern (described below) {294, 676, 1535}. As such, HPC is difficult to define at this time as a discrete entity, although lesions showing pericytic differentiation undoubtedly exist and were included in Stout's original descriptions {2036, 2040}.

The prototypical pericytic neoplasm is myopericytoma {825} (see page 138) and sinonasal HPC (see Tumours of the Upper Respiratory Tract) also appears to be pericytic in nature.

Epidemiology
The discrete subset of lesions remaining as HPC is rare. In light of the heterogeneity of lesions classified as HPC, there are no meaningful estimates of incidence. Myopericytoma appears substantially more common than the other discrete subset of lesions known as HPC which cannot currently be otherwise classified.

The discrete subset of soft tissue lesions known as HPC which currently justify retention of this nomenclature occur most often in middle-aged adults with an apparent female predominance.

Lesions formerly known as infantile HPC fall within the spectrum of infantile myofibromatosis {1412} (see respective section on page 59).

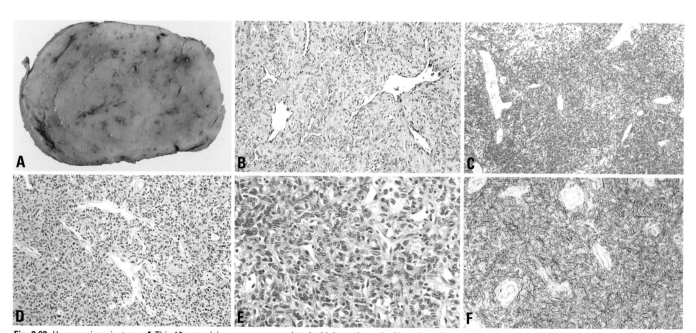

Fig. 2.63 Haemangiopericytoma. **A** This 12 cm pelvic mass was associated with hypoglycemia. Note the uniform, spongy cut surface. **B,C,D** Note the evenly distributed cellularity (in contrast to usual SFT) and the prominent branching vascular pattern. **E** Even in the more solid areas, tumour cells are arranged around numerous thin-walled vessels. Tumour cells are small with monomorphic nuclei and eosinophilic cytoplasm. **F** Diffuse positivity for CD34 is shared by the spectrum of lesions known as haemangiopericytoma and solitary fibrous tumour.

Sites of involvement

The subset of soft tissue lesions which, for the time being, are still named HPC, arise most often in deep soft tissue, particularly pelvic retroperitoneum. A smaller proportion of cases arise in the proximal limbs or limb girdles. Histologically comparable lesions also occur in the meninges (see WHO Blue Book on Tumours of the Nervous System).

Clinical features

Most tumours present as a slowly growing mass which, in the abdomen, may cause intestinal or urinary symptoms. Occasional cases, similar to SFT, are associated with hypoglycemia due to secretion of insulin-like growth factor {1671}.

Macroscopy

Convincing examples of so-called HPC in soft tissue tend to be well-circumscribed masses with a yellowish or tan cut surface and a fleshy or spongy consistency. Large vessels may be evident on the cut surface. Haemorrhage is common but necrosis is infrequent. Tumour size is variable but most cases are 5-15 cm in maximum diameter.

Histopathology

The discrete residual subset of so-called HPC closely resembles the cellular areas of SFT, albeit with the consistent presence of numerous, variably ectatic or compressed, thin-walled branching vessels often having a staghorn configuration. Tumour cells are usually closely packed, spindle-shaped to round, of uniform size, with small amounts of pale or eosinophilic cytoplasm with indistinct margins and small, bland often vesicular nuclei. Cytological pleomorphism is generally not a feature. In contrast to SFT, stromal hyalinization and varying cellularity are not usual features. The mitotic rate is highly variable. Some cases contain a prominent adipocytic component (such cases are known as lipomatous HPC – see below). These lesions also often show varying cellularity and are increasingly regarded as a variant of SFT. Tumours which very often were classified as HPC in the past include (among others) solitary fibrous tumour (p. 86), monophasic synovial sarcoma (p. 200), infantile myofibromatosis (p. 59), myopericytoma (p. 138), infantile fibrosarcoma (p. 98), deep fibrous histio-

cytoma (p. 114) and mesenchymal chondrosarcoma (p. 255).

Immunohistochemistry

The discrete subset of so-called HPC, comparable to SFT, shows fairly consistent positivity for CD34 and CD99, both of which are widely expressed in fibroblastic tumours. Endothelial markers are negative, as also (in most cases) are actin and desmin.

Ultrastructure

Most of the lesions reported as HPC have shown only undifferentiated spindle cell or fibroblastic features. Convincing evidence of true pericytic differentiation is not seen.

Genetics

Few cytogenetically investigated HPCs, located in the lung, tongue, brain, cerebellum, soft tissues, and intrabdominally, have been reported {1477}. The vast majority of cases have had near- or pseudodiploid karyotypes with the number of aberrations ranging from one to more than 20. The chromosome aberrations are quite disparate, but breakpoints in 12q13-15 and 19q13 have been identi-

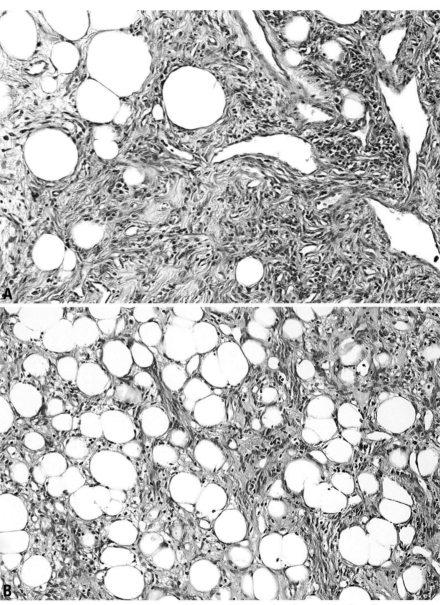

Fig. 2.64 Lipomatous haemangiopericytoma. **A** Many such lesions show features of solitary fibrous tumour in addition to containing numerous mature adipocytes. Note haemangiopericytoma-like branching vessels **B** An intimate admixture of bland spindle cells and mature adipocytes.

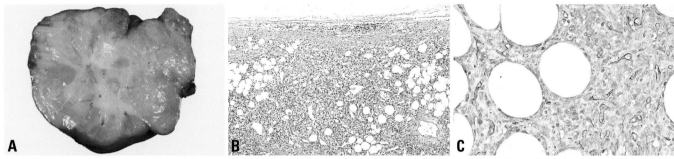

Fig. 2.65 Lipomatous hemangiopericytoma. **A** Gross appearance of a well circumscribed retroperitoneal lesion. Cut section shows fibrous bands dissecting the lesion from centre to periphery. **B** Similar to extrapleural solitary fibrous tumours, lipomatous hemangiopericytomas are well-delineated, often encapsulated masses. **C** Immunoreactivity of the tumour cells for CD34.

fied in almost half of the cases and one-fourth of the cases, respectively. In two cases, there was a balanced t(12;19)(q13;q13), in one case as the sole anomaly. Among the genomic imbalances, losses are predominating. Recurrent imbalances include loss of segments in 3p, 12q, 13q, 17p, 17q, 19q, and the entire chromosome 10, and gain of 5q sequences.

Prognostic factors

At least 70% (probably more) of HPCs pursue a benign clinical course, while the remainder are malignant. Histological criteria for malignancy are imprecise and prognostication in HPC has long been regarded as difficult. There have been no recent prognostic studies confined to the discrete subset of lesions which might nowadays be termed HPC. However, older data from major centres {598} suggest parameters similar to those used currently for SFT – specifically, 4 or more mitotic figures per 10 high power fields is the single feature most worrisome for malignancy. The presence of necrosis or nuclear pleomorphism, particularly in the context of a tumour >5 cm in diameter may also portend malignant behaviour.

Lipomatous haemangiopericytoma

Lipomatous haemangiopericytoma (LHPC) is an uncommon, slow-growing, almost non-recurring, non-metastasizing mesenchymal neoplasm composed of mature adipocytes and haemangiopericytoma-like areas {696,852,1556}. LHPC shares many features with SFT. Both lesions occur in similar clinical settings, although LHPC tends to predominate in males (M/F ratio 2:1) and to affect preferentially the deep soft tissues of the lower extremity (especially the thigh) and retroperitoneum. Morphologically, it is a well demarcated neoplasm consisting of a varying combination of patternless cellular areas, prominent haemangiopericytoma-like vessels, variably collagenized extracellular matrix, and lipomatous areas made of mature adipocytes. The non atypical tumour cells are consistently positive for CD99 and, less frequently, for CD34 (75%) and BCL2 (60%) {852}.

Inflammatory myofibroblastic tumour

C.M. Coffin
J.A. Fletcher

Definition
Inflammatory myofibroblastic tumour (IMT) is a distinctive lesion composed of myofibroblastic spindle cells accompanied by an inflammatory infiltrate of plasma cells, lymphocytes, and eosinophils. It occurs primarily in soft tissue and viscera of children and young adults.

ICD-O code   8825/1

Synonyms
Plasma cell granuloma {2008,2218}, plasma cell pseudotumour {1710}, inflammatory myofibrohistiocytic proliferation {2086}, omental mesenteric myxoid hamartoma {809}, inflammatory pseudotumour {1353,1750,2151,2301}. A closely related term is inflammatory fibrosarcoma {374,1392}.

Epidemiology
IMT is primarily a visceral and soft tissue tumour of children and young adults, although the age range extends throughout adulthood. The mean age is 10 years, and the median is 9 years {376, 380,960,1044,1750,2250}. Overall, IMT is most frequent in the first two decades of life. There is a slight female predominance.

Aetiology
The aetiology is unknown. The finding of human herpesvirus-8 DNA sequences and overexpression of human interleukin 6 and cyclin D1 has been recently report-

ed in 7 cases {806}. IMT has been reported following treatment for Wilms tumour {2207}.

Sites of involvement
IMT can occur throughout the body, and the most common sites are the lung, mesentery, and omentum {376,380, 1701}. Among extrapulmonary IMT, 43% arose in the mesentery and omentum {380}. Other sites include soft tissue, mediastinum, gastrointestinal tract, pancreas, genitourinary tract, oral cavity, skin, breast, nerve, bone, and central nervous system {30,203,722,960,998, 1044,1071,1434,1750,1912,1999,2086, 2130,2165,2209,2221,2250}.

Clinical features
The site of origin determines the symptoms of IMT. Pulmonary IMT is associated with chest pain and dyspnoea, but may be asymptomatic {1701}. Abdominal tumours may cause gastrointestinal obstruction. Dermatomyositis and obliterative phlebitis are uncommon

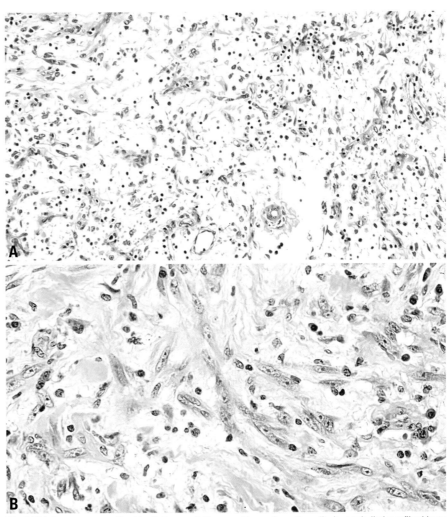

Fig. 2.67 Inflammatory myofibroblastic tumour. **A** The myxoid vascular pattern displays spindled myofibroblasts dispersed in a myxoid background with lymphocytes and plasma cells. **B** Spindled myofibroblasts and ganglion-like cells dispersed in a myxoid background with inflammatory reaction.

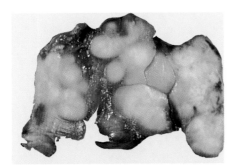

Fig. 2.66 Inflammatory myofibroblastic tumour presenting as a circumscribed, multinodular mass with a variegated cut surface.

manifestations {26,2297}. A mass, fever, weight loss, and pain are frequent complaints. In up to one-third of patients, a clinical syndrome occurs with fever, growth failure, malaise, weight loss, anaemia, thrombocytosis, polyclonal hyperglobulinemia, and elevated erythrocyte sedimentation rate {380,1999, 2043}. When the mass is excised, the syndrome disappears, and its reappearance heralds recurrence.

Imaging studies reveal a lobulated solid mass which may be inhomogeneous {277,458}. Calcifications are sometimes detectable {1071}.

Macroscopy
The gross appearance of IMT is a circumscribed or multinodular firm, white, or tan mass with a whorled fleshy or myxoid cut surface. Focal haemorrhage, necrosis, and calcification are seen in a

minority of cases. The mean diameter of extrapulmonary IMT is 6 cm with a range of 1-17 cm {380}. In some masses, a zonal appearance with a central scar and softer red or pink periphery is seen. Multinodular tumours are usually restricted to the same anatomic region and may be contiguous or separate.

Histopathology
The spindled myofibroblasts, fibroblasts, and inflammatory cells of IMT form three basic histological patterns {376,380}. Loosely arranged plump or spindled myofibroblasts in an oedematous myxoid background with abundant blood vessels and an infiltrate of plasma cells, lymphocytes, and eosinophils resemble granulation tissue, nodular fasciitis, or other reactive processes. A second pattern is characterized by a compact fascicular spindle cell proliferation with vari-

able myxoid and collagenized regions and a distinctive inflammatory infiltrate with diffuse inflammation, small aggregates of plasma cells or lymphoid nodules. This resembles a fibromatosis, fibrous histiocytoma, or a smooth muscle neoplasm. In some instances, the spindled myofibroblastic cells surround blood vessels or bulge into vascular spaces, similar to infantile myofibromatosis or intravascular fasciitis. Ganglion-like myofibroblasts with vesicular nuclei, eosinophilic nucleoli, and abundant amphophilic cytoplasm are often seen in these two patterns. The third pattern resembles a scar or desmoid-type fibromatosis, with plate-like collagen, lower cellularity, and relatively sparse inflammation with plasma cells and eosinophils. Coarse or psammomatous calcifications and osseous metaplasia are occasionally seen {1809}.

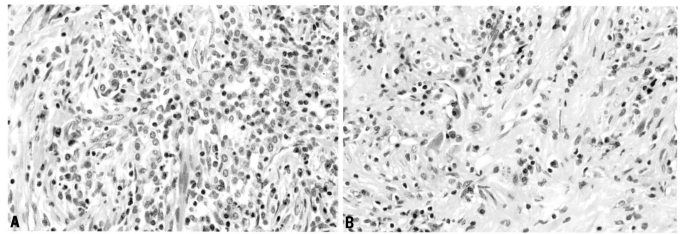

Fig. 2.68 Inflammatory myofibroblastic tumour. **A** The background contains collagen: the inflammatory infiltrate is focally dense. **B** Ganglion-like cells with vesicular nuclei and large eosinophilic nucleoli are dispersed within the fibroblastic-myofibroblastic and inflammatory proliferation.

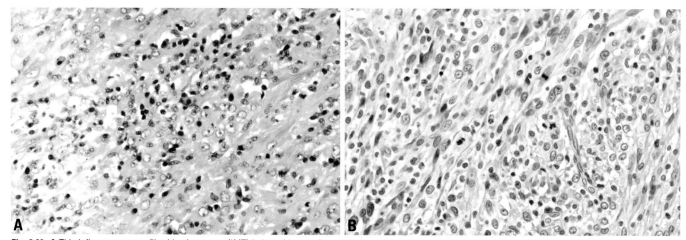

Fig. 2.69 **A** This inflammatory myofibroblastic tumour (IMT) behaved in a malignant fashion. It has large atypical vesicular nuclei and could be labelled 'inflammatory fibrosarcoma'. **B** Malignant transformation in IMT. In this example, the myofibroblasts are spindled to polygonal and show frequent mitoses and ganglion-like cells.

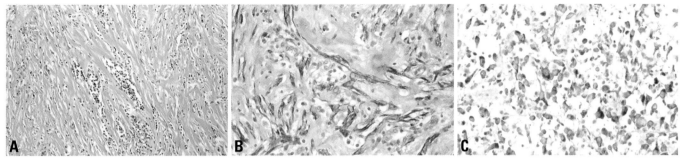

Fig. 2.70 Inflammatory myofibroblastic tumour. **A** The scar-like pattern contains abundant plate-like collagen with lower cellularity and relatively sparse inflammation. **B** Desmin is present in cytoplasm of myofibroblasts. **C** Cytoplasmic immunohistochemical reactivity for ALK (ALK1 antibody).

Highly atypical polygonal cells with oval vesicular nuclei, prominent nucleoli, and variable mitoses, including atypical forms, are seen in rare IMTs which undergo histologic malignant transformation {376,380,536}. Large ganglion-like cells and Reed-Sternberg-like cells are also seen {1475}. The round cell histiocytoid pattern may develop after multiple recurrences.

Immunophenotype
Strong diffuse cytoplasmic reactivity for vimentin is typical for virtually all IMT. Reactivity for smooth muscle actin and muscle specific actin varies from a focal to a diffuse pattern in the spindle cell cytoplasm, and desmin is identified in many cases {380,1750,2209}. Focal cytokeratin immunoreactivity is seen in about one-third of cases. Myogenin, myoglobin, and S100 protein are negative.

Immunohistochemical cytoplasmic positivity for ALK using a variety of monoclonal antibodies is detectable in approximately 50% of IMTs and correlates well with the presence of *ALK* rearrangements (occurring mainly in children) detectable by fluorescent in situ hybridization {326,378,396,838,2330}. However, ALK positivity is not specific for IMT. TP53 immunoreactivity is rare and has been reported in association with recurrence and malignant transformation {984}. IMT does not show immunoreactivity for CD117 (KIT).

Ultrastructure
IMT displays ultrastructural features of myofibroblastic and fibroblastic differentiation. Spindle cells with poorly developed Golgi, abundant rough endoplasmic reticulum, and extracellular collagen are seen, and some contain intracytoplasmic thin filaments and dense bodies {380,1392}.

Genetics
IMT are heterogeneous genetically, as is hardly surprising given the varied clinicopathological entities, which have been grouped in this category. IMT in children and young adults often contain clonal cytogenetic rearrangements that activate the *ALK* receptor tyrosine kinase gene in chromosome band 2p23 {838,1226, 2047}. By contrast, such rearrangements are uncommon in IMT diagnosed in adults beyond 40 years old {326,1226}. IMT with *ALK* genomic rearrangements show constitutive activation and overexpression of the ALK kinase domain, and both the *ALK* genomic rearrangements and ALK protein activation are restricted to the myofibroblastic component of the tumours {258,378,396,838,1226}. The inflammatory component is normal cytogenetically and does not express detectable ALK protein. A subset of IMT lack *ALK* oncogenic activation but contain chromosmal rearrangements targeting the *HMGIC* (also known as *HMGA2*) gene on chromosome 12 {1080}. Notably, certain of the ALK activation

mechanisms in IMT are also found in subsets of anaplastic large cell lymphomas {1212,2125}. Immunohistochemical detection of the ALK C-terminal end is undoubtedly the most efficient method for identifying ALK oncoproteins in IMT {378,396}. The specificity of this approach is conferred by the low-to-absent expression of native ALK proteins in nonneoplastic myofibroblasts. Therefore, the finding of strong C-terminal ALK expression provides strong evidence for an oncogenic activating mechanism.

Prognostic factors
Extrapulmonary IMT has a recurrence rate of approximately 25% related to location, resectability, and multinodularity {380}. Rare cases (<5%) also metastasize. Evidence suggests that a combination of atypia, ganglion-like cells, TP53 expression, and aneuploidy may help to identify IMT with a more aggressive potential {202,203,984,1163,1750}. Unfortunately it is difficult to predict on the basis of histopathological findings alone in an individual case whether recurrence or malignant transformation will occur. Although surgery is the principal treatment, regression and response to corticosteroids and nonsteroidal inflammatory agents have been noted in rare cases {374,376,1044,2048}.

Low grade myofibroblastic sarcoma

T. Mentzel
J.A. Fletcher

Definition
Low grade myofibroblastic sarcoma represents a distinct atypical myofibroblastic tumour often with fibromatosis-like features and predilection for the head and neck.

ICD-O code   8825/3

Synonym
Myofibrosarcoma.

Epidemiology
Given the lack of consensus on diagnostic criteria, myofibroblastic sarcomas in general are probably more common than currently believed, and include a variety of clinicopathological forms {1405}. Low grade myofibroblastic sarcoma represents a distinct entity that occurs predominantly in adult patients with a slight male predominance; more rarely children are affected {1414,1495,1969}.

Sites of involvement
Low grade myofibroblastic sarcoma shows a wide anatomic distribution, however, the extremities and the head and neck region, especially the tongue and the oral cavity, seem to be preferred locations {1414,1495}. Rare cases involving the salivary gland and the nasal cavity / paranasal sinus have been reported {201,1153}.

Clinical features
In most cases of low grade myofibroblastic sarcoma patients complain about a painless swelling or an enlarging mass. Pain or related symptoms have been more rarely reported. Clinically, local recurrences are common, whereas metastases only rarely occur and often after a prolonged time interval {1414}. Radiologically, these lesions have a destructive growth pattern.

Macroscopy
Grossly, most cases are described as a firm mass with pale and fibrous cut surfaces and mainly ill defined margins {1414}; a minority of neoplasms are well circumscribed with rather pushing margins {1495}.

Histopathology
Histologically, most cases of low grade myofibroblastic sarcoma are characterized by a diffusely infiltrative growth pattern, and, in deeply located neoplasms, tumour cells may grow between individual skeletal muscle fibres. Most cases are composed of cellular fascicles or show a storiform growth pattern of spindle-shaped tumour cells. Neoplastic cells have ill defined palely eosinophilic cytoplasm and fusiform nuclei that are either elongated and wavy with an evenly distributed chromatin, or plumper, more rounded and vesicular with indentations and small nucleoli. More rarely, hypocellular neoplasms with a more prominent collageneous matrix and focal hyalinization have been described. Importantly, neoplastic cells show at least focally moderate nuclear atypia with enlarged, hyperchromatic and irregular nuclei and a slightly increased prolif

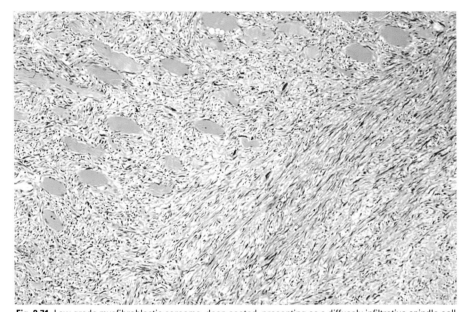

Fig. 2.71 Low grade myofibroblastic sarcoma, deep seated, presenting as a diffusely infiltrative spindle cell neoplasm with a fascicular arrangement of neoplastic cells.

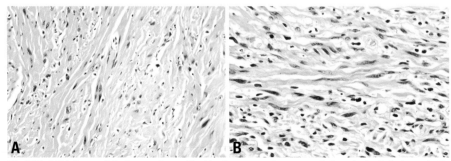

Fig. 2.72 A This hypocellular low grade myofibroblastic sarcoma is composed of atypical spindled neoplastic cells set in a prominent collegenous matrix. **B** Fusiform tumour cells in low grade myofibroblastic sarcoma contain ill defined, pale, eosinophilic cytoplasm and spindle-shaped nuclei that are either vesicular with small nucleoli and indentations or elongated and wavy, resembling neural differentiation.

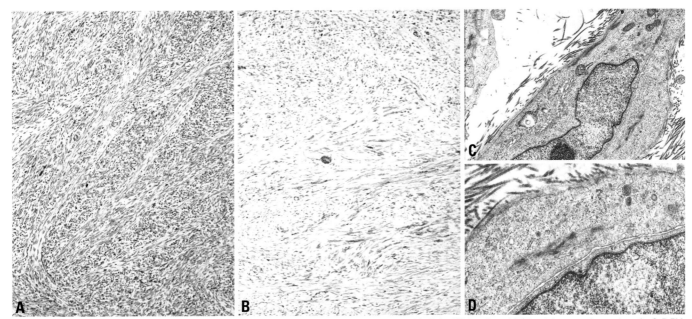

Fig. 2.73 Immunohistochemically, tumour cells in low grade myofibroblastic sarcoma often stain positively for **(A)** desmin and **(B)** for alpha-smooth muscle actin. **C, D** EM showing **(C)** a discontinuous basal lamina, **(D)** thin filaments with focal densities, subplasmalemmal attachment plaques, and micropinocytic vesicles.

erative activity. These neoplasms may contain numerous thin-walled capillaries. Lymphocytes and plasma cells are not a prominent feature.

Immunophenotype

Neoplastic cells in low grade myofibroblastic sarcoma have a variable immunophenotype: actin positive/desmin negative, actin negative/desmin positive, and actin positive/desmin positive cases. In addition, tumour cells may stain positively for fibronectin, and focal expression of CD34 and CD99 has been reported, whereas S100 protein, epithelial markers, laminin, and h-caldesmon are negative {1414}.

Ultrastructure

In contrast to smooth muscle cells, neoplastic cells in low grade myofibroblastic sarcoma contain indented and clefted nuclei, a variable amount of rough endoplasmic reticulum, and are surrounded by a discontinuous basal lamina. Unlike in fibroblasts, randomly oriented intermediate filaments and thin filaments with focal densities and subplasmalemmal attachment plaques, a discontinuous basal lamina and often micropinocytic vesicles are noted.

Genetics

Genetic aberrations have been described in only a few low grade myofibroblastic sarcomas. The preliminary reports are of karyotypes with a moderate number of chromosomal aberrations, substantially less complex than the karyotypes seen in most high grade myofibroblastic sarcomas {682}.

Prognostic factors

The presence of increased proliferative activity and tumour necrosis is associated with more aggressive behaviour {1495}.

Myxoinflammatory fibroblastic sarcoma

L.G. Kindblom
J.M. Meis-Kindblom

Definition
Myxoinflammatory fibroblastic sarcoma (MIFS) is a unique low grade sarcoma with myxoid stroma, inflammatory infiltrate and virocyte-like cells that predominantly involves the hands and feet.

ICD-O code   8811/3

Synonyms
Inflammatory myxohyaline tumour of the distal extremities with virocyte or Reed-Sternberg-like cells {1496}, acral myxoinflammatory fibroblastic sarcoma, inflammatory myxoid tumour of the soft parts with bizarre giant cells {1437}.

Epidemiology and aetiology
MIFS is rare and occurs primarily in adults with a peak incidence in the fourth and fifth decades. Males and females are equally affected.

The prominent acute and chronic inflammation seen in this lesion, presence of inclusion-like nucleoli in tumour cells, and history of a longstanding mass in many patients raise the possibility of an infectious aetiology. However, no evidence of CMV or EBV has been detected in MIFS using immunohistochemical and PCR techniques {1496}, and stains for bacteria, fungi and mycobacteria have been uniformly negative {1386}.

Clinical features
Two large series of this entity, including 44 and 51 cases, indicate a predilection for the distal extremities {1386,1496}. Two-thirds of tumours involve the hands and wrists and one-third the feet and ankles. The elbows and knees are rarely involved. Most patients have a relatively long history of a slowly growing, poorly defined mass that is occasionally associated with pain and decreased mobility. The preoperative diagnosis in most cases is benign and may include tenosynovitis, ganglion cyst, and giant cell tumour of tendon sheath.

Macroscopy
Most lesions are poorly defined and multinodular and frequently have alternating fibrous and myxoid zones. Tumour size ranges from less than 1 to 8 cm; median tumour size is 3–4 cm.

Morphology
The tumours typically infiltrate the subcutaneous fat and frequently involve the joints and tendons. Dermal invasion is often seen, whereas invasion of skeletal muscle is rare. Bone involvement has not been observed.

The most striking feature at low magnification is a prominent dense, mixed acute and chronic inflammatory infiltrate associated with alternating hyaline and myxoid zones in variable proportions. Aggregates of macrophages and uniform mononuclear cells with foci of haemosiderin deposition closely resemble pigmented villonodular synovitis. There are three main types of neoplastic cells seen in MIFS, including spindled cells, large polygonal and bizarre ganglion-like cells with huge inclusion-like nucleoli, and variably sized bubbly, multivacuolated lipoblast-like cells. These cells may be scattered singly or form coherent nodules.

Immunophenotype
The neoplastic cells are strongly positive for vimentin, variably positive for CD68 and CD34, and rarely positive for smooth muscle actin {1386}. Occasional cases show weak cytokeratin positivity. More importantly, they are negative for leukocyte common antigen, T and B-cell markers and CD30.

Ultrastructure
All three types of neoplastic cell display features of fibroblasts, including abundant rough endoplasmic reticulum and mitochondria, and a network of intermediate filaments occasionally forming densely packed perinuclear whorls {1386}.

The tumour cells simulating lipoblasts demonstrate cytoplasmic pseudoinclusions containing extracellular mucinous material.

Genetics
The only case for which cytogenetic information exists showed a t(1;10) together with loss of chromosomes 3 and 13 {1213}.

Prognostic factors
Reported rates of local recurrence vary widely, ranging from 20% to 70% {1386, 1496}. In one large series, repeated local recurrences with proximal extension eventually culminated in amputation in more than one-third of patients who had local recurrences {1386}. Differences in reported rates of local recurrence may be attributed to differences in primary surgical treatment, a high rate of misdiagnosis as a benign tumour, and differences in length of clinical follow-up.

Metastases to distant lymph nodes and lung occur but are exceedingly rare (<2% of all reported cases), based on currently available data {1386}.

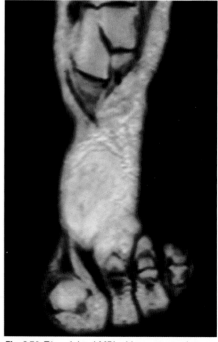

Fig. 2.74 T1-weighted MRI with contrast enhancement, showing an MIFS involving the dorsal foot.

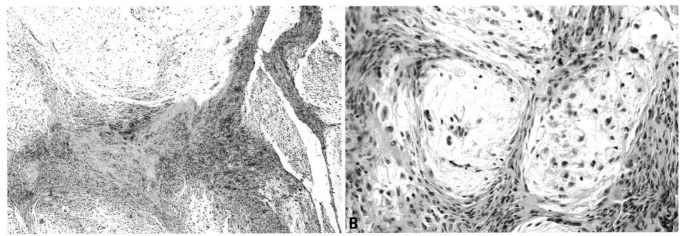

Fig. 2.75 Myxoinflammatory fibroblastic sarcoma (MIFS). **A, B** Note the alternating areas of myxoid tissue and more solidly cellular tissue containing inflammatory cells.

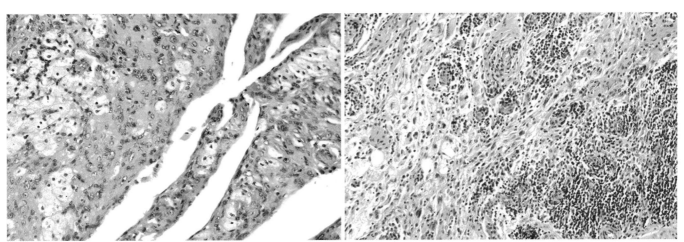

Fig. 2.76 Myxoinflammatory fibroblastic sarcoma (MIFS). Clusters of **(A)** macrophages and **(B)** lymphocytes may obscure the tumour cells.

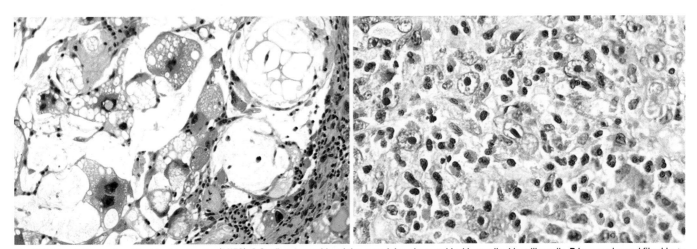

Fig. 2.77 Myxoinflammatory fibroblastic sarcoma (MIFS). **A** Confluent myxoid nodules containing pleomorphic, bizarre, lipoblast-like cells. **B** Large polygonal fibroblasts with inclusion-like nucleoli. Note the presence of prominent eosinophils.

Infantile fibrosarcoma

C.M. Coffin
J.A. Fletcher

Definition

Infantile fibrosarcoma (IFS) is histologically identical to classic fibrosarcoma of adults, but carries a much more favourable prognosis. It occurs in infants and young children, metastasizes rarely, and has a natural history similar to that of fibromatoses. IFS is morphologically and genetically related to congenital mesoblastic nephroma.

ICD-O code   8814/3

Synonyms

Congenital fibrosarcoma {214}, congenital-infantile fibrosarcoma {377}, juvenile fibrosarcoma {2038}, medullary fibromatosis of infancy, aggressive infantile fibromatosis, congenital fibrosarcoma-like fibromatosis, desmoplastic fibrosarcoma of infancy, medullary fibromatosis of infancy {40,1924}.

Epidemiology

IFS accounts for approximately 13% of fibroblastic-myofibroblastic tumours in children and adolescents {372} and 12% of soft tissue malignancies in infants {888}. 36%-80% of cases are congenital, and 36%-100% of cases occur in the first year of life {350,377,1017,1848,2001, 2038}. IFS is seldom encountered after 2 years of age {377} and in that context would require cytogenetic confirmation. There is a slight male predominance.

Aetiology

The aetiology is unknown. No definite predisposing factors, associated heredi-tary diseases, or causative agents have been demonstrated. Prenatal radiation, multiple congenital anomalies, congenital naevus, meningomyelocele, and Gardner syndrome have been reported in sporadic cases {377,628,847,915}.

Sites of involvement

The superficial and deep soft tissues of the extremities, especially distally, are the most common sites, accounting for 61% of cases overall {117,214,350, 377}. The trunk (19% of cases) and head and neck (16%) are other major sites. The mesentery and retroperitoneum are rarer sites of origin.

Clinical features

IFS presents as a solitary enlarging, non-tender mass or swelling in the soft tissues and grows rapidly {350,377,915, 2038}. The diameter may exceed 30 cm {377}. Congenital and infantile cases are often grotesquely large in proportion to the size of the child. The overlying skin is tense, erythematous, and ulcerated. Imaging studies reveal a large soft tissue mass with a heterogeneous enhancement pattern and variable osseous erosion {117,214,572}.

Macroscopy

IFS is a poorly circumscribed, lobulated mass that infiltrates adjacent soft tissue. Compression of adjacent tissue gives the appearance of a pseudocapsule, but the actual margins are irregular and infiltrative. The cut surface is soft to firm, fleshy, and grey to tan with variable areas of myxoid or mucinous change, cystic degeneration, haemorrhage, necrosis, and yellow-red discoloration {117,350,424,1808,2035,2038}.

Histopathology

The typical IFS is a densely cellular neoplasm composed of intersecting fascicles of primitive ovoid and spindle cells with a herringbone pattern or forming interlacing cords, sinuous bands or sheets of cells. Zonal necrosis and haemorrhage are frequent and may be associated with dystrophic calcifications {350,377,424,2038}. The cells show little pleomorphism. Giant cells are not usually seen. Collagen formation is variable, and mitotic activity is prominent. Most IFS contain scattered chronic inflammatory cells and may display focal extramedullary haematopoiesis. Histological variations include a focally prominent haemangiopericytoma-like pattern of irregular cavernous or clefted blood vessels, dilated blood vessels with fibrin thrombi, myxoid foci, or a predominant round or ovoid immature cellular proliferation with minimal collagen. Infiltrative growth results in entrapment of adipose tissue, skeletal muscle and other structures. Rarely, recurrent IFS displays features resembling a high grade pleomorphic sarcoma {1848}. Composite tumours with overlapping features of infantile myofibromatosis, infantile haemangiopericytoma, and infantile fibrosarcoma are occasionally encountered {2194}.

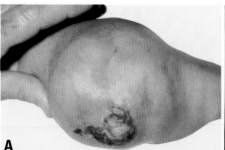 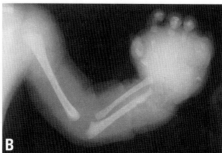 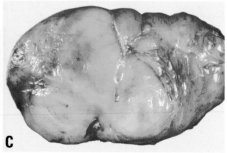

Fig. 2.78 Infantile fibrosarcoma (IFS). **A** IFS of the knee presenting as a large mass with purple discoloration and focal cutaneous ulceration. **B** X-ray of an large IFS of the hand. **C** IFS in soft tissue, displaying a fleshy, tan-white cut surface with focal haemorrhage, necrosis, and myxoid change.

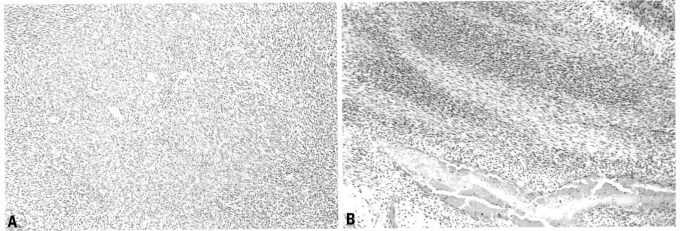

Fig. 2.79 Infantile fibrosarcoma. **A** Poorly formed fascicular growth pattern. **B** A herringbone pattern is present with variable collagen deposition.

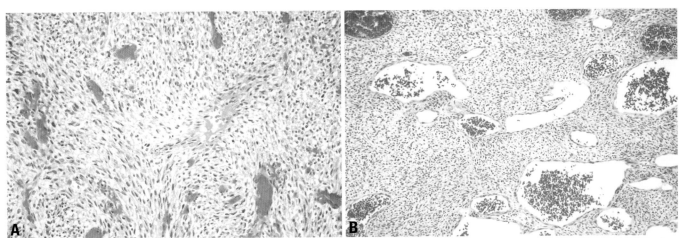

Fig. 2.80 Infantile fibrosarcoma. **A** Short interlacing fascicles, congested blood vessels, and zonal necrosis. **B** Dilated, irregularly branching blood vessels in IFS simulate haemangiopericytoma.

Immunophenotype

The immunohistochemical features of IFS have been reported by several groups with somewhat non-specific findings {377,1151,1933,2194,2278}. Vimentin immunoreactivity is found in 100%, but otherwise IFS is heterogeneous for markers such as neuron-specific enolase (35%), alpha-smooth muscle actin (33%), HHF35 actin (29%), and muscle-specific actin (30%). Fewer than 20% of cases are positive for desmin, S100 protein, CD34, CD57, CD68, factor XIIIa, and CAM5.2 cytokeratin.

Ultrastructure

IFS displays electron microscopic characteristics of fibroblasts and myofibroblasts, with a variable histiocytic component {82,424,807,810}. The cells have large nuclei, one or more nucleoli, dilated rough endoplasmic reticulum with dense material, variably abundant lysosomes, focal basement membrane-like material, and cytoplasmic filaments. In some cases, bundles of thin filaments are seen {1151}.

Genetics

Most infantile fibrosarcomas contain a chromosomal translocation t(12;15) (p13;q26) involving exchange of material between 12p and 15q, resulting in oncogenic activation of the *NTRK3* (a.k.a. *TRKC*) receptor tyrosine kinase gene {235,1142}. The mechanism of activation is a fusion of the 12p *ETV6* (a.k.a. *TEL*) gene to the 15q *NTRK3* gene, and the associated oncoprotein contains the N-terminal aspect of ETV6 fused to the NTRK3 kinase domain. The *ETV6/NTRK3* fusion mechanism is cytogenetically subtle, when assessed by conventional chromosome banding methods {1142, 1816}. However, *ETV6/NTRK3* rearrangement can be demonstrated readily by molecular cytogenetic methods or RT-PCR {16,80,235,553,1142,1816}. Trisomies for chromosomes 8, 11, 17 and 20 are nearly as characteristic as the *ETV6/NTRK3* fusion in infantile fibrosarcomas {1892}. These trisomies appear to be acquired after the *ETV6/NTRK3* fusion, and are perhaps responsible for inducing progression to a more mitotically-active neoplasm {1816}. Notably, a genetic profile similar to that in infantile fibrosarcoma is also seen in mixed-histology and cellular congenital mesoblastic nephroma. Therefore, the pathogenesis of congenital fibrosarcoma and congenital mesoblastic nephroma are doubtless closely related {1141,1816,1893}.

Prognostic factors

IFS has a favourable outcome when compared with adult fibrosarcoma. The mortality ranges from 4% to 25%, and the recurrence rate is 5% to 50% {350,377, 1017,18482001,2038}. Metastasis is rare in more recent series {350,377,2001}. No definitive morphological or genetic prognostic factors have been identified. Haemorrhage and involvement of vital structures by locally aggressive tumours may cause death {377}. Spontaneous regression and nonrecurrence of incompletely excised IFS have been reported {530,1101,1305,1708,2009,2278}. Although surgery is the mainstay of treatment, chemotherapy has been proven effective {371,1185,1195,1797,1938}.

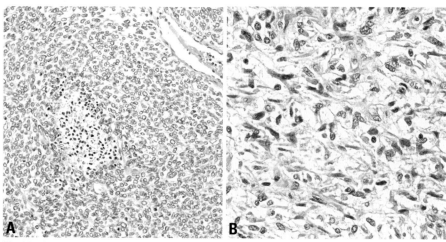

Fig. 2.81 Infantile fibrosarcoma (IFS). **A** A round cell pattern is a variant of IFS. **B** A myxoid focus in IFS contains primitive spindle and ovoid cells.

Adult fibrosarcoma

C. Fisher
E. van den Berg
W.M. Molenaar

Definition

Adult fibrosarcoma is a malignant tumour, composed of fibroblasts with variable collagen production and, in classical cases, a herringbone architecture. It is distinguished from infantile fibrosarcoma and from other specific types of fibroblastic sarcomas.

ICD-O code   8810/3

Epidemiology

The incidence of this tumour is difficult to assess because its diagnosis is partly one of exclusion, and because in recent years specific subtypes of fibrosarcoma (see page 47) have been defined. At most, it probably accounts for 1 to 3% of adult sarcomas {667}. Mixed patterns occur. Classical fibrosarcoma is most common in middle-aged and older adults, but an occasional tumour of this type is seen in childhood (see also section on infantile fibrosarcoma). The sex incidence is equal.

Sites of involvement

Fibrosarcomas involve deep soft tissues of extremities, trunk, head and neck. Fibrosarcoma has also been reported in visceral organs but the identity of these in older reports is questionable. Retroperitoneal fibrosarcoma is rare.

Clinical features

Fibrosarcoma presents as a mass with or without pain. In specific sites local symptoms relate to the effects of a mass. Hypoglycemia has been reported.

Aetiology

There are no specific predisposing factors. Some arise in the field of previous therapeutic irradiation, and rarely in association with implanted foreign material {6}, although the nature of these tumours in the older literature is not always certain. Tumours with the histological features of adult fibrosarcoma may arise in dermatofibrosarcoma (see WHO Tumours of Skin), solitary fibrous tumour (see page 86) and in well differentiated liposarcoma (see page 35), either in the primary or in recurrence, as a reflection of tumour progression.

Macroscopy

The typical fibrosarcoma is a circumscribed white or tan mass, variably firm in relation to the collagen content. Haemorrhage and necrosis can be seen in high grade tumours

Histopathology

The tumour is composed of spindle-shaped cells, characteristically arranged in sweeping fascicles that are angled in a chevron-like or herringbone pattern {2035}. Storiform areas can be seen. The cells have tapered darkly staining nuclei with variably prominent nucleoli and scanty cytoplasm. Mitotic activity is almost always present but variable. Higher grade tumours have more densely staining nuclei, and can display focal round cell change and multinucleated cells, but sarcomas with significant pleomorphism are classified as so-called malignant fibrous histiocytomas (undifferentiated pleomorphic sarcoma). The stroma has variable collagen, from a delicate intercellular network to paucicellular areas with diffuse or "keloid-like" sclerosis or hyalinization. Myxoid change and osteochondroid metaplasia can occur. Fibrosarcoma is usually more cellular than fibromatosis and has larger more hyperchromatic nuclei. However, fibromatosis-like areas can be seen in fibrosarcoma so that tumours should be carefully sampled.

Immunophenotype
Fibrosarcomas are positive for vimentin and very focally for smooth muscle actin, representing myofibroblastic differentiation. Some cases arising in dermatofibrosarcoma or solitary fibrous tumour are CD34 positive.

Ultrastructure
Fibrosarcoma is composed of fibroblasts with prominent rough endoplasmic reticulum and absence of myofilaments, external lamina or intercellular junctions. An occasional cell has peripheral filament bundles suggestive of myofibroblastic differentiation but tumours in which this is a prominent feature should be classified as myofibrosarcomas.

Genetics
Adult fibrosarcoma shows multiple chromosome rearrangements of a complex nature without characteristic anomalies

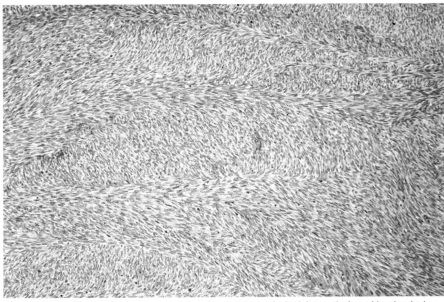

Fig. 2.82 Adult fibrosarcoma. Low power view shows the classical adult-type lesion with a herringbone growth pattern.

{436,1263,1477,2173}. However, two cases of adult fibrosarcoma showed involvement of the same 2q21-qter segment, leading to partial tri– or tetrasomy for 2q {1263}. Based on this finding and other reported cases, disruption of one or more genes in the 2q14-22 region might contribute to the pathogenesis of some adult fibrosarcomas.

Prognostic factors
There are no recent series of fibrosarcoma, which have utilised current definitions. In the older literature, for tumours regarded as fibrosarcoma, behaviour is related to grade and to general factors of tumour size and depth from surface. The probability of local recurrence relates to completeness of excision, with recurrence rates of 12-79% {1730,1731, 1914}.

Fibrosarcomas metastasize to lungs and bone, especially the axial skeleton, and rarely to lymph nodes. Metastasis occurs in 9-63% of patients and is time- and grade-dependent. 5 year survival is 39-54% {1731,1914}. Poor prognostic factors include high grade, high cellularity with minimal collagen, mitotic rates >20/10 hpf, necrosis, and little collagen.

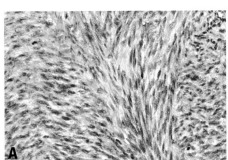 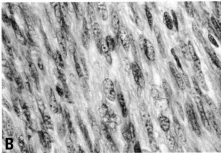 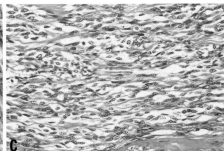

Fig. 2.83 Adult fibrosarcoma. **A** Cells are arranged in long intersecting fascicles with a herringbone pattern. **B** Short tapered spindle cells with scanty cytoplasm and mildly pleomorphic nuclei. **C** Tumour cells are separated by delicate intercellular collagen fibres.

Myxofibrosarcoma

T. Mentzel
E. van den Berg
W.M. Molenaar

Definition
Myxofibrosarcoma comprises a spectrum of malignant fibroblastic lesions with variably myxoid stroma, pleomorphism and with a distintinctively curvilinear vascular pattern.

ICO-O code   8811/3

Synonym
Myxoid malignant fibrous histiocytoma.

Epidemiology
Myxofibrosarcoma is one of the most common sarcomas in elderly patients with a slight male predominance. Although the overall age range is wide, these neoplasms affect mainly patients in the sixth to eighth decade, whereas they are exceptionally rare under the age of 20 years {1413,1422,2236}.

Sites of involvement
The majority of these tumours arise in the limbs including the limb girdles (lower > upper extremities), whereas they are seen only rarely on the trunk, in the head and neck area, and on the hands and feet {1413,1422,2236}. Origin in the retroperitoneum and in the abdominal cavity is extremely uncommon, and most lesions with myxofibrosarcoma-like features in these locations represent dedifferentiated liposarcomas {67,955,1389}. Notably, about two-thirds of cases develop in dermal/subcutaneous tissues, with the remainder occurring in the underlying fascia and skeletal muscle.

Clinical features
Most patients present with a slowly enlarging and painless mass. Local, often repeated recurrences occur in up to 50 to 60% of cases, unrelated to histological grade. In contrast, metastases and tumour associated mortality are closely related to tumour grade. Whereas none of the low grade neoplasms metastasizes, intermediate and high grade neoplasms may develop metastases in about 20 to 35% of cases. In addition to pulmonary and osseous metastases, lymph node metastases are seen in a small but significant number of cases {1413,1422,2236}. Importantly, low grade lesions may become higher grade in subsequent recurrences and hence acquire metastatic potential. The overall 5-year survival rate is 60-70%.

Macroscopy
Superficially located neoplasms typically consist of multiple, variably gelatinous or firmer nodules, whereas deep seated neoplasms often form a single mass with an infiltrative margin. In high grade lesions areas of tumour necrosis are often found.

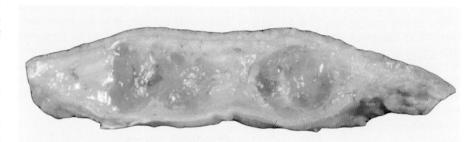

Fig. 2.84 Superficially located, low grade myxofibrosarcoma with multinodular growth pattern and gelatinous, myxoid cut surface.

Histopathology
Myxofibrosarcoma shows a broad spectrum of cellularity, pleomorphism, and proliferative activity; however, all cases share distinct morphological features, particularly multinodular growth with incomplete fibrous septa, and a myxoid stroma composed of hyaluronic acid. The low grade end of the morphological spectrum is characterized by hypocellular neoplasms composed of only few, non-cohesive, plump spindled or stellate tumour cells with ill defined, slightly eosinophilic cytoplasm and atypical, enlarged, hyperchromatic nuclei. Mitotic figures are infrequent in low grade lesions. A characteristic finding is the presence of prominent elongated, curvilinear, thin-walled blood vessels with a perivascular condensation of tumour cells and/or inflammatory cells (mainly lymphocytes and plasma cells). Frequently, so-called pseudolipoblasts (vacuolated neoplastic fibroblastic cells with cytoplasmic acid mucin) are noted. In contrast, high grade neoplasms are composed in large part of solid sheets and cellular fascicles of spindled and pleomorphic tumour cells with numerous, often atypical mitoses, areas of haemorrhage and necrosis. In many cases bizarre, multinucleated giant cells with abundant eosinophilic cytoplasm (resembling myoid cells) and irregular shaped nuclei are noted. However, high grade lesions also focally show features of a lower grade neoplasm with a prominent myxoid matrix and numerous elongated capillaries. The intermediate grade lesions are more cellular and pleomorphic relative to purely low grade neoplasms, but lack extensive solid areas, pronounced cellular pleomorphism and necrosis. Subcutaneous examples of myxofibrosarcoma commonly have very infiltrative margins, often extending beyond what is detected clinically.

Immunophenotype
Tumour cells stain positively for vimentin, and in a minority of cases some spindled or larger eosinophilic tumour cells express muscle specific actin and/or alpha-smooth muscle actin, suggestive of focal myofibroblastic differentiation; desmin, and so-called histiocytic markers (CD68, Mac 387, FXIIIa) are negative {1413}.

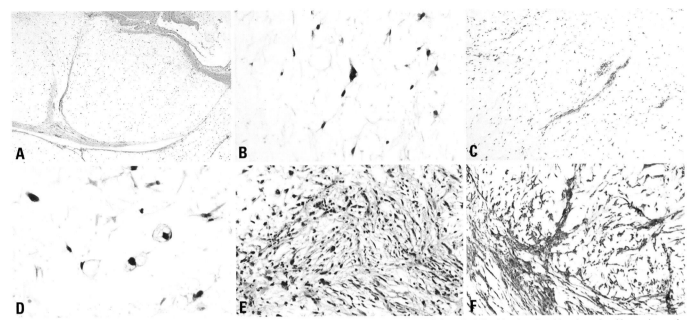

Fig. 2.85 A Low grade myxofibrosarcoma showing multinodular growth with a prominent myxoid matrix, **(B)** atypical fibroblastic cells with enlarged and hyperchromatic nuclei on a background of low cellularity, and **(C)** elongated, curvilinear blood vessels as well as pseudolipoblasts **(D)** are frequent findings in low grade myxofibrosarcoma. **E,F** Intermediate grade myxofibrosarcomas retain a myxoid stroma and characteristic vascular pattern, but are more cellular and pleomorphic than low grade lesions.

Ultrastructure

Although fibroblast-like, histiocyte-like, and myofibroblast-like cells, multinucleated giant cells and undifferentiated mesenchymal cells have been described in the past {732,1117,1209}, the majority of cells in myxoid areas show ultrastructural features of a fibroblastic differentiation (fusiform or oval tumour cells with elongated, occasionally clefted nuclei containing a prominent, often dilated rough endoplasmic reticulum) with secretory activity within a myxoid matrix {1413}.

Genetics

Cytogenetic aberrations have been detected in 25 cases diagnosed as myxoid MFH or myxofibrosarcoma {1477}. In general, the karyotypes tend to be highly complex, with extensive intratumoral heterogenity and chromosome numbers in the triploid or tetraploid range in the majority of cases {1317,1477,1486, 1635,1957}. No specific aberration has emerged, but ring chromosomes have been reported in five cases. In one case the ring chrosomome was shown to originate from 20q {1402}.
Genomic imbalances, as detected by comparative genomic hybridization (CGH), frequently include loss of 6p, and gain of 9q and 12q {1957}.

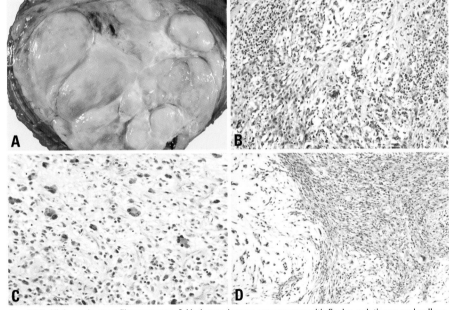

Fig. 2.86 High grade myxofibrosarcoma. **A** Variegated gross appearance with fleshy, gelatinous and yellow-orange areas of necrosis. **B** High grade myxofibrosarcoma with features of a high grade, MFH-like sarcoma and **(C)** frequent multinucleated giant cells with abundant eosinophilic cytoplasm. **D** Focally, areas of lower grade myxofibrosarcoma with a prominent myxoid matrix are usually present in high grade myxofibrosarcoma.

Prognostic factors

Whereas depth of the lesions and grade of malignancy do not influence the high rate of local recurrence, the percentage of metastases and tumour associated mortality are much higher in deep seated and high grade neoplasms {1413,1422, 2236}. A local recurrence within less than 12 months increases the tumour associated mortality {1413, 1422}. Proliferative activity, the percentage of aneuploid cells, and tumour vascularity are associated with the histological tumour grade, but no clear relation with the clinical outcome has been found {1409,1413}.

Low grade fibromyxoid sarcoma

A.L. Folpe
E. van den Berg
W.M. Molenaar

Definition
Low grade fibromyxoid sarcoma is a distinctive variant of fibrosarcoma, characterized by an admixture of heavily collagenized and myxoid zones, deceptively bland spindled cells with a whorling growth pattern and arcades of curvilinear blood vessels.

ICD-O code   8811/3

Synonyms
Hyalinizing spindle cell tumour with giant rosettes; fibrosarcoma, fibromyxoid type.

Epidemiology
Low grade fibromyxoid sarcomas are rare sarcomas, with fewer than 150 reported cases {304,507,563,619,621, 699,742,813,1053,1074,1217,1268, 1417,1552,1939,2077,2150,2296}. It is difficult, however, to estimate the exact incidence of low grade fibromyxoid sarcoma, as many tumours go unrecognized.
Low grade fibromyxoid sarcomas occur equally in men and women and typically affect young adults (median age at presentation 34 years). However, patients of any age may be involved and up to 19% of cases occur in patients younger than 18 years of age {699}.

Sites of involvement
Low grade fibromyxoid sarcomas typically occur in the proximal extremities or trunk, but may occur in unusual locations such as the head or retroperitoneum. The overwhelming majority of cases occur in a subfascial location. They are often large at the time of diagnosis.

Clinical features
Up to 15% of patients report a pre-biopsy duration of over 5 years. Low grade fibromyxoid sarcomas typically present as a painless deep soft tissue mass.

Histopathology
Classical low grade fibromyxoid sarcoma
Low grade fibromyxoid sarcomas show an admixture of heavily collagenized, hypocellular zones and more cellular myxoid nodules. Short fascicular and characteristic whorling growth patterns are seen, with the latter pattern often most apparent at the transition from collagenous to myxoid areas. The vasculature of low grade fibromyxoid sarcomas consists of both arcades of small vessels, and arteriole-sized vessels with perivascular sclerosis. The cells of low grade fibromyxoid sarcomas are very bland, with only scattered hyperchromatic cells. Mitoses are very scarce.

Approximately 10% of cases show areas with increased cellularity and nuclear atypia, similar to that seen in usual-type fibrosarcomas of intermediate grade.

Low grade fibromyxoid sarcoma with giant collagen rosettes
Approximately 40% of otherwise typical low grade fibromyxoid sarcomas show the focal presence of poorly formed collagen rosettes, consisting of a central core of hyalinized collagen surrounded by a cuff of epithelioid fibroblasts. In that subset of low grade fibromyxoid sarcomas where these collagen rosettes are particularly prominent and well formed, the term "hyalinizing spindle cell tumour with giant rosettes" has been applied {1217}. It has been recently shown that the behaviour of low grade fibromyxoid sarcomas with and without giant collagen rosettes are identical {699,2296}.

Immunohistochemistry and ultrastructure
Immunohistochemically, low grade fibromyxoid sarcomas typically express only vimentin, consistent with fibroblastic differentiation. Myofibroblastic differentiation, as reflected by focal smooth muscle actin expression may be seen on occasion. Low grade fibromyxoid sarco-

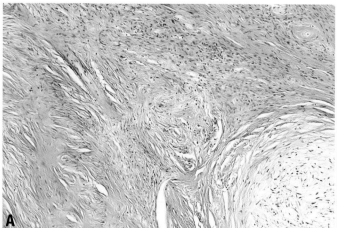
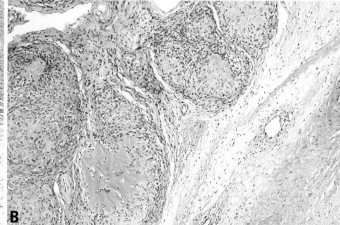

Fig. 2.87 A Low grade fibromyxoid sarcoma showing abrupt transition from hyalinized to myxoid nodules. **B** Low grade fibromyxoid sarcoma with numerous giant collagen rosettes (hyalinizing spindle cell tumour with giant rosettes).

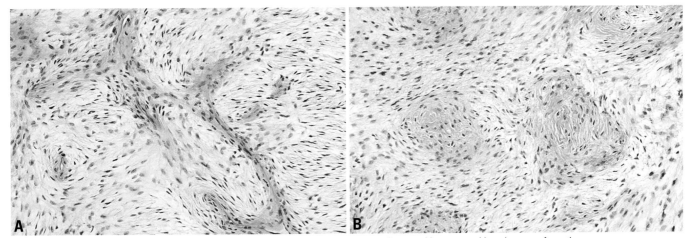

Fig. 2.88 A Low grade fibromyxoid sarcoma showing arcades of blood vessels. **B** Low grade fibromyxoid sarcoma with early rosette formation.

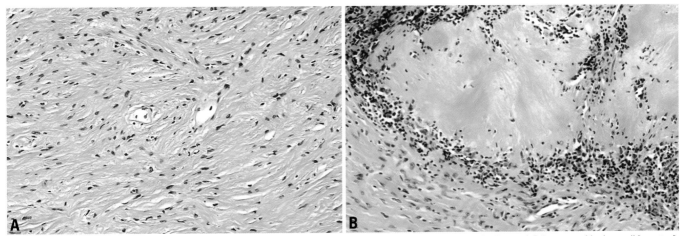

Fig. 2.89 A Low grade fibromyxoid sarcoma consisting of very bland spindle cells embedded in a densly collagenous background. **B** In cases with giant cell "rosettes", the tumour cells are arranged in cuffs around nodules of hyaline collagen.

mas almost never express desmin, S100 protein, cytokeratins, epithelial membrane antigen or CD34 {699,813,1552}. Ultrastructural studies have also shown almost exclusively fibroblastic differentiation both in classical low grade fibromyxoid sarcoma and in rosette-containing variants {1565}.

Genetics

Excluding cases published as "myxoid malignant fibrous histiocytoma" or "myxofibrosarcoma", only three low grade fibromyxoid sarcomas with chromosome aberrations have been reported {1477}. One had a balanced translocation as the sole aberration {1868}. The two others had supernumerary ring chromosomes, in one case shown by comparative genomic hybridization to consist of chromosome 7 and 16 material {1436}. Supernumerary ring chromosomes have been found in many other low grade mesenchymal tumours, including myxofibrosarcoma.

Prognostic factors

There has been a recent evolution in our understanding of the behaviour of low grade fibromyxoid sarcomas. Although the original series of Evans and Goodlad et al suggested that low grade fibromyxoid sarcomas were paradoxically aggressive sarcomas, with a local recurrence rate of 68%, a metastatic rate of 41% and a death rate of 18%, these were retrospective studies {621,813}. Almost all of the approximately 30 patients reported with low grade fibromyxoid sarcoma in these earlier studies were origi-

nally diagnosed with, and treated for a benign lesion. However, a recent large series of prospectively diagnosed low grade fibromyxoid sarcomas showed recurrences, metastases, and death from disease in only 9%, 6% and 2% of patients, respectively {699}, although, the median follow-up was only just over 4 years. However, low grade fibromyxoid sarcoma may metastasize many years after initial diagnosis and indefinite clinical follow-up is indicated for patients with this disease. Although the presence of small areas of higher grade fibrosarcoma within otherwise typical low grade fibromyxoid sarcoma has not been shown to be an adverse prognostic factor, the significance of larger high grade areas remains to be determined.

Sclerosing epithelioid fibrosarcoma

J.M. Meis-Kindblom   E. van den Berg
L.G. Kindblom   W.M. Molenaar

Definition
Sclerosing epithelioid fibrosarcoma (SEF) is a distinctive variant of fibrosarcoma, composed of epithelioid tumour cells arranged in nests and cords that are embedded within a sclerotic collagenous matrix, thus simulating a poorly differentiated carcinoma or sclerosing lymphoma.

ICD-O code   8810/3

Epidemiology
SEF is a very rare fibrosarcoma variant with a wide age spectrum (median age 45 years) and equal sex distribution {1388}. Approximately 25 additional cases of SEF have been reported {72, 86,347,629,791,1773} since the original series of 25 cases was published {1388}.

Sites of involvement
Most cases are located in the lower extremities and limb girdles, followed by the trunk, upper extremities, and the head and neck area. SEF is invariably deep-seated, frequently impinging upon but rarely invading underlying bone {72, 1388}.

Clinical features
Patients present with a mass of variable duration; in one-third of cases the mass has enlarged noticeably and is painful.

Macroscopy
Size is highly variable, ranging from 2 – 22 cm, with median size of 7-10 cm {72, 1388}. SEF is usually well circumscribed, lobulated or multinodular with a firm, whitish cut surface. Myxoid, cystic, and calcified areas may be seen as well {1388}. Necrosis is uncommon.

Histopathology
Overall, SEF is densely sclerotic, containing nests, strands and acini of small epithelioid cells with scant clear to eosinophilic cytoplasm and uniform oval, round or angulated bland nuclei having little mitotic activity. The abundant collagenous matrix is deeply acidophilic and variably arranged in thick fibrous bands, a delicate lace-like pattern, and fibrous, hyalinized zones reminiscent of a scar or fibroma. Less prominent spindled fascicular areas of conventional low grade fibrosarcoma and hypocellular myxoid zones resembling myxoma or myxofibrosarcoma are also seen, as well as degenerative myxoid cysts and foci of metaplastic bone and calcification. SEF often has a haemangiopericytoma-like vasculature. Despite being well delineated, vascular invasion may be seen along peripheral tumour margins.

Immunophenotype
Vimentin immunostains are consistently positive whereas stains for CD34, leukocyte markers, HMB45, CD68, desmin, GFAP, and TP53 are negative {72,1388}. Focal, weak immunostaining may be seen in a minority of cases with EMA, S100 protein and more rarely for cytokeratins {1388}.

Ultrastructure
The lesional cells display features of fibroblasts {72,1388}, including parallel arrays of rough endoplasmic reticulum filled with granular material and prominent networks of intermediate filaments that may form perinuclear whorls {1388}.

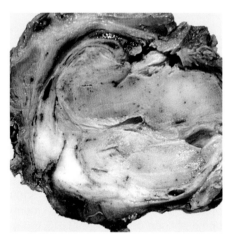

Fig. 2.90 Deep-seated, well circumscribed, extensively fibrous sclerosing epithelioid fibrosarcoma.

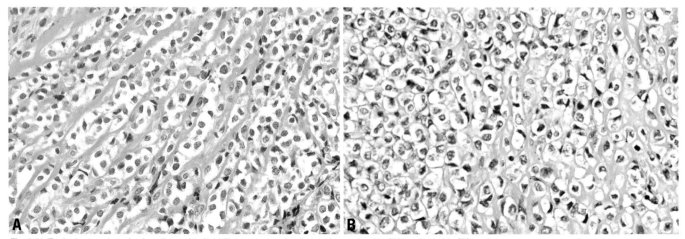

Fig. 2.91 Typical examples of sclerosing epithelioid fibrosarcoma showing cells arranged in (**A**) cords and in (**B**) nests.

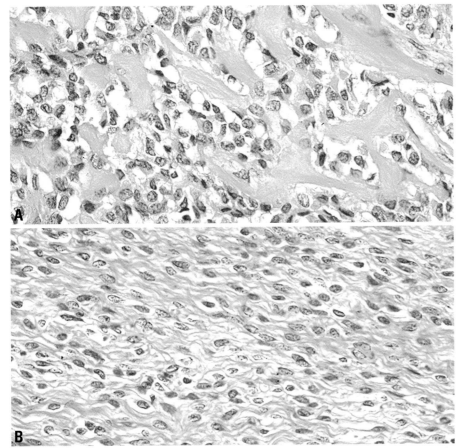

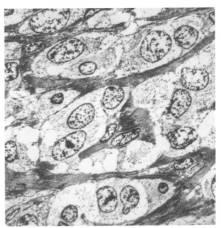

Fig. 2.93 EM features of sclerosing epithelioid fibrosarcoma. Epithelioid fibroblasts are arranged in cords and surrounded by abundant collagen.

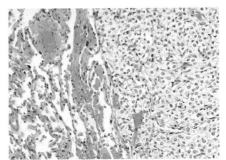

Fig. 2.94 Sclerosing epithelioid fibrosarcoma metastasis to the lung.

Fig. 2.92 A Sclerosing epithelioid fibrosarcoma (SEF) showing cells arranged in alveolae. **B** Area of low grade conventional fibrosarcoma in an SEF.

Genetics

A sclerosing epithelioid fibrosarcoma from a 14-year-old boy showed a complex karyotype with amplification of 12q13 and 12q15, including the *HMGIC* gene, and rearrangement of band 9p13, which has also been reported in a complex karyotype in a case of adult fibrosarcoma {791,1263}. A second case showed a different karyotype with involvement of Xq13, 6q15 and 22q13 {534}.

Prognostic factors

More than 50% of patients develop one or more local recurrences and more than 40% have metastases at median intervals of 5 and 8 years, respectively {1388}. Metastases are usually to lungs, pleura and bone. After 11 years, half of the patients are either dead of disease or have persistent or recurrent tumour {1388}. Somewhat higher rates of metastases and tumour death have recently been reported and may well be due to larger average tumour size, intracranial location, and potential referral bias {72}. Adverse prognostic factors include proximal tumour site, larger tumour size, male sex, local recurrences, and metastases {1388}.

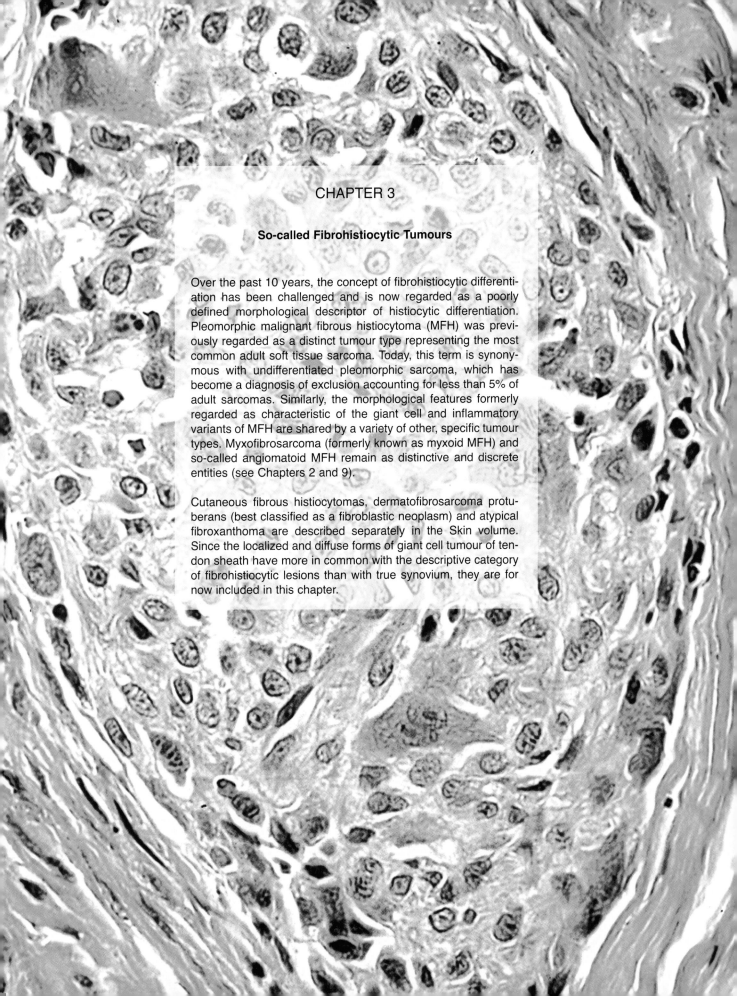

CHAPTER 3

So-called Fibrohistiocytic Tumours

Over the past 10 years, the concept of fibrohistiocytic differentiation has been challenged and is now regarded as a poorly
defined morphological descriptor of histiocytic differentiation.
Pleomorphic malignant fibrous histiocytoma (MFH) was previously regarded as a distinct tumour type representing the most
common adult soft tissue sarcoma. Today, this term is synonymous with undifferentiated pleomorphic sarcoma, which has
become a diagnosis of exclusion accounting for less than 5% of
adult sarcomas. Similarly, the morphological features formerly
regarded as characteristic of the giant cell and inflammatory
variants of MFH are shared by a variety of other, specific tumour
types. Myxofibrosarcoma (formerly known as myxoid MFH) and
so-called angiomatoid MFH remain as distinctive and discrete
entities (see Chapters 2 and 9).

Cutaneous fibrous histiocytomas, dermatofibrosarcoma protu-
berans (best classified as a fibroblastic neoplasm) and atypical
fibroxanthoma are described separately in the Skin volume.
Since the localized and diffuse forms of giant cell tumour of tendon sheath have more in common with the descriptive category
of fibrohistiocytic lesions than with true synovium, they are for
now included in this chapter.

Giant cell tumour of tendon sheath

N. de St. Aubain Somerhausen
P. Dal Cin

The term giant cell tumour of tendon sheath encompasses a family of lesions most often arising from the synovium of joints, bursae and tendon sheath {1027}. These tumours are usually divided according to their site (intra- or extra-articular) and growth pattern (localized or diffuse) into several subtypes, which differ in their clinical features and biological behaviour.

Definition

The localized type of giant cell tumour of tendon sheath is a circumscribed proliferation of synovial-like mononuclear cells, accompanied by a variable number of multinucleate osteoclast-like cells, foam cells, siderophages and inflammatory cells, most commonly occurring in the digits.

ICD-O code   9252/0

Synonyms

Tenosynovial giant cell tumour, localized type, nodular tenosynovitis.

Epidemiology

The localized form is frequent and the most common subset of giant cell tumours. Tumours may occur at any age but usually between 30 and 50 years, with a 2:1 female predominance {2163}.

Sites of involvement

Localized giant cell tumours occur predominantly in the hand where they probably represent the most common neoplasm. Approximately 85% of the tumours occur in the fingers, in close proximity to the synovium of the tendon sheath or interphalangeal joint. The lesions may infrequently erode or infiltrate the nearby bone {2160}, or rarely involve the skin.
Other sites include the wrist, ankle / foot, knee, and very rarely the elbow and the hip {1492,2163}.

Clinical features

The most common presenting symptom is that of a painless swelling. The tumours develop gradually over a long period and a preoperative duration of several years is often mentioned . Antecedent trauma is reported in a variable number of cases (from 1 to 50%) {1492,2163}.
Radiological studies usually demonstrate a well circumscribed soft tissue mass, with occasional degenerative changes of the adjacent joint or erosion of the adjacent bone {1046}.

Aetiology

Tenosynovial giant cell tumours initially were regarded as an inflammatory process based on animal models, the common history of trauma, the predilection for the first three fingers of the right hand {1492} and one X-inactivation study suggesting polyclonality {2295}. However, the finding of aneuploidy in some cases {7}, the demonstration of clonal chromosomal abnormalities {1774}, and the fact that these lesions are capable of autonomous growth strongly support a neoplastic origin.

Macroscopy

Grossly, most localized giant cell tumours are small (between 0.5 and 4 cm), although lesions of greater size may be found in large joints. Tumours are well circumscribed and typically lobulated, white to grey with yellowish and brown areas.

Histopathology

Tumours are lobulated, well circumscribed and at least partially covered by a fibrous capsule. Their microscopic appearance is variable, depending on the proportion of mononuclear cells, multinucleate giant cells, foamy macrophages, siderophages and the amount of stroma. Osteoclast-like cells, which contain a variable number of nuclei (from 3-4 to more than 50), are usually readily apparent but may be

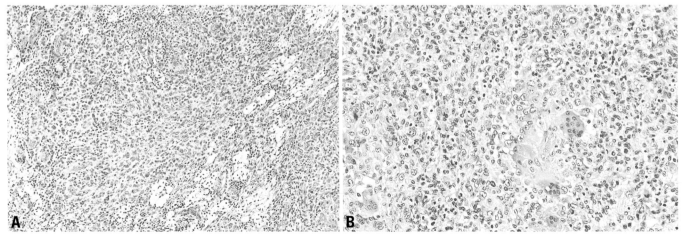

Fig. 3.01 Giant cell tumour of tendon sheath. **A** Typical admixture of histiocytoid cells, foamy cells and lymphocytes. In this case, giant cells are scanty. **B** Typical mononuclear histiocytoid cells with variably prominent eosinophilic cytoplasm and scattered osteoclastic giant cells.

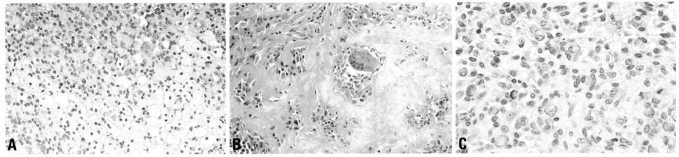

Fig. 3.02 Giant cell tumour of tendon sheath. **A** Most cases show focal collections of xanthoma cells, while others **(B)** show extensive stromal hyalinization. **C** Small, histiocyte-like cells with occasional nuclear grooves and larger cells with vesicular nuclei and abundant eosinophilic cytoplasm, frequently with a rim of haemosiderin.

inconspicuous in highly cellular tumours. Most mononuclear cells are small, round to spindle-shaped. They are characterized by pale cytoplasm and round or reniform, often grooved nuclei. They are accompanied by larger epithelioid cells with glassy cytoplasm and rounded vesicular nuclei. Xanthoma cells are frequent, tend to aggregate locally near the periphery of nodules and may be associated with cholesterol clefts. Haemosiderin deposits are virtually always identified. The stroma shows variable degrees of hyalinization and may occasionally have an osteoid-like appearance. Cleft-like spaces are less frequent than in the diffuse form {2163}. Mitotic activity usually averages 3 to 5 mitoses per 10 HPF but may reach up to 20/10 HPF {2295}. Focal necrosis is rarely seen.

Immunophenotype

Immunohistochemically, mononuclear cells are positive for CD68. Some cells may also express muscle-specific actin (HHF35). A subset of desmin-positive dendritic cells is reported in up to 50% of cases {705}.

Multinucleate giant cells express CD68, CD45 and markers such as tartrate resistant acid phosphatase {449,1590}.

Ultrastructure

Ultrustructural studies have revealed an heterogeneous cell population composed of a majority of histiocyte-like cells, accompanied by fibroblast-like cells, intermediate cells, foam cells and multinucleate giant cells {35,2163}.

Genetics

Cytogenetic aberrations have been described in 11 giant cell tumours of tendon sheath. A near- or pseudodiploid karyotype was seen in all cases, mostly with simple structural changes {1910}. The short arm of chromosome 1 is frequently involved, with a clustering of breakpoints to the region p11-p13 in 7/11 cases. A recurrent t(1;2)(p11;q35-36) has been identified, but several other translocation partners have been described, including 3q21, 5q31, and 11q11. In addition, two cases without 1p11-13 rearrangement had translocations involving 16q24, thus possibly representing an alternative primary cytogenetic change. Numerical changes seem to be rare. In particular, it should be noted that gain of chromosomes 5 and 7, which is common in the diffuse type giant cell tumour {1477}, has not been described in the localized form {1910}.

Prognostic factors

Localized giant cell tumour is a benign lesion with a capacity for local recurrence. Local excision is the treatment of choice. 4 to 30 % of cases recur {1504, 1757,1774} but these recurrence are usually non-destructive and are controlled by surgical reexcision. It has been suggested that recurrences develop most often in highly cellular tumours or lesions with a high mitotic count {1757,2298}.

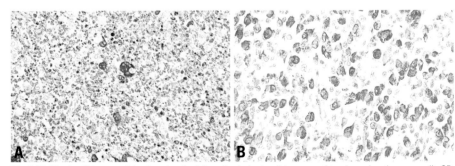

Fig. 3.03 Giant cell tumour of tendon sheath. **A** Localized giant cell tumours of tendons sheath are usually CD 68 positive. **B** Some cases of both localized and diffuse type contain numerous desmin-positive mononuclear cells, sometimes with dendritic cytoplasmic porcesses.

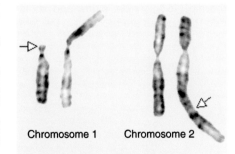

Chromosome 1   Chromosome 2

Fig. 3.04 Giant cell tumour of tendon sheath. Partial karyotype showing the characteristic t(1;2)(p13;q37) translocation. Arrows indicate breakpoints.

Diffuse-type giant cell tumour

N. de St. Aubain Somerhausen
P. Dal Cin

Definition

Diffuse-type giant cell tumour is a destructive proliferation of synovial-like mononuclear cells, admixed with multinucleate giant cells, foam cells, siderophages and inflammatory cells. The extraarticular form is defined by the presence of an infiltrative soft tissue mass, with or without involvement of the adjacent joint.

The very uncommon malignant giant cell tumour of tendon sheath is defined by the coexistence of a benign giant cell tumour with overtly malignant areas or by the recurrence of a typical giant cell tumour as a sarcoma.

ICD-O code   9251/0

Synonyms

Pigmented villonodular synovitis, pigmented villonodular tenosynovitis.

Epidemiology

Diffuse-type giant cell tumours tend to affect younger patients than their localized counterpart. The age of patients varies widely but most lesions affect young adults, under the age of 40. There is a slight female predominance {1523, 1984,2164}.

Sites of involvement

Intraarticular lesions affect predominantly the knee (75% of cases), followed by the hip (15%), ankle, elbow and shoulder. Rare cases are reported in the temporomandibular and spinal facet joints {782,1899}. Extraarticular tumours most commonly involve the knee region, thigh and foot. Uncommon locations include the finger, wrist, groin, elbow and toe {87, 1984,2164}.

Most extraarticular tumours are located in periarticular soft tissues but these lesions can be purely intramuscular or predominantly subcutaneous {2164}.

Clinical features

Patients complain of pain, tenderness, swelling or limitation of motion. Haemorrhagic joint effusions are common. The symptoms are usually of relatively long duration (often several years). Radiographically, most tumours present as ill defined peri-articular masses, frequently associated with degenerative joint disease and cystic lesions in the adjacent bone {542}. On magnetic resonance imaging, giant cell tumours show decreased signal intensity in both T1- and T2-weighted images {1036}.

Aetiology

Although these lesions have been regarded as reactive, the presence of clonal abnormalities {1910} and the capacity for autonomous growth are now widely regarded as evidence for a neoplastic origin.

Macroscopy

Diffuse-type giant cell tumours are usually large (often more than 5 cm), firm or sponge-like. The typical villous pattern of pigmented villonodular synovitis is usually lacking in extraarticular tumours. The latter have a multinodular appearance and a variegated colour, with alternation of white, yellowish and brownish areas.

Histopathology

Most tumours are infiltrative and grow as diffuse, expansile sheets. Their cellularity is variable: compact areas alternate with pale, loose, discohesive zones. Cleft-like spaces are common and appear either as artefactual tears or as synovial-lined spaces. Blood-filled pseudoalveolar spaces are seen in approximately 10% of cases.

In comparison with the localized form, osteoclastic giant cells are less common and may be absent or extremely rare in up to 20% of cases. They are irregularly distributed throughout the lesions and are more easily found around haemorrhagic foci.

The mononuclear component comprises two types of cells: small histiocyte-like cells, which represent the main cellular component, and larger cells. Histiocyte-like cells are ovoid or spindle-shaped, with palely eosinophilic cytoplasm. Their nuclei are small, ovoid or angulated, contain fine chromatin, small nucleoli and frequently display longitudinal grooves. Larger cells are rounded or sometimes show dendritic cytoplasmic processes. Their cytoplasm is abundant, pale to deeply eosinophilic, often contains a

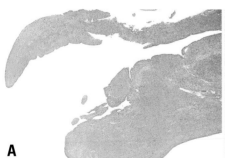 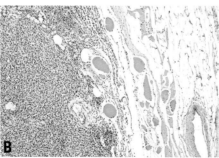 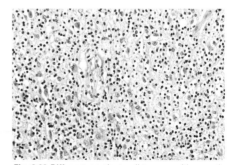

Fig. 3.05 A Villous appearance of an intra-articular diffuse-type giant cell tumour. **B** Low magnification of a completely extra-articular tumour showing infiltration of the muscular and adipose tissue.

Fig. 3.06 Diffuse-type giant cell tumour with prominent inflammatory component and numerous large dendritic cells with abundant cytoplasm.

peripheral rim of hemosiderin granules and occasionally shows a paranuclear eosinophilic filamentous inclusion. Nuclei are characterized by reniform or lobulated shape, thick nuclear membranes, vesicular chromatin and eosinophilic nuclei. The occasional predominance of these larger cells may obscure the typical features of giant cell tumour and lead to a diagnosis of sarcoma. Sheets of foam cells are frequently observed, usually in the periphery of lesions and variable amounts of haemosiderin are identified in most cases. Giant cell tumours may also contain a significant lymphocytic infiltrate. The stroma shows variable degrees of fibrosis and may appear hyalinized, although this is usually less marked than in the localized form.

Mitoses are usually identifiable and mitotic activity of more than 5 per 10 HPF is not uncommon {1984,2164,2239}.

There have been several reports of typical giant cell tumours recurring as a histologically malignant neoplasms and a few series included primary histologically malignant tumours of the tendon sheath resembling giant cell tumours {187,637,1555,1941,1984}. These neoplasms tended to show significantly increased mitotic rate (more than 20 mitoses / 10 HPF), necrosis, enlarged nuclei with nucleoli, spindling of mononucleated cells, the presence of abundant eosinophilic cytoplasm in histiocyte-like cells, and stromal myxoid change, although none of these features could be used in isolation as a criterion for malignancy {187,637,1984}.

In addition, two cases with banal histology which developed metastatic disease (in the lungs or lymph nodes) have been reported to date {1984,2239}.

Immunophenotype

The immunohistochemical and ultrastructural features of diffuse-type giant cell tumour are similar to those of the localized form. Mononuclear cells are positive for CD68 and other macrophage markers. Desmin stain highlights a population of cells with dendritic features in 35 to 40% of cases; these frequently correspond to the larger eosinophilic cells. Giant cells are positive for CD68 and CD45 {705,1590,1984}.

Genetics

Chromosomal aberrations have been described in 17 cases, all with a near- or

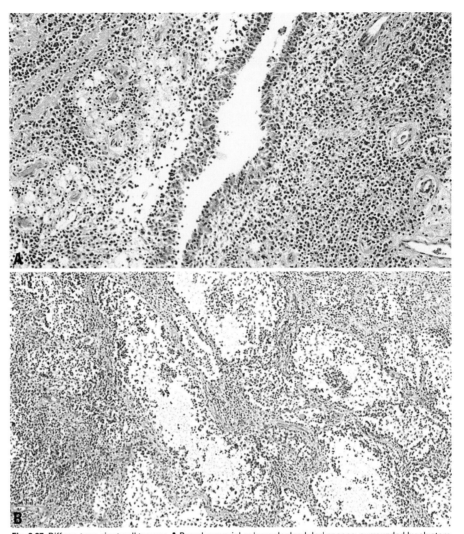

Fig. 3.07 Diffuse-type giant cell tumour. **A** Pseudosynovial or 'pseudoglandular' spaces, surrounded by clusters of xanthoma cells. **B** Pseudoalveolar spaces are commonly seen in diffuse-type giant cell tumours.

pseudodiploid karyotype. Rearrangements of the 1p11-13 region have been detected in eight of them, one had a t(1;2)(p22;q35-37), and one had involvement of band 16q24, suggesting a close cytogenetic relationship with the localized form of giant cell tumour {1910}. One difference, however, between these two entities, is that trisomies for chromosomes 5 and 7, usually as the sole anomalies, have been detected only in diffuse-type giant cell tumours {1477}. The sig-

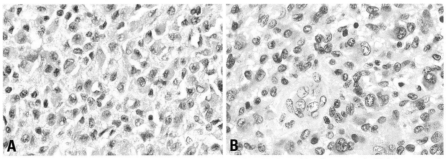

Fig. 3.08 Diffuse-type giant cell tumour. **A** Typical mononuclear histiocytoid cells, some of which have prominent eosinophilic cytoplasm. **B** Note frequent nuclear grooves in the histiocytoid cells. Some tumour cells have more prominent eosinophilic cytoplasm with haemosiderin granules.

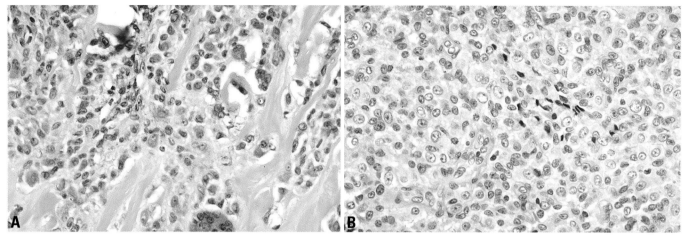

Fig. 3.09 Malignant diffuse-type giant cell tumour. Although there is usually at least focal morphological overlap with usual giant cell tumour (**A**), closer examination reveals increased cellularity and predominance of atypical large cells with prominent nucleoli (**B**).

nificance of trisomy 5 and 7 for tumour development in this context is questionable because the same aneuploidies are frequent also in synovial samples from patients with various forms of reactive synovial lesion {1429}.

Prognostic factors
Recurrences are common, often multiple and may severely compromise joint func-

tion. The recurrence rate has been estimated between 18 and 46 % for intraarticular lesions and between 33 and 50% of cases for extraarticular tumours {1899, 1984,2164,2239}. The risk of recurrence does not seem to be correlated with any histological parameter other than positive excision margins. Therefore, diffuse-type giant cell tumours should be regarded as locally aggressive but nonmetasta-

sizing neoplasms and wide excision is the treatment of choice.
Although the number of cases is limited, malignant giant cell tumours of tendon sheath showing obvious sarcomatous areas are potentially aggressive and may give rise to pulmonary metastasis {187, 1555,1941,1984}.

Deep benign fibrous histiocytoma

J.M. Coindre

Definition
A benign fibrous histiocytoma, which develops entirely within subcutaneous tissue, deep soft tissues or in parenchymal organs.

ICD-O code   8830/0

Epidemiology
Deeply located fibrous histiocytomas are rare. Based on the only published series, they represent less than 1% of fibrohistiocytic tumours {673}. Their exact frequency is difficult to determine because

some cases published as deep fibrous histiocytomas may represent solitary fibrous tumours {673,706}. They may develop at any age, but most affect adults over 25 years old, with a predominance in males.

Sites of involvement
The lower limb and the head and neck region are the most common sites. Most cases develop in subcutaneous tissue, but a few cases have been reported in muscle, mesentery, trachea and kidney {673,869,1147,1843}.

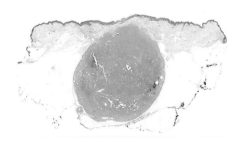

Fig. 3.10 Deep benign fibrous histiocytoma tends to be more circumscribed than the cutaneous form and pseudo-encapsulated.

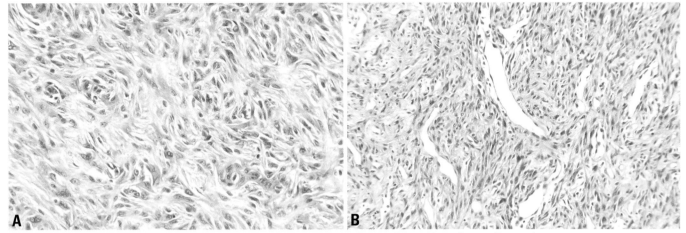

Fig. 3.11 Deep benign fibrous histiocytoma. **A** A monomorphic storiform pattern is usually seen. **B** Branching pericytoma-like vessels are common.

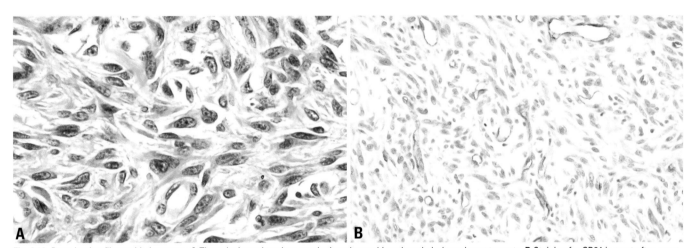

Fig. 3.12 Deep benign fibrous histiocytoma. **A** These lesions show less cytologic polymorphism than their dermal counterparts. **B** Staining for CD34 is most often negative.

Clinical features

Most lesions present as a painless and slowly enlarging mass.

Macroscopy

Contrary to the cutaneous form, deep lesions tend to be well circumscribed and pseudo-encapsulated with occasional areas of haemorrhage. Most lesions are 4 cm or more when resected.

Histopathology

Deep fibrous histiocytomas usually show a prominent storiform pattern, sometimes combined with haemangiopericytoma-like areas.
Contrary to conventional cutaneous lesions, most lesions show monomorphism and usually lack secondary elements such as foamy cells and giant cells but usually show scattered lymphocytes. Thus, they more closely resmble the cellular variant of cutaneous fibrous histiocytoma. The tumour cells are cytologically bland and generally spindle-shaped with elongated or plump vesicular nuclei and eosinophilic, ill defined cytoplasm. There is no nuclear pleomorphism or hyperchromasia, and mitoses, although commonly present, are usually less than 5 per 10 high power fields. The stroma may show myxoid change or hyalinization and rarely osteoclast-like giant cells or metaplastic ossification {673,1973}. Small foci of necrosis may be present.

Immunophenotype

Immunohistochemistry shows similar results as in cutaneous lesions with negativity for epithelial markers, desmin and S100 protein. Alpha smooth muscle actin may be positive in some parts of the lesion. CD34 is usually (but not always) negative, but, if positive, solitary fibrous tumour should be considered.

Prognostic factors

Deep fibrous histiocytoma may recur locally {673}, particularly if incompletely excised. No metastasis has been reported so far.

Plexiform fibrohistiocytic tumour

A.G. Nascimento
P. Dal Cin

Definition

Plexiform fibrohistiocytic tumour (PFT) is a mesenchymal neoplasm of children, adolescents, and young adults, characterized by fibrohistiocytic cytomorphology, and a multinodular growth pattern. It rarely metastasizes.

ICD-O code   8835/1

Epidemiology

PFT preferentially affects young individuals; mean age at presentation is approximately 14.5 years {603,1782}. The tumour occurs more often in female than in male patients, with reported female-to-male ratios ranging from 2.5:1 {603} to 6:1 {1782}. PFT has not been reported to occur with greater frequency in any particular race.

Sites of involvement

PFT involves the upper extremities in approximately 65% of cases {603,1782}, with the hands and wrists being affected in about 45% of cases {1782}. The lower extremities are involved in approximately 27% of cases {1782}. PFT rarely occurs in the head and neck region.

Clinical features

PFT usually presents as a small, poorly demarcated, painless dermal or subcutaneous mass that slowly enlarges for months to years {603,1782}. It is clinically characterized by slow growth, frequent local recurrence, and rare regional lymphatic and systemic metastasis {603, 1782}.

Macroscopy

PFT is usually a multinodular, firm, poorly circumscribed dermal or subcutaneous mass that rarely exceeds 3 cm.

Histopathology

PFT is composed of small nodules or elongated cellular clusters that are interconnected in a characteristic plexiform arrangement. Three distinct cell types are present in variable amounts: mononuclear histiocyte-like cells, spindle fibroblast-like cells, and multinucleate giant cells. The nodules and clusters are interconnected by spindle cells situated at the periphery of the nodules. Three histologic subtypes are recognized: a fibrohistiocytic subtype composed mainly of nodules of mononuclear histiocyte-like cells and multinucleated giant cells, a fibroblastic subtype composed mainly of elongated clusters and short fascicles of fibroblast-like cells, and a mixed subtype composed of both patterns in equal proportion. Cellular atypia and pleomorphism are minimal, mitotic count frequently is low, and necrosis is absent. Vascular invasion is observed in 10-20% of cases. The nodules and clusters are situated in subcutaneous tissue and deep dermis, but extension into skeletal muscle can occur. In pulmonary metastases, PFT presents as small fibrohistiocytic nodules in subpleural and peribronchiolar locations.

Immunophenotype

PFT displays immunoreactivity for vimentin, CD68 (KP1), and smooth muscle actin {62,783,962,1782,2340}. CD68 immunoreactivity is mainly displayed by multinucleated giant cells and mononu-

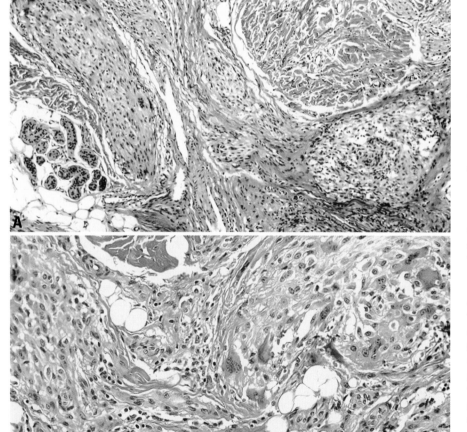

Fig. 3.13 A Plexiform fibrohistiocytic tumour is composed of a mixture of small nodules and elongated fascicles that interconnect with each other, forming a characteristic plexiform arrangement. **B** The fibroblastic subtype is composed mainly of elongated clusters and short fascicles of fibroblastlike cells, creating a picture resembling fibromatosis. Scattered multinucleated giant cells are present.

clear histiocyte-like cells {1782,2340}; the fibroblast-like cells stain only rarely with CD68. However, the fibroblast-like cells and occasional histiocytelike cells stain for smooth muscle actin {62,783, 962,2340}.

Ultrastructure

PFT cells have features of myofibroblasts and histiocyte-like cells {62,783,962}, such as abundance of lysosomes, prominent filopodia, and bundles of thin cytofilaments along the cytoplasmic membrane {62}.

Genetics

Only two plexiform fibrohistiocytic tumours with clonal chromosome aberrations have been reported, and no shared chromosome abnormalities were found {1767,1974}.

Prognostic factors

PFT has been associated with a local recurrence rate ranging from 12.5% {1782} to 37.5% {603}, a regional lymph node metastatic rate of 3/61 cases with follow-up {603,1782} and a systemic (lungs only, to date) metastatic rate of 3/61 cases {603}. Such significant metastatic rates likely reflect the bias of consultation practice. No clinicopathologic or genetic factors seem to influence the prognosis of patients with PFT {603, 1782}.

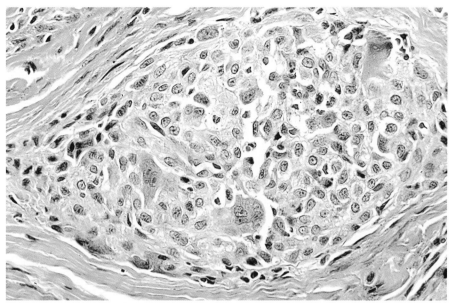

Fig. 3.14 The fibrohistiocytic subtype of plexiform fibrohistiocytic tumour is characterized by nodules of mononuclear histiocyte-like cells and multinucleated giant cells.

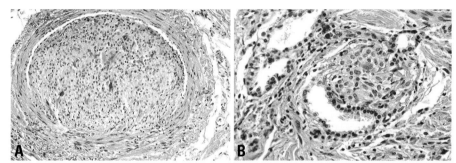

Fig. 3.15 Plexiform fibrohistiocytic tumour. **A** Vascular invasion is occasionally present in 10-20% of cases. **B** Small, peribronchiolar tumoural nodule in pulmonary metastasis of plexiform fibrohistiocytic tumour.

Giant cell tumour of soft tissue

A.G. Nascimento

Definition
Giant cell tumour of soft tissue (GCT-ST) is a primary soft tissue neoplasm that is clinically and histologically similar to giant cell tumour of bone; it very rarely metastasizes.

ICD-O code   9251/1

Synonyms
Osteoclastoma of soft tissue, giant cell tumour of low malignant potential.

Epidemiology
GCT-ST occurs predominantly in the fifth decade of life but can affect patients ranging in age from 5 to 89 years. GCT-ST affects both sexes in equal numbers. GCT-ST does not occur with greater frequency in any particular race {702,1591, 1608}.

Sites of involvement
GCT-ST usually occurs in superficial soft tissues of the upper and lower extremities (70% of tumours). Less frequently affected are the trunk (20%) and head and neck region (7%) {702,1591,1608}.

Clinical features
The tumours present as painless growing masses {1591,1608}, with an average duration of symptoms of 6 months {1608}. As in giant cell tumour of bone with soft tissue implants {397}, peripheral mineralization is exceedingly frequent

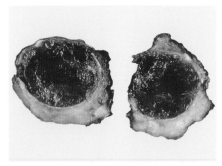

Fig. 3.16 Giant cell tumour of soft tissue, presenting as well circumscribed, mostly solid nodule with a fleshy, red-brown or grey cut surface.

in GCT-ST, yielding a characteristic radiographic appearance.

Aetiology
No aetiologic factors have been identified, but GCT-ST has occurred rarely in patients with Paget disease of bone {758} or after trauma {1608}.

Macroscopy
In the 3 major series of patients with GCT-ST reported to date {702,1591, 1608}, tumours ranged in size from 0.7 to 10 cm (mean, 3 cm). Seventy percent of the tumours involved subcutaneous adipose tissue or dermis; only 30% were situated below the superficial fascia. GCT-ST presents as a well circumscribed, mostly solid, nodular mass with a fleshy, red-brown or gray cut surface. Gritty regions of mineralized bone frequently are present at the periphery of the tumours {1591}.

Histopathology
At low magnification, approximately 85% of GCT-STs display a multinodular architecture, with the nodules ranging in size from microscopic dimensions to 15 mm {1608}. The cellular nodules are separated by fibroconnective tissue septa of varying thickness and containing haemosiderin-laden macrophages {1591}. The nodules are composed of a mixture of round to oval cells that are mononuclear and osteoclastlike giant cells that are multinucleated, with both cell types immersed in a richly vascularised stroma. The nuclei in the multinucleate cells are similar to the nuclei in the mononuclear cells.
Mitotic activity generally is present in every GCT-ST; typical mitoses range from 1 to 30 figures per 10 high-power fields {702,1591,1608}. Atypia, pleomorphism, and tumoural giant cells are absent, and necrosis is found rarely {702,1591, 1608}. Metaplastic bone formation is present in approximately 50% of the tumours; frequently it is in the form of a peripheral shell of woven bone.

Secondary cystic changes and the formation of blood-filled lakes, changes that are similar to aneurysmal bone cystic changes, are present in approximately 30% of tumours. Unquestionable foci of vascular invasion are part of the histological picture in about 30% of tumours {702,1608}. Additional histological features include stromal haemorrhage (50%) and regressive changes in the form of marked stromal fibrosis and clusters of foamy macrophages (70%).

Immunophenotype
GCT-STs display immunoreactivity for vimentin, CD68, and smooth muscle actin {702,1591,1608}. CD68 strongly marks the multinucleated giant cells; the mononuclear cells show focal staining only. Smooth muscle actin stains a few mononuclear cells and does not mark the multinucleated giant cells. Rarely, tumours react focally with antibodies against keratin and S100 protein {1608}.

Prognostic factors
In patients with clinical follow-up ranging from 34 to 45 months, GCT-ST was associated with a local recurrence rate of 12% and very rare metastasis and death {702,1591,1608}. Incomplete surgical excision is apparently followed by local recurrence {702}. No clinicopathologic factors are currently predictive of metastatic behaviour associated with GCT-ST {702,1591,1608}.

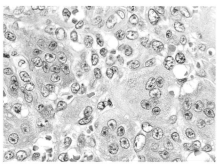

Fig. 3.17 Cellular nodules in giant cell tumour of soft tissue contain a mixture of round / oval mononuclear and multinucleate osteoclast-like giant cells.

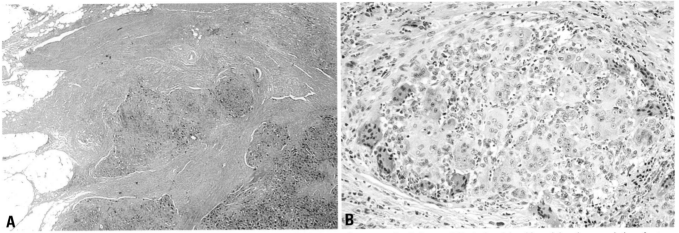

Fig. 3.18 A A multinodular growth pattern is present in approximately 85% of giant cell tumours of soft tissues. **B** Typical nodule with peripheral accumulation of osteo-clast-like giant cells.

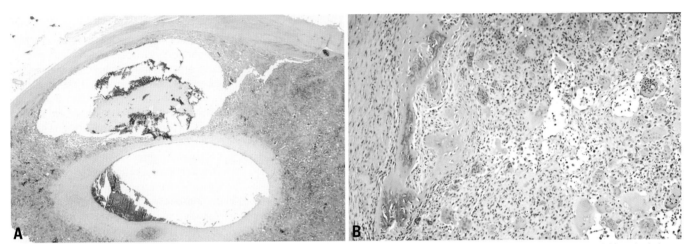

Fig. 3.19 A Secondary cystic changes, similar to aneurysmal bone cystic changes, occur in approximately 30% of giant cell tumours of soft tissue. **B** Metaplastic bone, frequently in the form of a peripheral shell of woven bone, is present in approximately 50% of giant cell tumours of soft tissue.

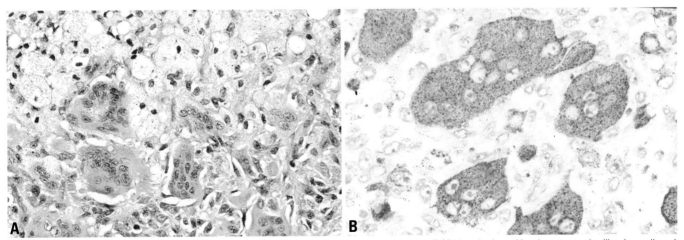

Fig. 3.20 A Clusters of foam macrophages reflecting regressive change in a giant cell tumour of soft tissue. **B** CD68 marks the multinucleate, osteoclastlike giant cells and a few of the mononuclear cells in giant cell tumours of soft tissue.

Pleomorphic malignant fibrous histiocytoma / Undifferentiated high grade pleomorphic sarcoma

C.D.M. Fletcher
E. van den Berg
W.M. Molenaar

Definition

The term pleomorphic malignant fibrous histiocytoma is now reserved for a small group of undifferentiated pleomorphic sarcomas. Both terms may be used synonymously. Current technology does not show a definable line of differentiation.

ICD-O code   8830/3

Synonyms

Fibroxanthosarcoma {1088}; malignant fibrous histiocytoma, storiform or fibroblastic type; malignant fibrous xanthoma.

Historical annotation

For many years, pleomorphic malignant fibrous histiocytoma (MFH) has been regarded as the prototypical form of MFH and the most common soft tissue sarcoma in adults {599,2233,2237}. Originally defined, based on morphology and tissue culture analysis, as a pleomorphic spindle cell malignant neoplasm showing fibroblastic and facultative histiocytic differentiation, it is now widely accepted that the morphologic pattern known as so-called pleomorphic MFH may be shared by a wide variety of poorly differentiated malignant neoplasms {675}. It is also now agreed that these tumours show no evidence of true histiocytic differentiation. This diagnostic term is now reserved (by those who still use it) for the much smaller group of pleomorphic sarcomas which, by current technology, show no definable line of differentiation {2243}. As a consequence, the apparent incidence of pleomorphic MFH has fallen sharply over the past 10 years and it is possible that this term may disappear altogether at such time as criteria for the diagnosis of pleomorphic sarcomas showing fibroblastic or myofibroblastic differentiation can be reproducibly defined.

Epidemiology

The group of pleomorphic (MFH-like) sarcomas collectively represent the most common types of sarcoma in patients over age 40. The overall incidence among adults approximates to 1-2 cases per 100,000 patients annually and the incidence increases with age {861}.

Most undifferentiated high grade sarcomas occur in patients over age 40 with peak incidence in the 6th and 7th decades. Rare examples may be encountered in adolescents and young adults. There is a male predominance of approximately 1.2:1.

Sites of involvement

Most undifferentiated high grade pleomorphic sarcomas occur in the extremities (especially the lower limb) and less often the trunk. The majority of cases arise in deep (subfascial) soft tissue, while less than 10% are primarily subcutaneous. A notable exception among pleomorphic sarcomas is dedifferentiated liposarcoma (see p. 38) which is most common in the retroperitoneum.

Clinical features

Undifferentiated high grade pleomorphic sarcomas are typically large deep-seated tumours which show progressive, often rapid enlargement. Only those which grow very rapidly tend to be painful. Around 5% of patients have metastases at presentation, most often to lung. Although little is known about aetiology of these lesions, a subset of pleomorphic sarcomas (<2-3%) arise at the site of prior radiation therapy {1224} and very rare cases arise at the site of chronic ulceration or scarring.

Macroscopy

Most undifferentiated high grade pleomorphic sarcomas are well circumscribed, expansile masses which may appear pseudoencapsulated. Tumour size varies and, to some extent, depends on location with subcutaneous lesions often measuring <5 cm, while retroperitoneal tumours often exceed 20 cm. Most tumours measure between 5 and 15 cm in maximum diameter. Cut surface is variable and may include pale fibrous or fleshy areas, admixed with zones of necrosis, haemorrhage or myxoid change. Aside from an adjacent well-differentiated component in dedifferentiated liposarcoma, there are no distinctive macroscopic features which correlate reliably with line of differentiation.

Histopathology

Undifferentiated high grade sarcoma is a diagnosis of exclusion following thorough sampling and judicious use of ancillary diagnostic techniques. Tumours in the general category of high grade pleomorphic (MFH-like) sarcomas are very heterogeneous in appearance and also in cellularity, since some cases have an extensive fibrous stroma. These tumours have in common marked cytological and nuclear pleomorphism, often with bizarre tumour giant cells, admixed with spindle cells and often rounded histiocyte-like cells (which may have foamy cytoplasm) in varying proportion {675}. A storiform growth pattern and stromal chronic inflammatory cells are common. The spindle cell component most often appears fibroblastic, myofibroblastic or smooth muscle-like. Tumours showing myogenic differentiation (pleomorphic leiomyosarcoma or rhabdomyosarcoma), as well as carcinoma and melanoma with MFH-like morphology, often have more copious eosinophilic cytoplasm and prominent large polygonal cells. The presence of fascicular spindle cell areas may suggest smooth muscle or nerve sheath differentiation (which needs to be proved immunohistochemically or ultrastructurally). Thorough

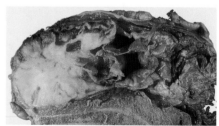

Fig. 3.21 Undifferentiated high grade pleomorphic sarcomas are typically deep-seated and large, with a variable cut surface; this case shows fleshy solid areas, necrosis and cystic change.

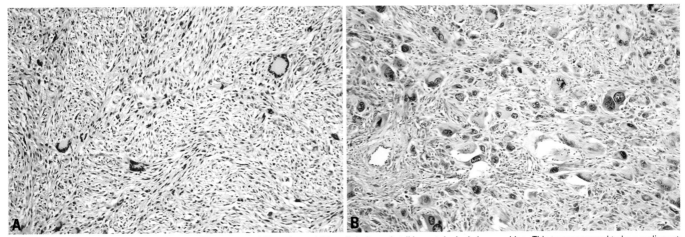

Fig. 3.22 Undifferentiated high grade pleomorphic sarcoma. **A** Note the variable cellularity and striking cytological pleomorphism. This tumour proved to be a malignant peripheral nerve sheath tumour. **B** In other areas this lesion turned out to be pleomorphic liposarcoma with prominent lipoblasts.

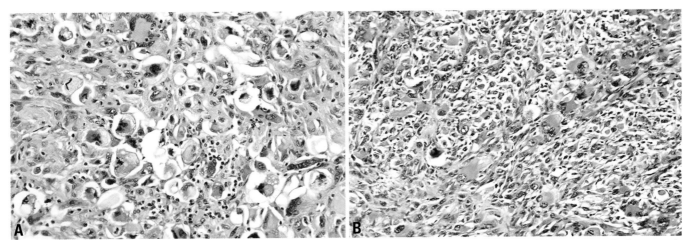

Fig. 3.23 Undifferentiated high grade pleomorphic sarcoma. **A** Note the anaplastic cytomorphology in this unclassified sarcoma. **B** Many tumour cells show a prominent eosinophilic cytoplasm and this case proved to be pleomorphic leiomyosarcoma.

sampling is critical in all cases to check for the presence of lipoblasts or 'malignant' osteoid.

Immunohistochemistry

The widespread introduction of immuno-histochemistry has been one of the major factors in demolition of the MFH concept. Most high grade pleomorphic sarcomas show a definable line of differentiation, foremost among which are the pleomorphic variants of leiomyosarcoma, liposarcoma, rhabdomyosarcoma and myxofibrosarcoma, after carcinomas, melanomas and lymphomas have been excluded {675}. Immunohistochemistry was critical in helping to separate the latter non-mesenchymal malignancies. Controversy exists as to the extent of immunopositivity required for a given antigen to define a specific line of differentiation but diagnostic criteria have

been proposed for the different pleomorphic sarcomas and these appear to be reproducible {683,1425}. The presence of just rare cells showing positivity for epithelial or myogenic antigens most often has little significance and does not, of itself, exclude this diagnosis. It is now accepted that histiocytic antigens (such as alpha-1-antitrypsin, alpha-1-antichymotrypsin, lysozyme and CD68) play no useful role in the diagnosis of pleomorphic sarcomas.

Ultrastructure

Electron microscopic findings depend upon the specific type of tumour giving rise to the pleomorphic MFH pattern. Inevitably almost all tumours in this category are poorly differentiated so only a minority of tumour cells may show ultrastructural features of a specific lineage. Many tumour cells show relatively undif-

ferentiated, non-specific fibroblast-like or histiocyte-like features.

Genetics

The genetic aspects of malignant fibrous histiocytomas (MFH) are difficult to evaluate because of the shifting diagnostic criteria used throughout the years. Bearing these shortcomings in mind, cytogenetic aberrations have been detected in more than 50 cases published as storiform or pleomorphic MFH or MFH NOS {1477}. Only a few cases of giant cell or inflammatory MFH have been investigated. In general, the karyotypes tend to be highly complex, with extensive intratumoral heterogenity and chromosome numbers in the triploid or tetraploid range in the majority of cases {1317,1477,1486,1635,1957}. Also nearhaploid karyotypes have been reported in a few cases {92}. No specific structur-

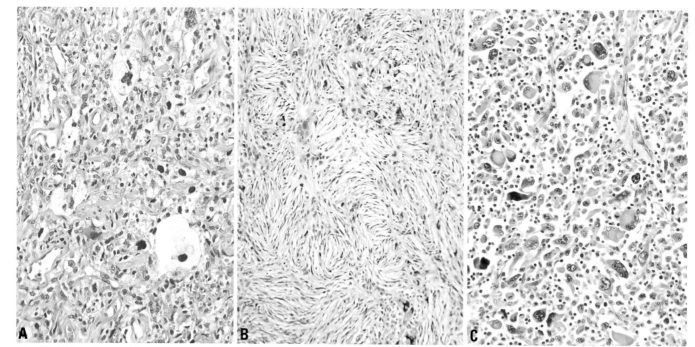

Fig. 3.24 A Many pleomorphic sarcomas contain large bizarre cells with foamy cytoplasm, which in the past were mistakenly regarded as histiocytic in nature. **B** A storiform growth pattern is a common feature shared by many of these undifferentiated high grade pleomorphic sarcomas, irrespective of lineage. **C** The presence of polygonal cells with prominent eosinophilic cytoplasm usually suggests myogenic, epithelial or less often melanocytic differentiation. This case proved to be a pleomorphic rhabdomyosarcoma.

al or numerical aberrations have emerged, but telomeric associations, ring chromosomes, and/or dicentric chromosomes are frequent. Such chromosomal abnormalities are, however, common also in other fibrohistiocytic lesions {1854}. Due to the presence of numerous marker chromosomes in most cases, the distribution of genomic imbalances is impossible to asses reliably from cytogenetic data.

Genomic imbalances, as detected by comparative genomic hybridization (CGH), frequently include loss of 2p24-pter and 2q32-qter, and chromosomes 11, 13 and 16 {1219,1311,1651,1957, 2094}, as well as gain of 7p15-pter, 7q32, and 1p31.

Several proto-oncogenes mapping to chromosome region 12q13-15 appear to participate in the development of MFH-like pleomorphic sarcomas: *SAS*, *MDM2*,

CDK4, *DDIT3* (a.k.a. *CHOP*), and *HMGIC* (a.k.a *HMGA2*) have all been reported to be amplified in MFH {172,1772,1842}. In an amplicon at 8p23.1 a candidate gene designated *MASL1* has been found {1842}.

Alterations (mutations and/or deletions) of *TP53*, *RB1* and *CDKN2A* have been suggested to play a critical role in pleomorphic sarcoma development {341, 1772,1957,2097,2326}, but no clear relationship with clinical outcome has yet been found. The significance of *HRAS* mutations and their relationship with other genetic changes, such as *TP53* and *MDM2* gene status, remain to be clarified {221,1790,2269}.

Prognostic factors

High grade pleomorphic sarcomas are aggressive with an overall 5-year survival probability of only 50-60% {861,2233}.

However, it has become clear that there are prognostic subgroups among the lesions formerly categorised as pleomorphic MFH {683}. For example, dedifferentiated liposarcoma has a metastatic rate of only 15-20%, high grade myxofibrosarcoma has a metastatic rate of around 30-35%, while pleomorphic myogenic sarcomas (leiomyosarcoma or rhabdomyosarcoma) are especially aggressive with much more frequent metastasis and shorter relapse-free survival {1679}. The clinical and therapeutic benefits of subclassifying pleomorphic sarcomas are only just beginning to be appreciated, hence the approach to subclassification and grading of pleomorphic sarcomas is likely to evolve.

Giant cell malignant fibrous histiocytoma / Undifferentiated pleomorphic sarcoma with giant cells

C.D.M. Fletcher

Definition
Formerly defined as a variant of malignant fibrous histiocytoma (MFH) with prominent osteoclastic giant cells, it is now appreciated that this morphologic pattern may be shared by a variety of tumour types. The term giant cell MFH is currently reserved for undifferentiated pleomorphic sarcomas with prominent osteoclastic giant cells.

ICD-O code   8830/3

Synonyms
Malignant giant cell tumour of soft parts, malignant osteoclastoma, giant cell sarcoma.

Historical annotation
Although formerly defined as a variant of malignant fibrous histiocytoma (MFH) with prominent osteoclastic giant cells {599} (and frequently known as malignant giant cell tumour of soft parts/tissues {61,848}) it is now appreciated that this morphologic pattern may be shared by a variety of tumour types (most notably giant cell tumour of soft tissues, extraskeletal osteosarcoma, leiomyosarcoma and osteoclast-rich carcinoma) {961}. It is difficult to define giant cell MFH as a discrete entity and this diagnosis is gradually disappearing from common usage in soft tissue pathology.

Epidemiology
All of the lesions previously subsumed under this heading are very uncommon. Arguably giant cell tumour of soft tissues (see page 118) is the most frequent. Almost all of the tumours which adopt the pattern known as so-called giant cell MFH occur in older adults with no sex predilection. Rare examples of giant cell tumour of soft tissue occur in children and adolescents.

Sites of involvement
With the exception of giant cell tumour of soft tissues (which shows a predilection for subcutaneous tissue) {702,1591, 1608}, most tumours in this general category occur in deep soft tissue of the limbs or trunk. Organs in which giant cell-rich or osteoclastoma-like carcinomas are most common include pancreas, thyroid, breast and kidney.

Clinical features
Most tumours in this general category present as an enlarging, painless, deep-seated mass without distinctive features.

Macroscopy
With the exception of giant cell tumour of soft tissues, most tumours in this general category are high grade and thus tend to be large tumours with haemorrhage and necrosis. Tumour size is variable but superficially located examples are smaller than those in deep soft tissue.

Histopathology
The features shared by tumours previ-

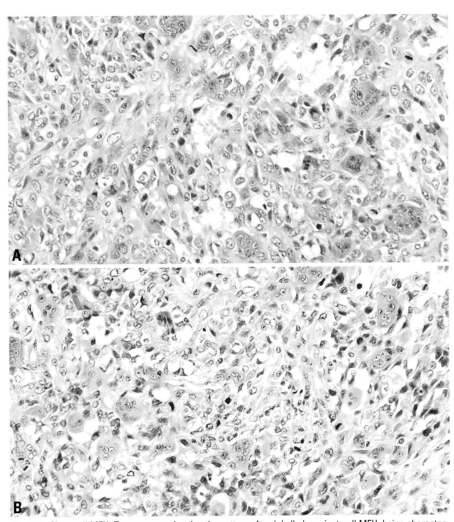

Fig. 3.25 Giant cell MFH. Two tumours showing the pattern often labelled as giant cell MFH, being characterized by atypical spindle-shaped and more epithelioid cells admixed with prominent osteoclastic giant cells. The example on top (**A**) proved to be anaplastic carcinoma of thyroid, while the lower one (**B**) was a soft tissue osteosarcoma.

ously labelled as giant cell MFH include variably pleomorphic ovoid-to-spindle-shaped cells and a prominent stromal osteoclastic giant cell reaction. In most (but not all) lesions the giant cell component lacks cytological features of malignancy, but some tumours diagnosed as giant cell MFH were notable for the presence of numerous bizarre multinucleate tumour giant cells.

Aside from these similar (shared) features, morphology is largely determined by the specific tumour type. Giant cell-rich soft tissue osteosarcoma (see page 182) definitionally shows variably prominent 'malignant' osteoid being laid down by cytologically atypical cells {355}. Giant cell tumour of soft tissues (see page 118) usually has a multinodular growth pattern and cytologically resembles giant cell tumour of bone {702, 1591, 1608}. Leiomyosarcoma with prominent osteoclastic giant cells has at least small areas with conventional smooth muscle cytomorphology and a fascicular growth pattern {1411}. Other sarcoma types may occasionally show prominent osteoclastic giant cells {1415}.

Immunohistochemistry

Leiomyosarcoma with prominent osteoclastic giant cells usually shows positivity for smooth muscle actin and desmin in the fascicular spindle cell component. Unequivocal positivity for keratin is a diagnostic requirement for osteoclastoma-like or giant cell-rich carcinoma, with the exception of those cases showing obvious morphologic transition to usual carcinoma.

Prognostic factors

Undifferentiated high grade sarcomas with prominent osteoclastic giant cells behave similarly to other pleomorphic

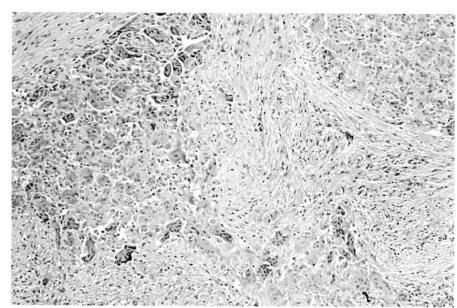

Fig. 3.26 Giant cell MFH may resemble giant cell tumour of soft tissue, which has a multinodular growth pattern, was often formerly labelled as giant cell MFH.

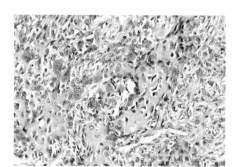

Fig. 3.27 Giant cell-rich soft tissue osteosarcoma. This osteoclast-rich spindle cell malignant neoplasm contains seams of osteoid produced by cytologically malignant cells.

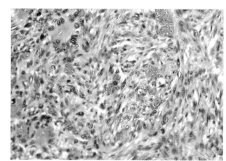

Fig. 3.28 Leiomyosarcoma mimicking so-called giant cell MFH. Note with prominent osteoclastic giant cells and the eosinophilic fascicular spindle cell component..

sarcomas. Among neoplasms simulating giant cell MFH, extraskeletal osteosarcoma and leiomyosarcoma are much more aggressive than giant cell tumour of soft tissues.

Inflammatory malignant fibrous histiocytoma / Undifferentiated pleomorphic sarcoma with prominent inflammation

J.M. Coindre

Definition
A malignant neoplasm characterized by numerous xanthomatous cells, morphologically both benign and malignant, admixed with atypical spindle cells and acute and chronic inflammatory cells. Originally regarded as a variant of so-called malignant fibrous histiocytoma (MFH), differentiation in these tumours is poorly understood and their morphology may be shared by both mesenchymal and epithelial neoplasms. The term inflammatory MFH is now reserved for undifferentiated pleomorphic sarcomas with a prominent histiocytic and inflammatory infiltrate.

ICD-O code   8830/3

Synonyms
Xanthomatous MFH, malignant fibrous xanthoma, xanthosarcoma.

Epidemiology
This is the rarest and the least documented type of MFH, with only two published series of 7 and 8 cases {1096,1198} and a few case reports. There is no apparent gender predominance, and patients are usually more than 40 years old.

Sites of involvement
The most common site is the retroperitoneum but intra-abdominal and deep soft tissue locations have also been observed.

Clinical features
In addition to symptoms and imaging features of a large retroperitoneal tumour, inflammatory MFH may be associated with fever, weight loss, leukocytosis, eosinophilia, and leukaemoid reaction. Analysis of tumour extracts and immunohistochemistry suggested that production of specific cytokines by tumour cells is responsible for the systemic symptoms {1401,2076}.

Aetiology
There is no aetiology known for inflammatory MFH, but one post-radiation case has been reported {735}.

Macroscopy
This tumour is usually large and often displays a yellow colour due to large collections of xanthoma cells.

Histopathology
Inflammatory MFH is characterized by sheets of benign xanthoma cells with numerous inflammatory cells including neutrophils, eosinophils and a minor component of lymphocytes and plasma cells. Some cases show only a few or no xanthoma cells but are predominantly composed of neutrophils and eosinophils. There are scattered atypical large cells, with one or more irregular, hyperchromatic nuclei with prominent nucleoli. These cells may be rare and difficult to find and occasionally resemble Reed-Sternberg cells. Occasionally atypical cells are xanthomatized and typically display phagocytosis of neutrophils. These cells may be set in a hyalinized collagenous background. In most cases, there are typical areas of pleomorphic MFH-like sarcoma with spindle and pleomorphic cells arranged in a haphazard growth pattern. Like pleomorphic MFH, inflammatory MFH is a diagnosis of exclusion and could represent an inflammatory dedifferentiated component shared by different neoplasms such as carcinomas, lymphomas, leiomyosarcomas, inflammatory myofibroblastic tumours and liposarcomas {956,961}. Among these, dedifferentiated liposarcoma is the most common simulant.

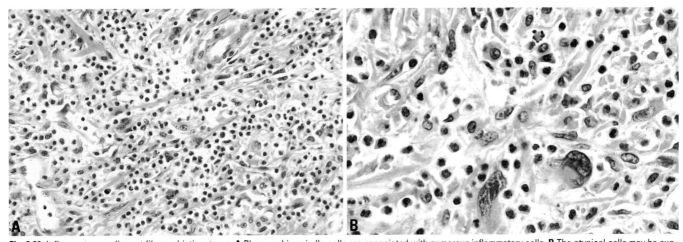

Fig. 3.29 Inflammatory malignant fibrous histiocytoma. **A** Pleomorphic spindle cells are associated with numerous inflammatory cells. **B** The atypical cells may be suggestive of a lymphoid neoplasm.

Therefore inflammatory MFH areas may often be associated with areas of more specific tumours which should be carefully looked for.

Immunophenotype
Immunohistochemistry is useful for showing a specific line of differentiation such as epithelial, lymphoid or smooth muscular. In the other cases, the neoplastic cells express vimentin, occasionally CD68, but are negative for CD15, CD20, CD30, CD43 and CD45 {1096}.

Ultrastructure
The tumour cells do not differ ultrastructurally from tumour cells of pleomorphic MFH.

Genetics
Genetic analysis may be particularly useful for identifying a possible dedifferentiated liposarcoma or other simulants such as anaplastic large cell lymphoma.

Prognostic factors
From a review of the literature {961} and a small series {1198}, it appears that two-thirds of patients died of their tumour with persistent or recurrent disease. About one fourth of patients developed distant metastasis. As in other retroperitoneal sarcomas, this poor prognosis is probably related to the extent of the tumour and its inaccessibility to proper surgery at the time of the diagnosis.

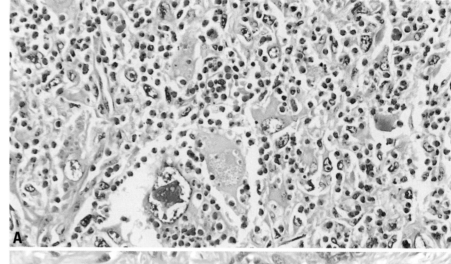
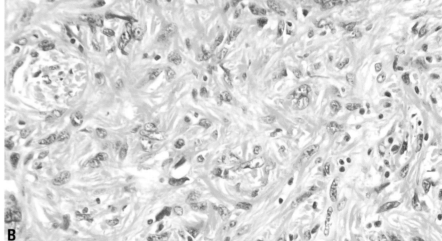

Fig. 3.30 Inflammatory malignant fibrous histiocytoma. **A** Note the striking cytophagocytosis. **B** Pleomorphic MFH-like areas with collagenous stroma are common.

CHAPTER 4

Smooth Muscle Tumours

Smooth muscle tumours arising at non-cutaneous, non-uterine locations have been the focus of a considerable conceptual shift in recent years and this is ongoing. Specifically, it has been uncertain whether or not there exist benign leiomyomas of deep soft tissue, but these lesions are now becoming better recognized and defined. The vast majority of so-called smooth muscle tumours arising in the gastrointestinal tract, mesentery and omentum are, in fact, gastrointestinal stromal tumours defined by the presence of activating *KIT* mutations and expression of KIT protein. These lesions, described in the Digestive System volume, also account for most cases formerly classified as epithelioid smooth muscle tumours, or smooth muscle tumours of uncertain malignant potential.

During the past decade, it has been recognized, mainly through immunohistochemistry, that soft tissue leiomyosarcoma is more common than formerly believed and that a rare but histologically distinct subset of these lesions is related to Epstein Barr virus infection in immunocompromised patients.

Pilar leiomyoma and cutaneous leiomyosarcoma are described in the Skin volume. Smooth muscle tumours of the external genitalia (vulvovaginal region, scrotum and nipple), as well as leiomyomatosis peritonealis disseminata, are described in the respective WHO Blue Books.

Angioleiomyoma

H. Hashimoto
B. Quade

Definition
A frequently painful, benign subcutaneous or deep dermal tumour composed of mature smooth muscle bundles which surround and intersect between vascular channels. These tumours form a morphological continuum with myopericytoma and myofibroma.

ICD-O code   8894/0

Synonyms
Angiomyoma, vascular leiomyoma.

Epidemiology
Angioleiomyoma is a relatively common neoplasm. In the largest series reported by Hachisuga et al., 562 cases of angioleiomyoma accounted for approximately 4.4 % of a total of 12,663 cases of benign soft tissue tumours {863}.

Sites of involvement
Most angioleiomyomas occur in the extremities, especially the lower extremity, and other sites include the head and the trunk {1309}. The tumours are usually located in the subcutis and less often in the deep dermis. Most of the solid histological subtype (see below) develop in the lower extremity, and most of the cavernous subtype in the upper extremity {863}. Tumours of the venous type develop more often in the head than do the other subtypes. In contrast to pilar leiomyoma (see volume on Skin Tumours), almost all angioleiomyomas are solitary.

Clinical features
Angioleiomyomas occur more frequently in women {555, 1500}, although tumours located in the upper extremity and the head appear more frequent in men than in women {863}. The lesions usually develop between the fourth and sixth decades of life.

Most angioleiomyomas present as a small, slowly enlarging mass usually of several years' duration. Pain is the most characteristic subjective complaint in about half of patients with angioleiomyoma {555}. In some patients the pain is exacerbated by wind, cold, pressure, pregnancy, or menses.

Macroscopy
Angioleiomyomas are sharply demarcated, spherical, grey-white or brown nodules, and most are less than 2 cm in diameter. Tumours of the solid type are smaller than those of the other two types.

Histopathology
Angioleiomyomas may be separated into three subtypes according to the dominant histological pattern: solid, venous and cavernous. Smooth muscle cells of angioleiomyoma are mature and well differentiated. Mitotic figures are usually absent or very rare. In tumours of the solid type smooth muscle bundles are closely compacted, and intersect with one another. Vascular channels in this type of tumour are large in number but usually small in size and slit-like. Tumours of the venous type have vascular channels of venous type with thick muscular walls, and lesional smooth muscle bundles are not so compact. The outer layers of the smooth muscle in the vascular walls blend with intervascular smooth muscle bundles. Tumours of the cavernous type are composed of dilated vascular channels with small amounts of smooth muscle, and the muscular walls of these vessels are difficult to distinguish from intervening smooth muscle bundles. Although two different histological patterns are seen occasionally in the same tumour, one of the above histological subtypes is generally identified as the dominant histology. According to this subclassification, the angioleiomyomas reported by Hachisuga et al. were separated into 374 cases (66%) of the solid type, 127 (23%) of the venous type, and 61 (11%) of the cavernous type {863}. Rarely, the nuclei of smooth muscle cells are enlarged and hyperchromatic, probably displaying degenerative nuclear atypia {307,1076,1344}. Areas of hyalinization, calcification, myxoid change, haemorrhage, and small groups of mature fat cells may be seen {863}. Because there is no evidence of any relationship between those fat-containing angioleiomyomas and renal or retroperitoneal angiomyolipomas, nor with tuberous sclerosis, they should not be labelled "subcutaneous angiomyolipoma".

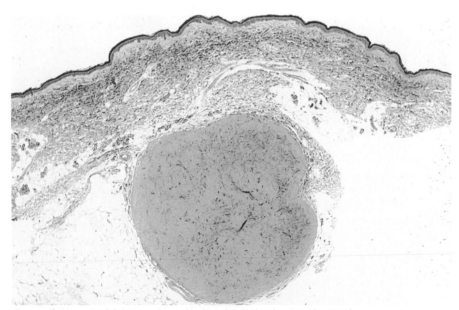

Fig. 4.01 Solid type angioleiomyoma located in the subcutis showing sharp demarcation.

Immunohistochemistry

Most cells are positive for alpha-smooth muscle actin, desmin, vimentin and collagen type IV. According to a study by Hasegawa et al., in more than half of cases, small nerve fibres positive for both S100 protein and PGP9.5 are seen within the capsule of tumours and tumour stroma {899}. The peculiar pain of angioleiomyomas is possibly mediated by these nerve fibres. In contrast to renal and retroperitoneal angiomyolipoma, angioleiomyomas (including the fat-containing examples) are consistently negative for HMB45.

Genetics

Cytogenetic data exist for only four angioleiomyomas from different sites. All had near-diploid karyotypes, but no consistent abnormality has been detected among them {926,936,1567, 1989}.

Prognostic factors

Angioleiomyoma is benign. Simple local excision is adequate treatment, and recurrence after excision is exceptional.

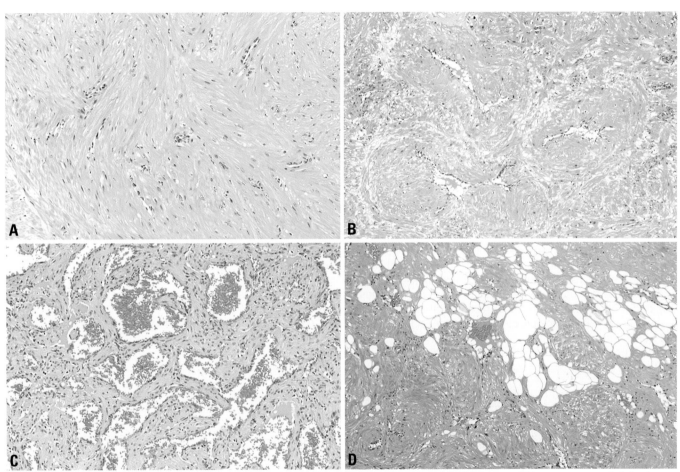

Fig. 4.02 A Angioleiomyomas are typically composed of monomorphic well differentiated smooth muscle cells. **B** Solid type angioleiomyoma composed of closely compacted vascular and muscle elements. **C** Cavernous type angioleiomyoma showing dilated vascular channels with little muscular thickening of the walls. **D** Angioleiomyoma with groups of mature fat cells.

Leiomyoma of deep soft tissue

H. Hashimoto
B. Quade

Definition

A very rare type of leiomyoma that occurs in the deep somatic soft tissue or retroperitoneum/abdominal cavity.

ICD-O code   8890/0

Epidemiology

The existence and diagnostic criteria of leiomyomas of deep soft tissue have been controversial, and only sporadic cases reports of leiomyomas arising in the deep soft tissue have been reported, except for the recent three large series by Kilpatrick et al. {1106}, Billings et al. {196}, and Paal and Miettinen {1636}, respectively.

Sites of involvement

The extremities are the most common site in the deep somatic soft tissue. They arise in the deep subcutis or skeletal muscle. Pelvic retroperitoneum and abdominal cavity, including the mesentery and omentum, are other deep soft tissues where leiomyomas may occur. They are always distinct from the uterus and independent soft tissue primaries rather than parasitic leiomyomas of the uterus.

Clinical features

Leiomyomas of the deep somatic soft tissue affect both sexes equally, whereas leiomyomas of the retroperitoneum or abdominal cavity occur almost exclusively in women {196,1636}. Most patients in both groups are young adults or middle-aged. Many lesions are calcified, so they may be detected radiographically.

Macroscopy

Leiomyomas of the deep soft tissue are well circumscribed, grey-white tumours. The greatest diameter of 11 leiomyomas of the deep somatic soft tissue reported by Kilpatrick et al. ranged 2.5 – 15 cm (mean 7.7 cm), and most measured 5 cm or more, exceeding the usual size of angioleiomyomas {1106}. Twenty retroperitoneal and 3 abdominal leiomyomas reported by Billings et al. ranged in size 3.2-37 cm (mean 14 cm) {196}. The greatest diameter of 51 retroperitoneal leiomyomas reported by Paal and Miettinen ranged 2.5 - 31 cm (mean 16.2 cm), and the tumour weight ranged 28 - 5400 g (mean 1600 g) {1636}. Myxoid change is common.

Histopathology

Leiomyomas of deep soft tissue are composed of cells that closely resemble normal smooth muscle cells because they have eosinophilic cytoplasm with haematoxylin and eosin, fuchsinophilic, red-staining cytoplasm with Masson's trichrome technique and bland, uniform blunt-ended, cigar-shaped nuclei. They are arranged in orderly intersecting fascicles. They are highly differentiated, possess little or no atypia and, at most, an extremely low level of mitotic activity. In limb lesions and intra-abdominal lesions in males, mitoses number less than 1/50 HPF. In peritoneal / retroperitoneal lesions in females (showing positivity for hormonal receptors) mitoses may number up to 5/50 HPF. Necrosis should not been present in deep leiomyoma. Most lesions are paucicellular, and degenerative or regressive changes, such as fibrosis, hyalinization, calcification and myxoid change, are common in large leiomyomas. Ossification, focal epithelioid change, clear cell change and fatty differentiation {1393} are also occasionally seen. If the fatty change is prominent, such tumours should be termed myolipoma (see page 29). The significance of focal degenerative nuclear atypia is as yet not fully defined and should always prompt a careful search for mitoses and additional sampling.

Immunohistochemistry

Tumour cells are always positive for actin, desmin and h-caldesmon at least focally. S100 protein is negative. Billings et al. reported that all six of the retroperitoneal leiomyomas tested were positive for progesterone receptors and five of six were positive for oestrogen receptors, probably indicating that the tumours arise from hormonally sensitive smooth muscle {196}, whereas none of the somatic leiomyomas {196} or retroperitoneal leiomyosarcomas {1636} expressed either hormone receptor protein.

Prognostic factors

Tumours categorized as leiomyomas of the deep soft tissue should be cured by complete excision. If they recur, the recurrence should be nondestructive. Long-term follow-up did not reveal metastases, but one of 29 patients reported by Billings et al {196} and two of 36 patients reported by Paal and Miettinen {1636} had local recurrence; however, none of the patients with recurrence demonstrated disease progression in follow-up.

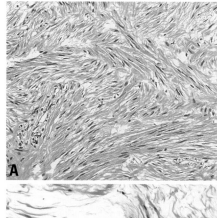

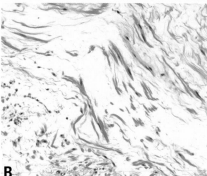

Fig. 4.03 A Leiomyoma of the retroperitoneum composed of interlacing fascicles of bland smooth muscle cells. **B** Leiomyoma of the retroperitoneum showing myxoid change.

Leiomyosarcoma

H.L. Evans
J. Shipley

Definition
Leiomyosarcoma is a malignant tumour composed of cells showing distinct smooth muscle features.

ICD-O code   8890/3

Epidemiology
Soft-tissue leiomyosarcoma usually occurs in middle-aged or older persons, although it may develop in young adults and even in children {1839, 2066}. Leiomyosarcoma forms a significant percentage of retroperitoneal (including pelvic) sarcomas {906,1749,1754,1945, 2268} and is the predominant sarcoma arising from larger blood vessels {166, 1095,1243,2192}. Aside from these locations, it is a comparatively less common sarcoma, accounting for perhaps 10-15% of limb sarcomas. The sex incidence depends on tumour location, with women forming a clear majority of patients with retroperitoneal and inferior vena cava leiomyosarcomas but not of those with leiomyosarcomas in other soft tissue sites.

Sites of involvement
The most common location of soft tissue leiomyosarcoma is the retroperitoneum, including the pelvis. Another distinctive subgroup consists of leiomyosarcomas that arise in large blood vessels, most commonly the inferior vena cava and the large veins of the lower extremity. Arterial origin occurs but is rare; sarcomas of the pulmonary artery and other large arteries generally do not have the features of leiomyosarcoma and are better classified as intimal sarcomas (see page 223). Leiomyosarcomas involving nonretroperitoneal soft tissue sites constitute a third group {423,642,903,2039}. These are found most frequently in the lower extremity but may develop elsewhere. Intramuscular and subcutaneous localizations occur in approximately equal proportion, and some of these tumours show evidence of origin from a small to medium sized (unnamed) vein. Leiomyosarcomas also develop in the dermis, but these are discussed in the volume on tumours of the skin.

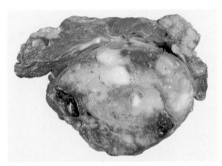

Fig. 4.04 Leiomyosarcoma. This high grade lesion (19 cm) from the quadriceps muscle shows extensive necrosis and haemorrhage.

Clinical features
Soft tissue leiomyosarcoma generally presents as a mass lesion. With retroperitoneal tumours, pain may also be present. The symptoms produced by leiomyosarcoma of the inferior vena cava depend on the portion involved. When the tumour is in the upper portion, it obstructs the hepatic veins and produces the Budd-Chiari syndrome, with haepatomegaly, jaundice, and ascites.

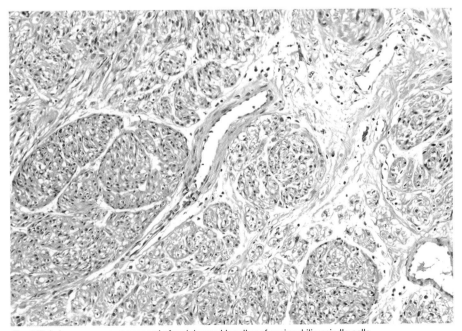

Fig. 4.05 Leiomyosarcoma composed of nodules and bundles of eosinophilic spindle cells.

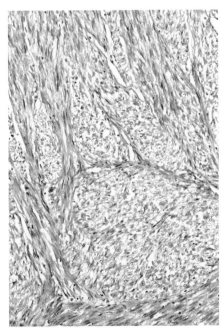

Fig. 4.06 Leiomyosarcoma with typical intersecting groups of spindle cells.

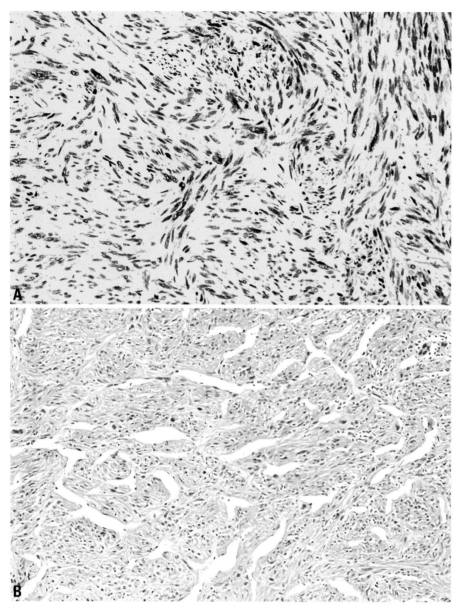

Fig. 4.07 Leiomyosarcoma **(A)** showing fascicles which intersect at 90° and, in another case **(B)**, showing a pericytoma-like vascular pattern.

Location in the middle portion may result in blockage of the renal veins and consequent renal dysfunction, whereas involvement of the lower portion may cause leg oedema. The latter may also occur with leiomyosarcomas of the large veins of the lower extremity.

Imaging studies of leiomyosarcoma demonstrate a nonspecific soft tissue mass but are helpful in delineating the relationship to adjacent structures, particularly in the retroperitoneum.

In the instance of leiomyosarcoma of vein origin, venogram may demonstrate an intraluminal component.

Aetiology

The cause of soft tissue leiomyosarcoma is unknown. The predominant occurrence of retroperitoneal and inferior vena cava leiomyosarcomas in women raises the question of hormonal influence, but this is unclear.

Macroscopy

Leiomyosarcoma of soft tissue typically forms a fleshy mass, with colours varying from grey to white to tan. A whorled character may be evident to some degree. Larger examples often display haemorrhage, necrosis, or cystic change. The tumour border

frequently appears well circumscribed, although obvious infiltrativeness may also be found. In the retroperitoneum there may be extension into adjacent organs.

Histopathology

The typical histological pattern of leiomyosarcoma is that of intersecting, sharply marginated groups of spindle cells. This pattern may be less well defined in areas of some tumours, and occasionally there is a focal storiform, palisaded, or haemangiopericytoma-like arrangement. The tumours are usually compactly cellular, but fibrosis or myxoid change may be present; in the latter instance, a retiform or microcystic pattern may result. Hyalinized, hypocellular zones and coagulative tumour necrosis are frequent in larger leiomyosarcomas. Rarely there is abundant chronic or acute inflammation {1421}.

The tumour cell nuclei are characteristically elongated and blunt-ended and may be indented or lobated. Nuclear hyperchromatism and pleomorphism are generally notable, although they may be focal, mild, or occasionally absent. Mitotic figures can usually be found readily, although they may be few or patchy; and atypical mitoses are often seen. The cytoplasm varies from typically eosinophilic to pale, and in the former instance is often distinctly fibrillar. Cytoplasmic vacuolation is frequently apparent, particularly in cells cut transversely. Epithelioid cytomorphology, multinucleated osteoclastlike giant cells {1411}, very prominent chronic inflammatory cells {1421}, and granular cytoplasmic change {1573} are unusual findings that are normally present in only part of a tumour when identified. Occasional soft tissue leiomyosarcomas contain areas with a nonspecific, poorly differentiated, pleomorphic appearance in addition to typical areas {1594}. These could be regarded as "dedifferentiated leiomyosarcomas" although this term is not in common use. Rarely, an osteosarcomalike or rhabdomyosarcomatous component is associated with leiomyosarcoma (see "malignant mesenchymoma").

Immunophenotype

SMA, desmin and h-caldesmon are positive in a great majority of soft tissue leiomyosarcomas. However, none of

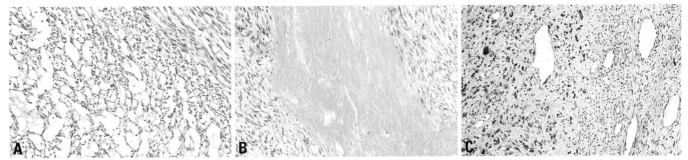

Fig. 4.08 Leiomyosarcoma showing **(A)** a myxoid, reticular appearance, **(B)** necrosis and hyalinization, and **(C)** abrupt transition to more pleomorphic tumour indicative of dedifferentiation.

these is absolutely specific for smooth muscle (or indeed muscle in general), and positivity for two of these markers is more supportive of leiomyosarcoma than positivity for one alone. "Dedifferentiated" areas may be negative for SMA and desmin, but total negativity for both in a tumour would cast great doubt on the diagnosis of leiomyosarcoma. Stains that may be positive, at least focally, include keratin, EMA, CD34, and S100 protein. KIT (CD117) is normally negative, in contrast to gastrointestinal stromal tumours. In general, the diagnosis of soft tissue leiomyosarcoma should not be made on the basis of immunostains in the absence of appropriate morphologic features.

Ultrastructure

Soft tissue leiomyosarcomas usually demonstrate at least some of the ultrastructural features of normal smooth muscle cells, namely cytoplasmic filaments with densities, cell junctions, pinocytotic vesicles, and basement membrane. However, any, or occasionally, all of these may be focal or absent, and the findings may be nonspecific. It is particularly important to note that filaments with densities are present in myofibroblasts and can occur in other cells. Electron microscopy is not generally needed for the diagnosis of soft tissue leiomyosarcoma, and ultrastructural observations should always be correlated with the light microscopic appearance.

Genetics

Cytogenetics

Karyotypes from around 100 leiomyosarcomas have been reported {1477}. Most karyotypes are complex and no consistent aberrations have been noted

{2215}. Frequently lost chromosome regions include 3p21-23, 8p21-pter, 13q12-13, 13q32-qter, whereas the 1q21-31 region is often gained {1314}. No striking differences among different subtypes have been identified {1314}. Comparative genomic hybridization (CGH) has confirmed frequent numerical changes, including gain of material from chromosomes 1, 15, 17, 19, 20, 22 and X and loss from 1q, 2, 4q, 9p, 10, 11q, 13q and 16, and has identified regions of amplification, e.g., 1q21, 5p14-pter, 12q13-15, 13q31, 17p11 and 20q13) {2215}. Tumour size-related changes have been observed, such as an association of gain of 16p and 17p with smaller tumours and gain of 6q and 8q with larger tumours {577}.

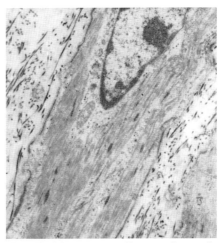

Fig. 4.09 Leiomyosarcoma. Tumour cells contain prominent longitudinal filament bundles with focal densities. Note also the external lamina.

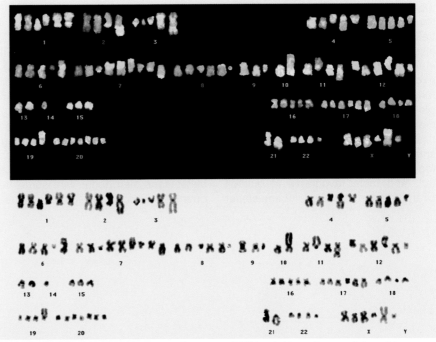

Fig. 4.10 24-colour karyotype and corresponding reverse DAPI-banded image from a soft tissue leiomyosarcoma showing multiple copies of chromosomes and many rearranged chromosomes.

Molecular genetics

The *RB1* gene has been implicated, which is consistent with loss of chromosome 13 material {2042}. Analysis of the genes and proteins in the Rb-cyclinD pathway (*RB1, CDKN2A, CCND1,* and *CCND3*) has revealed frequent abnormalities in leiomyosarcomas {488}. Involvement of *TP53* and *MDM2* appears less frequent than in other sarcoma types {488,692}, although such abnormalities have been suggested to correlate with a poorer prognosis in leiomyosarcomas {1668}. Amplification at a number of loci suggest candidate genes in these regions including *MDM2, GLI, CDK4* and *SAS* at 12q13-15, the *FLF* and *PRUNE* genes at 1q21, and the critical region involved in Smith-Magenis syndrome at 17p11.2 {579,692,708, 709,712,1627}.

Prognostic factors

Soft tissue leiomyosarcomas are capable of both local recurrence and distant metastasis. Regional (or other) lymph node metastasis is rare. The most important prognostic factors by far are tumour location and size, which are strongly interrelated. Retroperitoneal leiomyosarcomas are fatal in the great majority of cases; they are typically large (over 10 cm), often difficult or impossible to excise with clear margins, and prone to both local recurrence and metastasis. Leiomyosarcomas of large vessels also tend to have a poor prognosis, although local control rates are higher except for those in the upper inferior vena cava, and very small examples (1-2 cm) may be less prone to metastasize. Nonretroperitoneal soft tissue leiomyosarcomas are generally smaller than those in the retroperitoneum, more amenable to local control, and more favourable in outlook overall. In some studies, intramuscular

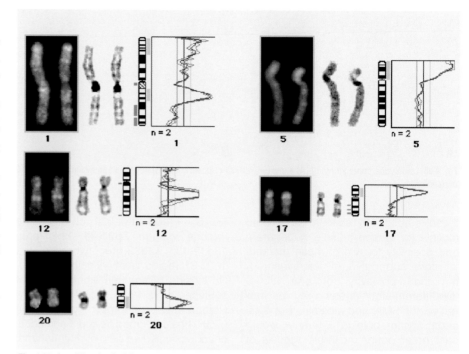

Fig. 4.11 Amplification in leiomyosarcomas identified by CGH analysis. CGH images, reverse DAPI-banded chromosomes and corresponding profiles of the red to green fluorescence intensities are shown and indicate amplification at 1q21-q25, 5p, 12q13-q21, 17q11.2-q12 and 20q, respectively.

rather than subcutaneous location {903} and larger tumour size {642, 1479} were related to increased metastasis and poorer patient survival within this group. Histological grading as well as osseous and vascular involvement are reliable prognostic indicators.

Local recurrences and metastases of soft tissue leiomyosarcoma usually become manifest within the first few years after diagnosis but may appear as much as 10 years later. For retroperitoneal leiomyosarcomas, the most common sites of metastases are the lungs and liver, whereas the lungs are the dominant location when the primary tumour is nonretroperitoneal. Metastases also occur with some frequency in skin, soft tissue, and bone.

Smooth muscle tumours in immunocompromised patients

Smooth muscle tumours in immunocompromised individuals, to this point described only in single case reports and small series, form a distinctive subgroup. These usually involve parenchymal organs rather than soft tissue, occur predominantly in children and young adults who are HIV positive {323,1368,1811, 2179} or post-transplant, and are associated with Epstein-Barr virus. The tumours may be multifocal, and at least in some instances this appears to represent true multicentricity rather than metastasis {1811,1985}. Histologically, they range from bland to mitotically active, may have a variable lymphocytic infiltrate of uncertain significance and may show a perivascular growth pattern.

CHAPTER 5

Pericytic (Perivascular) Tumours

Pericytic / perivascular neoplasms have traditionally been dominated by haemangiopericytoma. However, it is now recognized that the latter diagnostic category subsumes a wide variety of tumour types which share the presence of thin-walled branching blood vessels. If such lesions are otherwise classified, there remains only a small group of spindle cell lesions designated as haemangiopericytoma, although they have no evident relationship to pericytes, and may be more closely related to solitary fibrous tumour (see Chapter 2).

The lesions now remaining in this pericytic / perivascular category all show evidence of differentiation towards myoid / contractile perivascular cells and all share the characteristic tendency to grow in a circumferential perivascular fashion. Currently, the term 'myopericytoma' is preferred to avoid confusion with the ill defined former terminology.

Important advances have been made in predicting biological potential of glomus tumours and in understanding the close relationship between myopericytoma, myofibroma / myofibromatosis, and so-called infantile haemangiopericytoma, which essentially form a single morphological continuum. Their myoid nature and shared features with angioleiomyoma explain their more logical alignment with smooth muscle tumours rather than vascular tumours in this new classification.

Sinonasal haemangiopericytoma, which appears to be a truly pericytic lesion, is described in the Respiratory System volume.

Glomus tumours

A.L. Folpe

Definition
Glomus tumours are mesenchymal neoplasms composed of cells that closely resemble the modified smooth muscle cells of the normal glomus body.

ICD-O codes
Glomus tumour	8711/0
Glomus tumours of uncertain malignant potential	8711/1
Malignant glomus tumour	8711/3

Epidemiology
Glomus tumours are rare, accounting for less than 2% of soft tissue tumours {1946}. Multiple lesions may be seen in close to 10% of patients. Malignant glomus tumours are exceedingly rare, comprising less than 1% of glomus tumours {697}.

Glomus tumours typically occur in young adults but may occur at any age. No sex predilection is seen, except in subungual lesions, which are far more common in women {2079,2177}.

Sites of involvement
The vast majority of glomus tumours occur in the distal extremities, particularly the subungual region, the hand, the wrist and the foot {2246}. Rare tumours have however been reported in almost every location, including the stomach {885}, penis {1132}, mediastinum {952}, nerve {293}, bone {1815} and lung {751}. Glomus tumours almost always occur in the skin or superficial soft tissues, although rare cases occur in deep soft tissue or viscera. Malignant glomus tumours are usually deeply seated, but may be cutaneous {697}.

Clinical features
Cutaneous glomus tumours are typically small (<1 cm), red-blue nodules that are often associated with a long history of pain, particularly with exposure to cold or minor tactile stimulation.

Deeply seated or visceral glomus tumours may have either no associated symptoms or symptoms referable to the involved organ.

Histopathology
Typical glomus tumours
Typical glomus tumours are subcategorized as "solid glomus tumour", "glomangioma", and "glomangiomyoma" depending on the relative prominence of glomus cells, vascular structures and smooth muscle. Glomus cells are small, uniform, rounded cells with a centrally placed, round nucleus and amphophilic to lightly eosinophilic cytoplasm. Each cell is surrounded by basal lamina, seen best on PAS or toluidine blue histochemical stains. Occasionally cases show oncocytic {1967} or epithelioid change {1737}.

Solid glomus tumours are the most common variant, comprising approximately 75% of cases {2242}. They are composed of nests of glomus cells surrounding capillary sized vessels. The stroma may show hyalinization or myxoid change. Small cuffs of glomus cells are often seen around small vessels located outside of the main mass. Glomangiomas, comprising approximately 20% of glomus tumours, are characterized by dilated veins surrounded by small clusters of glomus cells. Glomangiomas are the most common type of glomus tumour in patients with multiple or familial lesions. Glomangiomyomas, the least common subtype of typical glomus tumour, are characterized by an overall architecture similar to solid glomus tumour or glomangioma and by a transition from typical glomus cells to elongated cells resembling mature smooth muscle. In some glomus tumours a branching, haemangiopericytoma-like vasculature is present and such cases have been designated "glomangiopericytoma" {825}.

Glomangiomatosis
Glomangiomatosis is an extremely rare variant of glomus tumour with an overall architectural resemblance to diffuse angiomatosis (see page 161) {697, 823, 1294}. Glomangiomatosis is distinguished from angiomatosis by the presence of multiple nodules of solid glomus tumour investing the vascular walls. It is benign despite its infiltrative growth.

Symplastic glomus tumours
Symplastic glomus tumours show striking nuclear atypia in the absence of any other worrisome feature (e.g., large size, deep location, mitotic activity, necrosis) {697}. The marked nuclear atypia that characterizes these tumours is believed to be a degenerative phenomenon. All cases reported to date have behaved in a benign fashion.

Malignant glomus tumours (glomangiosarcomas) and glomus tumours of uncertain malignant potential
Histologically malignant glomus tumours are exceedingly rare and clinically malignant ones (e.g., metastatic) rarer yet. Prior to 2000, fewer than 20 histologically malignant and 2 clinically malignant tumours had been reported {21,54,247,823,885,952,953,1575, 2219,2220, 2255}. Criteria for the diagnosis of malignancy in glomus tumours were only recently elaborated {697}. The diagnosis of "malignant glomus tumour" should be reserved for tumours showing: 1) Size >2 cm and subfascial or visceral location; 2) Atypical mitotic figures; or 3) Marked nuclear atypia and any level of mitotic activity. These features frequently co-vary in a given case. A component of pre-existing benign-appearing glomus tumour is often but not always present. There are two types of malignant glomus tumour.

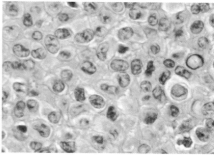

Fig. 5.01 Glomus tumour. Note the typical rounded cytomorphology and well defined cell membranes.

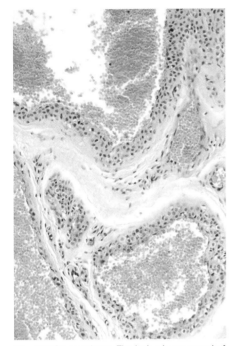

Fig. 5.02 Glomangioma. The lesion is composed of dilated vascular spaces, the walls of which contain several layers of glomus cells.

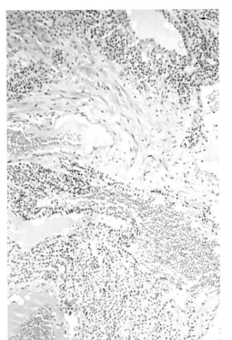

Fig. 5.03 Glomangioma, composed of dilated vascular spaces, the walls of which contain several layers of glomus cells.

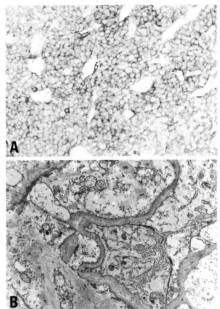

Fig. 5.04 Glomus tumour. **A** Tumour cells show consistently strong immunoreactivity for smooth muscle actin. **B** Ultrastructure showing prominent external lamina, pinocytotic vesicles and intracytoplasmic actin microfilaments.

In the first type, the malignant component resembles a leiomyosarcoma or fibrosarcoma. In the second type, the malignant component retains an overall architectural similarity to benign glomus tumour and consists of sheets of highly malignant appearing round cells. Immunohistochemical demonstration of smooth muscle actin and pericellular type IV collagen is required for the diagnosis of this second type of malignant glomus tumour, in the absence of a clear-cut benign precursor. Malignant glomus tumours are highly aggressive with metastases in approximately 40% of cases, resulting in the death of the patient {697}. Glomus tumours not fulfilling criteria for ma-

lignancy, but having at least one atypical feature other than nuclear pleomorphism should be diagnosed as "*glomus tumours of uncertain malignant potential*".

Immunohistochemistry
Glomus tumours of all types typically express smooth muscle actin and have abundant pericellular type IV collagen production. H-caldesmon is also positive. Other markers, including desmin, CD34, cytokeratin and S100 protein are usually negative {697}.

Ultrastructure
Ultrastructurally glomus cells have short interdigitating cytoplasmic processes,

bundles of thin actin-like filaments with dense bodies and occasional attachments plaques to the cytoplasmic membrane and prominent external lamina {1449}.

Genetics
Multiple familial glomus tumours appear to have an autosomal dominant pattern of inheritance {164,884,1363}. An association between subungual glomus tumours and neurofibromatosis type I has been reported {1109,1602,1867}. The gene for multiple inherited glomus tumours has been linked to chromosome 1p21-22 {229,297}. The genetic events underlying sporadic glomus tumours are not known.

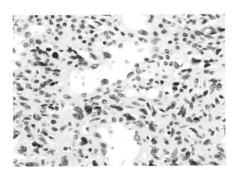

Fig. 5.05 Symplastic glomus tumour with prominent nuclear atypia but without mitotic activity.

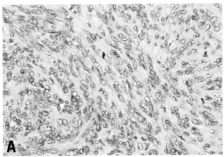
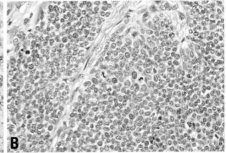

Fig. 5.06 A Malignant glomus tumour, spindle cell type. **B** Malignant glomus tumour, round cell type. Note the brisk mitotic activity.

Myopericytoma

M.E. McMenamin

Definition
Myopericytoma is a benign, generally subcutaneous tumour that is composed of oval-to-spindle shaped myoid appearing cells with a striking tendency for concentric perivascular growth. It is believed that the lesional cells show apparent differentiation towards perivascular myoid cells or myopericytes. Myopericytoma forms a morphological continuum with myofibroma, angioleiomyoma and so-called infantile haemangiopericytoma.

ICD-O code   8713/1

Synonyms
In the past, myopericytoma may have been diagnosed as a solitary myofibroma or "haemangiopericytoma."

Epidemiology
Myopericytoma arises most commonly in mid adulthood; however, lesions can arise at any age. Familial cases have not been reported.

Sites of involvement
Myopericytoma generally arises in subcutaneous tissue. There is a predilection for lesions to involve the distal extremities; however, tumours can also arise at other sites, including the proximal extremities and neck. It is likely that a wider site distribution will be described with increased recognition of this tumour.

Clinical features
Myopericytoma generally presents as a painless, slow-growing subcutaneous nodule that can be present for years. Some lesions are painful. Myopericytoma most commonly arises as a solitary lesion but multiple lesions are not infrequent. Multiple lesions generally arise metachronously and usually involve a particular anatomic region such as a foot.

Macroscopy
Myopericytoma tends to be a well circumscribed nodule measuring less than 2 cm in diameter.

Histopathology
Myopericytomas are unencapsulated and most lesions are fairly well circumscribed. Lesions are composed of relatively monomorphic oval-to-spindle shaped myoid appearing cells that show striking multilayered concentric growth around lesional blood vessels. The cells have eosinophilic or amphophilic cytoplasm. Lesions can be solidly cellular; however some cases have prominent myxoid stroma. In occasional cases, the spindle cells fall apart in the intervascular regions. In many cases, blood vessels outside the

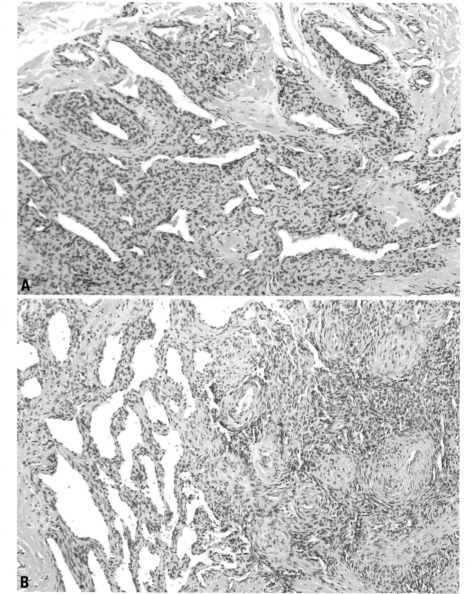

Fig. 5.07 Myopericytoma. **A** Typical proliferation of tumour cells around blood vessels at the periphery of this poorly circumscribed example. **B** Prominent gaping thin-walled blood vessels (left) and formation of whorls of spindle cells.

lesion also show concentric perivascular proliferation of spindle cells. Lesional blood vessels tend to be numerous and can be variable in size. In some cases, numerous thin walled branching or gaping blood vessels are present. Fasicular or whorled arrangements of spindle cells with abundant eosinophilic cytoplasm, embedded in myxoid stroma, are present in some cases. These areas are similar to the myoid whorls of myofibromatosis/ myofibroma and invagination or bulging of these areas into the lumina of lesional blood vessels is frequently seen. Subendothelial proliferation of lesional cells in vessel walls is frequently seen and, indeed, myopericytoma can be located entirely within the lumen of a vein. Some myopericytomas have a component of cells with glomus-type features including cuboidal shape, distinct cell borders, clear to eosinophilic cytoplasm and central round nuclei and the term *glomangiopericytoma* can be used in such cases. In reality a spectrum of lesions exists that includes myofibromatosis, myofibroma, infantile haemangiopericytoma, glomangiopericytoma and myopericytoma {295,825}. Rarely, lesions show marked hyalinization, cystic change or focal metaplastic bone. Mitoses are not conspicuous (generally much less than 1/10 HPF). Coagulative necrosis has been described in a glomangiopericytoma; however, this appears to be a very unusual finding {825}.

Immunophenotype

The spindle cells in myopericytomas are positive for smooth muscle actin (SMA). SMA staining is generally diffusely positive, but can be only focally positive, generally in a perivascular distribution.

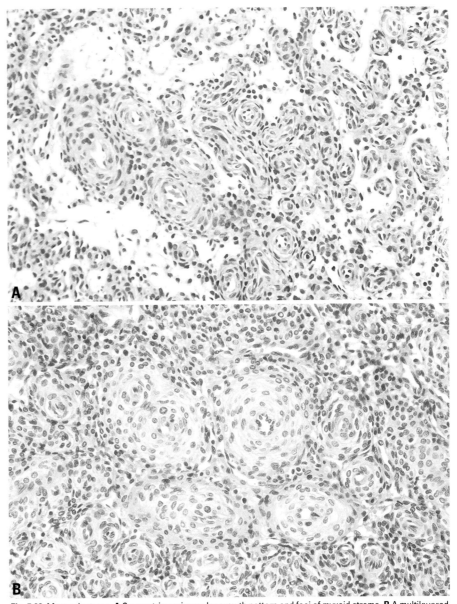

Fig. 5.08 Myopericytoma. **A** Concentric perivascular growth pattern and foci of myxoid stroma. **B** A multilayered concentric proliferation of spindle cells with myoid features around blood vessels.

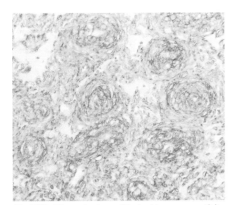

Fig. 5.09 Myopericytoma. Marked immunoreactivity for smooth muscle actin accentuates the perivascular growth pattern.

Occasional cases are focally desmin positive {825}. Focal CD34 staining by lesional cells occurs in some cases. Lesional cells are negative for S100 protein and most cases are negative for cytokeratin.

Prognostic factors

Most myopericytomas do not recur following excision. Recurrence may be related to poor circumscription of a lesion. Sometimes it is difficult to know whether a myopericytoma has recurred or whether a new lesion has developed in the same anatomic area. Very rare malignant myopericytomas exist {1383}.

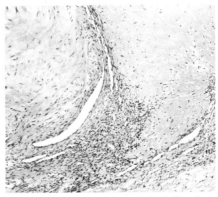

Fig. 5.10 Myopericytoma. A whorl of spindle cells in myxoid stroma bulges into the lumen of a blood vessel reminiscent of myofibromatosis / myofibroma.

CHAPTER 6

Skeletal Muscle Tumours

Extracardiac rhabdomyomas take several forms, may affect adults or children and are very rare. They are clinically benign and usually have no great biologic significance once they have been accurately diagnosed.

Malignant tumours showing skeletal muscle differentiation are very uncommon, but retain importance as they represent the largest subset of soft tissue sarcomas in infants and children. Because of the important prognostic differences, much emphasis has been placed in recent years on the more accurate and reproducible distinction between the embryonal and alveolar variants of rhabdomyosarcoma. Validation of this distinction (and important support for the existence of a solid variant of alveolar rhabdomyosarcoma) has come particularly from cytogenetic and molecular genetic analysis. With increasing and more reliable use of immunostains, rhabdomyosarcoma in adults is no longer regarded as exceptionally rare. In this age group it is most often represented by the pleomorphic subtype.

Rhabdomyoma

S.B. Kapadia
F.G. Barr

Rhabdomyoma (RM) is a benign mesenchymal tumour with skeletal muscle differentiation that is classified into cardiac and extracardiac types based on location {1978}. Cardiac RM will be dealt with in the WHO classification of heart tumours. Extracardiac RM is further classified into adult and fetal types, depending on the degree of differentiation, and has a predilection for the head and neck {515,1063,1065,1155,2274}. Rarely, RM may occur in the genital tract (genital RM). Unlike cardiac RM, there is no association with tuberous sclerosis {1065,1978,2274}.

ICD-O code   8900/0

Adult rhabdomyoma

Definition
Adult rhabdomyoma (A-RM) is a rare benign mesenchymal tumour with mature skeletal muscle differentiation and a predilection for the head and neck region.

ICD-O code   8904/0

Sites of involvement
The head and neck region (90%) is the most common site, mainly the upper aerodigestive mucosa (pharynx, oral cavity, and larynx) and soft tissue of neck {1065}.

Clinical features
The median age is 60 years (range 33 to 80 years) with a 3:1 male predominance {1065}. Symptoms include upper airway obstruction and mucosal or soft tissue mass (median duration 2 years, range 2 weeks to 3 years); in 10% the mass is asymptomatic {1065}. A-RM is often solitary (70%), but may be multinodular (26%) with discrete nodules in the same anatomic area or, rarely, multicentric (4%) {1065}.

Macroscopy
The mass (median size 3 cm, range 1.5 to 7.5 cm) is circumscribed deep tan to red-brown, soft, and nodular or lobulated {1065}.

Histopathology
A-RM is well circumscribed but unencapsulated and composed of lobules of closely packed uniform large polygonal cells in a scant stroma {1065}. The cells have abundant, eosinophilic, granular or vacuolated cytoplasm ("spider" cells) with well defined borders, and vesicular, small, round, centrally or peripherally located nuclei, at times with prominent nucleoli. Haphazardly arranged rod-like cytoplasmic inclusions and cross striations are seen focally. The glycogen-rich cytoplasm is periodic acid-Schiff (PAS)-positive, diastase sensitive. Phosphotungstic acid-hematoxylin, Masson trichrome or immunohistochemical stains highlight the cytoplasmic cross striations as well as the crystalline or rod-like inclusions {1065}.

Immunophenotype
The skeletal muscle differentiation is easily demonstrated on immunohistochemical stains with cytoplasmic positivity for MSA, desmin and myoglobin in all cases {368,616,880,933,1063,1065,2274}. Focal or rare positivity may be seen for vimentin, SMA and S100 protein. GFAP, cytokeratin, EMA, and CD68 stains are negative {1065}.

Ultrastructure
Electron microscopy demonstrates cytoplasmic myofilaments, Z-bands and glycogen granules {142,368,933,1155}.

Prognostic factors
Complete excision is the recommended treatment. In one study, follow-up showed local recurrence (42%) in the same anatomic site, from 2-11 years after diagnosis, often after incomplete

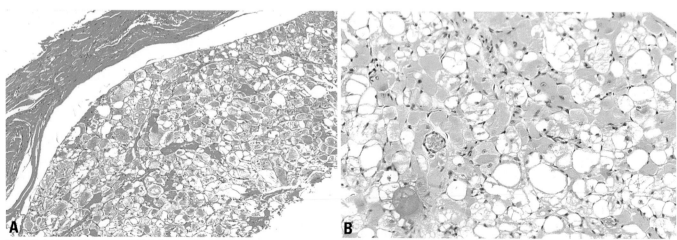

Fig. 6.01 Adult rhabdomyoma. **A** Well circumscribed mass composed of large polygonal cells with eosinophilic vacuolated cytoplasm and surrounded by normal skeletal muscle. **B** Higher magnification shows large, polygonal cells with abundant granular and vacuolated cytoplasm.

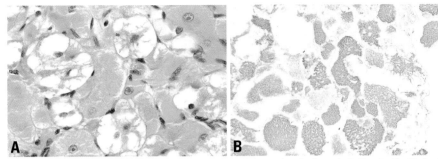

Fig. 6.02 Adult rhabdomyoma. **A** Vesicular nuclei and prominent round nucleoli are the hallmark of "spider" cells. **B** Cytoplasmic immunopositivity for myoglobin.

excision {1065}. A-RM may recur after many years or on more than one occasion, but lacks aggressive behaviour or malignant potential.

Fetal rhabdomyoma

Definition
Fetal rhabdomyoma (F-RM) is a rare benign mesenchymal tumour that exhibits immature skeletal muscle differentiation and a predilection for the head and neck.

ICD-O code   8903/0

Sites of involvement
More than 90% of F-RM occur in the soft tissue or mucosal sites of the head and neck although, rarely, other sites may be involved {409,485,1064,1620}. "Classic" F-RM has a predilection for the postauricular soft tissue {485,1064}, and those with "intermediate" differentiation tend to occur in soft tissue of face or in mucosal sites, but both subtypes may occur at any site in head and neck {1064}.

Clinical features
The median age is 4 years (range, 3 days-58 years) with a 2.4:1 male predominance {1064}. In one study, 10/24 cases (42%) were <1 year old, 6 (25%) were congenital, and 11 (46%) occurred in patients >15 years of age.
The median size is 3.0 cm (range 1-12.5 cm). F-RM presents as a well defined solitary mass involving soft tissue or mucosa (median duration 8 months, range 3 days to 19 years) {1064}. Some cases are associated with naevoid basal cell syndrome.

Macroscopy
F-RM presents as a solitary, circumscribed, soft, gray-white to tan-pink mass with a glistening cut surface. In mucosal sites F-RM is polypoid.

Histopathology
F-RM is circumscribed but unencapsulated. "Classic" immature F-RM is composed of bland primitive spindled cells associated with delicate fetal myotubules haphazardly arranged in abundant myxoid stroma. "Intermediate" F-RM (also referred to as "juvenile" or "cellular") displays a wider spectrum of differentiation or more advanced maturation between that of the "classic" F-RM and A-RM {485, 515, 1064, 1155, 1620}. Interlacing large strap-like striated muscle cells, broad fascicles of delicate spindled rhabdomyoblasts simulating a smooth muscle tumour, or ganglion-like rhabdomyoblasts may be seen {1064}. Nuclear atypia and necrosis are absent in F-RM. Mitoses are usually absent, but in one study 5/24 F-RM had had 1-14 mitoses/50HPF {1064}. The relationship of the latter cases to well differentiated embryonal rhabdomyosarcoma is unclear. Lack of prominent nuclear atypia is the most important criterion separating F-RM from rhabdomyosarcoma {1064}.

Immunophenotype
A skeletal muscle immunophenotype is demonstrated in all cases, with strong positivity for MSA, myoglobin and

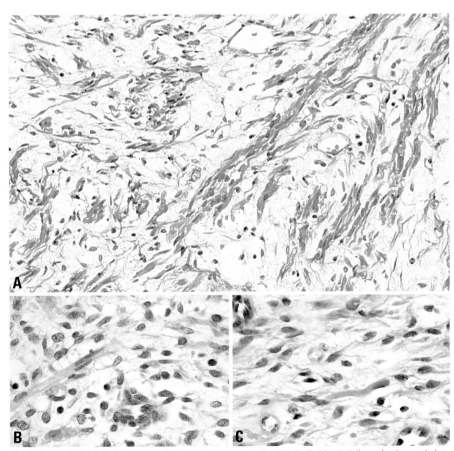

Fig. 6.03 Classic fetal rhabdomyoma. **A** Tumour is composed of cytologically bland, delicate fetal myotubules. **B** Primitive spindle cells in a myxoid stroma. **C** Occasional delicate rhabdomyoblasts display cross striations.

desmin {1064}. Focal reactivity may also be noted for SMA, S100 protein, GFAP, and vimentin {1064}. Vimentin staining is variable and often weak. Cytokeratin, CD68, and EMA are negative {1064}.

Ultrastructure
Electron microscopy demonstrates thick and thin myofilaments with Z-bands and glycogen within cytoplasm of immature rhabdomyoblasts {485}.

Genetic susceptibility
Multiple cases of fetal rhabdomyoma have been reported in patients with nevoid basal cell carcinoma syndrome {818}. This syndrome is caused by mutations in the tumour suppressor gene *PTCH* {524,866,1043}. *PTCH* encodes an inhibitory receptor in the sonic hedgehog signaling pathway, and germline mutations often lead to protein truncation and functional inactivation {2264}. Though rhabdomyomas have not been specifically examined, the wild-type allele is often eliminated by an allelic loss mechanism in other tumours found in this syndrome {755}.

Prognostic factors
Complete excision of the mass is the recommended treatment. In one study, follow-up available in 15 cases (median duration 49 months, range 2 months-52 years) showed local recurrence in only 1 case, at 3 months after excision, probably due to incomplete excision {1064}. None of the tumours metastasized.

Genital rhabdomyoma

Definition
Genital rhabdomyoma (G-RM) is a rare benign mesenchymal tumour with an advanced degree of skeletal muscle differentiation and a predilection for the vagina, almost exclusively in middle-aged women.

ICD-O code   8905/0

Sites of involvement
Most cases present as polyps in the vagina, vulva or cervix {322,750,803, 1066,1240,1283,2049}. Rare G-RM have been described in males in the parates-ticular region or epididymis {2085, 2225}.

Clinical features
The mean age is 42 years (range 30-48 years) {1066}. The mass may be asymptomatic or known to be present for 4-5 years {1066}. Vaginal RM is a well

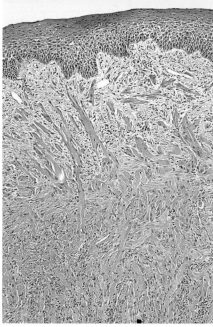

Fig. 6.05 Intermediate fetal rhabdomyoma. Submucosal mass shows broad strap-like rhabdomyoblasts with abundant eosinophilic cytoplasm.

defined, solitary mass with the clinical appearance of a benign vaginal polyp.

Macroscopy
The polypoid vaginal mass (median size 2 cm, range 1-3 cm) is covered by smooth mucosa. A pedicle (0.6-1.5 cm long) is seen in some cases.

Histopathology
The polypoid unencapsulated mass is composed of a haphazard arrangement of bland, interlacing, broad strap-like or round striated muscle cells embedded in a fibrous stroma containing dilated vascular channels {1066}. The cells have abundant eosinophilic glycogen-rich cytoplasm that displays uniform advanced maturation with cross striations and longitudinal myofibrils seen in many cells. One (or more) uniform, centrally located round vesicular nucleus contains prominent round nucleoli. Vaginal RM lacks the vacuolated "spider" cells seen in A-RM, and the prominent myxoid stroma and primitive spindle cells or delicate fetal-type rhabdomyoblasts seen in "classic" F-RM. They show more rhabdomyoblastic maturation than the "classic" F-RM and are analogous to some "intermediate" mucosal F-

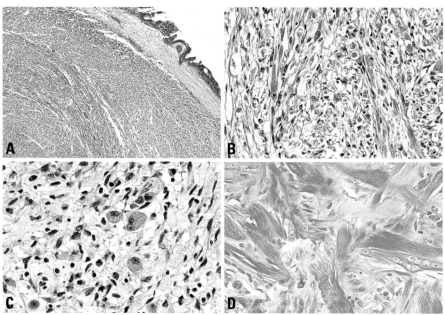

Fig. 6.04 Intermediate fetal rhabdomyoma. **A** Mucosal lesion showing more advanced rhabdomyoblastic maturation than the "classic" type. **B** Fascicles of spindled rhabdomyoblasts simulating smooth muscle cells. **C** Note round ganglion cell-like rhabdomyoblasts. **D** Cytoplasmic cross striations are highlighted by Masson trichrome stain.

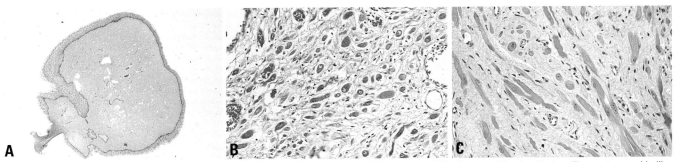

Fig. 6.06 Vaginal rhabdomyoma. **A** Whole mount shows a polypoid configuration and a fibrous stroma. **B** Medium magnification displays fibrous stroma with dilated vessels and round or strap-like rhabdomyoblasts with abundant eosinophilic cytoplasm. **C** Cellular details of rhabdomyoblasts.

RM of the head and neck. However, they lack the more variable cellular morphology and architecture of head and neck "intermediate" F-RM {1066}.

Immunophenotype
The skeletal muscle differentiation of G-RM is confirmed in all cases on immunohistochemical stains which show diffuse cytoplasmic positivity for MSA, myoglobin and desmin {1066, 1283, 2049, 2085, 2225}. The SMA, vimentin, cytokeratin, S-100, GFAP, Leu 7, EMA and CD 68 stains are negative {1066}.

Ultrastructure
Electron microscopy confirms the striated muscle origin of the striated rhabdomyoblasts in G-RM {803,1240, 2085}.

Prognostic factors
Local excision is adequate treatment. Follow-up available in four vaginal RM in one study (median duration 11 years, range 2 to 20 years) revealed no recurrence after excision and no evidence of tumour at other sites {1066}. G-RM lacks aggressive behaviour or any malignant potential.

Embryonal rhabdomyosarcoma

D.M. Parham
F.G. Barr

Definition

A primitive, malignant soft tissue sarcoma that recapitulates the phenotypic and biological features of embryonic skeletal muscle. The term embryonal rhabdomyosarcoma encompasses the spindle cell, botryoid, and anaplastic variants.

ICD-O codes

Embryonal rhabdomyosarcoma	8910/3
Spindle cell rhabdomyosarcoma	8912/3
Botryoid rhabdomyosarcoma	8910/3
Anaplastic rhabdomyosarcoma	8910/3

Synonyms

Myosarcoma, malignant rhabdomyoma, rhabdomyosarcoma, rhabdopoietic sarcoma, rhabdosarcoma, embryonal sarcoma.

Epidemiology

Rhabdomyosarcomas comprise the single largest category of soft tissue sarcomas in children and adolescents, occurring in 4.6/million U.S. children <15 years of age {860}. Embryonal rhabdomyosarcomas constitute the most common subtype of rhabdomyosarcoma, occurring in 3.0/million U.S. children <15 years of age {860}. Children less than ten years of ages are typically affected; among patients <15 years of age, only 17% of embryonal rhabdomyosarcoma arise in adolescents {860}. The greatest proportion (46%) of embryonal rhabdomyosarcomas occur in children less than 5 years of age. Five per cent of rhabdomyosarcomas affect infants {1746}, and a few are congenital {1011}. Embryonal rhabdomyosarcoma also constitutes important histological variant in adults {610, 910}, albeit such cases are rare.

In the U.S., embryonal rhabdomyosarcomas show a slight male:female predominance (1.2:1) {860}. Seventy per cent of U.S. rhabdomyosarcomas occur in non-Hispanic whites, compared to 14% in African-Americans, 10% in Hispanics, and 4.5% in Asians {846}, and incidence rates are higher in whites {1664}. Incidence figures in Europe resemble those in the U.S., with a similar male excess, whereas incidence rates appear somewhat lower in eastern and southern Asia {1664}.

Sites of involvement

Although embryonal rhabdomyosarcomas contain cells that are histologically identical to developing striated muscle, less than 9% arise within the skeletal musculature of the extremities. The greatest proportion occur within head and neck (about 47%), followed by the genitourinary system (about 28%) {1550}. Common locations in the genitourinary tract include the urinary bladder, prostate, and paratesticular soft tissues. Typical sites of origin in the head and neck include the soft tissues intrinsic to or surrounding the orbit and eyelid, oropharynx, parotid, auditory canal and middle ear, pterygoid fossa, nasopharynx, nasal passages and paranasal sinuses, tongue, and cheek. Besides these two general regions, embryonal rhabdomyosarcomas occur in the biliary tract, retroperitoneum, pelvis, perineum, and abdomen and have been reported in various visceral organs, such as the liver, kidney, heart, and lungs. Embryonal rhabdomyosarcomas may involve the soft tissues of the trunk and appendicular skeleton but much less frequently than alveolar rhabdomyosarcomas (see below). Primary origin in the skin also rarely occurs.

Spindle cell and botryoid variants of rhabdomyosarcoma involve a relatively limited repertoire of organs. Spindle cell rhabdomyosarcomas most commonly arise in the scrotal soft tissues, with the remainder mostly involving head and neck regions {316}. Spindle cell rhabdomyosarcoma also occurs in adults, usually in non-paratesticular locations {1818}. By definition, botryoid rhabdomyosarcomas must arise beneath a mucosal epithelial surface, limiting it to organs such as the urinary bladder, biliary tract, pharynx, conjunctiva, or auditory canal.

Clinical features

Coincident with the diversity of their anatomic origins, embryonal rhabdomyosarcomas produce a variety of clinical symptoms, generally related to mass effects and obstruction {1829}.

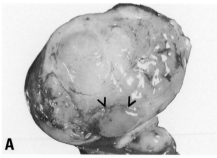
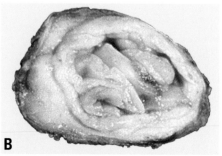
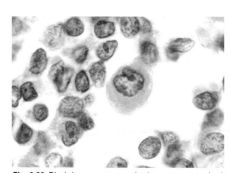

Fig. 6.07 A Large embryonal rhabdomyosarcoma involving the paratesticular soft tissues. The tumour forms a fleshy, pale tan mass with compression of the adjacent testis (arrows). **B** Botryoid rhabdomyosarcoma presenting as polypoid mucosal excrescences, obliterating the lumen of the gall bladder.

Fig. 6.08 Rhabdomyosarcoma. In the centre, a typical rhabdomyoblast, with an eccentric oval nucleus, central nucleolus, and eosinophilic cytoplasm.

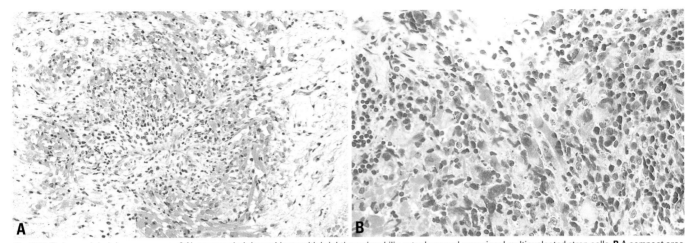

Fig. 6.09 Embryonal rhabdomyosarcoma. **A** Numerous rhabdomyoblasts with brightly eosinophilic cytoplasm and occasional multinucleated strap cells. **B** A compact area with rhabdomyoblastic differentiation adjacent to an area with loose, mucoid stroma.

Hence, head and neck lesions can cause proptosis, diplopia, sinusitis, or unilateral deafness, depending on their location. Similarly, genitourinary lesions may produce a scrotal mass or urinary retention, and biliary tumours may cause jaundice. Otherwise, the symptoms are generally those of a rapidly growing soft tissue mass.

Imaging studies are primarily used in delineating the extent of lesions for staging and prior to definitive surgery. Computed tomography and magnetic resonance imaging are most useful for these purposes, although ultrasonography can be used as a screening modality. Images generally recapitulate those of an expansile soft tissue mass in various organs, with heterogenous signals reflecting the variable vascularity, myx-

oid stroma, and necrosis. Of particular note is the striking appearance of botryoid lesions, which create a cluster of tumour nodules of variable size, typically within hollow viscera such as the urinary bladder or gall bladder.

Aetiology

Embryonal rhabdomyosarcomas may result from sporadic or inherited mutations, as discussed below. Generally this occurs as a variation of the Knudson-Strong two-hit hypothesis, which theoretically may involve loss of heterozygosity or aberrant gene methylation as well as DNA mutations. Malignant transformation of rhabdomyomas very rarely causes rhabdomyosarcoma. Carcinogens causing rhabdomyosarcomas in humans have not

been identified but have been found in studies of mice {2124} and zebrafish {2012}.

Macroscopy

Like most primitive pediatric neoplasms, embryonal rhabdomyosarcomas form poorly circumscribed, fleshy, pale tan masses that directly impinge upon neighbouring structures. Spindle cell and botryoid variants display additional distinctive features. Spindle cell rhabdomyosarcomas, like other spindle cell lesions, form firm, fibrous tumours with tan-yellow, whorled cut surfaces. Botryoid tumours, as the name implies, have a characteristic polypoid appearance with clusters of small, sessile or pendunculated nodules that abut an epithelial surface.

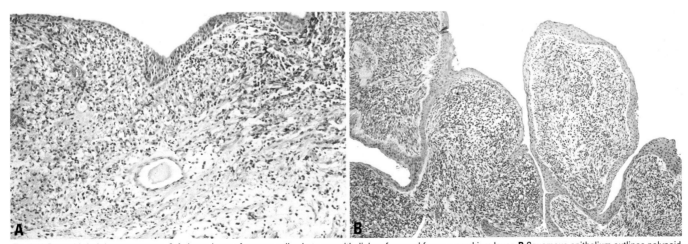

Fig. 6.10 Botryoid rhabdomyosarcoma. **A** A dense layer of tumour cells abuts an epithelial surface and forms a cambium layer. **B** Squamous epithelium outlines polypoid masses of tumour cells.

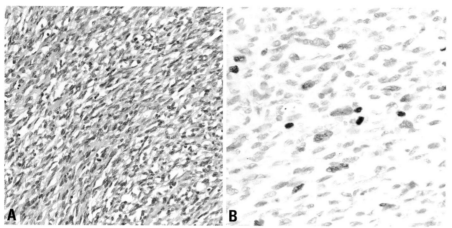

Fig. 6.11 Spindle cell rhabdomyosarcoma. **A** The fascicular architecture of this paratesticular tumour may readily be mistaken for other forms of spindle cell sarcoma. **B** Some tumour cells show nuclear immunopositivity for myf-4 (myogenin).

Histopathology

Analogous to embryonic skeletal muscle, embryonal rhabdomyosarcomas are composed of primitive mesenchymal cells in various stages of myogenesis, i.e. rhabdomyoblasts. Stellate cells with lightly amphophilic cytoplasm and central, oval nuclei represent the most primitive end of this spectrum. As these cells differentiate, they progressively acquire more cytoplasmic eosinophilia and elongate shapes, manifested in descriptive terms such as "tadpole", "strap", and "spider" cell. Bright eosinophilia, cytoplasmic cross striations, and multinucleation indicate terminal differentiation, and myotube forms may be evident. Differentiation tends to be more evident following chemotherapy, as differentiated elements become the predominant cell population, separated by therapy-induced necrosis and fibrosis {379}.

The histological architecture of embryonal rhabdomyosarcoma also resembles embryonic muscle, which forms aggregates of myoblasts amid loose, myxoid mesodermal tissues {1549}. Similarly, alternating areas of dense, compact cellularity and loose, myxoid tissues constitute embryonal rhabdomyosarcomas. The amount of loose and dense cellularity varies from case to case: an abundant, mucoid stroma containing scattered rhabdomyoblasts and resembling myxomas predominates in some examples, and compact aggregates of densely arrayed spindle cells form other tumours.

The botryoid variant of embryonal rhabdomyosarcoma contains linear aggregates of tumour cells that tightly abut an epithelial surface. This feature, known as a "cambium layer", typifies these tumours. Botryoid rhabdomyosarcomas also contain variable numbers of polypoid nodules, often with an abundant, loose, myxoid stroma that can appear deceptively benign.

Densely arrayed whorls or fascicles of spindle cells constitute the spindle cell variant of embryonal rhabdomyosarcoma. These spindle cells often resemble smooth muscle cells, with blunted central nuclei and tapered ends, but cytoplasmic cross striations, if present, and/or bright eosinophilia indicate striated muscle differentiation, which should be confirmed by immunohistochemistry. Spindle cell rhabdomyosarcomas may have a storiform architecture similar to fibrous histiocytoma or a wavy character like neurofibroma.

The presence of enlarged, atypical cells with hyperchromatic nuclei defines the anaplastic variant of rhabdomyosarcoma {1149}. This feature may be seen in both embryonal and alveolar tumours but is more prevalent in the former. Bizarre, multipolar mitoses are also often present. Anaplastic features can be focal or diffuse. Focal anaplasia indicates the presence of only single, dispersed anaplastic cells, whereas diffuse anaplasia indicates the presence of clone-like clusters of anaplastic cells.

Immunophenotype

Markers of skeletal muscle differentiation typify embryonal rhabdomyosarcomas {1653}. The presence of these markers correlates with the degree of tumour cell differentiation, as it does in embryogenesis. Thus, only vimentin is present in the cytoplasm of the most primitive cells, and desmin and actin are acquired by developing rhabdomyoblasts. Differentiated cells exhibit myoglobin, myosin, and creatine kinase M, markers that correspond to terminal differentiation. A variety of less commonly used muscle markers, such as titin, dystrophin, and acetylcholine receptor antigens alsocharacterize rhabdomyosarcomas. Muscle markers such as desmin and muscle-specific actin (HHF-35) are shared by cells with a myogenic phenotype, including smooth muscle, cardiac muscle, myofibroblasts, myoepithelial cells, pericytes, and some mesothelial cells.

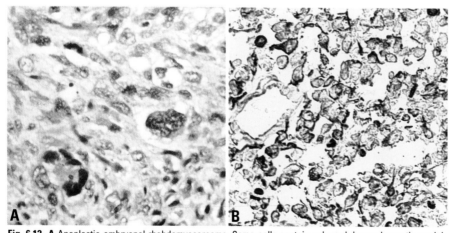

Fig. 6.12 A Anaplastic embryonal rhabdomyosarcoma. Some cells contain enlarged, hyperchromatic nuclei. **B** Desmin stain of rhabdomyosarcoma. Scattered tumour cells contain strongly positive cytoplasmic tails.

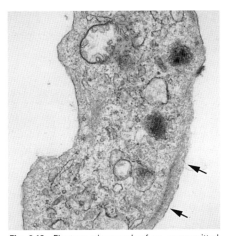

Fig. 6.13 Electron micrograph of an uncommitted mesenchymal cell in rhabdomyosarcoma. There are no features of myoblastic differentiation. Note the subplasmalemmal microfilaments (arrows).

Antibodies against MyoD1 and myogenin are highly specific and sensitive for rhabdomyosarcoma and are currently used as standard antibodies for diagnosis {321}. However, one must note that only nuclear staining is specific and that non-specific cytoplasmic MyoD positivity is common in heat-retrieved, paraffin-embedded tissues {2214}.

Occasional aberrant staining with a variety of immunohistochemical markers has been noted. Aberrantly expressed markers include cytokeratin, S100 protein, neurofilaments, and B cell proteins such as CD20 and immunoglobulins {384, 1450, 1709}. Smooth muscle actin and neuron-specific enolase staining occurs more frequently (in 10% and 30% of rhabdomyosarcomas, respectively) {1652, 1653}.

Ultrastructure

Rhabdomyosarcomas exhibit a range of ultrastructural characteristics corresponding to those of developing striated muscle, primarily bundles of 5 and 15 nm thick and thin filaments punctuated by abortive Z-bands. Parallel arrays of 15 nm filaments and ribosomes (myosin-ribosome complexes) comprise the earliest diagnostic stage {609}. Earlier cells show non-specific features of primitive mesenchyme, such as discontinuous basal lamina, phagocytosed collagen, and ergastoplasm {520}. These uncommitted cells may contain lipid or subplasmalemmal microfilaments. Leptomeric fibrils may be seen on occasion.

Genetics

Molecular analyses of polymorphic loci revealed allelic loss in chromosomal region 11p15 in most embryonal rhabdomyosarcomas {1160,1915}. The finding of growth suppression when chromosomal fragments containing the 11p15 region were introduced into embryonal rhabdomyosarcoma cells further supports the premise that there is a tumour suppressor gene within this region {1152,1278}. Furthermore, inherited alterations of the 11p15 region occur in Beckwith-Wiedemann syndrome {1251}, a heterogeneous overgrowth syndrome with an increased risk for development of several cancers, including embryonal rhabdomyosarcoma. Expression studies have indicated that several 11p15 genes, such as *IGF2*, *H19*, and *CDKN1C*, are expressed from one of the two alleles in a parent-of-origin specific process termed imprinting. These combined findings suggest a model in which an imprinted tumour suppressor gene is inactivated during embryonal rhabdomyosarcoma tumourigenesis by allelic loss of the active allele and retention of the inactive allele.

Cytogenetic studies of embryonal rhabdomyosarcoma have found complex structural and numerical chromosomal changes, often including extra copies of chromosomes 2, 8, and 13 {816, 2210}. Rearrangements of the 1p11-q11 and 12q13 regions have also been noted in a fraction of cases. Subsequent comparative genomic hybridization analyses of genome-wide copy number changes confirmed chromosomal gains and identified several regions of loss, such as chromosome 16, in embryonal rhabdomyosarcoma subsets {260, 2223}. These analyses also indicated that genomic amplification was generally rare in embryonal rhabdomyosarcoma, except for its subset with anaplastic features {259}. Finally, directed analyses of known oncogenes and suppressor genes identified inactivating mutations of *TP53* {648} and *CDKN2A* {1009} and activating mutations of *RAS* family genes in subsets of embryonal rhabdomyosarcoma {2041}. These various genetic alterations may indicate

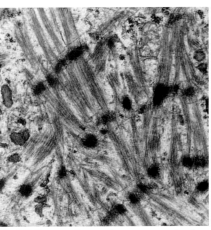

Fig. 6.14 Electron microscopic appearance of embryonal rhabdomyosarcoma showing well-formed Z-bands.

variable collaborating events that occur during embryonal rhabdomyosarcoma tumourigenesis.

Prognostic factors

Prognosis can be determined by stage, histological classification, age, and site of origin. Staging is accomplished by clinical evaluation (IRSG Stage) or surgicopathological evaluation (IRSG Group) {1755}. Younger patients tend to have a more favourable prognosis. Histological classification in paediatric patients predicts outcome independent of age, stage, and location, with embryonal tumours having a better prognosis than alveolar tumours {1755}. Spindle cell and botryoid variants have a superior outcome as a group. However, the rare spindle cell lesions in adults are more aggressive {1818} and, in fact, histological subtype in adults with rhabdomyosarcoma appears to have no prognostic relevance. Embryonal rhabdomyosarcomas with diffuse anaplasia may have a worse outcome than the other subsets of embryonal rhabdomyosarcoma {1149}. Parameningeal and extremity tumours tend to have a bad outcome compared to other locations, whereas orbital and paratesticular tumours tend to have a better one.

Tumour cell ploidy predicts outcome in some reports, with hyperdiploid embryonal rhabdomyosarcomas having a better outcome. However, this phenomenon has not been universally confirmed and does not appear to be an independent variable {478,1107,1928}.

Alveolar rhabdomyosarcoma

D.M. Parham
F.G. Barr

Definition

Alveolar rhabdomyosarcoma is a primitive, malignant, round cell neoplasm that cytologically resembles lymphoma and which shows partial skeletal muscle differentiation.

ICD-O code   8920/3

Synonyms

Rhabdomyoblastoma, rhabdomyopoietic sarcoma, monomorphous round cell rhabdomyosarcoma.

Epidemiology

Alveolar rhabdomyosarcomas occur at all ages, but they do not show a predilection for younger children and more often occur in adolescents and young adults; very rare cases may be congenital. The median ages of affected patients was 6.8 and 9.0 years in reports from the International Society of Pediatric Oncology (SIOP) {291}, and the Intergroup Rhabdomyosarcoma Study (IRS) {1550}. They occur less frequently than embryonal rhabdomyosarcomas (21% of rhabdomyosarcomas in the IRS report; 19% in the SIOP report). The male:female ratio is approximately even. No geographic or racial predilection is reported.

Sites of involvement

Alveolar rhabdomyosarcomas commonly arise in the extremities, where 39% were reported in the the Kiel Paediatric Tumour registry {887}. The Armed Forces Institute of Pathology series indicates that there is no favoured site of origin {596}. Additional sites of involvement include the paraspinal and the perineal regions and the paranasal sinuses. Mixed embryonal/alveolar tumours may arise in areas favoured by embryonal rhabdomyosarcomas, such as the urogenital tract and orbit, but generally these are unusual sites of origin {887}.

Clinical features

Alveolar rhabdomyosarcomas typically present as rapidly growing extremity masses. Paranasal lesions may present with proptosis or cranial nerve deficits. Perirectal tumours can cause constipation. Paraspinal lesions can cause nerve root abnormalities, such as paresthesia, hypesthesia, or paresis. Imaging is best accomplished by nuclear magnetic resonance, which reveals an infiltrative, expansile, soft tissue mass. Rare tumours present as disseminated lesions with no obvious primary and resemble leukaemia {613}.

Alveolar rhabdomyosarcomas tend to be high stage lesions at presentation {1158, 1756}.

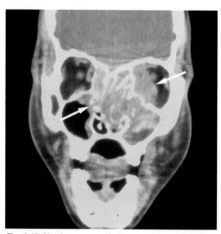

Fig. 6.15 Nuclear magnetic image of a cranial alveolar rhabdomyosarcoma. The expansile lesion destroys the nasal and paranasal bone and extends into the orbit and parameningeal tissues (arrows).

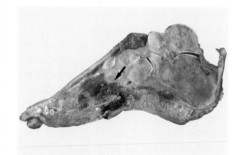

Fig. 6.16 Sagittal section of foot containing alveolar rhabdomyoasarcoma. An infiltrative, haemorrhagic mass arises in the soft tissue of the plantar and metatarsal soft tissues (arrows).

Macroscopy

Alveolar rhabdomyosarcomas form expansile, rapidly growing soft tissue tumours with a fleshy, grey tan quality. They contain variable amounts of fibrous tissue.

Histopathology

Three major histological subtypes comprise alveolar rhabdomyosarcoma: those with typical features, those with a solid pattern, and those with mixed embryonal and alveolar features {1549}. All alveolar rhabdomyosarcomas exhibit round cell cytological features reminiscent of lymphomas but with primitive myoblastic differentiation. Morphologic features vary, depending on the presence or absence of fibrous stroma and embryonal histology. Typical alveolar rhabdomyosarcomas produce fibrovascular septa that separate the tumour cells into discrete nests. These nests contain central clusters of cells with loss of cohesion around the periphery. Tumour cells align the septa in a picket fence pattern. Giant cells with rhabdomyoblastic differentiation are common. Occasional cases show clear cell morphology and may mimic clear cell carcinoma or liposarcoma.

Solid variant alveolar rhabdomyosarcomas lack the fibrovascular stroma and form sheets of round cells with variable rhabdomyoblastic differentiation (often little). Occasional small nests may be seen, particularly with larger samples. The cytologic features do not differ from typical lesions {2138}.

Mixed embryonal / alveolar rhabdomyosarcomas contain foci with embryonal histology, i.e., myxoid stroma and spindle cell myoblasts as well as areas with alveolar histology. The alveolar foci usually contain nests with fibrous stroma, although highly cellular solid foci resembling lymphoma may occur.

Immunophenotype

Alveolar rhabdomyosarcomas stain with antibodies against muscle proteins, as described under "Embryonal rhab-

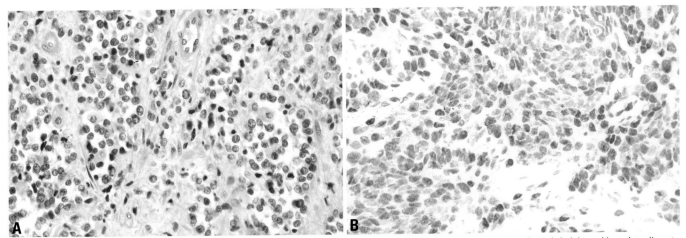

Fig. 6.17 A Typical alveolar rhabdomyosarcoma. Collagenous fibrovascular septa divide mixtures of undifferentiated tumour cells and rhabdomyoblasts into discrete nests. **B** Myogenin stain of alveolar rhabdomyosarcoma. Many tumour cell nuclei show strong immunopositivity.

domyosarcoma" (see above), although primitive tumours may have focal or lack positivity. MyoD-related stains, especially myogenin, typically show a diffuse, strong nuclear staining pattern {516}.

Genetics

Cytogenetic analyses demonstrated recurrent translocations that are consistently and specifically associated with alveolar rhabdomyosarcoma. A t(2;13)(q35;q14) was found in the majority of alveolar rhabdomyosarcoma cases and a t(1;13)(p36;q14) was noted in a smaller subset of cases {125}. These translocations juxtapose the *PAX3* or *PAX7* genes on chromosomes 2 and 1, respectively, with the *FKHR* gene on chromosome 13, to generate chimeric genes which encode PAX3/FKHR and PAX7/FKHR fusion proteins {127,456,

759}. PAX3 and PAX7 are related members of the paired box family of transcription factors whereas FKHR is a member of the forkhead transcription factor family. The PAX3/FKHR and PAX7/FKHR fusion products contain the PAX3/PAX7 DNA binding domain and the FKHR transcriptional activation domain, and function as potent transcriptional activators {162, 163}. In addition to this functional change, the translocations also alter the expression and subcellular localization of regulatory pathways to generate high levels of these chimeric proteins that are constitutively present in the nucleus {455, 495}. These changes maximize the ability of these chimeric proteins to activate downstream transcriptional targets, and are postulated to exert oncogenic effects by altering control of proliferation, apoptosis, and differ-

entiation {170,605,1097,1211}

As part of an effort to find other genetic alterations that collaborate with the gene fusion events in alveolar rhabdomyosarcoma tumourigenesis, comparative genomic hybridization studies of ARMS cases identified a variety of amplification events {814}. The most frequent amplification events in alveolar rhabdomyosarcoma, each occurring in roughly one-third of cases, involve chromosomal regions 12q13-15 and 2p24. The 12q13-15 region contains many growth-related genes such as the *GLI*, *CDK4*, and *MDM2*, whereas the 2p24 region harbours the *MYCN* oncogene, which is amplified in several tumour categories, such as neuroblastoma. Other less frequent amplicons occur at chromosomal regions 13q31, 2q34-qter, 15q24-26, and 1p36. The *PAX7/FKHR* fusion gene is

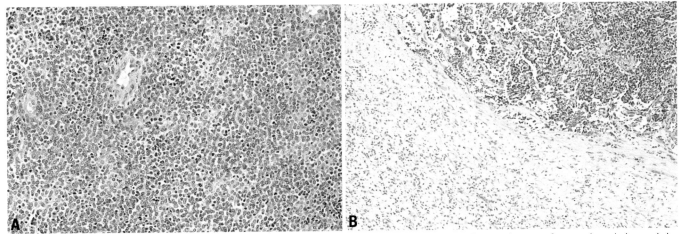

Fig. 6.18 A Solid variant alveolar rhabdomyosarcoma. Sheets of undifferentiated rhabdomyosarcoma cells without fibrovascular septa. Cytogenetic analysis revealed a t(2;13) translocation, characteristic of alveolar rhabdomyosarcoma. **B** Mixed alveolar-embryonal rhabdomyosarcoma. A discrete, highly cellular focus of alveolar rhabdomyosarcoma contrasts with the adjacent loose embryonal histology.

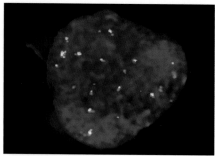

Fig. 6.19 1460 Alveolar rhabdomyosarcoma. Interphase fluorescence in situ hybridization (FISH) analysis showing amplification of the *PAX7/FKHR* fusion gene (juxtaposed red and green signals) by 1;13 translocation breakpoint-flanking probes.

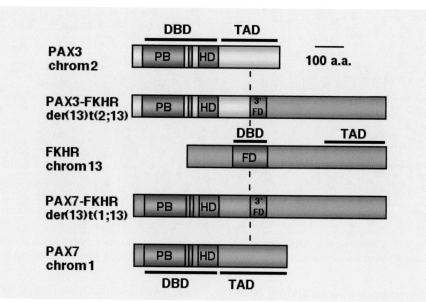

Fig. 6.20 Wild-type and fusion products associated with the 2;13 and 1;13 translocations. The paired box, octapeptide, homeobox and fork head domain are shown as grey boxes. Transcriptional domains (DNA binding domain - DBD, transcriptional activiation domain - TAD) are indicated as solid horizontal bars. The translocation fusion point is shown as a vertical dashed line.

amplified in the majority of ARMS cases with the 1;13 translocation in contrast to the less frequent amplification of the *PAX3/FKHR* fusion in alveolar rhabdomyosarcoma with the 2;13 translocation {128}.

The subset of alveolar rhabdomyosarcomas not displaying a typical *PAX/FKHR* gene fusion is genetically heterogeneous, with some cases showing alternative fusions with other genes or unusual fusion products and some possibly being true fusion-negative cases {129}.

Prognostic factors

Alveolar rhabdomyosarcomas are high grade neoplasms that are inherently more aggressive than embryonal rhabdomyosarcomas {1755}. Surgicopathological staging (IRS grouping) is predictive of outcome. With mixed embryonal / alveolar tumours, site may also be predictive, as described under "Embryonal rhabdomyosarcoma", although, in general these mixed lesions behave the same as the alveolar subtype. Age predicts outcome of rhabdomyosarcomas in general {1200}. Preliminary data indicate that genetic fusions predict outcome, with *PAX7/FKHR* positive tumours behaving in a more benign fashion than *PAX3/FKHR* positive ones {1085}.

Pleomorphic rhabdomyosarcoma

E. Montgomery
F.G. Barr

Definition

Pleomorphic rhabdomyosarcoma is a high grade sarcoma occurring almost exclusively in adults and consisting of bizarre polygonal, round, and spindle cells which display evidence of skeletal muscle differentiation. No embryonal or alveolar component should be identified.

ICD-O code   8901/3

Epidemiology

These lesions occur almost exclusively in adults, are more common in men and present at a median age in the 6th decade {675,746,748,753,1897}.
Exceptional cases may be seen in children but their existence has been disputed {1550}.

Sites of involvement

These tumours usually occur in the deep soft tissues of the lower extremities but have been reported in a wide variety of other locations {37,389,675,746,748, 753,1149,1897}.

Clinical features

Most patients present with a rapidly-growing painful swelling {748}. On imaging, lesions are isointense to skeletal muscle on T1 weighted images and heterogeneous on T2 images. Necrotic foci are readily identifiable in many cases.

Macroscopy

Tumours are well circumscribed, usually large (5-15 cm), and often surrounded by a pseudocapsule. The cut surface is whitish and firm with variable haemorrhage and necrosis.

Histopathology

These are pleomorphic sarcomas composed of undifferentiated round to spindle cells and an admixture of polygonal cells with densely eosinophilic cytoplasm in spindle, tadpole, and racquet-like contours. Some observers have classified adult lesions into "classic" (pleomorphic rhabdomyoblasts in sheets), "round cell", and "spindle cell" patterns {748}. Cross striations are vanishingly rare. The presence of pleomorphic polygonal rhabdomyoblasts on routine hematoxylin and eosin stains coupled with immunohistochemical evidence of at least one skeletal muscle-specific marker by immunohistochemistry is required for diagnosis {675,748,753}.

Immunophenotype

Pleomorphic rhabdomyosarcomas, like other rhabdomyosarcoma types, express myoglobin, MyoD1, skeletal muscle myogenin, fast (skeletal muscle) myosin, and desmin. They variably express muscle specific actin, smooth muscle actin, and myogenin {517, 675, 746, 748, 753, 1149, 1897, 2251}. Interestingly, myoD1 and myogenin seem to show more limited positivity than in paediatric rhabdomyosarcomas. They lack epithelial markers and S100 protein.

Ultrastructure

By ultrastructure, rudimentary sarcomere formation is the key criterion. Such sarcomeres consist of Z-bands or irregular masses of Z-band material with converging thick (16nm) and thin (8nm) filaments {748, 1897}.

Genetics

Only six pleomorphic rhabdomyosarcomas with chromosome aberrations have been reported. All had highly complex karyotypes, and in none of them could a t(1;13) or t(2;13) translocation be detected {1477}.

Prognostic factors

The prognosis for these tumours is poor and reliable prognostic factors have yet to be developed. In two series with follow-up, 28/38 patients (74%) died of disease {748, 753}.

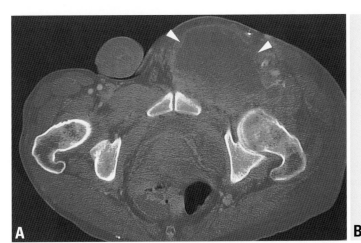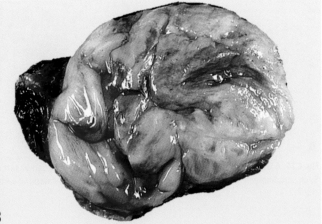

Fig. 6.21 A CT without contrast enhancement of a recurrent pleomorphic rhabdomyosarcoma. The tumour is similar in consistency to the adjacent skeletal muscles. **B** This mass, which displays zones of necrosis, was excised from the thigh of a 56-year-old man. The lesion extended into the pelvis and recurred quickly following the initial resection.

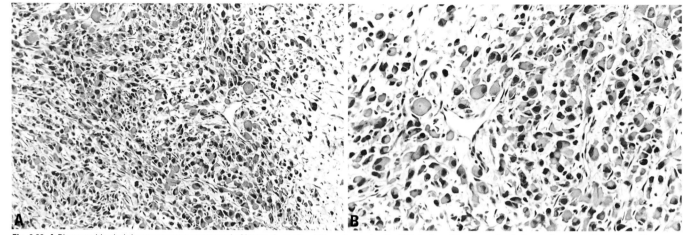

Fig. 6.22 A Pleomorphic rhabdomyosarcoma composed of intensely eosinophilic polygonal cells. **B** Note the wide range of cell shapes from round to tadpole-like.

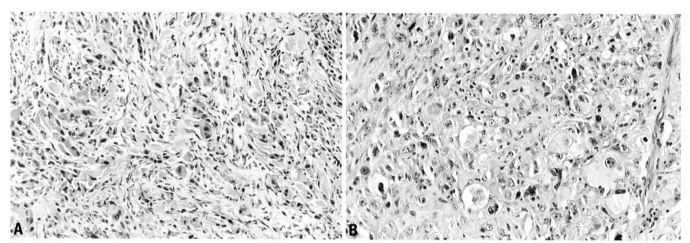

Fig. 6.23 A Pleomorphic rhabdomyosarcoma composed of spindled and polygonal cells. **B** Bizarre nuclei and abundant cytoplasm are seen in this example of pleomorphic rhabdomyosarcoma.

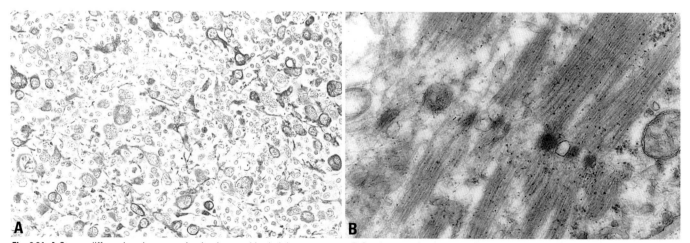

Fig. 6.24 A Strong diffuse desmin expression in pleomorphic rhabdomyosarcoma. **B** On electron microscopy, rudimentary sarcomere formation is the key criterion. Such sarcomeres consist of Z-bands or irregular masses of Z-band material with converging thick (16 nm) and thin (8 nm) filaments.

CHAPTER 7

Vascular Tumours

Benign vascular tumours are very common and most frequently occur in the skin (see WHO classification of skin tumours). At all sites, it is often difficult to determine whether benign vascular lesions are malformations, true neoplasms or, in some cases, reactive processes. Similarly, it remains essentially impossible to reliably distinguish blood vessel endothelium from lymphatic endothelium, which probably reflects the close functional and embryogenetic relationship between these cell types.

Changes and advances since the 1994 WHO classification include the characterization of various newly recognized entities, particularly in the categories of intermediate malignancy, including the kaposiform, retiform and composite types of haemangioendothelioma. Use of the term 'haemangioendothelioma' remains problematic since, in the past, this term has been used variably for benign, intermediate and malignant lesions. In current practice, the term usually connotes intermediate malignancy, except in the context of epithelioid haemangioendothelioma, the metastatic rate of which is high enough (albeit much lower than conventional angiosarcoma) to justify its classification as malignant.

Angiosarcomas in soft tissue are now more frequently recognized, in large part to the realization that many such tumours have epithelioid cytomorphology at deep soft tissue locations, including the pleural and peritoneal cavities.

Haemangiomas

E. Calonje

Synovial haemangioma

Definition
Synovial haemangioma (SH) is a benign proliferation of blood vessels arising in a synovium-lined surface, including the intra-articular space and bursa. Similar lesions occurring within the tendon sheath do not fall into this diagnostic category.

Epidemiology
SH is very rare. Most patients are children or adolescents and there is a predilection for males {509}.

Sites of involvement
The most common site by far is the knee, followed much less commonly by the elbow and hand.

Clinical features
The tumour presents as a slowly growing lesion often associated with swelling and joint effusion {509}. Recurrent pain is a frequent symptom. In about one third of cases pain is not a feature. Magnetic resonance imaging is the best radiological technique to identify the lesion particularly with regards to the extent of involvement {835}.

Aetiology
The presentation of most lesions at a young age suggests that SH is a form of vascular malformation. Trauma is unlikely to be of relevance in the pathogenesis.

Macroscopy
Numerous congested, variably dilated vessels of different calibre can be seen and the tumour can be fairly circumscribed or diffuse.

Histopathology
The tumour often has the appearance of a cavernous haemangioma with multiple dilated thin-walled vascular channels. A smaller percentage of cases have the appearance of either a capillary or arteriovenous haemangioma. The vascular channels are located underneath the synovial membrane and are surrounded by myxoid or fibrotic stroma. Haemosiderin deposition can be prominent. Secondary villous hyperplasia of the synovium is present in some cases.

Prognostic factors
Small lesions are usually easy to remove completely with no risk of local recurrence. When more diffuse involvement of the joint is present, complete excision can be difficult to achieve.

Intramuscular angioma

Definition
Intramuscular angioma (IA) is defined as a proliferation of benign vascular channels within skeletal muscle and it is associated in most instances with variable amounts of mature adipose tissue.

ICD-O code   9132/0

Synonyms
Intramuscular haemangioma, intramuscular angiolipoma.

Epidemiology
Although relatively uncommon, IA is one of the most frequent deep-seated soft tissue tumours. The age range is wide but adolescents and young adults are most commonly affected (in up to 90% of cases) {44,152,651}. Lesions have often been present for many years and it is therefore likely that many examples are congenital. There is an equal sex incidence.

Sites of involvement
IA most commonly affects the lower limb, particularly the thigh, followed by the head and neck, upper limb and trunk. Rare cases can present in the mediastinum and retroperitoneum.

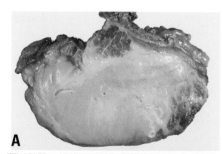
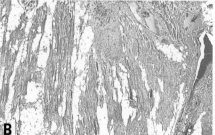

Fig. 7.02 Intramuscular haemangioma. **A** This lesion was excised from the rectus abdominis muscle of a young adult female. Note the poorly circumscribed margins and prominent fatty stroma. **B** Extensive replacement of the muscle by dilated vascular channels with focal thrombosis. Note the prominent adipocytic component.

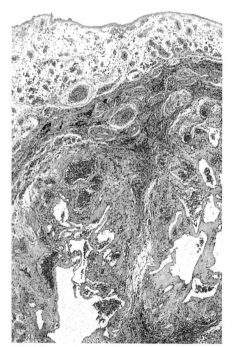

Fig. 7.01 Synovial haemangioma. A mixture of cavernous and capillary vascular channels underlie the synovium.

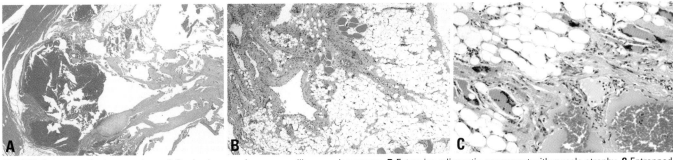

Fig. 7.03 Intramuscular haemangioma. **A** Predominance of cavernous-like vascular spaces. **B** Extensive adipocytic component with muscle atrophy. **C** Entrapped muscle fibres with hyperchromatic, reactive nuclei.

Clinical features

The typical presentation is that of a slowly growing mass which is often painful, particularly after exercise. Pain is mainly present in tumours located in the limbs. Radiological examination often reveals the presence of calcification secondary to phleboliths or metaplastic ossification.

Aetiology

It is likely that these lesions are malformations and there is no relation to trauma.

Macroscopy

Tumours are often large and there is diffuse infiltration of the involved muscle. Variably sized vascular channels with thrombosis and haemorrhage are usually readily seen. The appearance of the tumour can be solid and yellowish as a result of the presence of adipose tissue. Lesions also appear solid when capillaries predominate.

Histopathology

IA has been traditionally classified according to the vessel size into small (capillary), large (cavernous) and mixed. This is not practical, however, as most tumours contain a mixture of vascular channels frequently including lymphatics. IA usually consists of large thick-walled veins, a mixture of cavernous-like vascular spaces and capillaries or a prominent arteriovenous component. Tumours purely composed of capillaries have a predilection for the head and neck area and those with a predominant cavernous lymphatic component are seen mainly on the trunk, proximal upper limb and head. Variable amounts of mature adipose tissue are almost always present and may be very prominent. This explains why IA was sometimes known in the past as angiolipoma {1264}. Atrophy of muscle fibres secondary to the infiltra-

tive nature of the tumour often results in degenerative/reactive sarcolemmal changes with hyperchromatic nuclei.

Prognostic factors

The rate of local recurrence is high (between 30 to 50%) and therefore wide local excision is recommended.

Venous haemangioma

Definition

Venous haemangioma (VH) is composed of veins of variable size, often having thick muscular walls. Intramuscular angiomas and angiomatosis can be composed almost exclusively of veins but are usually intermixed with other vessel types. These subtypes are described under their respective headings.

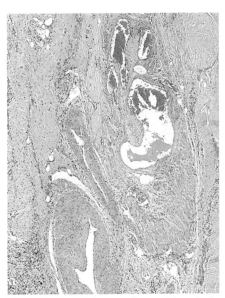

Fig. 7.04 Venous haemangioma with typically numerous prominent thick-walled veins.

ICD-O code   9122/0

Epidemiology

Pure VHs are rare and mainly present in adults.

Sites of involvement

Tumours present in the subcutaneous or deeper soft tissues with predilection for the limbs.

Clinical features

VH often presents as a long-standing slowly growing tumour. Radiological examination often shows the presence of calcification due to phleboliths.

Aetiology

The clinical evolution and clinicopathological features suggest that these lesions represent vascular malformations.

Macroscopy

VH is ill defined and consists of dilated congested vascular spaces with areas of haemorrhage.

Histopathology

VH typically consists of large thick-walled vessels, which are variably dilated and commonly display thrombosis with occasional formation of phleboliths. Widely dilated vessels can show attenuation of their walls, mimicking a cavernous haemangioma.

Elastic stains reveal the absence of an internal elastic lamina. This aids in the distinction from an arteriovenous haemangioma.

Prognostic factors

Deep-seated tumours are difficult to excise and can recur locally but subcutaneous tumours do not show a tendency to recur.

Arteriovenous haemangioma

Definition
Arteriovenous haemangioma (AVH) is a non-neoplastic vascular lesion characterized by the presence of arteriovenous shunts. There are two distinctive variants {63,1825}: deep-seated and cutaneous (cirsoid aneurysm or acral arteriovenous tumour; see WHO classification of skin tumours).

When these lesions involve multiple tissue planes, they are termed angiomatosis (see page 161). AVH should not be confused with juvenile, cutaneous (cellular) haemangiomas as they do not regress spontaneously.

ICD-O code   9123/0

Synonym
Arteriovenous malformation.

Epidemiology
Deep-seated AVH is uncommon and affects children and young adults.

Sites of involvement
AVH affects predominantly the head and neck followed by the limbs.

Clinical features
Angiography is an essential tool to confirm the diagnosis and establish the extent of the disease. Lesions are often associated with a variable degree of arteriovenous shunting and this can be severe enough to induce limb hypertrophy, heart failure, and consumption coagulopathy (Kasabach-Merritt syndrome). Pain is also a frequent symptom and superficial cutaneous changes mimicking Kaposi sarcoma clinically and histologically can be seen (pseudo-Kaposi sarcoma or acroangiodermatitis) {2046}. The presence of shunting can be confirmed clinically by auscultation.

Macroscopy
Tumours are ill defined and contain variable numbers of small and large blood vessels, many of which are dilated.

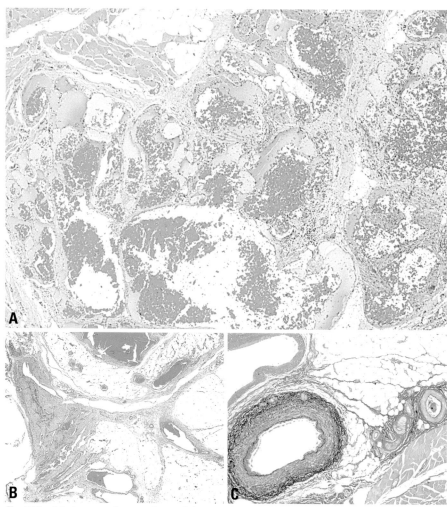

Fig. 7.05 Arteriovenous haemangioma. **A** In some cases, cavernous vascular spaces predominate. **B** Extensive infiltration of the subcutaneous tissue by large vessels. **C** An elastic stain is useful to determine the type of vessels (elastic van Gieson).

Histopathology
This diagnosis always requires clinico-pathological and radiological correlation. AVH is characterized by large numbers of vessels of different size, which include veins and arteries with the former largely outnumbering the latter. Areas resembling a cavernous or capillary haemangioma are frequent, as are thrombosis and calcification. Recognition of arteriovenous shunts is difficult and requires examination of numerous serial sections. Fibrointimal thickening in veins is a useful diagnostic clue.

Elastic stains are helpful in distinguishing between arteries and veins. Negative GLUT-1 staining may facilitate distinction from juvenile haemangioma {1582}.

Prognostic factors
Treatment is difficult because of the degree of involvement, which has to be determined by angiographic examination. Local recurrence is common because of the difficulties in achieving complete excision.

Epithelioid haemangioma

J.F. Fetsch

Definition
A benign vascular tumour with well formed but often immature vessels, the majority of which are lined by plump, epithelioid (histiocytoid) endothelial cells with amphophilic or eosinophilic cytoplasm and a large nucleus with an open chromatin pattern and central nucleolus. Subcutaneous examples are usually associated with a muscular artery. Most cases have a prominent inflammatory component.

ICD-O code   9125/0

Synonyms
Angiolymphoid hyperplasia with eosinophilia {314, 661, 1059, 1384, 1612, 1805, 2248}, nodular angioblastic hyperplasia with eosinophilia and lymphofolliculosis {158}, subcutaneous angioblastic lymphoid hyperplasia with eosinophilia {1769} and inflammatory angiomatoid nodule.

Epidemiology
Epithelioid haemangioma affects a wide age range, peaking in the third through fifth decades {661, 1612}. Females appear to be affected more commonly than males.

Sites of involvement
The most frequently affected sites are the head, especially the forehead, preauricular area, and scalp (often in the distribution of the superficial temporal artery), and the distal portions of the extremities, especially the digits {661,1612}.

Clinical features
The majority of patients present with a mass of a year or less in duration. However, some examples have been reported to be present for as many as 15 years before excision {661,1612}. The process is usually uninodular, but multinodularity (generally in contiguous areas) is encountered with some frequency. Most examples affect the subcutis, with dermal examples being less frequent, and deep-seated cases being rare {661, 1612}. Rare cases arise from a large vessel. The most frequent preoperative clinical impressions are an epidermal cyst or angioma {1612}.

Aetiology
There remains considerable controversy as to whether epithelioid haemangioma (angiolymphoid hyperplasia with eosinophilia) is a reactive lesion or a true neoplasm. Features that lend support for a reactive process include: 1) a predilection for superficial soft tissue sites that overlie bone and have minimal soft tissue padding, coupled with a compelling history of trauma in up to 10% of cases {661,1612}, 2) a tendency for subcutaneous examples to be well delineated and symmetrically organized around a larger vessel that may have evidence of damage (e.g., fibro-intimal proliferation, a disrupted elastic lamina, or mural disruption), 3) a pronounced inflammatory reaction, and 4) some morphologic evidence supporting lesional maturation over time. However, the alternative view that this is a true benign neoplasm with self-limiting biologic potential cannot be dismissed, especially in view of the local recurrence rate.

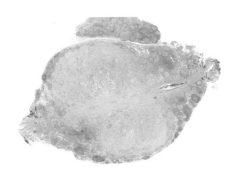

Fig. 7.06 Subcutaneous epithelioid haemangioma, showing circumscription, a peripheral lymphoid reaction, and symmetrical growth around a muscular artery.

Macroscopy
These lesions are usually 0.5–2.0 cm in size, with rare examples exceeding 5 cm {1612}. Apart from size, the gross characteristics of this process are not well-described. Many examples may have a rather nonspecific nodular appearance. Some examples with retained blood may have an appearance suggestive of a haemangioma. Occasionally, subcutaneous examples may resemble a lymph node because of circumscription and a peripheral lymphoid reaction.

Histopathology
Subcutaneous examples of epithelioid haemangioma are characterized by a prominent proliferation of small, capillary-sized vessels lined by plump, epithelioid endothelial cells. The vessels typically have an immature appearance and they may lack a well defined lumen, but they are well formed with single cell layering of the endothelium and an intact myopericytic/smooth muscle layer. The endothelial cells have amphophilic or eosinophilic cytoplasm that is sometimes vacuolated, and they contain a single, relatively large, nucleus with an open chromatin pattern, and often, a central nucleolus. The process is usually well demarcated from the surrounding soft tissue, and commonly, it is associated with (sometimes centred around) a larger vessel, usually a muscular artery. An inflammatory milieu rich in eosinophils and lymphocytes is present in the overwhelming majority of cases, and many examples are bordered by a prominent lymphoid reaction with follicle formation. It is common to encounter epithelioid endothelial cells within the lumen of the larger vessel, either replacing part of the normal endothelial lining or "coating" fibrin fronds, as seen in papillary endothelial hyperplasia. Cross-sections of the larger vessel may also reveal epithelioid

endothelial-lined channels that transgress the vessel wall and communicate with the surrounding vascular proliferation.

Dermal examples of epithelioid haemangioma also feature a proliferation of small vessels, lined by epithelioid endothelial cells, set in an inflammatory milieu rich in lymphocytes and eosinophils. However, in this location, the vessels often have a more mature appearance with a well canalized lumen, and the endothelial cells are somewhat less plump, frequently more cobblestone or hobnail-like in appearance. Also, dermal examples are less circumscribed and often lack lymphoid follicles. Finally, these superficial lesions are not usually associated with a larger central vein or muscular artery.

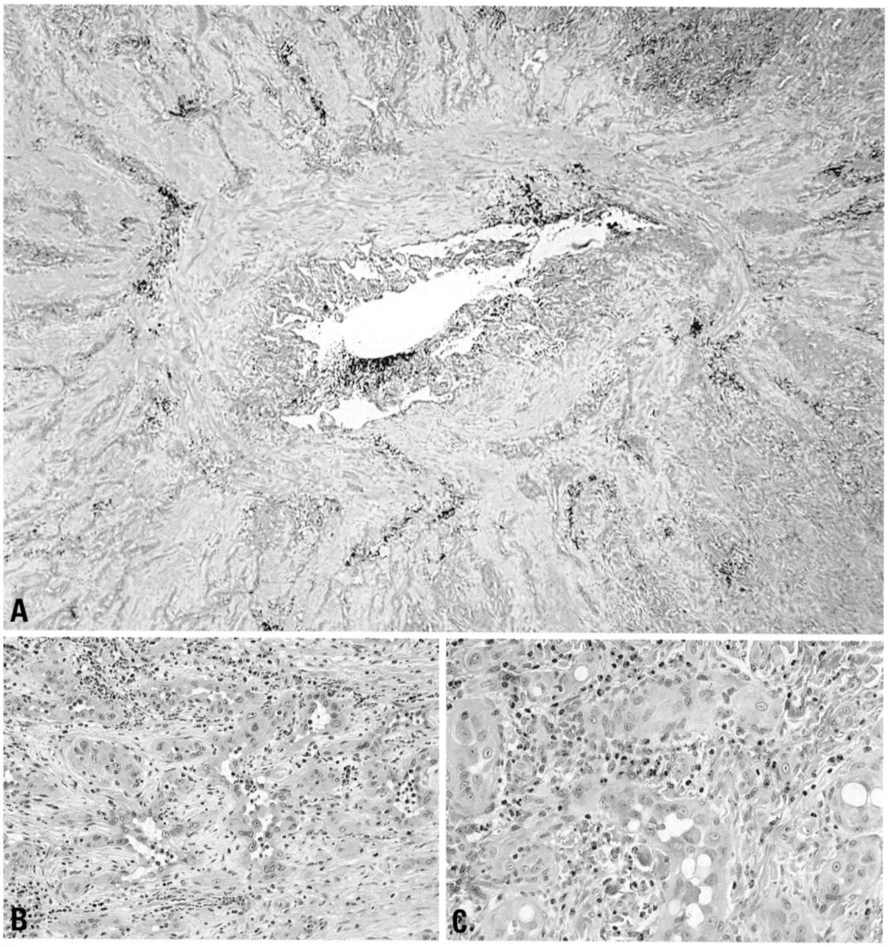

Immunophenotype

The epithelioid endothelial cells of epithelioid haemangioma are immunoreactive for CD31 and factor VIIIrAg. Immunoreactivity for CD34 is also present, though often to a lesser degree. Infrequently, limited keratin expression may be detected. Immunostaining for alpha-smooth muscle actin or musclespecific actin is helpful in demonstrating an intact myopericytic layer around the immature vessels. Actin-positive myopericytes are generally present to a much lesser extent in malignant vascular tumours such as epithelioid haemagioendothelioma and epithelioid angiosarcoma.

Prognostic factors

Complete local excision and follow-up are optimal management for epithelioid haemangioma. Local recurrence is reported to occur in up to one-third of patients {1612}. Whether this is due to persistence of an underlying vascular anomaly (e.g., an arteriovenous shunt) that incites regrowth or an indication of true neoplastic potential is unresolved. Metastases do not occur. There is one report of apparent regional lymph node seeding that had no adverse affect on patient outcome with 5 years follow-up {1769}.

Fig. 7.07 Epithelioid haemangioma. **A** Involvement of a muscular artery. Note the presence of an intraluminal component, and the immature, but well formed, vessels around the artery. **B,C** Immature vessels, lined by epithelioid endothelial cells. Note the presence of an inflammatory infiltrate rich in lymphocytes and eosinophils.

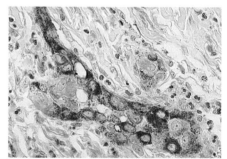

Fig. 7.08 Epithelioid haemangioma. The epithelioid endothelial cells are strongly reactive for factor VIIIrAg.

Angiomatosis

S.W. Weiss

Definition
Angiomatosis is a diffuse form of haemangioma that affects a large segment of the body in a contiguous fashion, either by vertical extension, to involve multiple tissue planes (e.g. skin, subcutis, muscle, bone), or by crossing muscle compartments to involve similar tissue types (e.g. multiple muscles). This definition implies that the diagnosis is a combined clinical and pathological one.

Synonyms and historical annotation
Vascular malformation, arteriovenous malformation, and venous malformation have been employed as synonyms for angiomatosis. These earlier terms underscore the prevailing view that angiomatosis probably represents congenital malformations (rather than neoplasms) which make their appearance during childhood. The term "infiltrating angiolipoma"; used to refer to intramuscular lesions composed of both a mature vascular and fatty component, has also been used for angiomatosis.

Epidemiology
Approximately two-thirds of cases develop within the first two decades of life and nearly all are apparent by age 40 years.

Females are affected with slightly greater frequency than males {1758}.

Sites of involvement
Over one half of cases occur in the lower extremities, followed by the chest wall, abdomen, and upper extremity.

Clinical features
Patients present with diffuse persistent swelling of the affected part, which occasionally waxes and wanes in size and is affected by strenuous activity. Only rarely is significant arteriovenous shunting leading to gigantism observed. Plain films of the affected region show an ill defined mass which on CT scan can sometimes be identified as vascular due to the presence of serpinginous densities corresponding to tortuous veins.

Macroscopy / Histopathology
The lesions are ill defined masses which vary from a few centimeters to 10-20 cm. in diameter. Although they vary in colour, many may have a fatty appearance, due to the presence of mature adipose tissue. Angiomatosis may assume one of two patterns. The more common pattern is that of a melange of venous, cavernous and capillary-sized vessels scattered haphazardly throughout soft tissue. The venous vessels contain irregularly attenuated walls from which clusters of smaller vessels herniate in bouquet-like arrangement. In the second pattern the lesion resembles an infiltrating capillary haemangioma. Large amounts of mature fat frequently accompany both types. Although the first pattern is highly characteristic of angiomatosis, the diagnosis should not be made on this pattern alone, but on the combination of these changes in association with the clinical features {2240}.

Rare lesions with prominent glomus cells are classified as glomangiomatosis (see page 136).

Clinical behaviour
Although angiomatosis is considered a benign lesion, nearly 90% of cases persist (often mistakenly interpreted as true local recurrence). In some studies nearly 50% of patients develop multiple recurrences. Metastasis or malignant transformation has not been reported {510,978,1758}.

These recurrence rates probably reflect incomplete excisions in the face of extensive disease.

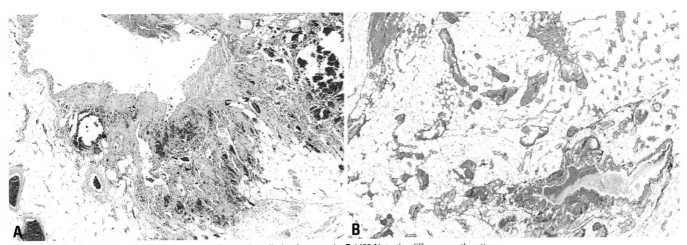

Fig. 7.09 Angiomatosis showing (**A**) clusters of small vessels radiating from a vein. **B** 1436 Note the diffuse growth pattern.

Lymphangioma

A. Beham

Definition
A benign, cavernous / cystic vascular lesion composed of dilated lymphatic channels. Lymphangioma circumscriptum and progressive lymphangioma are described in the WHO classification of skin tumours.

ICD-O code   9170/0

Synonym   Cystic hygroma.

Epidemiology
Lymphangiomas are common paediatric lesions, which most often present at birth or during first years of life {47,375,671, 1045}. Some cases may be identified in Turner syndrome (and other malformative syndromes) and may be found in abortuses {375}. Cavernous/cystic lymphangioma of head and neck represents the most frequent subtype.

Sites of involvement
Cystic lymphangiomas are mostly located in the neck, axilla and groin, whereas the cavernous type occurs additionally in the oral cavity, upper trunk, limbs and abdominal sites including mesentery and retroperitoneum {47}.

Clinical features
The lesions present as rather circumscribed painless swellings, which are soft and fluctuant at palpation, and can show displacement of surrounding organs at mediastinal or intraabdominal sites. Imaging procedures like ultrasonography display their cystic nature, angiography shows poor vascularization and CT scan reveals multiple, homogeneous, nonenhancing areas.

Aetiology
Early or even congenital appearance in life and lesional architecture are in favour of developmental malformations, with genetic abnormalities playing an additional role.

Macroscopy
Cavernous / cystic lymphangiomas correspond to a multicystic or spongy mass, the cavities of which contain watery to milky fluid.

Histopathology
Cavernous/cystic lymphangiomas are characterized by thin-walled, dilated lymphatic vessels of different size, which are lined by a flattened endothelium and frequently surrounded by lymphocytic aggregates. The lumina may be either empty or contain proteinaceous fluid, lymphocytes and sometimes erythrocytes. Larger vessels can be invested by a smooth muscle layer, and long-standing lesions reveal interstitial fibrosis and stromal inflammation. Stromal mast cells are common and haemosiderin deposition is frequently seen.

Immunophenotype
The endothelium demonstrates variable expression of FVIII-rAg, CD31 and CD34 {704}.

Ultrastructure
The endothelium of thin-walled vessels is not enveloped by a basement membrane and no pericytes are attached to it, thus directly contacting with the interstitium. With increasing caliber the vessels may acquire pericytes and smooth muscle cells, respectively.

Genetics
Cystic lymphangiomas ("cystic hygroma") of the neck are often associated with Turner syndrome {289,339}.

Prognostic factors
Recurrences are due to incomplete surgical removal, whereas malignant transformation does not occur. Lymphangiomas of the neck/axilla sometimes extend to the mediastinum and may be of vital significance by compromising trachea, esophagus etc. Abdominal lesions can lead to intestinal obstruction.

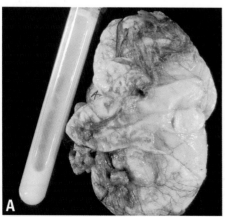
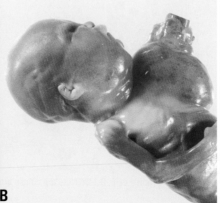
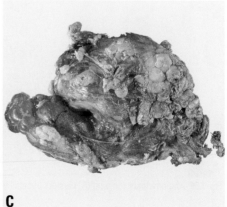

Fig. 7.10 A Cystic lymphangioma, collapsed. The adjacent tube shows the milky lymph removed from the lesion. **B** Cystic lymphangioma in the lower neck of a fetus with Turner syndrome. **C** Large, partly cystic lymphangioma from mesentery and partially covered by adipose tissue.

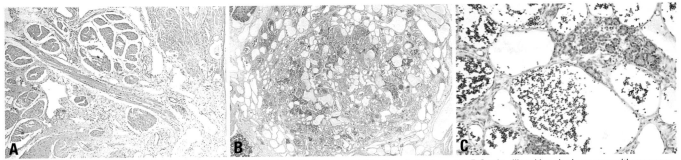

Fig. 7.11 Lymphangioma. **A** Multiple, cystic or ectatic, thin-walled lymphatic spaces infiltrating skeletal muscle. **B** Cystic, dilated lymphatic spaces with accompanying stromal lymphocytic aggregates, infiltrating the parotid gland in a sieve-like manner. **C** Thin-walled spaces of varying diameter, containing lymph and / or lymphocytes, and lined by flattened endothelium.

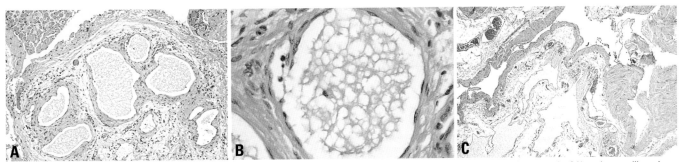

Fig. 7.12 Cavernous lymphangioma. **A** Note the prominent smooth muscle in the vessel walls. **B** There is no endothelial multilayering or atypia. **C** Note the cyst-like enlargments of lymphatic vessels.

Kaposiform haemangioendothelioma

W.Y.W. Tsang

Definition
Kaposiform haemangioendothelioma is a locally aggressive, immature vascular neoplasm, characterized by a predominant Kaposi sarcoma-like fascicular spindle cell growth pattern.

ICD-O code   9130/1

Synonyms
Kaposi-like infantile haemangioendothelioma {2135}, haemangioma with Kaposi sarcoma-like features {1554}.

Epidemiology
This is a rare tumour with no known racial predilection.

Site of involvement
The tumour most commonly occurs in the retroperitoneum {2135,2352} and the skin {1300,1554,2204}, but it can also occur in the head and neck region, mediastinum, and deeper soft tissues of the trunk and extremities {1418,2270,2352}.

Clinical features
Kaposiform haemangioendothelioma typically occurs in infancy and first decade of life, but adult cases are increasingly recognized {1300,1418}. Retroperitoneal tumours usually present as abdominal mass, ascites, intestinal obstruction, and jaundice. Deep soft tissue lesions produce single or multiple masses and may involve the underlying bone and rarely regional lymph nodes (variably interpreted as either local extension or local metastasis) {1300}. Cutaneous lesions present as ill defined violaceous plaques. Consumption coagulopathy (Kasabach-Merritt syndrome) may complicate the larger tumours due to activation of clotting pathways within the tumour vasculature.

Aetiology
There is no known association with HIV infection or HHV8.

Macroscopy / Histopathology
Cutaneous lesions appear as ill defined,

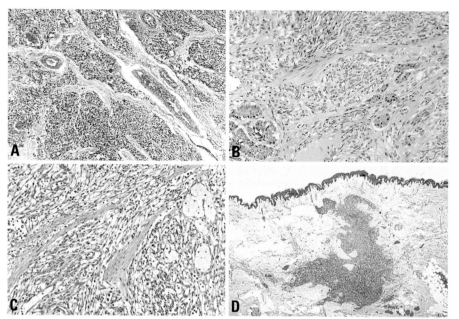

Fig. 7.13 Kaposiform haemangioendothelioma. **A** Subcutaneous lesion showing well developed lobular architecture. **B** Retroperitoneal lesion in a young infant with destructive infiltration of the pancreas. **C** Higher magnification shows loosely arranged spindle cells forming vascular slits mixed with some dilated capillaries. **D** Cutaneous kaposiform haemangioendothelioma with irregular, infiltrative tumour growth in the dermis.

be tumour lo-bules resembling cellular haemangioma or capillary haemangioma. There are often adjacent foci resembling lymphangiomatosis. Fibrin thrombi and fragmented red cells can be found in the slit-like spaces and the capillaries. There may be haemorrhage, haemosiderin deposition and rare hyaline globules.

Immunophenotype
The spindle cells are usually negative for Factor VIII-related antigen, but positive for CD34 and CD31, especially those lining vascular slits. Muscle-specific actin highlights variable numbers of spindle cells, suggesting the presence of pericytes in at least some areas.

Ultrastructure
Ultrastructural hallmarks of endothelial cells are poorly developed in the spindle cells and represented by poorly formed lumens and discontinuous basal lamina. Weibel-Palade bodies may be totally absent.

Prognostic factors
Kaposiform haemangioendothelioma shows no tendency for spontaneous regression {1300}. The prognosis varies with the site and size of the lesion. Outlook is poor for large tumours occurring in infancy complicated by Kasabach-Merritt syndrome, especially when occurring in intraabdominal sites. Lesions in the somatic soft tissue are curable by complete excision, and recurrence appears to be rare.

violaceous plaques. Soft tissue tumours are greyish to reddish, multi-nodular, and may coalesce and encase surrounding structures.

Microscopically, the tumour grows in the form of infiltrative vague lobules separated by fibrous septa. It consists predominantly of criss-crossing spindle cell fascicles interspersed with capillaries. The fascicles are curved or straight, and may be compact with few interspersed spaces or more loosely arranged, containing slit-like, sieve-like or crescent-shaped vascular lumens. Nuclear atypia and mitotic activity are usually inconspicuous. Rarely, the spindle cell fascicles may blend with round "glomeruloid" solid nests of polygonal / epithelioid endothelial cells which possess abundant eosino-philic cytoplasm. The interspersed capillaries are lined by flat or plump endothelial cells, and there can

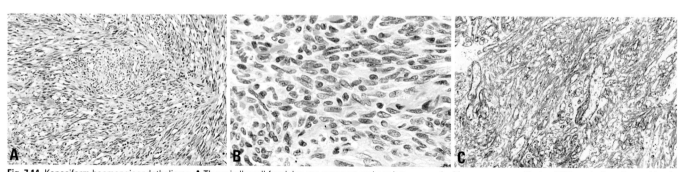

Fig. 7.14 Kaposiform haemangioendothelioma. **A** The spindle cell fascicles are compact and are interspersed with numerous capillaries. **B** The spindle cells are bland-looking. **C** The spindle cells and capillaries show strong reactivity with CD31.

Retiform haemangioendothelioma

E. Calonje

Definition
Retiform haemangioendothelioma (RH) is a locally aggressive, rarely metastasizing vascular lesion, characterized by distinctive arborizing blood vessels lined by endothelial cells with characteristic hobnail morphology. These tumours appear to be closely related to papillary intralymphatic angioendothelioma.

ICD-O code   9135/1

Synonym
Hobnail haemangioendothelioma.

Epidemiology
RH is uncommon. Since its original description in 1994, only 20 cases have been reported {296,734,1419}. The age range is wide but it usually affects young adults with no sex predominance.

Sites of involvement
The tumour involves predominantly the skin and subcutaneous tissue and shows predilection for the distal extremities, particularly the lower limb.

Clinical features
RH presents as a red/bluish slowly growing plaque or nodule usually less than 3 cm in maximum dimension. A case with multiple lesions has been described {556}. Exceptional cases occur in the setting of previous radiotherapy or pre-existing lymphoedema {296}.

Macroscopy / Histopathology
Macroscopic examination reveals diffuse induration of the dermis with frequent involvement of the underlying subcutaneous tissue. Scanning magnification reveals characteristic elongated and narrow arborizing vascular channels with a striking resemblance to the normal rete testis. Although this pattern is usually readily apparent, if the vascular channels are small or collapsed, then the retiform architecture might be difficult to recognize. Monomorphic hyperchromatic endothelial cells with prominent protuberant nuclei and characteristic tombstone or hobnail appearance line the blood vessels. These cells have scanty cytoplasm, which seems to

blend with the underlying stroma. Pleomorphism is absent and mitotic figures are rare. A prominent stromal and often intravascular lymphocytic infiltrate is present in around half of the cases. The stroma surrounding the tumour tends to be sclerotic. Focal solid areas composed of sheets of endothelial cells are often identified. Vacuolated cells are uncommonly seen. Monomorphic endothelial spindle-shaped cells are also a rare feature and were described in the single metastatic lymph node reported {296}. In some cases there are intravascular papillae with hyaline collagenous cores similar to those seen in papillary intralymphatic angioendothelioma. Retiform haemangioendothelioma can be one of the components of a composite haemangioendothelioma (see page 168).

Immunophenotype
The neoplastic cells in RH stain for vascular markers including CD31, CD34 and VWF (von Willebrand factor). Staining for CD34 is often stronger than that of other vascular markers. Most of the lymphocytes in the infiltrate stain for pan-T cell markers including CD3. Only a minority of the lymphocytes stain for the B cell marker CD20. The latter are only found in the stroma surrounding the vascular channels. In general experience these lesions are HHV-8 negative.

Prognostic factors
Multiple local recurrences (in up to 60% of cases), often over a period of many years, are the rule unless wide local excision is performed {296}. So far only one patient has been reported to develop a metastasis to a regional lymph node. A further patient developed a local soft tissue metastasis from a primary in the right big toe {1419}. To date, no patients have been described to develop distant metastasis or to die from this disease.

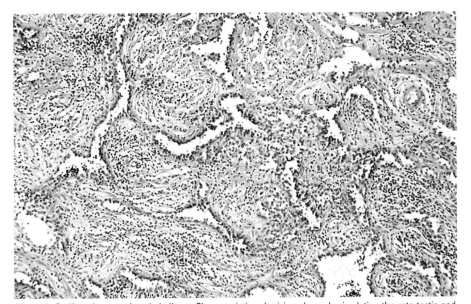

Fig. 7.15 Retiform haemangioendothelioma. Characteristic arborizing channels simulating the rete testis and with a prominent stromal lymphocytic infiltrate.

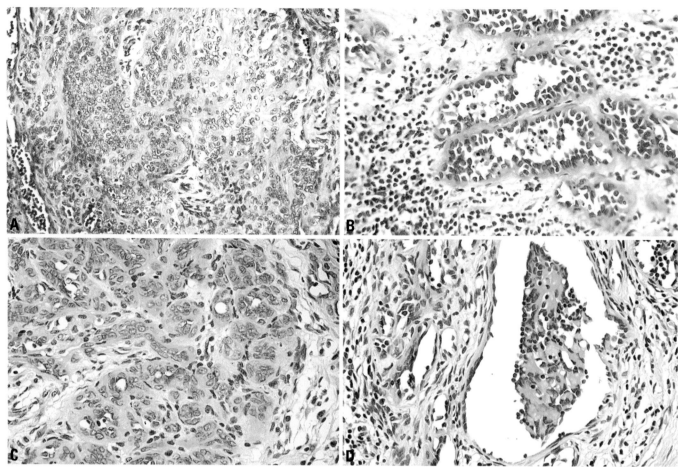

Fig. 7.16 Retiform haemangioendothelioma. **A** Focal areas with a more solid growth pattern are frequent. **B** Typical hobnail endothelial cells with prominent nuclei. **C** Vacuolated cells and **(D)** intraluminal papillae with collagenous cores similar to those seen in Dabska's tumour are seen in some cases.

Papillary intralymphatic angioendothelioma

E. Calonje

Definition
Papillary intralymphatic angiothe-lioma (PILA) is a locally aggressive, rarely metastasizing vascular lesion characterized by lymphatic-like channels and papillary endothelial proliferation. These tumours appear to be closely related to retiform haemangioendothelioma.

ICD-O code   9135/1

Synonyms
Dabska tumour, malignant endothelial papillary angioendothelioma, hobnail haemangioendothelioma.

Epidemiology
PILA is very rare and has predilection for infants and children.
Around 25% of cases present in adults {635}. Sex incidence is similar.

Sites of involvement
Most cases involve the limbs and fewer cases present on the trunk.

Clinical features
PILAs present as a slowly growing asymptomatic cutaneous plaque or nodule.

Macroscopy
Tumours are ill defined and usually involve the dermis and subcutaneous tissue. The vascular nature of the lesion is not immediately apparent and haemorrhage is rare. Cystic spaces can be identified in some instances.

Histopathology
If strict diagnostic criteria are used, tumours can be described as composed of dilated, thin-walled vascular spaces often resembling a cavernous lymphangioma {635}. In rare cases the vascular channels are smaller and more irregular. Formation of prominent intraluminal papillary tufts with hyaline cores lined by hobnail endothelial cells is a characteristic finding.
The endothelial cells lining the spaces have scant pink cytoplasm and a prominent nucleus with little or no cytological atypia and a typical hobnail or matchstick appearance. The hyaline cores contain basement membrane material synthesized by tumour cells. A variable number of lymphocytes are seen within and around the vascular channels. Mitotic figures are rare.

Immunophenotype
Staining for vascular markers including CD31, von Willebrand factor and CD34 is usually positive. The finding of strong expression of vascular endothelial growth facto receptor-3 (VEGFR-3) by tumour cells in lesions with hobnail endothelial cells has been regarded as suggestive of lymphatic differentiation {635,704}. However, the specificity of this marker as an indicator of lymphatic origin is doubtful.

Prognostic factors
In the original series, a tendency for local recurrence and regional lymph node metastasis was suggested {419}. Furthermore, at least one of the patients in the original series died of disease. However, follow-up in 8 of the 12 cases reported recently reported neither local recurrences nor metastatic spread {635}. Therefore, the issue about the malignant potential of this tumour remains unsolved pending further studies. It is advisable to excise lesions widely when feasible.

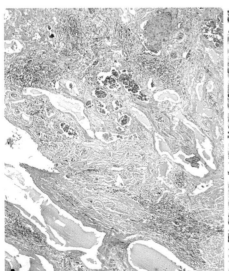
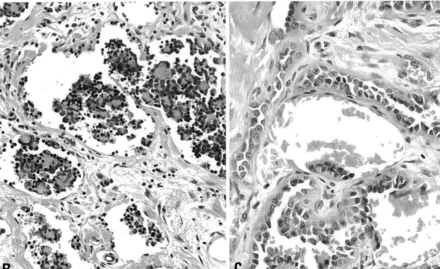

Fig. 7.17 Papillary intralymphatic angioendothelioma. **A** Cavernous lymphangioma-like spaces. **B** Numerous intravascular papillae with collagenous cores. **C** Note the characteristic hobnail epithelium.

Composite haemangioendothelioma

B.P. Rubin

Definition
Composite haemangioendothelioma is defined as a locally aggressive, rarely metastasizing neoplasm with vascular differentiation, containing an admixture of histologically benign, intermediate and malignant components.

ICD-O code   9130/1

Epidemiology
Composite haemangioendothelioma is an extremely rare and recently described neoplasm with less than 10 cases reported in the English language literature {1543,1776}. Histologically similar lesions were previously reported {373}. The gender distribution is approximately equal and the majority of cases occur in adults, although a single case which first developed in infancy has been described {1776}.

Sites of involvement
Most cases have shown a predilection for the distal extremities, especially the hands and feet, with the exception of a single case which arose in the tongue.

Clinical features
25% of patients with composite haemangioendothelioma have a history of lymphoedema. Lesions are usually long-standing (2-12 years) and have a reddish-blue, variably nodular appearance.

Macroscopy
Composite haemangioendothelioma presents as an infiltrative, uninodular or multinodular mass (individual nodules measure 0.7–6 cm), or as an area of ill defined "swelling". Some of the lesions are associated with reddish purple skin discoloration, suggestive of the diagnosis of a vascular neoplasm.

Histopathology
Composite haemangioendothelioma is a poorly circumscribed, infiltrative lesion, centered in the dermis and subcutis. It possesses a complex admixture of histologically benign and malignant vascular components that vary greatly in their relative proportions. These lesions are unified by a similar admixture of the different components which include epithelioid haemangioendothelioma, retiform haemangioendothelioma, spindle cell haemangioma, "angiosarcoma-like" areas, and benign vascular lesions (arterio-venous malformation, and lymphangioma circumscriptum). Another interesting feature, seen in several cases, is the presence of large numbers of vacuolated endothelial cells which impart a pseudolipoblastic appearance. The "angiosarcoma-like" areas are characterized by a low grade angiosarcomatous appearance composed of complex dissecting vascular channels with endothelial atypia and relatively few mitotic figures. The biological significance of such lesions should be determined in larger studies. Exceptionally, the "angiosarcoma-like" area in a single case had the appearance of high grade angiosarcoma characterized by a solid growth pattern and numerous mitotic figures. The biological potential of lesions such as the latter remains to be determined through study of larger case numbers. Lesions are positive for vascular markers (CD31, CD34, and von Willebrand Factor).

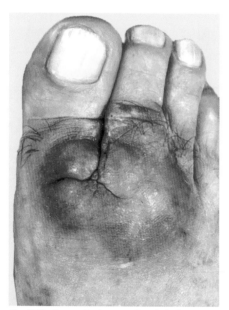

Fig. 7.18 Composite haemangioendothelioma presenting as a bluish-purple multinodular mass.

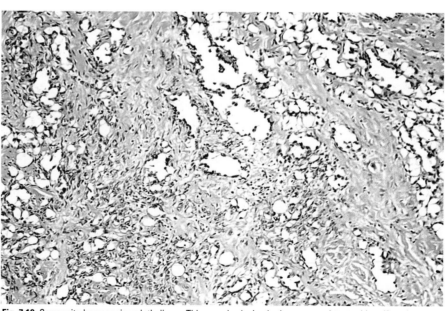

Fig. 7.19 Composite haemangioendothelioma. This complex lesion had areas consistent with retiform haemangioendothelioma as well as more solid areas consistent with epithelioid haemangioendothelioma.

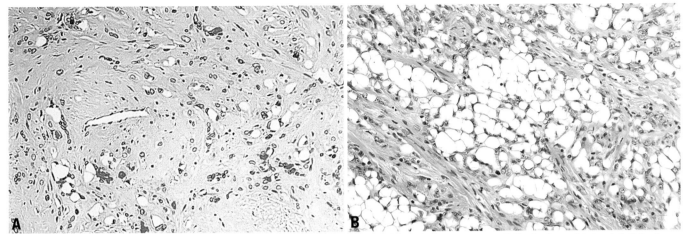

Fig. 7.20 Composite haemangioendothelioma. **A** Typical appearance of the epithelioid haemangioendothelioma component. **B** Sheets of vacuolated endothelial cells are not unusual.

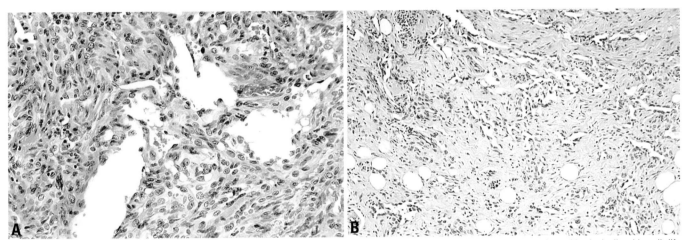

Fig. 7.21 Composite haemangioendothelioma. **A** Several lesions have areas consistent with spindle cell haemangioma. **B** Areas consistent histologically with well-differentiated angiosarcoma.

Prognostic factors

Half of the lesions recurred locally between 4 and 10 years after excision of the primary mass, often with multiple recurrences. In the patient with the tongue lesion, metastasis occurred to a submandibular lymph node and to the soft tissue of the thigh at 9 and 11 years after excision of the primary, respectively. Thus, the behaviour appears to be much less aggressive than conventional angiosarcoma.

Kaposi sarcoma

J. Lamovec
S. Knuutila

Definition

Kaposi sarcoma (KS) is a locally aggressive endothelial tumour that typically presents with cutaneous lesions in the form of multiple patches, plaques or nodules but may also involve mucosal sites, lymph nodes and visceral organs. The disease is uniformly associated with human herpes virus 8 (HHV-8) infection.

ICD-O code   9140/3

Synonyms

Idiopathic multiple pigmented sarcoma of the skin, angiosarcoma multiplex, granuloma multiplex haemorrhagicum, Kaposi disease.

Epidemiology

Four different clinical and epidemiological forms of KS are recognized: 1. *classic indolent form* occurring predominantly in elderly men of Mediterranean/East European descent, 2. *endemic African KS* that occurs in middle-aged adults and children in Equatorial Africa who are not HIV infected, 3. *iatrogenic KS* appearing in solid organ transplant recipients treated with immunosuppressive therapy and also in patients treated by immunosuppressive agents, notably corticosteroids, for various diseases {2127}, 4. *acquired immunodeficiency syndrome-associated KS* (AIDS KS), the most aggressive form of the disease, found in HIV-1 infected individuals, that is particularly frequent in homo- and bisexual men. The relative risk of acquiring KS in the latter patients is >10,000 {800}; it

has been reduced with the advent of highly active antiretroviral therapy (HAART) {194}.

Aetiology

The long sought-after infectious agent of KS was identified in 1994 by Chang et al. and was named KS-associated herpesvirus (KSHV) or human herpesvirus (HHV8) {332, 1505}. The virus is found in KS cells of all epidemiological-clinical forms of the disease and is detected in the peripheral blood before the development of KS {763,2258}; the disease itself is the result of the complex interplay of HHV8 with immunologic, genetic and environmental factors {587,1144}.

Sites of involvement

The most typical site of involvement by KS is the skin. During the course of the disease or initially, mucosal membranes (e.g. oral mucosa), lymph nodes and visceral organs may be affected, sometimes without skin involvement. The involvement of a wide variety of tissues and organs has been described {1008}, although KS is very rarely, if ever, seen in skeletal muscles, brain and kidney.

Clinical features

Classic type of KS is characterized by the appearance of purplish, reddish blue or dark brown macules, plaques and nodules that may ulcerate. They are particularly frequent in distal extremities and may be accompanied by lymphoedema. The disease is usually indolent, lymph node and visceral involvement occurs

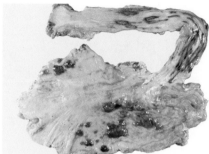

Fig. 7.22 Esophageal and gastric involvement in visceral Kaposi sarcoma (KS).

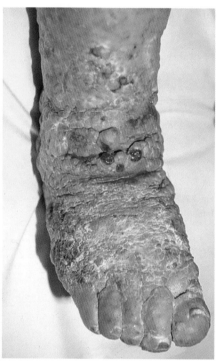

Fig. 7.23 Advanced skin lesions in classic KS.

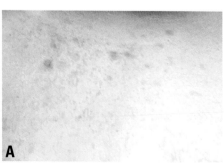
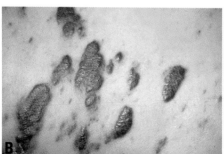
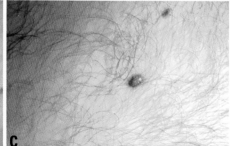

Fig. 7.24 Cutaneous Kaposi sarcoma (KS). **A** Patch lesion. **B** Plaque stage lesion. **C** Nodular stage lesion.

Table 7.01
Epidemiological-clinical types of Kaposi sarcoma.

Type	Risk groups	Skin lesions--predilection sites	Visceral involvement	Course
Classic	Elderly men of Mediterranean/ East European descent	Lower legs	Rare	Indolent
Endemic	Middle-aged men and children in Equatorial Africa	Extremities	Fairly common – adults Frequent – children (lymph nodes)	Indolent – adults Aggressive – children
Iatrogenic	Immunosuppressed patients (post-transplant, other diseases)	Lower legs	Fairly common	Indolent or aggressive
AIDS-associated	Younger, mainly homo- and bisexual HIV-1 infected men	Face, genitalia, lower extremities	Frequent	Aggressive

infrequently. Classic KS may be associated with haematopoetic malignancies.

In the *endemic form of KS*, the disease may be localized to skin and shows a protracted course. A variant of endemic disease, a lymphadenopathic form in African children is rapidly progressive and highly lethal.

Iatrogenic KS is relatively frequent. It develops in a few months to several years after the transplantation of solid organs or immunosuppressive treatment for a variety of conditions. The disease may resolve entirely upon withdrawal of immunosuppressive treatment although its course is somewhat unpredictable {2127}. Patients who develop visceral lesions may succumb to their disease {1684}.

AIDS-related KS is the most aggressive type of KS. In the skin, lesions are most common on the face, genitals, and lower extremities; oral mucosa, lymph nodes, gastro-intestinal tract and lungs are frequently involved. Lymph node and visceral disease without muco-cutaneous lesions may occur. The disease commonly behaves aggressively.

While skin lesions and lymphadenopathy are obvious signs of the disease in various types of KS, the spread into visceral organs may be silent or symptomatic depending on the extent and particular location of the lesions.

Macroscopy

The lesions in the skin (patches, plaques, nodules) range in size from very small to several centimeters in diameter. The involvement of the mucosa, soft tissues, lymph nodes and visceral organs pres-

ents as haemorrhagic nodules of various sizes that may coalesce.

Histopathology

Microscopic features of all four different epidemiological-clinical types of KS do not differ. Early lesions of the skin disease are uncharacteristic and present with subtle vascular proliferation {1827}. In *patch stage*, vascular spaces are increased in number, of irregular shape, and may dissect collagen fibres in the upper reticular dermis. They often run parallel to the epidermis. The vascular

proliferation is often perivascular and periadnexal. Endothelial cells lining the spaces are flattened or more oval, with little atypia. Pre-existing blood vessels may protrude into the lumen of new vessels. Admixed are sparse lymphocytes and plasma cells; frequently, extravasated erythrocytes and deposits of hemosiderin surround the vascular structures. Slits lined by attenuated endothelial cells between collagen bundles are also seen. In some cases, there is a proliferation of spindle or oval endothelial cells around pre-existing blood vessels in the dermis.

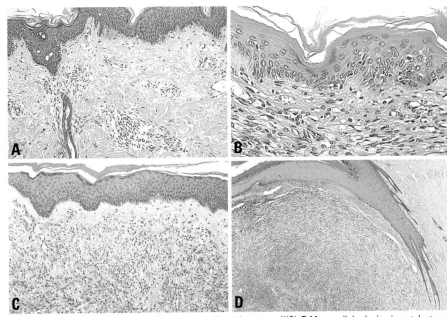

Fig. 7.25 A Early lesion (patch stage) in cutaneous Kaposi sarcoma (KS). **B** More cellular lesion in patch stage of cutaneous KS. **C** Marked spindle cell and and vascular proliferation with extravasation of erythrocytes in early plaque stage. **D** Nodular KS of the skin; a collar of epidermis surrounds a densely cellular spindle cell tumour.

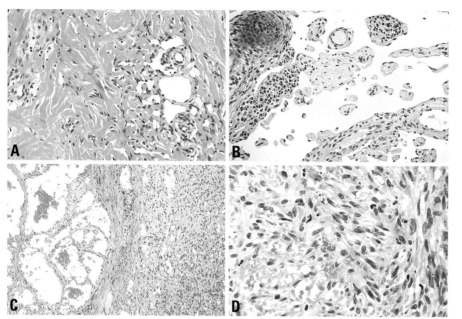

Fig. 7.26 A Irregular jagged vascular spaces in KS, dissecting collagen fibers of the dermis. **B** Lymphangioma-like lesions are uncommon and morphologically deceptive. Note the accompanying plasma cells. **C** Angiomatous component in KS lesion of the skin (plaque stage). **D** High power view of nodular KS lesion; several hyaline bodies are seen.

Slit-like spaces, lymphocyte and plasma cell infiltration and extravasated erythrocytes are also observed.

In *plaque stage*, all characteristics of patch stage are exaggerated. There is more extensive angio-proliferation with vascular spaces showing jagged outlines. Inflammatory infiltrate is denser and extravascular red cells and siderophages are numerous. Hyaline globules (likely representing destroyed red blood cells) are frequently found.

Nodular stage is characterized by well defined nodules of intersecting fascicles of spindle cells with only mild atypia and numerous slit-like spaces containing red cells. Peripherally, there are ectatic blood vessels. Many spindle cells show mitoses. Hyaline globules are present inside and outside the spindle cells. Some patients, usually with endemic nodular type KS, develop lesions which closely resemble lymphangioma.

In lymph nodes, the infiltrate may be uni- or multifocal and the lymph node may be entirely effaced by tumour. Early lesions may be subtle, showing only increased number of vascular channels accompanied by plasma cell infiltration {1287}. In visceral organs, the lesions tend to respect architecture of the organs involved and spread along vascular structures, bronchi, portal areas in the liver, etc., and from these sites they involve surrounding parenchyma {631, 1008}.

Immunohistochemistry

The lining cells of clearly developed vascular structures are usually positive for vascular markers, while the spindle cells consistently show positive reaction for CD34 and commonly for CD31 but are factor VIII negative. All cases, irrespective of epidemiologic subgroup, are HHV-8 positive. The new marker FLI1, a nuclear transcription factor, appears to be expressed in almost 100% of different vascular tumours, including KS {695}.

Genetics

Little is known about cytogenetic and molecular alterations in Kaposi sarcoma, but growth factors, such as VEGF/VPF and FGF most probably play an essential role in transformation {1250,1853}.

Cell lines and primary tumours have been reported to have chromosome aberrations {311,1715,1838}, including gain of 8q and 1q and loss of 3p, and rearrangements of 7q22, 8p11, 13q11 and 19q13. A comparative genomic hybridization (CGH) study of seven cases could not confirm these findings, but showed recurrent gains at 11q13 {1130}. Further investigation suggested that the target genes in the amplified area are *FGF4* and *FGF3* (a.k.a. *INT2*). Also *KRAS2* and *TP53* rearrangements were reported {1553,1904}.

Prognostic factors

The evolution of disease depends on the epidemiological-clinical type of KS and on its clinical extent. It is also modified by treatment that includes surgery, radio- and chemotherapy. Cases with widespread visceral involvement are commonly poorly responsive to treatment.

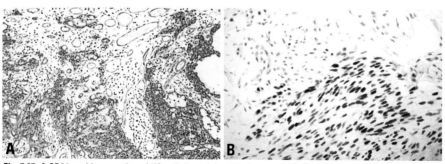

Fig. 7.27 A CD34 positive reaction of KS cells in nodular skin disease. **B** Nuclear immunopositivity for HHV-8 is a consistent finding in all histologic types and clinical subsets of Kaposi sarcoma.

Other intermediate vascular neoplasms

B.P. Rubin
W.Y.W. Tsang
C.D.M. Fletcher

The Working Group also considered two other tumours for possible inclusion in the new WHO classification – *polymorphous haemangioendothelioma* and *giant cell angioblastoma* – but decided that available data are insufficient to allow definitive classification of these lesions. Specifically, very few cases have been reported to date, there are as yet no clear diagnostic criteria and there are uncertainties regarding biological potential.

Giant cell angioblastoma, of which 4 cases have been reported, arises in soft tissue of infants, is comprised of nodular aggregates of histiocytoid cells arranged around bland angiomatous vessels and may show persistent growth {808,2193}.

As yet, it is not certain that this is primarily an endothelial tumour.

Polymorphous haemangioendothelioma, of which less than ten cases have been reported, may primarily involve soft tissue or lymph nodes, affects adults, has complex and worrisome morphologic features and metastasizes in some cases {327,1537,1771}.

Epithelioid haemangioendothelioma

S.W. Weiss
J.A. Bridge

Definition
Epithelioid haemangioendothelioma is an angiocentric vascular tumour with metastatic potential, composed of epithelioid endothelial cells arranged in short cords and nests set in a distinctive myxohyaline stroma.

ICD-O code   9133/3

Synonyms
Intravascular bronchioloalveolar tumour, angioglomoid tumour, myxoid angioblastomatosis.

Epidemiology
Epithelioid haemangioendothelioma is a rare vascular tumour although its precise incidence has never been determined. The lesion occurs in nearly all age groups with the exception of the early childhood years and affects the sexes equally {1407, 2238, 2245}.

Sites of involvement
The tumour develops as a solitary tumour in either superficial or deep soft tissue of the extremities. Nearly one half to two-thirds originate from a vessel, usually a small vein. In exceptional cases the lesion may arise from a large vein or artery in which case it presents as an entirely intraluminal mass.

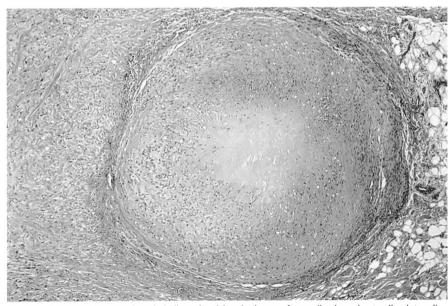

Fig. 7.28 Epithelioid haemangioendothelioma involving the lumen of a small vein and extending into adjacent tissue. Origin from a vessel is evident in approximately 30% of cases.

Clinical features

The tumour develops as an often painful nodule in either superficial or deep soft tissue. Because of its origin from a vessel there may be associated symptoms of oedema or thrombophlebitis. Deeply situated tumours may be associated with focal ossification which can be detected on plain films. Although an association with oral contraceptives has been raised with respect to hepatic forms of the disease, no such association has been documented with soft tissue variants.

Macroscopy

In its classic form, epithelioid haemangioendothelioma arises as a fusiform intravascular mass which may resemble an organizing thrombus except for the fact that it appears matted down and infiltrative of surrounding structures.

Histopathology

In small or early tumours, the lesion expands the originating vessel, preserving its architecture as its extends centrifugally into soft tissue. The lumen is filled with necrotic debris and dense collagen. Tumours are composed of short strands, cords, or solid nests of rounded to slightly spindled eosinophilic endothelial cells which have been referred to as "epithelioid" or "histiocytoid." These cells display endothelial differentiation primarily at the cellular level as evidenced by intracytoplasmic lumina (vacuoles) containing erythrocytes which distort or

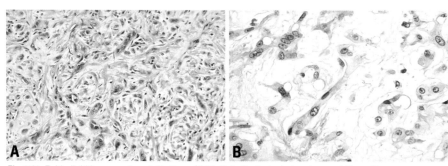

Fig. 7.29 Epithelioid haemangioendothelioma (**A,B**). Note the typical strand or cord-like pattern.

blister their contours. Seldom do they produce multicellular vascular channels as may be seen in epithelioid hemangiomas. The cells appear quite bland with little or no mitotic activity. The neoplastic epithelioid endothelial cells are embedded in a distinctive, sulfated acid-rich matrix which varies from a light blue (chondroid-like) to a deep pink (hyaline) colour. Metaplastic bone is occasionally present within large deep lesions and some cases contain prominent osteoclastic giant cells.

Approximately one third of epithelioid haemangioendotheliomas show atypical histologic features which confer a more aggressive course. These include marked nuclear atypia, mitotic activity (>1/10 HPF), spindling of the cells, and necrosis. These features justify the designation "malignant epithelioid haemangioendothelioma". Some cases represent a morphological continuum with epithelioid angiosarcoma.

Immunohistochemistry / Ultrastructure

A variety of vascular antigens can be identified within epithelioid haemangioendothelioma but CD31, CD34 and FLI1 are more sensitive and more reliable markers than von Willebrand factor. Focal cytokeratin expression is noted in about 25-30% of cases. By electron microscopy the neoplastic cells are situated on a distinct basal lamina, possess surface-oriented pinocytotic vesicles, and occasional Weibel-Palade bodies. They differ from normal endothelium by the abundance of intermediate (vimentin) filaments.

Genetics

An identical translocation involving chromosomes 1 and 3 [t(1;3)(p36.3;q25)] has been reported in two of three cytogenetically analysed soft tissue epithelioid haemangioendotheliomas, possibly representing a characteristic rearrangement for this entity {232,1403}.

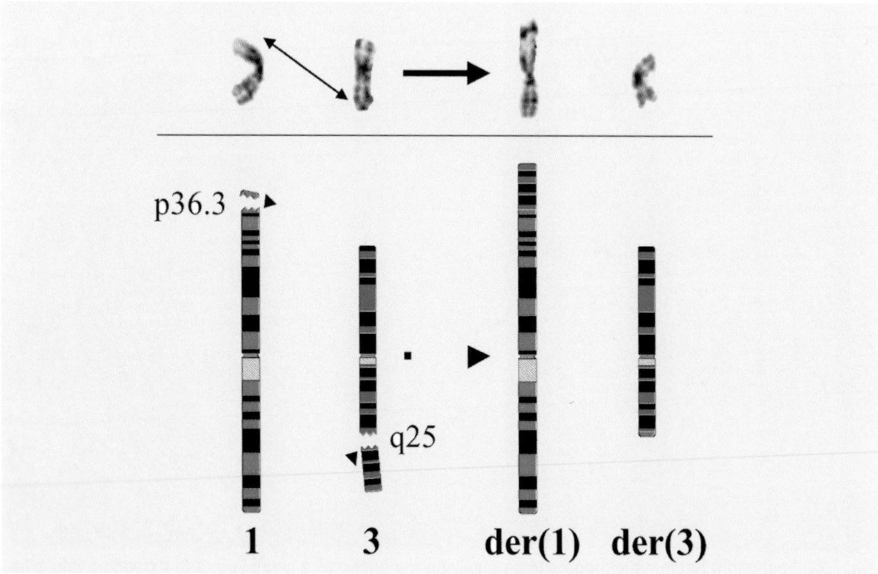

Prognosis and prognostic factors

The behaviour of epithelioid haemangioendothelioma is intermediate between haemangiomas and conventional (high grade) angiosarcomas, although the actual mortality figures are greatly influenced by inclusion of cases with atypical or malignant features in any given series. Based on studies which include both classic and malignant epithelioid haemangioendotheliomas {1407,2238,2245} the local recurrence rate is 10-15%, metastatic rate 20-30%, and mortality 10-20%. Separate analysis of classic epithelioid haemangioendothelioma lacking atypical histological features has a metastatic rate of 17% and mortality of 3% {2245}. Atypical morphological features (described above) correlate with an increased risk of metastases.

Fig. 7.30 Partial G-banded karyotype illustrating the t(1;3)(p36.3;q25) in epithelioid haemangioendothelioma.

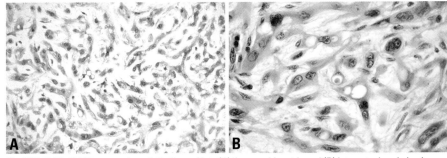

Fig. 7.31 Epithelioid haemangioendothelioma. Note **(A)** the myxoid matrix and **(B)** intracytoplasmic lumina.

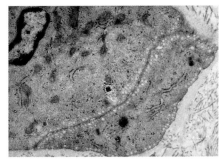

Fig. 7.32 Ultrastructure showing a prominent linear arrangement of pinocytotic vesicles and electron dense Weibel-Palade bodies.

Angiosarcoma of soft tissue

S.W. Weiss
J. Lasota
M.M. Miettinen

Definition
Angiosarcoma is a malignant tumour the cells of which variably recapitulate the morphologic and functional features of normal endothelium.

ICD-O code   9120/3

Synonyms
Lymphangiosarcoma, haemangiosarcoma, haemangioblastoma, malignant haemangioendothelioma, malignant angioendothelioma.

Incidence
Angiosarcomas are rare sarcomas the majority of which develop as cutaneous tumours sometimes associated with lymphedema (see Skin volume). Less than one quarter present as a deep soft tissue mass {1387, 2244}.

Epidemiology
Unlike cutaneous angiosarcomas, soft tissue angiosarcomas are more evenly distributed throughout the decades with a peak incidence in the 7th decade. Angiosarcomas occurring in childhood, however, are very rare.

Sites of involvement
Most lesions occur in the deep muscles of the lower extremities (about 40%) followed by the arm, trunk and head and neck. A significant proportion arise in the abdominal cavity. Rarely the lesions are multifocal.

Clinical features
Soft tissue angiosarcomas develop as enlarging masses which in one third of patients are also associated with other symptoms such as coagulopathy, anaemia, persistent haematoma, or bruisability. In very young patients high output cardiac failure from arteriovenous shunting or even massive haemorrhage may be observed. About one third of patients develop these tumours in association with certain pre-existing conditions suggesting several pathogenetic mechanisms in the development of this form of angiosarcoma. For example, soft tissue angiosarcomas have been reported within benign or malignant nerve sheath tumours associated with neurofibromatosis (NF1), adjacent to synthetic vascular grafts or other foreign material, in rare benign haemangiomas, in

patients with Klippel-Trenaunay and Maffucci syndromes, and following radiation for various types of malignancies.

Macroscopy / Histopathology
These lesions are multinodular haemorrhagic masses that range in size from a few centimeters to several centimeters in diameter. They vary in appearance from spindle to epithelioid neoplasms. Thus, at one extreme an angiosarcoma may resemble a fibrosarcoma or Kaposi sarcoma or at the other extreme an undifferentiated carcinoma. Angiosarcomas with either one of these extreme appearances may be very difficult to diagnose on light microscopy without the benefit of ancillary studies (see below). Generally angiosarcomas in soft tissue have both epithelioid and spindled areas with an emphasis on the former. Epithelioid areas are made up of large rounded cells of relatively high nuclear grade which are arranged in sheets, small nests, cords or rudimentary vascular channels. The diagnosis of angiosarcoma is suspected on light microscopy by identifying cells forming rudimentary vascular channels. Unlike normal vascular channels, these

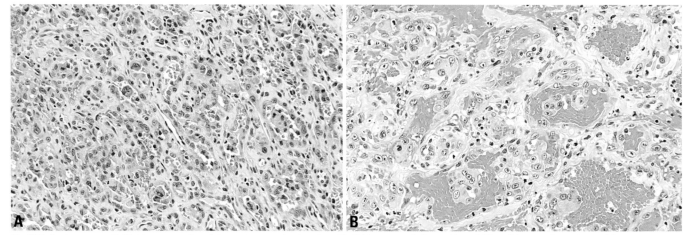

Fig. 7.33 Angiosarcoma (**A,B**). Many cases in soft tissue have predominantly epithelioid cytomorphology with variably solid or vasoformative architecture.

neoplastic channels are irregular in shape, freely intercommunicate with one another in a sinusoidal fashion, and infiltrate surrounding tissues in a destructive fashion. In some areas the vessels may be lined by a single attenuated layer of neoplastic endothelium resembling a haemangioma while in other areas the vascular channels are lined by a surfeit of neoplastic endothelium forming intraluminal buds, projections or papillae. Extensive haemorrhage is a characteristic feature of most tumours, and, in the extreme case, a haemorrhagic soft tissue angiosarcoma may masquerade as a chronic haematoma.

The majority of soft tissue angiosarcomas are high grade tumours characterized by cells of high nuclear grade displaying mitotic activity. In occasional cases, however, areas with low grade, sometimes epithelioid morphology may be observed. These areas can be noted, but the overall diagnosis should usually reflect the diagnosis of a high grade angiosarcoma.

Epithelioid angiosarcoma
Epithelioid angiosarcoma is a variant of angiosarcoma composed predominantly or exclusively of large rounded "epithelioid" endothelial cells with abundant amphophilic or eosinophilic cytoplasm and large vesicular nuclei {681}. Architecturally the cells are arranged in the patterns described above. Although these lesions may occur as cutaneous tumours, most segregate in deep soft tissue. Many cases express cytokeratin along with endothelial markers. Their principal significance is the close mimicry they provide with carcinoma.

Immunohistochemistry
Immunohistochemistry is an important adjunctive procedure in the diagnosis of angiosarcoma, particularly for poorly differentiated forms in which vascular channel formation is difficult to identify. Angiosarcomas express to a greater or lesser degree the usual vascular antigens including von Willebrand factor, CD31, and CD34. Although von Willebrand factor is the most specific of the vascular markers, it is also the least sensitive, often present in only a minority of angiosarcomas as focal weak staining. CD31, on the other hand, combines both relative specificity with excellent sensitivity and is positive in approximately 90% of angiosarcomas of all types {477, 2244}. Cytokeratin is present in about one third of soft tissue angiosarcomas, particularly in the epithelioid forms, reflecting the fact that cytokeratin cannot be used as an absolute discriminant between angiosarcoma and carcinoma. Although not regarded as "first line" antigens, in the diagnosis of angiosarcomas,

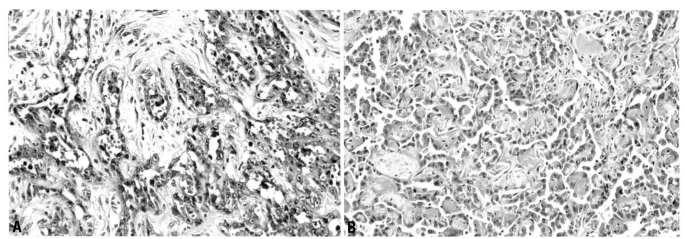

Fig. 7.34 Angiosarcoma (**A,B**). These lesions show more obvious vasoformative growth with complex anastomosing channels.

laminin and Type IV collagen can be detected around neoplastic vascular channels and, therefore, can been used to accentuate vascular channel formation not readily apparent by light microscopy. Actin likewise identifies pericytes which partially invest the vascular channels in angiosarcomas. In general experience angiosarcomas are consistently HHV-8 negative.

Ultrastructure

In better differentiated areas of angiosarcoma, clusters of neoplastic cells surrounded by basal lamina and occasional pericytes can be identified. The neoplastic cells are joined by junctional attachments and possess abundant intermediate filaments, sparse to moderate rough endoplasmic reticulum mitochondria and Golgi apparatus, and have surface oriented pinocytotic vesicles. Weibel-Palade bodies, a specific tubular organelle of normal endothelium, are only rarely identified {1387}.

Genetics

Genetic studies of soft tissue angiosarcomas are scant and limited to isolated cases.

Almost all reported angiosarcoma karyotypes have shown complex cytogenetic aberrations {320,787,929,1120, 1489,1896,2293,2349}. The only exception is a karyotype obtained from angiosarcoma arising in cavernous haemangioma, showing trisomy 5 and loss of the Y as the sole cytogenetic abnormalities {1321}. No consistent, recurring chromosomal abnormality has yet been identified. However, some cytogenetic changes reported in tumours

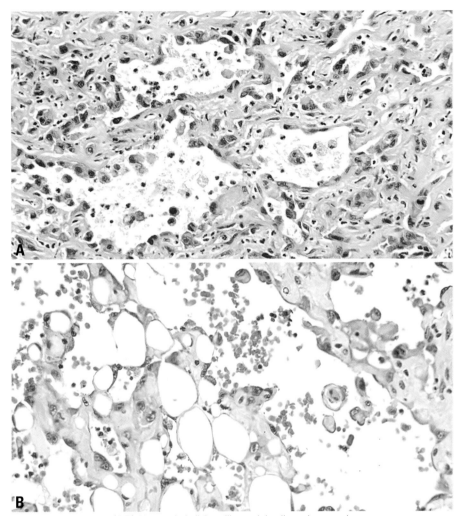

Fig. 7.35 Angiosarcoma **(A,B).** Note endothelial papillae and the dissecting growth pattern.

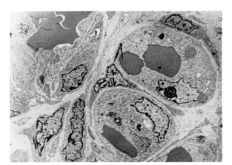

Fig. 7.36 High grade angiosarcoma with epithelioid features showing an ill-formed vessel lined by plump endothelial cells and containing erythrocytes.

from different locations revealed similarities. Among the most common changes were gains of 5pter-p11, 8p12-qter, 20pter-q12 and losses of 4p, 7p15-pter, -Y and abnormalities involving 22q {320, 787, 929, 1120, 1321, 1896, 2293, 2349}.

Flow cytometric DNA studies have shown diploid, tetraploid and aneuploid patterns {521, 614, 739}. No significant correlation between clinical outcome and DNA ploidy pattern has been reported {521,614,739}.

Association between exposure to thorium dioxide or vinyl chloride and development of liver angiosarcoma is well known. Specific KRAS2 and TP53 mutations were identified in these tumours {963, 1330,1331,1527,1734,1981,2129}. Similar KRAS2 and TP53 mutations were

also reported in sporadic skin / soft tissue and parenchymal angiosarcomas {1527,1734,1981,2344}. An alteration of the TP53 / MDM2 pathway with elevated expression of TP53 and MDM2 proteins was documented in 60% of angiosarcomas {2344}.

Prognostic factors

Soft tissue angiosarcomas are highly aggressive tumours. Local recurrences develop in about one fifth of patients and one half may be expected to die within the first year after diagnosis with metastatic disease in the lung followed by lymph node, bone, and soft tissue. The features which have been statistically correlated with poor outcome include older age, retroperitoneal location, large size, and high Ki-67 values {1387}.

CHAPTER 8

Chondro-Osseous Tumours

In the current classification, only soft tissue chondroma and extraskeletal osteosarcoma are retained under this heading. Myositis ossificans and fibro-osseous pseudotumour are now regarded as variants of nodular fasciitis (see Chapter 3) and fibrodysplasia ossificans progressiva appears to be a non-neo-plastic process. Extraskeletal myxoid chondrosarcoma, despite its name, is now realized to show little evidence of cartilaginous differentiation and has therefore been provisionally placed in the Miscellaneous category.

In contrast to its more common osseous counterpart, (see page 264), extraskeletal osteosarcoma is a rare tumour occurring mainly in adults and a significant subset of these lesions arise at the site of prior irradiation. The prognosis is much worse than that for primary osteosarcoma of bone, in part due to differences in delivery of (and response to) chemotherapy.

Soft tissue chondroma

S. Nayler
S. Heim

Definition
Soft tissue chondromas are benign soft tissue tumours occurring in extra-osseous and extra-synovial locations, predominantly composed of adult type hyaline cartilage, devoid of other differentiated elements, except osseous, fibrous and / or myxoid stroma.

ICD-O code   9220/0

Synonyms (Variants)
Extraskeletal chondroma (fibrochondroma, myxochondroma, osteochondroma), chondroma of soft parts.

Epidemiology
The majority of patients are middle-aged, with the reported age range from infancy {762} to 79 years {351, 428, 982}. There is a slight male predominance {351, 428}.

Sites of involvement
The majority of tumours (~64%) occur in the region of the fingers {351}. The remainder of cases occur in the hands, toes and feet, with origin in the trunk, head and neck region {1056} being extremely uncommon. Rare examples have been described in the skin {57, 218}, upper aero-digestive tract {1040, 1244,2211}, dura {281} and, exceptionally, the fallopian tube {2005}.

Clinical features
Most tumours are solitary and present as painless lumps arising in the vicinity of tendons and joints. By definition they are not attached to intraarticular synovium or periosteum. Radiologically they are well demarcated, lobulated neoplasms with central and peripheral calcifications, often curvilinear in nature {120,2347}. Diagnosis can be made on magnetic resonance imaging {2294}.

Macroscopy
Grossly soft tissue chondromas are well circumscribed, lobulated neoplasms. They exhibit a cartilaginous cut surface, although myxoid areas and cystic change may be noted. They rarely exceed 20 to 30 mm in maximal diameter.

Histopathology
Microscopically typical chondromas are composed of lobules of mature, adult hyaline cartilage {1087}. Chondrocytic cells are identified in lacunae, often growing in clusters. When these cells are numerous this variant may be labelled a chondroblastic chondroma {1255}. Prominent fibrosis warrants a designation of fibrochondroma, whilst those tumours with prominent ossification or myxoid change may be classified as osteochondromas {1780} or myxochondromas, respectively {2241}. A chondroblastoma-like variant has also been described

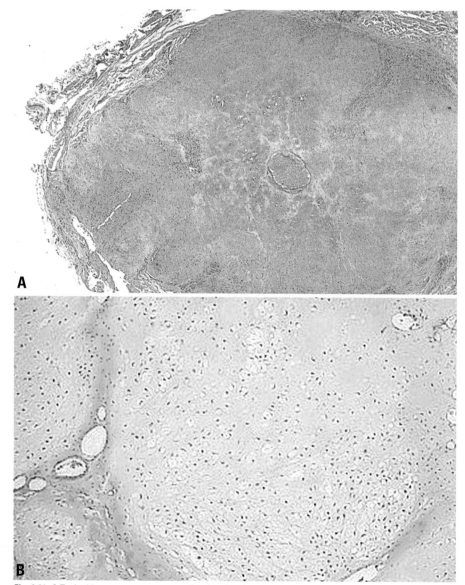

Fig. 8.01 A Typical low power appearance showing the circumscribed lobulated growth pattern. **B** Soft tissue chondroma, consisting of lobules of mature hyaline cartilage.

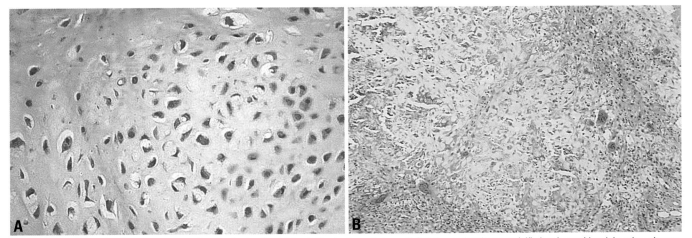

Fig. 8.02 A Soft tissue chondroma, mature cartilage wells showing mild variation in size and shape. **B** Soft tissue chondroma, calcified variant, with calcium deposits surrounding cartilage cells.

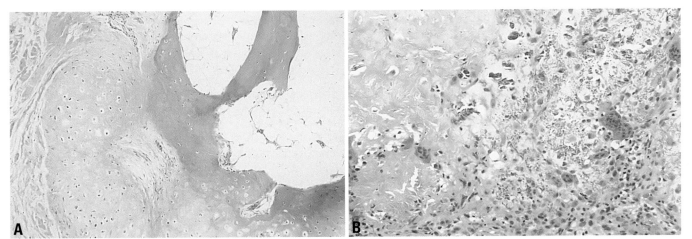

Fig. 8.03 Soft tissue chondroma. **A** Intralesional ossification is quite often seen. **B** Some cases, especially those which are classified, show a striking histiocytic reaction at the periphery.

{315,1012}. One-third of cases may demonstrate extensive calcification, which may mask the cartilaginous appearance of the tumour, particularly in the centre of the tumour lobules. Typical chondroblastic areas are usually discernible at the periphery of the lobules in such cases. Rare tumours may have abundant myxoid matrix with plump immature cells resembling a myxoid chondrosarcoma; however, typical chondroblastic areas are discernible in the periphery of the tumour lobules. Up to 15 percent of cases may show an adjacent granuloma-like reaction {2314} with peripherally situated epithelioid and multinucleated giant cells, surrounding each lobule.

The individual cells are usually small and normochromic. Some tumours cells may be variable in size and shape, with prominent nuclear hyperchromasia and nucleomegaly. Sparse mitoses may be seen, but abnormal mitotic figures are never observed.

Immunophenotype
As with normal cartilaginous cells, the cells of soft tissue chondromas are positive with S100 protein {2314}.

Ultrastructure
Electron microscopy shows typical features of cartilage cells, with abundant rough endoplasmic reticulum, free ribosomes and short irregular microvillous processes surrounded by aggregates of calcium crystals {351}.

Genetics
Only four soft tissue chondromas have shown clonal chromosomal abnormalities {266, 437, 1316, 2105}, and there is no indication of a non-random, let alone specific, aberration pattern.

Prognostic features
Extraskeletal chondromas are benign tumours, although 15 to 20 percent may recur locally {351}. In most instances local excision is curative {351,428,1775}. Transformation to chondrosarcoma, although not uncommon with osseous and synovial cartilaginous tumours, has not been described in extraskeletal chondromas.

Extraskeletal osteosarcoma

A.E. Rosenberg
S. Heim

Definition

Extraskeletal osteosarcoma (EO) is a malignant mesenchymal tumour of soft tissue composed of neoplastic cells that recapitulate the phenotype of osteoblasts and synthesize bone. Some EOs also contain cellular elements that differentiate along chondroblastic and fibroblastic cell lines. Accordingly, all EOs contain neoplastic bone but may also have cartilaginous and fibroblastic components. By definition, no other lines of differentiation are evident.

ICD-O code   9180/3

Synonym

Soft tissue osteosarcoma.

Epidemiology

Extraskeletal osteosarcoma is a rare neoplasm that accounts for 1-2% of all soft tissue sarcomas and approximately 2-4% of all osteosarcomas {119,1284, 1994}. It typically arises during mid and late adulthood with most patients in the 5th-7th decades of life at the time of diagnosis. Males are affected more frequently than females at a ratio of 1.9:1 {119,355,663,1231,1257,1284,1994}.

Sites of involvement

The majority of EOs arise in the deep soft tissues and fewer than 10% are superficial, originating in the dermis or subcutis. The single most common location is the thigh (approximately 50% of cases); other frequent sites include the buttock, shoulder girdle, trunk, and retroperitoneum {119,355,663,1231,1257,1284,1994}.

Clinical features

Most patients present with a progressively enlarging mass that maybe associated with pain. Plain radiographs, CT and MRI usually reveal a large deep-seated soft tissue mass with variable mineralization. By definition these tumours do not arise from bone, but may secondarily involve the periosteum, cortex or medullary canal.

Aetiology

The majority of EOs develops de novo but up to 10% are associated with previous radiation or well-documented trauma. Radiation-induced EO usually develops at least 4 years following radiation for another malignancy {355, 1231, 1257, 1994}.

Macroscopy

Extraskeletal osteosarcomas range in size from 1-50 cm (mean 8-10 cm) and are circumscribed, tan-white, haemorrhagic and focally necrotic gritty masses. The tumour bone is frequently most prominent in the centre of the lesion. In a small number of cases (less than 10%) they exhibit extensive haemorrhagic cystic change.

Histopathology

All of the major subtypes of osteosarcoma that arise in bone may be seen in EO. The most common is the osteoblastic variant, followed by the fibroblastic, chondroid, telangiectatic, small cell, and well differentiated types {119, 355, 663, 1231, 1257, 1284, 1994, 2322}. The tumour cells are spindle or polyhedral cells that are cytologically atypical, are mitotically active and frequently demonstrate atypical mitotic figures. Common to all variants is the presence of neoplastic bone, intimately associated with tumour cells, which may be deposited in a lacy, trabecular or sheet-like pattern. The bone is usually most prominent in the centre of the tumour with the more densely cellular areas located in the periphery a pattern that is the reverse of myositis ossificans (see page 52). In the osteoblastic variant, the tumour cells resemble malignant osteoblasts and bone matrix is abundant. Spindle cells arranged in a herringbone or storiform patterncharacterize the fibroblastic subtype and malignant cartilage predominates in the chondroid variant. Telangiectatic EOs contain numerous large blood filled spaces lined by malignant cells. Sheets of small round cells that mimic Ewing sarcoma or lymphoma are typical of the small cell variant. The extremely rare well differentiated subtype contains abundant bone deposited in well formed trabeculae, surrounded by a minimally atypical spindle cell component similar to parosteal osteosarcoma.

Immunophenotype

Several studies indicate that the immunophenotype of EO is similar to osteosarcoma arising in bone {632, 640, 893, 1257}. EOs are uniformly positive for vimentin, 68% express smooth muscle actin, 25% desmin, 20% S100 protein (including cells in non-cartilaginous areas), 52% EMA, 8% keratin, and 0% PLAP {893, 1257}. Osteocalcin is theoretically the most specific antigen for EOs and it is expressed in the malignant cells and matrix in 82% and 75% of cases, respectively {632}. CD99 is expressed in all types of osteosarcoma.

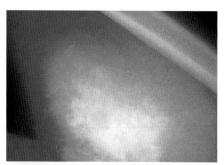

Fig. 8.04 Plain X-ray showing large mineralized mass in posterior thigh.

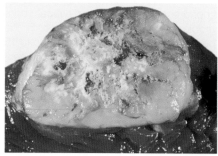

Fig. 8.05 EO composed of white gritty centre with surrounding soft tan tissue.

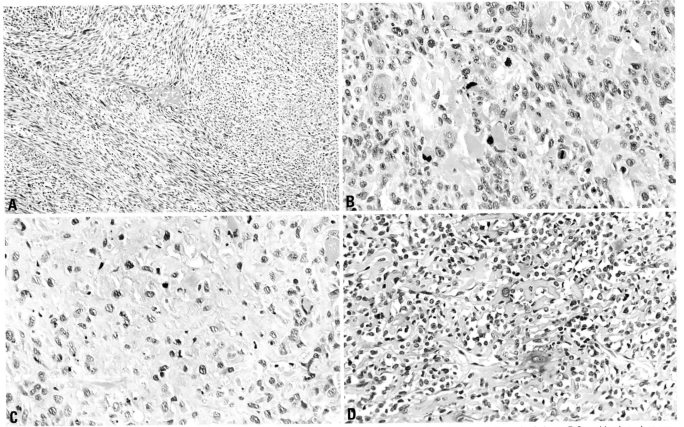

Fig. 8.06 Extraskeletal osteosarcoma. **A** Fibroblastic variant. Fascicles of malignant spindle cells surround a small amount of neoplastic bone. **B** Osteoblastic variant consisting of cytologically malignant cells associated with lace-like tumour bone. Note numerous mitoses. **C** Chondroblastic variant. Cellular malignant hyaline cartilage merging peripherally with tumour bone. **D** Small cell variant composed of sheets of malignant small round cells associated lace-like tumour bone and small islands of neoplastic cartilage.

Ultrastructure

The neoplastic cells of EO vary in appearance. The cells and nuclei are usually large with irregular contours and the cytoplasm contains rough endoplasmic reticulum that may be dilated, as well as a well-developed Golgi complex and filaments {1766}. Desmosomes or tight junctions are rare or absent. Collagen predominates in the extracellular space and electron dense crystals of hydrox-

yapetite are present in areas of bone deposition.

Genetics

Only three cases with clonal chromosomal aberrations have been reported. In two tumours {1319, 1425}, highly complex aberration patterns were seen, whereas the third {1485} had a moderately hyperdiploid karyotype with relatively few chromosomal abnormalities.

So far, therefore, nothing indicates that systematic genetic differences exist between osteosarcomas of bone and soft tissues.

Prognostic factors

Extraskeletal osteosarcoma has a very poor prognosis and approximately 75% of patients die of disease within 5 years of diagnosis {119, 355, 663, 1231, 1257, 1284, 1994}. Morphologic features purported to be associated with a better outcome include small size (<5 cm), histological subtype (fibroblastic, chondroblastic) and diminished proliferative activity as measured by Ki-67 index {119, 355, 1231, 1257}. However, the utility of these prognostic factors has not been confirmed in independent studies. The well differentiated variant may behave in a more indolent fashion; however, too few cases have been reported to draw definitive conclusions regarding their biologic potential.

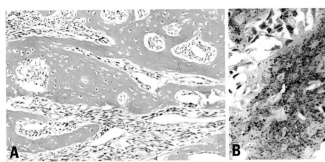

Fig. 8.07 A Well differentiated extraskeletal osteosarcoma with abundant trabeculae of woven bone, surrounded by a bland spindle cell component. **B** Tumour cells and stromal osteoid show immunoreactivity for osteocalcin (ABC method).

CHAPTER 9

Tumours of Uncertain Differentiation

In the past, tumours in this category were often labelled as being of 'uncertain histogenesis'. However, a histogenetic concept for mesenchymal neoplasms is no longer regarded as tenable and there is little or no evidence that connective tissue tumours arise from their normal cellular counterparts. Instead we now think in terms of line of differentiation, which is determined by patterns of gene expression. For tumours in this category, in most cases we have no clear idea as to the line of differentiation (or normal cellular counterpart) that these lesions are recapitulating. Conversely, in some cases (e.g., mixed tumour, synovial sarcoma and clear cell sarcoma), we can identify a line of differentiation but we are unable to define a cellular counterpart in normal mesenchymal tissues.

Principal changes and advances in the category since the 1994 WHO classification are the addition of several newly-recognized entities, including pleomorphic hyalinizing angiectatic tumour, mixed tumour / myoepithelioma in soft tissue and PEComa, as well as the allocation of the angiomatoid fibrous histiocytoma and extraskeletal myxoid chondrosarcoma to this category. As the occurrence of divergent differentiation in a variety of other sarcoma types has become better defined, the category of malignant mesenchymoma seems gradually to be disappearing.

Extraskeletal Ewing sarcoma / peripheral primitive neuroecto-dermal tumour, now acknowledged to be a single definable entity with a variable degree of neuronal differentiation, is described in the Bone section of this volume.

Intramuscular myxoma

G. Nielsen
G. Stenman

Definition

Intramuscular myxoma is a benign soft tissue tumour characterized by bland spindle shaped cells embedded in hypovascular, abundantly myxoid stroma. Intramuscular myxomas may have areas of hypercellularity and increased vascularity ("cellular myxoma"). Mazabraud syndrome is the combination of intramuscular myxoma(s) and skeletal fibrous dysplasia.

ICD-O code   8840/0

Epidemiology

Intramuscular myxoma has a predilection for females and most patients are 40 to 70 years of age at the time of diagnosis.

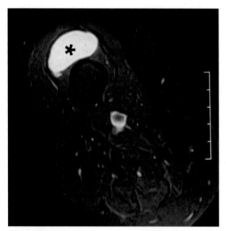

Fig. 9.01 Intramuscular myxoma. MRI reveals a well-circumscribed, hyperintense tumour (∗) adjacent to the tibia.

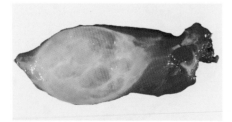

Fig. 9.02 Intramuscular myxoma showing a gelatinous mass with internal septa. The tumour appears well-circumscribed, but closer inspections shows some infiltration of the surrounding skeletal muscle.

Sites of involvement

The most frequent sites affected are the large muscles of the thigh, shoulder, buttocks and upper arm.

Clinical features

Patients usually complain of a painless soft tissue mass. Angiographic studies reveal a poorly vascularized tumour {1119}. Magnetic resonance imaging studies show that the tumour is bright on T2-weighted images and has low signal intensity relative to skeletal muscle on T1-weighted images {1171,1900}.

Macroscopy

Grossly, the tumours have a gelatinous, lobulated cut surface. They can measure up to 20 cm {904}, however most tumours are between 5 and 10 cm in greatest diameter. Although intramuscular myxomas may appear well circumscribed, closer inspection often reveals ill defined borders with the tumour merging with the surrounding skeletal muscle. Fluid filled cystic spaces may be present.

Histopathology

The classic intramuscular myxoma is composed of uniform and cytologically bland spindle and stellate shaped cells with tapering eosinophilic cytoplasm and small nuclei {591,1448}. The cells are separated by abundant myxoid extracellular stroma containing very sparse capillary sized blood vessels. The stroma may be vacuolated and may show cystic change. In some areas a fibrous capsule may surround the tumour. Sections from the interface of the tumour and the surrounding skeletal muscle frequently shows infiltration between muscle fibres or around individual skeletal muscle cells, which may be atrophic. Areas of increased cellularity are present in many intramuscular myxomas and they can occupy 10 to 90% of the tumour {1562, 2182}. Increased number of cells, and more numerous collagen fibres and blood vessels characterize these areas and, if this pattern predominates, then

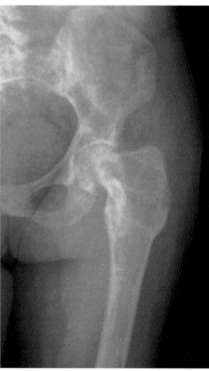

Fig. 9.03 X-ray from a patient with Mazabraud syndrome. AP view of the entire femur and pelvis shows multifocal lytic lesions with thin sclerotic margins involving the wing of the ilium, the acetabulum, the pubis and the femur which shows "shepherd's crook deformity".

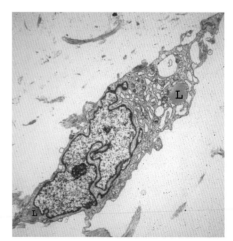

Fig. 9.04 Intramuscular myxoma. EM shows predominantly fibroblastic differentiation; the cells have abundant dilated rough endoplasmic reticulum and occassional intracytoplasmic lipid droplets (L).

the term *'cellular myxoma'* may be used {2182}. Mitoses, pleomorphism, hyperchromasia or necrosis are not present even in the most cellular areas {1562, 2182}. The vessels in these hypercellular regions are capillary sized but occasional thick walled vessels with smooth muscle in their walls are also present.

Immunophenotype
Immunohistochemically the cells stain for vimentin and show variable staining for CD34, desmin and actin. There is no staining for S100 protein.

Ultrastructure
The tumour cells have the features of fibroblasts or myofibroblasts with prominent secretory activity. The cells contain well-developed dilated rough endoplasmic reticulum, Golgi complexes, free ribosomes, pinocytotic vesicles and occasional filaments. Also seen are more primitive appearing mesenchymal cells and histiocyte-like cells. Intracytoplasmic lipid droplets can be seen {904}.

Genetics
The only published case with abnormal karyotype displayed a hyperdiploid clone with trisomy 18 as the sole anomaly {1389}. Molecular genetic analysis has shown that point mutations of the *GNAS1* gene (a.k.a. $G_s\alpha$) seem to be common in intramuscular myxomas {1605}. Mutations in codon 211 (Arg -> His and Arg -> Cys) were detected in five of six intramuscular myxomas with (Mazabraud syndrome) and without fibrous dysplasia of bone {630}. *GNAS1* encodes the a-subunit of the guanine nucleotide binding protein, i.e. the G-protein that stimulates the formation of cAMP. Activating *GNAS1* mutations in codon 211 have previously also been found in certain endocrine tumours {2328}, McCune-Albright syndrome {1903}, as well as in isolated fibrous dysplasia of bone {1935}.

Prognostic factors
Conventional intramuscular myxoma is usually a non-recurrent tumour. The cellular variant has a small risk of local non-destructive recurrence {2182}.

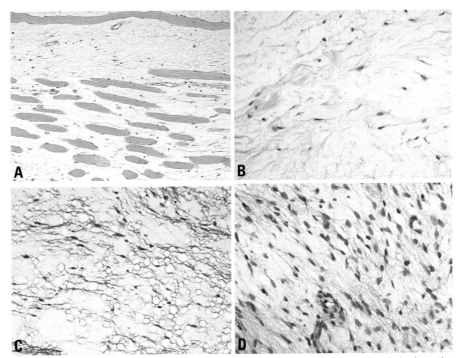

Fig. 9.05 A Intramuscular myxoma. At the periphery, the tumour infiltrates the surrounding skeletal muscle. **B** Intramuscular myxoma. Typically, bland spindle cells are separated by abundant extracellular myxoid matrix. **C** Intramuscular myxoma. The extracellular matrix in intramuscular myxoma may show prominent frothy appearance, mimicking lipoblasts. **D** Cellular myxoma. The cells within the cellular area are bland and do not demonstrate cytological atypia, mitoses or pleomorphism (same case as Fig. 9.06).

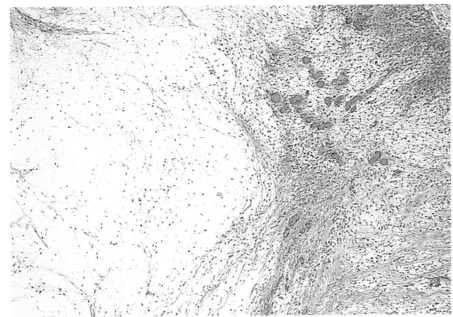

Fig. 9.06 Cellular myxoma. Classic intramuscular myxoma (left) merging with cellular myxoma (right). The former is hypocellular and hypovascular whereas the latter demonstrates increased cellularity and vascularity.

Juxta-articular myxoma

G. Nielsen
G. Stenman

Definition

Juxta-articular myxoma is a rare, benign soft tissue tumour that usually arises in the vicinity of a large joint, has histological features resembling a cellular myxoma, and is frequently associated with ganglion-like cystic changes.

ICD-O code   8840/0

Synonyms

Some lesions described in the literature as parameniscal cyst, periarticular myxoma, cystic myxomatous tumour around the knee, meniscal cyst and myxoid lesion associated with ganglion cysts probably represent examples of juxta-articular myxoma {41}.

Epidemiology

In the largest series the patients ranged in age from 16 to 83 years (median 43 years) {1394}; a tumour arising in a 9-year-old girl has also been reported {446}.

Sites of involvement

The majority of lesions (88%) occur in the vicinity of the knee joint. Other locations include the elbow region, shoulder region, ankle and hip.

Clinical features

The patients present with a swelling or a mass that can be painful or tender. The duration of symptoms ranges from weeks to years. Radiographic studies show a soft tissue mass that has similar imaging characteristics as intramuscular myxoma {1121}. However, the presence of haemosiderin or fibrous tissue within the lesion might suggest the possibility of pigmented villonodular synovitis or a low grade sarcoma {446}.

Macroscopy

The tumour is myxoid, slimy and gelatinous, frequently with cystic areas. The tumours range in size from 0.6 to 12 cm (mean 3.8 cm; median 3.5 cm).

Histopathology

Histologically, it is reminiscent of the cellular form of intramuscular myxoma and is composed of bland appearing spindle cells embedded in a hypovascular myxoid stroma. Although areas of increased cellularity are often present, mitotic figures are absent or very rare. Cystic, ganglion-like spaces, are seen in 89% of cases. These cystic spaces are lined by a layer of delicate fibrin or thicker layer of collagen. The periphery of the tumour is ill defined and infiltrates adjacent tissues. Areas of haemorrhage, haemosiderin deposition, chronic inflammation, organizing fibrin and fibroblastic reaction may be seen, especially in recurrent tumours.

Immunophenotype

Same as intramuscular myxoma.

Ultrastructure

Same as intramuscular myxoma.

Genetics

Clonal chromosome abnormalities have been reported in a single case of juxta-articular myxoma {1908}. The tumour contained two unrelated clones distinguished by an inv(2)(p15q36) and +7, t(8;22)(q11-12;q12-13), respectively. Juxta-articular myxomas lack mutations of the GNAS1 gene, in contrast to intramuscular myxomas {1604}.

Prognostic factors

In the series by Meis and Enzinger {1394} 10 of 29 (34%) tumours locally recurred: five recurred once, two recurred twice, two recurred three times and one recurred four times. Malignant transformation has not been reported.

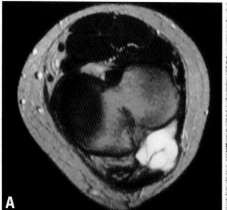
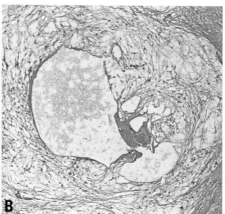
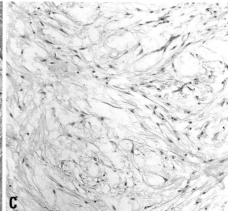

Fig. 9.07 Juxtaarticular myxoma. **A** MRI of a tumour located adjacent to the knee joint, showing a homogeneous bright signal, similar to intramuscular myxoma. **B** A cystic area filled with myxoid material is surrounded by more cellular proliferation. The cystic, ganglion like space, is lined by an eosinophilic layer of fibrin. **C** Note the bland appearance of the spindle cells.

Deep 'aggressive' angiomyxoma

J.F. Fetsch
G. Stenman

Definition

A soft tissue neoplasm with a predilection for pelvic and perineal regions and a tendency for local recurrence. It is composed of small stellate and spindle cells in a myxoedematous stroma with entrapped regional structures.

ICD-O code   8841/0

Epidemiology

Deep 'aggressive' angiomyxoma has a strong predilection for adult females in the third through sixth decades of life with a peak incidence in the fourth decade {330, 656, 826}. Elderly or postmenopausal women are only rarely affected, and the diagnosis should be viewed with suspicion in prepubertal girls. One purported example has been reported in an 11-year-old female, but the illustrations are more consistent with a superficial angiomyxoma {2260}. The tumour has also been described rarely in males with a median age at presentation in the sixth decade {367,1000,2136}.

Sites of involvement

Pelvicoperineal, inguinoscrotal, and retroperitoneal regions.

Clinical features

Most patients with deep 'aggressive' angiomyxoma present with a slow-growing mass in the pelvicoperineal region that is either asymptomatic or associated with regional pain, dyspareunia, or a pressure-like sensation {656}. The true

tumour size is often significantly underestimated by physical examination with the most common clinical impressions being a Bartholin gland cyst, vaginal cyst, hernia or lipoma. Because the bulk of the tumour is often concealed within the deep soft tissues and the process generally does not cause rectal, urethral, vaginal, or vascular obstruction, the majority of examples are quite large at the time of resection.

The imaging characteristics of this tumour are well described {1629}. CT demonstrates a hypoattenuating or isoattenuating mass that tends to grow around pelvic floor structures, usually without causing significant disruption of the vaginal or rectal musculature. A high signal intensity is noted with T2-weighted MR images. Both T2-weighted MR and enhanced CT images also frequently demonstrate a swirled or layered internal structure. These techniques are invaluable for assessing tumour extent and determining the best surgical approach.

Macroscopy

Gross examination usually reveals a large mass, often greater than 10 cm and sometimes larger than 20 cm {656,

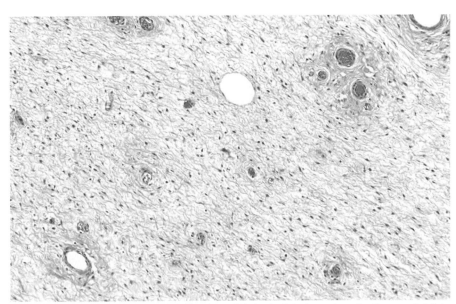

Fig. 9.09 Deep 'aggressive' angiomyxoma. Note low cellularity, hyalinized vessels, and uniform small stellate and spindle cells.

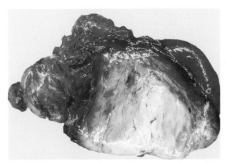

Fig. 9.08 Deep 'aggressive' angiomyxoma with whitish surface showing fibrous bands in a myxoid matrix.

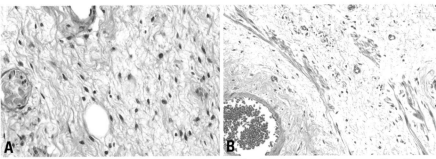

Fig. 9.10 Deep 'aggressive' angiomyxoma. **A** Small tumour cells without nuclear atypia, scattered in a fibromyxoid background. **B** Aggressive angiomyxoma with myoid cells in close proximity to vessels.

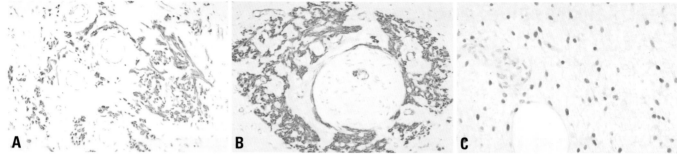

Fig. 9.11 Deep 'aggressive' angiomyxoma. Desmin **(A)** and smooth muscle actin **(B)** immunoreactivity in the myoid element. **C** Nuclear immunoreactivity for oestrogen receptor protein.

2024}. Small tumours under 5 cm in size are less frequent. The lesions frequently have a lobular contour with adherence to fat, muscle, and other regional structures. A soft, firm, or rubbery consistency may be present, and a glistening, myxooedematous, pink or reddish-tan cut surface is usually evident. Cystic change has occasionally been noted.

Histopathology
The tumours are of low to moderate cellularity and are composed of relatively uniform, small, stellate and spindled cells, set in a loosely collagenous, myxooedematous matrix with scattered vessels of varying caliber and entrapped regional structures. The tumour cells have scant, pale, eosinophilic cytoplasm with poorly defined borders and relatively bland nuclei with an open chromatin pattern and a single, small, centrally located nucleolus. Multinucleated cells may rarely be observed. Mitotic figures are infrequent. A characteristic finding that is seen in most cases is the presence of loosely organized islands of well-developed myoid (myofibroblastic or true smooth muscle) cells around the larger

nerve segments and vessels. Although the tumour name implies abundant myxoid matrix, these neoplasms are usually only weakly positive for mucosubstances, a finding that suggests oedema fluid is a major component of the noncollagenous stroma.

Immunophenotype
The tumour cells of deep 'aggressive' angiomyxoma usually show diffuse immunoreactive for vimentin, moderate to diffuse (nuclear) immunoreactivity for oestrogen and progesterone receptor protein, and variable levels of immunoreactivity for actins and CD34 {656,826, 1369}. Desmin positivity can be identified in almost all cases. Immunoreactivity for S100 protein is absent.

Ultrastructure
Ultrastructural evaluation has revealed cells with fibroblastic, myofibroblastic, and smooth muscle features {150, 1965, 2024}.

Genetics
Cytogenetic studies have revealed clonal chromosome abnormalities in five

cases of deep 'aggressive' angiomyxoma, all affecting the female genital tract {1081, 1586}. Four tumours had abnormalities involving chromosome 12, including one case with monosomy 12 and three cases with structural rearrangements of 12q13-15. Molecular analyses of two of the cases with rearrangement of 12q13-15 identified *HMGIC* (a.k.a. *HMGA2*) as the target gene {1081,1586}. In one case the rearrangement resulted in a fusion gene in which the first three exons of *HMGIC* were fused to ectopic sequences derived from a novel gene in 12p11.2 and in the other case the translocation breakpoint was located 3' of the gene leading to deregulation of *HMGIC* expression.

Prognostic factors
Deep 'aggressive' angiomyxoma has a local recurrence rate of approximately 30% {150, 330, 656, 826, 2024}, and such recurrences are usually controlled by a single re-excision. Thus, these tumours are less aggressive than was originally believed. These lesions have no metastatic potential.

Pleomorphic hyalinizing angiectatic tumour of soft parts

S.W. Weiss

Definition
Pleomorphic hyalinizing angiectatic tumour of soft parts (PHAT) is a non-metastasising tumour of uncertain lineage, characterized by clusters of ectatic, fibrin-lined, thin-walled vessels, which are surrounded by a mitotically inert, spindled, pleomorphic neoplastic stroma containing a variable inflammatory component.

Synonyms
There are no recognized synonyms for this distinctive lesion. Prior to the original description of this lesion in 1996 {1972} these lesions were undoubtedly misdiagnosed as schwannomas because of the ectatic vessels or as so-called malignant fibrous histiocytoma because of the degree of atypia.

Epidemiology
PHAT is characteristically a tumour arising in adults without gender predilection.

Sites of involvement
Over half of the cases arise in the subcutaneous tissues of the lower extremity, but may also occur in the subcutis of the chest wall, buttock and arm. Only a minority develop in deep soft tissues and none to date have been reported in body cavities.

Clinical features
These tumours arise as slowly growing masses which have been present for several years before coming to medical attention. Clinically they are diagnosed as haematomas, Kaposi sarcoma or a variety of benign lesions.

Macroscopy / Histopathology
The tumours are lobulated infiltrating masses which vary from white-tan to maroon in colour. They are characterized by clusters of thin-walled ectatic vessels scattered throughout a sheet-like proliferation of spindle cells. The vessels, which range in size from small microscopic structures to macroscopic ones, tend to occur in distinct clusters. They are lined by endothelium which is lifted off the vessel wall by a subjacent coat of thick amorphous hyaline material which is largely fibrin. This material extends through the vessel wall into the surrounding stroma entrapping the neoplastic cells and resulting in areas of stromal hyalinization. Organising thrombus is frequently present within the vessels. The stromal cells are plump spindled and rounded cells with hyperchromatic pleomorphic nuclei often containing intranuclear cytoplasmic inclusions. Despite the level of atypia, mitotic activity is usually scant (<1 mitosis/50 HPF). A variable component of mast cells, lymphocytes, plasma cells and eosinophils may infiltrate the tumours. Psammoma bodies are occasionally present.

These tumours consistently express vimentin and occasionally CD34. Some cases show epithelial membrane antigen positivity. Notably they do not express S100 protein, making that antigen important in their distinction from schwannoma. Other antigens such as actin, desmin, cytokeratin, von Willebrand factor, and CD31 are also negative.

Clinical behaviour
About 50% of these tumours recur locally, but metastasis has not been recorded. Generally recurrences are non destructive in their growth.

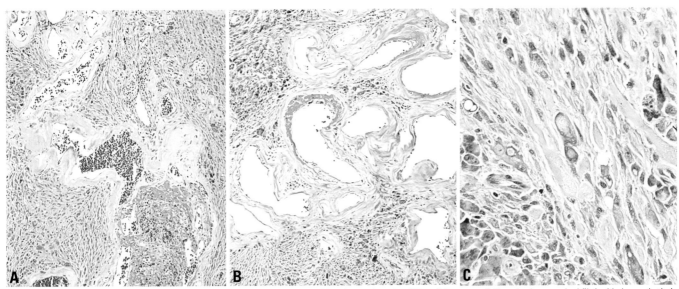

Fig. 9.12 Pleomorphic hyalinizing angiectatic tumour of soft parts. **A** Note the dilated vessels and solidly cellular areas. **B** Vessels show marked fibrinoid change in their walls. **C** Spindle cell component shows pleomorphic cells with intranuclear inclusions..

Ectopic hamartomatous thymoma

J.K.C. Chan

Definition
Ectopic hamartomatous thymoma is a benign tumour of the lower neck showing an admixture of spindle cells, epithelial islands and adipose cells suggesting branchial pouch origin.

ICD-O code   8587/0

Sites of involvement
The tumour occurs exclusively in the superficial or deep soft tissues of the supraclavicular, suprasternal or presternal region {83,328,615,660,935,1442,1806,1834,2341}.

Clinical features
The tumour affects adults with a median age of 43 years and marked male predilection (male to female ratio 8:1) {328,935,2341}. The patients present with a long-standing mass lesion.

Macroscopy
The well circumscribed tumour usually measures a few cm in diameter, but some tumours can be much larger. It shows grey-white to yellowish solid cut surfaces which may be punctuated by small cysts.

Histopathology
The tumour shows haphazard blending of spindle cells, epithelial islands and adipocytes, which are present in highly variable proportions. The spindle cells exhibit fascicular or lattice-like growth, and possess bland-looking elongated nuclei with pointed ends and light-staining cytoplasm. Some spindle cells can have a myoid appearance due to the presence of eosinophilic cytoplasm. The epithelial component takes the form of squamous islands, syringoma-like tubules, anastomosing networks, simple

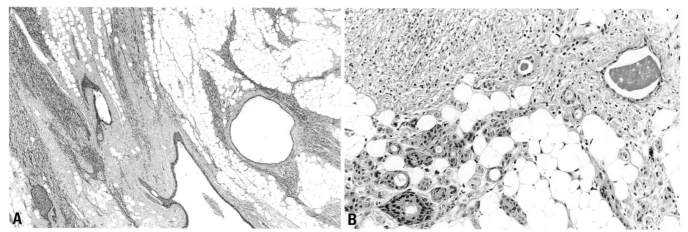

Fig. 9.13 Ectopic hamartomatous thymoma. **A** Haphazard blending of spindle cells, epithelial islands and adipose cells. Some cysts are also seen. **B** The epithelium sometimes takes the form of glandular structures. Note the presence of intermingled adipose cells.

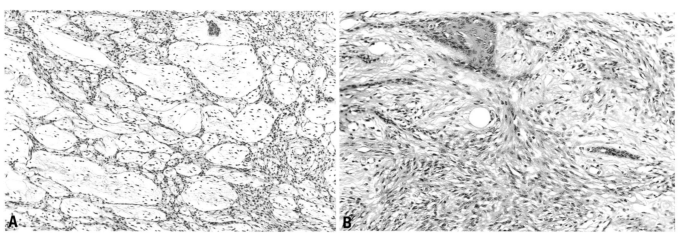

Fig. 9.14 Ectopic hamartomatous thymoma. **A** The spindle cells commonly exhibit lattice-like growth, reminiscent of atrophic thymus. **B** Characteristically elongated strands of epithelium merge into spindle cells. The epithelium commonly shows squamous differentiation.

glandular structures and cysts. The epithelial islands are surrounded by a fibrous sheath or merge imperceptibly into the spindle cells.

Immunophenotype

Both the epithelial and spindle cell components stain diffusely and strongly for cytokeratin, in particular high molecular weight cytokeratin, indicating that the spindle cells are epithelial in nature. In some cases, a proportion of the spindle cells are immunoreactive for myoid markers such as actin or myoglobin, but not desmin {83,1442,1834,2341}. Staining for CD34 remarkably highlights the smaller stromal cells between the fascicles of spindle cells as well as some spindle cells.

Ultrastructure

The spindle cells exhibit tonofilaments and desmosomes.

Prognostic factors

This benign lesion does not recur after excision. In the rare examples reported to show malignant change, there has not been recurrence or metastasis {1442}. Such cases focally feature closely packed glands lined by highly atypical cells, but there is no frank invasion beyond the parent tumour.

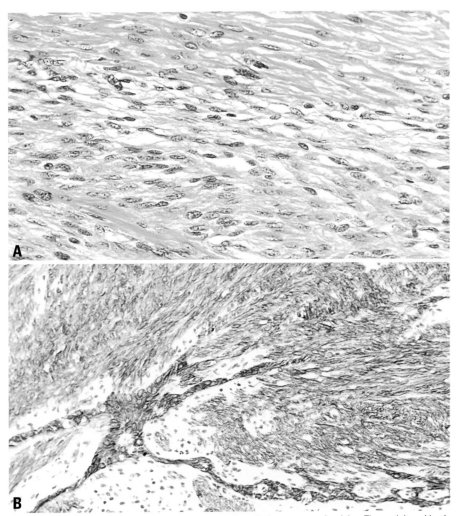

Fig. 9.15 Ectopic hamartomatous thymoma. **A** The spindle cells form compact fascicles. The nuclei are bland-looking, often with pointed ends. Some cells have deeply eosinophilic cytoplasm, suggestive of a myoid phenotype. **B** Immunostaining for cytokeratin highlights both the epithelial strands and the spindle cells. The immunonegative smaller stromal cells in between are strongly positive for CD34 (not shown).

Angiomatoid fibrous histiocytoma

J.C. Fanburg-Smith
P. Dal Cin

Definition

Angiomatoid fibrous histiocytoma (AFH) generally affects children and young adults. It has a partially myoid phenotype and low metastatic potential. This tumour should not be confused with, and is not identical to, aneurysmal fibrous histiocytoma of skin.

ICD-O code   8836/1

Synonym

Angiomatoid malignant fibrous histiocytoma.

Epidemiology

Originally described by Enzinger in 1979 {593}, AFH comprises 5% of tumours designated as "malignant fibrous histiocytoma" and approximately 0.3% of all soft tissue tumours. Although AFH has a wide age range from birth {81} to 71 years old {638}, it is predominantly a tumour of children and young adults, with a mean age of 20 years. In larger series, there is a slight female predilection {404, 638}, whereas other series show a male predominance {593,1700}.

Sites of involvement

The extremities are the most common site for AFH, followed by the trunk and head and neck. Sixty-six percent of lesions {638} occur in areas where normal lymph nodes may be found, i.e. antecubital fossa, popliteal fossa, axilla, inguinal area, supraclavicular fossa, and anterior and posterior neck.

Clinical features

AFH is mainly a slow-growing tumour of the deep dermis and subcutis and may often simulate a haematoma. Some patients report antecedent trauma to the area; pain is generally not a symptom. Occasional associated systemic signs of fever, anaemia, and weight loss suggest cytokine production by the tumour, similar to haematopoietic tumours such as fibroblastic reticulum cell sarcoma {59}, another suggestion of the possible relationship of AFH to this entity. MRI of AFH may reveal fluid-fluid levels, indicating haemorrhage, similar to that seen for aneurysmal bone cyst {1522}.

Macroscopy

The median size for AFH is 2.0 centimeters, range 0.7 to 12.0 centimeters {404, 593,638}. Its firm consistency and circumscribed, tan-grey appearance grossly resembles a lymph node. On cut surface, it is often multinodular with blood-filled cystic spaces and a red-

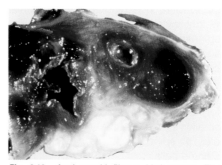

Fig. 9.16 Angiomatoid fibrous histiocytoma. The macroscopic appearance resembles haematoma or haemorrhage within a lymph node.

brown appearance, denoting haemosiderin, occasionally simulating a haematoma or cystic haemorrhage within a lymph node.

Histopathology

The four key morphologic features of AFH may be found in varying proportions: (1) a multinodular proliferation of eosinophilic, histiocytoid or myoid cells, (2) pseudoangiomatoid spaces, (3) a thick fibrous pseudocapsule, and (4) a pericapsular lymphoplasmacytic infiltrate. The latter three features may variably be absent or not apparent on the submitted histologic sections. Always present are the spindled or epithelioid

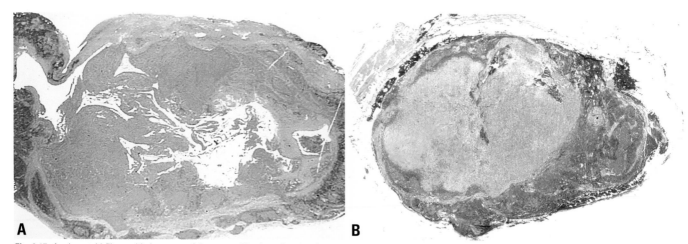

Fig. 9.17 Angiomatoid fibrous histiocytoma. **A** Low magnification microscopic appearance of the tumour shown in Fig. 9.16, showing cystic dilation, partially filled with blood and surrounded by lymphoid tissue. **B** Another example demonstrating typical morphological features: fibrohistiocytic and lymphoid proliferation, angiomatoid blood filled cystic spaces, and pseudocapsule all simulating a tumour within a lymph node.

cells, generally uniform with ovoid vesicular nuclei and often arranged in nodules. The pseudoangiomatoid spaces are not lined by endothelium but rather are cystic spaces within the tumour, filled with blood. The lymphoplasmacytic infiltrate and occasional germinal centre formation make this tumour simulate a lymph node tumour histologically; however, the infiltrate is often outside of the pseudocapsule and subcapsular sinuses or hilar lymphatics of a lymph node are absent in AFH. Cannon-ball-like growth pattern and myxoid change is sometimes observed. Cellular pleomorphism and increased mitotic activity may be identified, particularly in the spindled tumours, but does not correlate with outcome {404}.

Immunophenotype

AFH is positive for desmin in 50% of cases, often also with scattered desmin positive cells within the lymphoid proliferation {403,638,674,898,1971}.

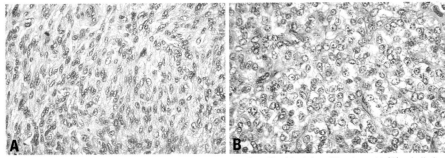

Fig. 9.18 Angiomatoid fibrous histiocytoma. Fibrohistiocytic (myofibroblastic) proliferation with **(A)** spindled or **(B)** epithelioid morphology.

Approximately 40% of cases show EMA positivity and many examples show staining for CD68. Yet strong evidence for histiocytic, smooth muscle or skeletal muscle phenotype are absent. Half of the cases may be positive for the nonspecific marker CD99 {638,898}. The tumour cells are uniformly negative for other reticulum cell tumour markers (CD21, CD35), S100 protein, HMB-45, keratins, CD34, and vascular-specific markers (CD31, Factor VIIIrag).

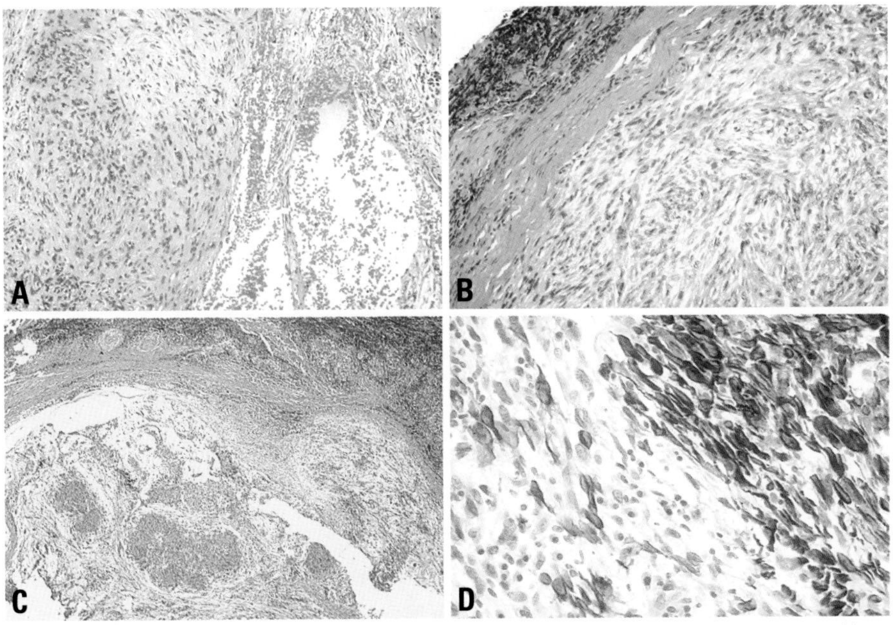

Ultrastructure

Published ultrastructural data have been conflicting and inconclusive with regard to the line of differentiation in tumour cells, perhaps in part due to sampling error.

Genetics

Only one angiomatoid MFH with chromosome aberrations has so far been reported {2222}. Complex rearrangements involving chromosomes 2, 12, 16 and 17, as well as a del(11)(q24) were observed. Further molecular investigation revealed that the *FUS* (a.k.a. *TLS*) gene, mapping to chromosome band 16p11, was fused with the *ATF1* gene, located in band 12q13. The translocation thus generates a chimeric FUS/ATF1 protein, similar to the EWS/ATF1 chimeric protein seen in clear cell sarcomas with a t(12;22)(q13;q12).

Prognostic factors

AFH has overall indolent behaviour with 2-11% local recurrences {404, 638} and less than 1% metastases, generally non-fatal to regional lymph nodes {638} and rare deaths due to late distant metastases {403, 404, 593, 1700}. While local recurrence may be higher with infiltrating margins, location on the head and neck, and deep intramuscular location {404}, there are no known clinical, morphological, or genetic factors that predict metastasis. Wide local excision is the treatment of choice for primary tumours {404, 638}.

Fig. 9.19 Angiomatoid fibrous histiocytoma. **A** Pseudoangiomatoid blood-filled cystic spaces without endothelial lining. **B** Fibrous pseudocapsule surrounds lymphoplasmacytic and fibrohistiocytic (myofibroblastic) components and the absence of subcapsular sinus or hilar lymphatics are evidence against a true lymph node process. **C** Occasional cannon ball-like growth pattern of myofibroblastic cells with myxoid change. **D** Desmin immunoreactivity is seen in approximately half of cases.

Ossifying fibromyxoid tumour

B.P. Rubin
G. Stenman

Definition
Ossifying fibromyxoid tumour is a rare neoplasm of uncertain lineage, with cords and trabeculae of ovoid cells embedded in a fibromyxoid matrix, often surrounded by a partial shell of lamellar bone. Occasionally, this lesion may acquire a malignant phenotype.

ICD-O codes
Ossifying fibromyxoid tumour   8842/0
Ossifying fibromyxoid tumour
(malignant)   8842/3

Epidemiology
Males (64%) are affected more frequently than females. Lesions tend to occur in adults with patient age ranging from 14-79 years with a median age of 50 years.

Sites of involvement
Approximately 70% of cases arise in the extremities {602}. Other sites of involvement include the trunk, head and neck, oral cavity, mediastinum, and retroperitoneum {602,1513,2111}.

Clinical features
Most patients present with a small, painless, subcutaneous mass, often attached to the underlying tendons, fascia, or skeletal muscle. Lesions are usually of longstanding duration and have been present from 1 to 20 or more years (median 4 years). Radiological studies characteristically, but not invariably reveal a well circumscribed, lobulated mass, with irregular calcifications within the mass, surrounded by an incomplete ring of calcification {602,1873}. Erosion of underlying bone and periosteal reaction has also been noted in some cases {602,1873}.

Macroscopy
Most lesions range from 3-5 cm in greatest dimension with a median size of about 4 cm. Occasional examples are large, measuring up to 17 cm or larger {602}. Ossifying fibromyxoid tumours are well circumscribed, nodular or multinodular, and typically covered by a thick fibrous pseudocapsule with or without a shell of bone. On cut section, they are white to tan in colour, and either firm, hard, or rubbery in texture.

Histopathology
Ossifying fibromyxoid tumour is composed of lobules of uniform, round to fusiform-shaped cells arranged in nests and cords, and set in a variably fibromyxoid stroma. Approximately 80% of lesions are surrounded by an incomplete shell of metaplastic (hypocellular) lamellar bone, while the other 20% of cases lack a shell of bone (non-ossifying variant) {602, 1444,1894,2273}. The neoplastic cells are monomorphous with round-to-ovoid

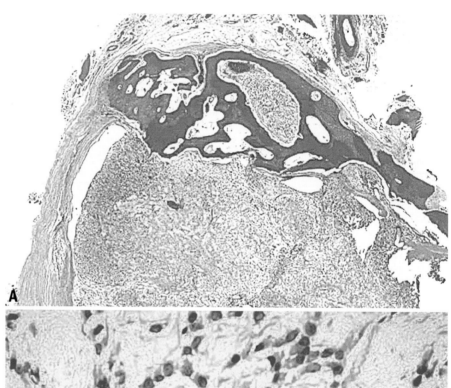

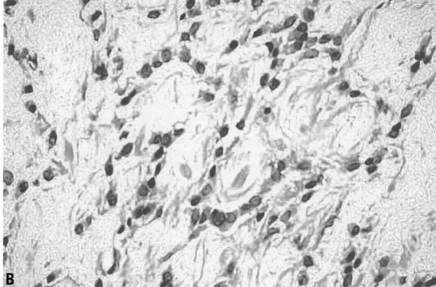

Fig. 9.20 Ossifying fibromyxoid tumour. **A** This lesion is partially surrounded by lamellar bone and partially by a thickened fibrous pseudocapsule. **B** Anastomosing cords of cells set in a myxoid matrix.

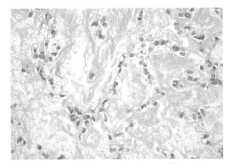

Fig. 9.21 Ossifying fibromyxoid tumour. The cells are monomorphous and have vesicular nuclei with inconspicuous nucleoli, and scant eosinophilic cytoplasm.

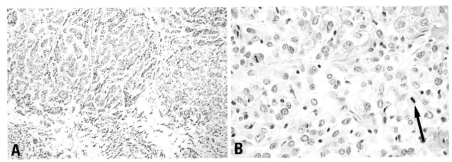

Fig. 9.22 Atypical / malignant ossifying fibromyxoid tumour. **A** Cellular areas and centrally placed osteoid. **B** Cells have enlarged nuclei and more prominent, sometimes multiple, nucleoli. Note the mitotic activity (arrow).

nuclei and inconspicuous nucleoli, and a scant amount of eosinophilic cytoplasm. Mitotic activity is usually less than 1 per 10 high power fields. The stroma is quite variable and can be predominantly myxoid (alcian blue positive, hyaluronidase sensitive) or collagenous/hyalinized with a prominent vasculature which can exhibit perivascular hyalinization. Calcifications and/or nodules of metaplastic cartilage are occasionally identified.

Rare examples of ossifying fibromyxoid tumour are hypercellular and/or have increased numbers of mitotic figures and deposition of tumour osteoid by neoplastic cells randomly, or more frequently, within the centre of the lesions. One such case showed features reminiscent of osteosarcoma {602}. These lesions have been termed "atypical" or "malignant" (for those tumours that metastasise) {1104}. Furthermore, these "atypical" or "malignant" ossifying fibromyxoid tumours tend to have a much less complete shell of bone than conventional examples.

Immunophenotype

Ossifying fibromyxoid tumours (including atypical and malignant examples) are typically positive for vimentin and S100 protein (70%), often show desmin positivity and may also express Leu-7, neuron-specific enolase, glial fibrillary acidic protein and smooth muscle actin (rare)

{602, 669, 1104, 1444, 1894, 2273, 2319}. Rare cases show focal keratin positivity.

Ultrastructure

The cytoplasm contains prominent rough endoplasmic reticulum, often with cisternal dilatations, moderate numbers of mitochondria, and numerous microfilaments, often clustered in the perinuclear area {533, 669, 1444}. Ribosome-lamellar complexes have also been described {669}. Many cells have a partial reduplicated external lamina, and occasional cells have complex, sometimes interdigitating cell processes.

Genetics

A single case of ossifying fibromyxoid tumour has been analysed cytogenetically {2003}. The tumour had a hypodiploid karyotype distinguished by a der(6;14)(p10;q10) and an add(12)(q24).

Prognostic factors

Follow-up data is available in 41 cases of ossifying fibromyxoid tumour from the largest series {602}. Recurrences were noted in 11 cases (27%), sometimes multiple. One patient had a presumed metastasis to the contralateral thigh (in contrast to a second primary lesion) 20 years after excision of the primary {602}. The histological and clinical features of

the majority of the recurrent tumours were identical to the non-recurrent tumours. However, increased mitotic activity (8-10 mitotic figures per 10 high power fields) and increased cellularity were noted in some of the recurrent lesions. These latter lesions would probably be regarded as "atypical" or "malignant" ossifying fibromyxoid tumours by some. Clinical follow-up in the 3 cases reported as "atypical" or "malignant" with significant follow-up, revealed local recurrence in one case 2 years after excision of the primary, and pulmonary metastasis at the time of presentation followed by a local recurrence and additional pulmonary metastasis 25 months later in the other {1104}.

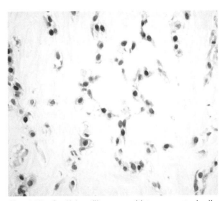

Fig. 9.23 Ossifying fibromyoxoid tumours typically show diffuse immunoreactivity for S100 protein.

Mixed tumour / Myoepithelioma / Parachordoma

S.E. Kilpatrick
J. Limon

Definition
Mixed tumours are well circumscribed lesions displaying epithelial and / or myoepithelial elements in varying proportions, within a hyalinized to chondromyxoid stroma. Those tumours, comprised mostly of myoepithelial cells, closely resembling those observed in pleomorphic adenoma, and lacking obvious ductal differentiation, are designated myoepitheliomas. Parachordomas closely resemble mixed tumours / myoepitheliomas and are best considered within this spectrum.

ICD-O codes
Mixed tumour, not otherwise
specified   8940/1
Mixed tumour, malignant, not
otherwise specified   8940/3
Myoepithelioma   8982/1
Parachordoma   9373/1

Synonym
Ectomesenchymal chondromyxoid tumour.

Epidemiology
The actual incidence of this group of tumours is difficult to estimate, as they have only recently been adequately characterized. Mixed tumours/myoepitheliomas and parachordomas are usually found in adults, average age 35 years {694,1104}. A significant number of patients, possibly up to 20%, are children less than 10 years of age. There may be a slight male predominance but data are limited.

Sites of involvement
The vast majority of cases arise in the subcutaneous or deep subfascial soft tissues of the extremities (upper > lower extremities). Less commonly, localization within the head and neck and trunk regions is observed. Rare reports have documented mixed tumours arising from bone, all involving the extremities {475}.

Clinical features
Most patients present with superficial to subfascial, painless swellings, ranging from a few weeks to several years duration. Localized pain is rarely reported.

Histopathology
Histologically, mixed tumours of soft tissue show the same morphologic spec trum observed in their salivary gland counterparts. Varying proportions of uniform-appearing, epithelioid cells with eosinophilic to clear cytoplasm, arranged in nests, cords, and ductules, and/or spindled cells, are embedded in a

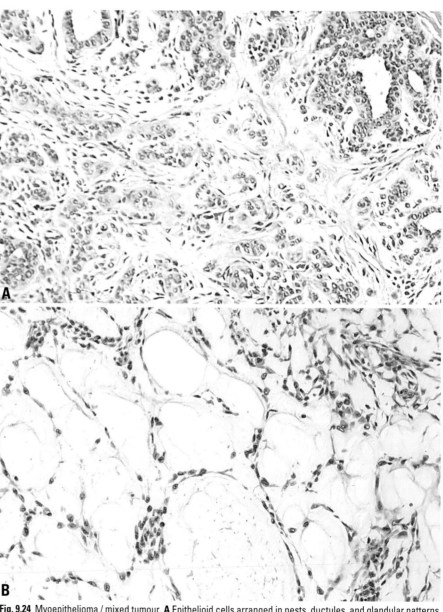

Fig. 9.24 Myoepithelioma / mixed tumour. **A** Epithelioid cells arranged in nests, ductules, and glandular patterns within a partially myxoid stroma. **B** Many cases have a reticular growth pattern, reminiscent of myxoid chondrosarcoma.

hyalinized to chondromyxoid matrix {1104, 1439}. Divergent differentiation, including squamous, adipocytic, and bone and cartilaginous metaplasia, may be observed. From a strict histologic perspective, myoepitheliomas differ from mixed tumours in that they typically lack a definite ductal component. Additionally, the myoepithelial cells range from plasmacytoid forms to spindle cells. Intracytoplasmic hyaline inclusions, a feature previously described in rare cases of chondroid syringoma of the extremities, are rarely observed, sometimes imparting a "rhabdoid" like appearance {654,1104}. Parachordomas closely resemble mixed tumours with the exception that cytoplasmic vacuolation may be a prominent feature in the former {420,694}. Mitotic activity tends to be scant, <2 mitoses per 10 high power fields and nuclear pleomorphism is generally minimal. Similar to salivary gland lesions, dedifferentiation into frank carcinoma or sarcoma is seen in occasional cases.

Immunophenotype

Despite a broad morphologic spectrum, greater than 95% of cases express cytokeratin, vimentin, and S100 protein {1104,1439}. Less consistently, positivity for calponin, smooth muscle actin, glial fibrillary acidic protein, desmin, and epithelial membrane antigen are observed.

Genetics

Three cases with clonal aberrations have been published {694,1669,2114}. Two tumours had a hypodiploid and one a hyperdiploid modal chromosome number. Loss of material from 17p was detected in all three cases.

Prognostic factors

The majority of mixed tumours / myoepitheliomas / parachordomas behave in a benign fashion. However, a minority may locally recur and metastasise, resulting in death {1104}. At present, there are no morphological features reliably predictive of prognosis, other than those few lesions which show frankly malignant histological features.

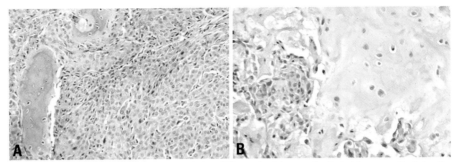

Fig. 9.25 Mixed tumour. **A** Osseous metaplasia within a mixed tumour dominated by myoepithelial cells. **B** Lobules of immature hyaline cartilage adjacent to nests of myoepithelial cells.

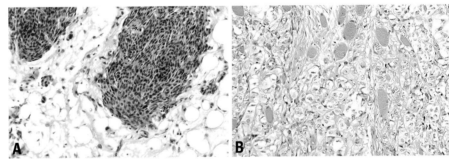

Fig. 9.26 Mixed tumour. **A** Parachordomas are often dominated by large, variably vacuolated eosinophilic epithelioid cells. **B** Rarely, cells may exhibit "rhabdoid" features and intracytoplasmic hyaline inclusions.

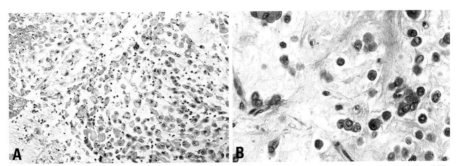

Fig. 9.27 Myoepithelioma. **A** In this case, monomorphic spindle-shaped myoepithelial cells lie adjacent to an area with variable adipocytic differentiation. **B** This lesion from the thigh shows features of carcinoma arising in the context of a myoepithelioma / mixed tumour. Note the marked atypia of the epithelioid cells.

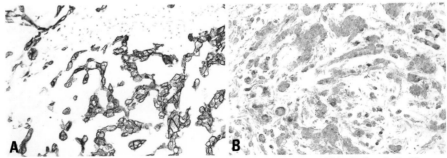

Fig. 9.28 Myoepithelioma. **A** Almost all cases show at least some immunopositivity for keratin, in this case AE1/AE3. Fewer cases stain for epithelial membrane antigen. **B** Most cases are also immunopositive for S100 protein.

Synovial sarcoma

C. Fisher
D.R.H. de Bruijn
A. Geurts van Kessel

Synovial sarcoma (SS) is a morphologically, clinically and genetically distinct entity, that may occur at any site. It does not arise from or differentiate toward synovium, which, unlike SS, lacks epithelial differentiation and has different histochemistry. No origin from or continuity with, pre-existing epithelium has ever been identified. Because of its epithelial features, it has been proposed that SS be renamed carcinosarcoma or spindle cell carcinoma of soft tissue {1451}. However, the term SS is generally recognized and has proven useful.

Definition
Synovial sarcoma is a mesenchymal spindle cell tumour which displays variable epithelial differentiation, including glandular formation and has a specific chromosomal translocation t(X;18) (p11;q11).

ICD-O codes
Synovial sarcoma	9040/3
Synovial sarcoma, spindle cell	9041/3
Synovial sarcoma, biphasic	9043/3

Synonyms
Older synonyms such as tendosynovial sarcoma, synovial cell sarcoma, malignant synovioma, and synovioblastic sarcoma should be abandoned.

Epidemiology
SS accounts for 5 to 10% of soft tissue sarcomas {1168}. They are reported from birth to 89 years but occur mainly in young adults and more commonly in males; 90% of cases occur before 50, and most between 15 and 35 years.

Sites of involvement
SS is unrelated to synovium and <5% originate within a joint or bursa. Over 80% arise in deep soft tissue of extremities, especially around the knee and the tumour frequently arises adjacent to joints or tendon sheaths. Around 5% arise in the head and neck region; however, any site can be affected {79,668, 690,1018}.

Clinical features
There is usually a mass with or without pain. In specific sites local symptoms, e.g. dysphagia, relate to effects of a mass. Growth is often slow, averaging 2-4 years, and 20-year histories are known. Some tumours have radiologically detectable irregular calcification that is occasionally massive.

Aetiology
There are no specific predisposing factors. One example was associated with a metal implant used in hip replacement {1215}, and another with previous therapeutic irradiation for Hodgkin disease {2171}. SS has a chromosomal translocation that is presumably relevant in pathogenesis (see below).

Macroscopy
The typical SS is 3-10 cm in diameter, and circumscribed (when slowly growing) or infiltrative. The tumour is tan or grey, and soft when lacking fibrous stroma. It is frequently multinodular, and can be multicystic. Necrosis is seen in poorly differentiated (PD) SS.

Histopathology
Histologically, SS is biphasic or monophasic. *Biphasic SS* has epithelial and spindle cell components, in varying proportions. The epithelial cells have ovoid nuclei and abundant cytoplasm. They form glands with lumina (containing epithelial mucin) or papillary structures with one or (rarely) more layers of uniform cells. The glandular component can predominate {1312} with large closely packed glands and a scanty spindle component that can be overlooked, allowing misinterpretation as adenocarcinoma. The epithelial component can also form solid cords, nests or rounded clusters. Squamous metaplasia, sometimes with keratinization, occurs in about 1% of cases {1474}. The spindled (not "stromal") tumour cells are uniform and relatively small, with ovoid, pale-staining nuclei and inconspicuous nucleoli. Cytoplasm is sparse and cell borders are indistinct, so that nuclei appear to overlap. Mitoses can be scarce, except in poorly differentiated SS. The spindle cell component often occurs alone as *monophasic SS*. Typically

Table 9.01
Unusual Sites of Occurrence of Synovial Sarcoma.

Head and Neck	Intra-abdominal
Orofacial	Mesentery
Tongue	Retroperitoneum
Tonsil	Intrathoracic
Larynx	Mediastinum
Trachea	Pleura
Parapharynx	Lung
Abdominal wall	Heart
Vulva	Oesophagus
Penis	Intraneural
Kidney	Intra-osseous
Prostate	Intra-articular
Skin	Intracranial
Intravascular	Third ventricle

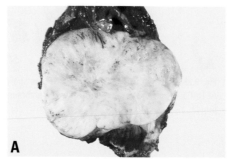 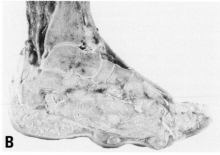

Fig. 9.29 A Biphasic synovial sarcoma of thigh showing a white-tan, firm cut surface. **B** Surgical specimen of a monophasic synovial sarcoma of the foot, showing a destructive lesion with a white-tan cut surface.

there are densely cellular sheets or vague fascicles, with occasional nuclear palisading Many tumours display, at least focally, a prominent haemangiopericytomatous vascular pattern. Extensive sampling can sometimes reveal an epithelial component but this is not necessary for diagnosis.

Stromal collagen is usually wiry and scanty but some tumours have foci of dense fibrosis, especially after irradiation. Myxoid change is usually focal (and rarely diffuse and predominant {1167}), with alternating hypocellular and more cellular areas, and microcyst formation. Mast cells can be abundant.

Purely glandular monophasic SS theoretically exists but is indistinguishable from adenocarcinoma without cytogenetics. SS composed of plump epithelioid cells has sometimes been termed *monophasic epithelial SS*, but examples with rhabdoid cells are included with PD SS.

Calcifying SS. About one third of SS show focal tumoural calcification, with or without ossification. When extensive the prognosis is improved {2191}. Some have antecedent trauma. Most are biphasic {2191}, with calcification in glandular lumina, but they can be monophasic with a deceptively bland or hypocellular spindle component. In ossifying SS, the osteoid has a lace-like pattern mimicking osteosarcoma, and the bone is lamellar and trabecular {1456}. Separately, metaplastic bone or cartilage can occur in the stroma.

Poorly differentiated SS. Areas with high cellularity, numerous mitoses and often necrosis are present in many SS but in some tumours (perhaps 20% of all SS) these predominate {703,2170}. There are typically sheets of darkly staining ovoid or rounded cells like those in other small

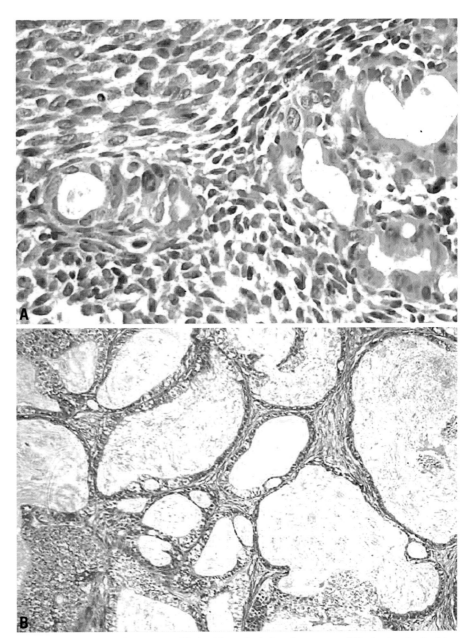

Fig. 9.30 A Biphasic synovial sarcoma with glandular and spindle cell component. **B** Predominantly glandular synovial sarcoma. Variably-sized mucin-secreting glands with a scanty spindle cell component.

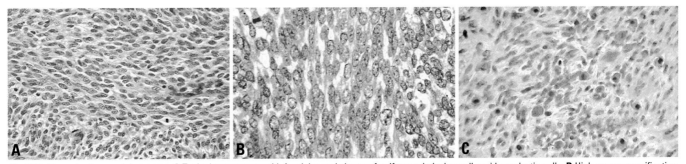

Fig. 9.31 Monophasic synovial sarcoma. **A** Typical appearance with fascicles and sheets of uniform, relatively small ovoid neoplastic cells. **B** High power magnification of the spindle component. **C** Mast cells may be abundant in the spindle cell component.

round cell tumours, especially PNET. The cells are sometimes larger with more cytoplasm, and can appear rhabdoid. Rarely, the rather uniform spindle cells of MSS can be somewhat pleomorphic. PDSS have the same immunophenotype and genetic abnormalities as regular SS {2170}.

Immunophenotype

About 90% of all SS express cytokeratins (CK), in the epithelial component and in rare cells in the spindle cell component. In MSS, CK-positive cells are seen singly, or in cords, nests or sheets; this can be focal and not present in every block. Several CK subtypes are expressed including cytokeratins 7 and 19 {1443}; these are absent from malignant peripheral nerve sheath tumour {1977} and Ewing Sarcoma / PNET {1303}, which is diagnostically useful. Epithelial membrane antigen (EMA) is expressed more often and more widely than CK, especially in the poorly-differentiated subtype. It outlines glandular lumina, and slit-like spaces in solid epithelial areas, and the surface of single cells or small nests in MSS. Some cases are EMA+ but CK-, or vice versa so that both markers should be used.

S100 protein may be detectable (in nuclei and cytoplasm) in 30% of synovial sarcomas including MSS {854}. CD99 is positive in 62% of SS, in the cytoplasm of epithelial cells and with membrane staining on spindle cells, mimicking that in ES/PNET {492}. BCL2 protein is diffusely expressed in all SS, especially in spindle cells {2060}. However, CD34 is usually negative. Amongst muscle markers, calponin is found in most SS. Desmin is absent, but occasionally in MSS there is focal positivity for muscle specific or smooth muscle actin. Vimentin is present in the spindle cells of SS.

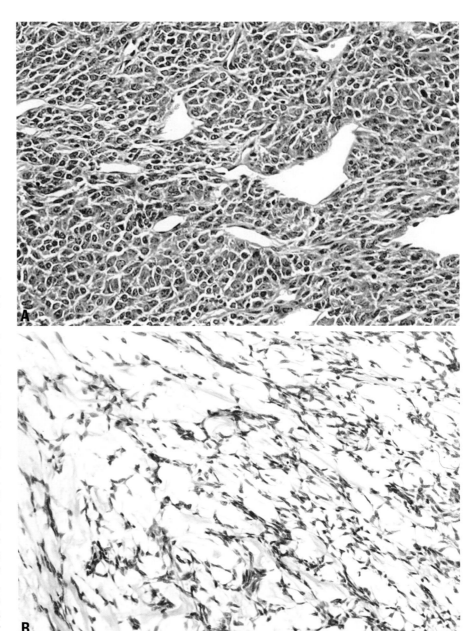

Fig. 9.33 A A haemangiopericytomatous vascular pattern is seen in many monophasic synovial sarcomas. **B** In myxoid synovial sarcoma spindle-shaped tumour cells are widely dispersed in a myxoid stroma.

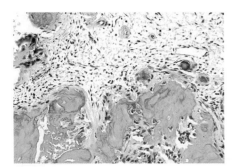

Fig. 9.32 Ossifying synovial sarcoma showing irregular bone formation within the tumour and scant neoplastic spindle cells.

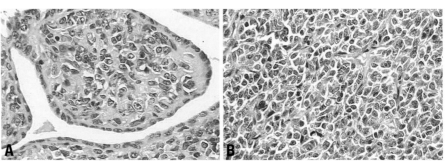

Fig. 9.34 Poorly differentiated **(A)** biphasic and **(B)** monophasic synovial sarcoma.

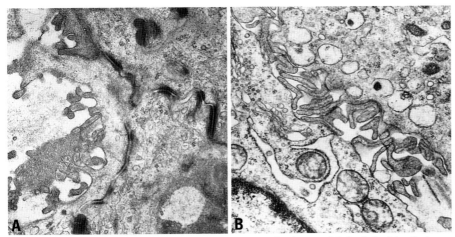

Fig. 9.35 A Electron microscopy of a biphasic synovial sarcoma showing a well defined glandular-like lumen with few projecting microvilli, amorphous intraluminal material and desmosomal junctional complexes. **B** Monophasic synovial sarcoma with abortive lumina and projecting microvilli.

Ultrastructure

The epithelial component is similar to adenocarcinoma {665}. External lamina encloses groups of cells containing intermediate filaments including tonofilaments. Cells are joined by a terminal bar complex and have surface microvilli protruding into the glandular lumen. In MSS, the cells are featureless and rarely have prominent RER indicative of fibroblasts. There are very occasional intercellular gaps, into which protrude short or long processes. Short segments of external lamina associated with single cells can

rarely be found. Transitions between the spindle and the epithelial component are not seen. Calcifying examples show intramitochondrial needle-like calcifications {2280}.

Genetics

Cytogenetics

The t(X;18)(p11;q11) is the cytogenetic hallmark of synovial sarcoma, being present in more than 90% of the 150 cases that have been reported {1477}. Variant, more complex translocations have been described. In one-third of the

tumours it is the sole aberration, whereas the others also have secondary changes, in particular –3, +7, +8, and +12.

Molecular genetics

The genes affected by the t(X;18) have been isolated: *SS18* (a.k.a. *SYT* or *SSXT*), from chromosome 18, and *SSX1*, *SSX2* and *SSX4* from the X chromosome {360, 408,471,472,1966}. Several studies have indicated that the t(X;18) translocation arises exclusively in synovial sarcomas. FISH and (real-time) RT-PCR have been employed widely for the rapid diagnosis of synovial sarcoma {197,473, 973,1004, 1570,1784,1942}. Of at least 350 synovial sarcomas analysed for the presence of *SS18/SSX* fusions, two-thirds showed an *SS18/SSX1* fusion, one-third an *SS18/SSX2* fusion and three separate cases an *SS18/SSX4* fusion {543,543a, 1855}.

The human *SS18* gene is expressed ubiquitously {466,469} and codes for a 55 kDa protein (418 amino acids). The *SSX* gene family encompasses at least five members, encoding 188 amino acid proteins with high sequence homologies. In most SS18/SSX fusion proteins identified, the C-terminal 8 amino acids of SS18 are replaced by the last 78 amino acids of SSX. The consequence of this is that the QPGY domain of SS18 is interrupted and that the KRAB domain of SSX

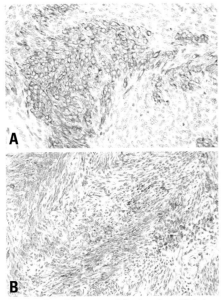

Fig. 9.36 Synovial sarcoma. **A** Cytokeratin positivity in a case of monophasic synovial sarcoma. **B** EMA is a more sensitive immunohistochemical marker than keratin in monophasic and poorly differentiated lesions.

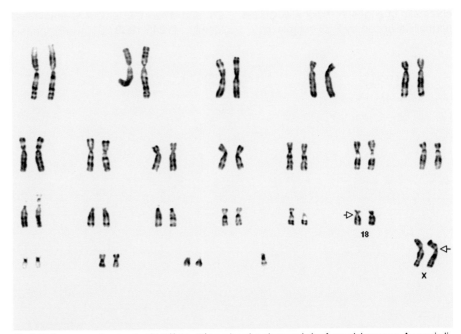

Fig. 9.37 Karyogram showing the t(X;18)(p11;q11) translocation characteristic of synovial sarcoma. Arrows indicate breakpoints.

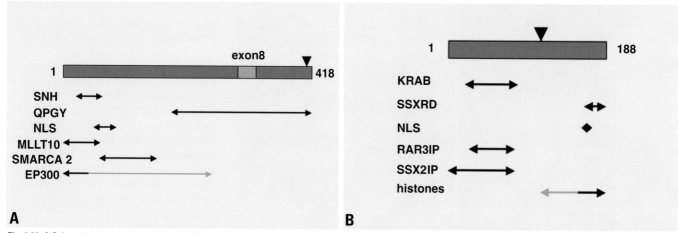

Fig. 9.38 A Schematic representation of the SS18 protein which is affected by the t(X;18) translocation. Marked as doubleheaded arrows are the SNH and QPGY domains, as well as the domain responsible for nuclear localization (NLS). Also marked as doubleheaded arrows are the SS18 domains which are responsible for the interactions with MLLT10, SMARCA2 and EP300. Additionally, the most frequent breakpoint in synovial sarcoma (arrowhead) and the the alternatively spliced exon 8 are indicated. **B** Schematic representation of an SSX protein. Marked as doubleheaded arrows are the KRAB and SSX repression domain (SSXRD), as well as the nuclear localization signal (NLS). Also marked as doubleheaded arrows are the domains which are responsible for the interactions with RAB3IP, SSX2IP and core-histones. The arrowhead denotes the most frequent breakpoint in synovial sarcoma.

is lost in the fusion protein. Since the other interaction domains of SS18 are retained, the SS18-SSX protein may still interact with the SWI/SNF complex and EP300. Several lines of evidence have indicated that interruption of the SS18 QPGY domain may lead to a loss of function for this domain {252,2106}. This loss may also be caused by aberrant folding through the addition of SSX sequences and/or through aberrant targeting of the whole complex {467,468}. Such aberrant targeting may lead to SWI/SNF mediated chromatin changes in regions which are normally silenced by PcG complexes.

Prognostic factors

Up to 50% of SS recur, usually within 2 years, but sometimes up to 30 years after diagnosis {2242}. Some 40% metastasise, commonly to lungs and bone and also regional lymph nodes. Adequate local excision with postoperative radiotherapy can control local recurrence.

5 year survival is 36-76%, and 10 year survival is 20-63% {2242}. The best outcomes are in childhood patients, in tumours which are <5 cm in diameter, have <10 mitoses / 10 hpf and no necrosis, and when the tumour is eradicated locally {1245,1958,2010}. Prognosis

does not differ between monophasic and biphasic tumours, or in relation to immunophenotype. However, cases with the *SS18/SSX2* variant gene, which is mostly found in MSS, have a better prognosis {71,1077,1569}.

PDSS is aggressive, and metastasises in a high percentage of cases. The presence of rhabdoid cells or of more than 50% necrosis, are adverse prognostic factors; in one series, 50% died with a mean survival of 33 months {2171}. The calcifying variant fares better with survival of 83% after five years, and 66% after 10 years {2191}.

Epithelioid sarcoma

L. Guillou
Y. Kaneko

Definition
A distinctive sarcoma of unknown lineage showing predominantly epithelioid cytomorphology, affecting mainly adolescents and young adults. This tumour may be misdiagnosed as a benign lesion, especially as a benign granulomatous process.

ICD-O code   8804/3

Epidemiology
Epithelioid sarcoma (ES) was first recognized as a distinctive entity in 1970 by Enzinger {592}. It occurs in young adults mainly between 10 and 39 years of age (median: 26 years) {336}. Male patients outnumber females by about 2:1 {336,1723}, especially in the second through fifth decades of life.

Sites of involvement
The flexor surface of the fingers, hand, wrist, and forearm are most commonly involved, followed by knee and lower leg, proximal extremities, ankle, feet and toes {336}. The trunk (including genital areas) and head and neck regions are seldom involved by classical epithelioid sarcoma.

Clinical features
When superficially located, ES usually presents as firm, slowly growing painless nodules or plaque-like lesions, solitary or multiple. Ulceration of the skin may occur. Deep-seated lesions are often attached to tendons, tendon sheaths, and / or aponeuroses.

Aetiology
Unknown. A history of trauma is reported in 20% {336} to 25% {1723} of cases.

Macroscopy
In its classical «distal» form, ES usually presents as small, indurated, ill defined, dermal and/or subcutaneous nodules, or larger, variably necrotic masses involving tendons and/or fascia. The cut surface shows a whitish lesion with often a yellow to brown centre due to necrotic and/or haemorrhagic changes. The size of the superficial nodules varies from a few millimeters to 5 cm; deep-seated tumours tend to be larger (up to 15 cm) {336}.

Histopathology
The conventional «distal» form of ES shows a characteristic nodular growth pattern and is composed of a mixed proliferation of eosinophilic epithelioid and spindle cells exhibiting slight nuclear atypia, vesicular nuclei and small nucleoli. Transition between the two cell types is gradual and intercellular collagen deposition usually marked. Frequently, tumour nodules undergo central necrosis resulting in a pseudogranulomatous appearance, simulating a benign necrobiotic process such as a rheumatoid nodule or granuloma annulare. Deep-seated and fascial-based tumours often form scalloped or garland-like structures admixed with areas of necrosis {336}. Pseudoangiosarcomatous features due to cell disaggregation, dystrophic calcifications and bone formation (10-20% of cases), and accompanying chronic inflammation are possible additional features {336}. Perineural and perivascular infiltration are commonly seen. The number of mitoses is usually low, often less than 5 per 10 hpf. A «fibroma-like» variant of ES has been described and shows a predominantly spindle cell proliferation with minimal cytological atypia set in an

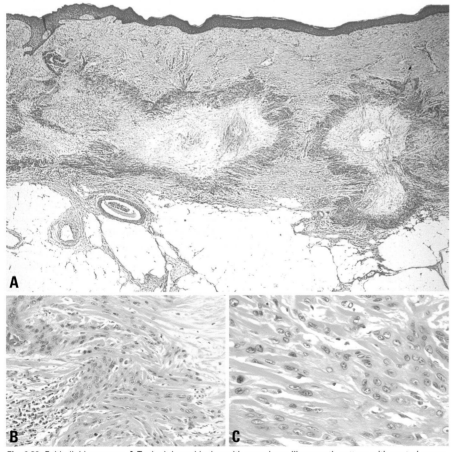

Fig. 9.39 Epithelioid sarcoma. **A** Typical dermal lesion with granuloma-like growth pattern with central necrosis. **B** Tumour cells with a tendency for palisading around central necrotic areas. **C** Cellular details showing abundant ill defined eosinophilic cytoplasm, opened chromatin nuclei, and readily apparent central nucleoli.

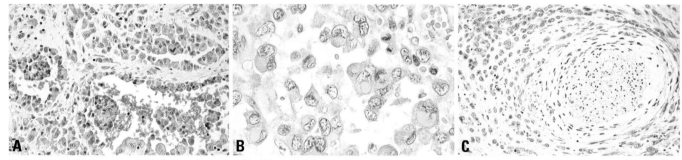

Fig. 9.40 Epithelioid sarcoma. Epithelioid angiosarcoma-like (**A**) and rhabdoid features (**B**), as well as perineural invasion (**C**) are common in conventional epithelioid sarcoma.

abundant collagen-rich extracellular matrix {1446,1473}.

Immunophenotype

Immunohistochemically, ES is characteristically immunoreactive for vimentin and epithelial markers: low- and high-molecular-weight cytokeratins, keratin 8 {1446}, keratin 19 {1446} and/or EMA {432,1324, 1397,1446,1888}. Half of the cases are also positive for CD34 {1446,2172}; occasional reactivity for muscle-specific and smooth muscle actins, neuron specific enolase, and S100 protein has also been reported {1446,1888}.

Ultrastructure

Tumour cells show a spectrum of differentiation ranging from epithelial-appearing cells characterized by well formed desmosome-like intercellular junctions, intracytoplasmic aggregates of intermediate filaments (tonofilaments) and/or surface microvilli, to uncommitted fibroblast-like mesenchymal cells {666}.

Genetics

Cytogenetic studies of epithelioid sarcoma are limited to 8 primary or metastatic tumours and 3 cell lines {398,445,480, 646,934,1021,1487,1770,1987,1990, 2029}. Six tumours were from typical sites, including the forearm or elbow, and five from atypical sites. Various chromosome deletions and gains, none of which is specific for epithelioid sarcoma, were found in the 11 tumours: 8p-/i(8)(q10) in five tumours, -4, +7/+7p, -9/9p- or 9q-, -13, -16/16p- or 16q-, -18/18p-, and +20 in four tumours, and 1p-, 7q-, +8q, and −22/22q- in three tumours. The only recurrent breakpoints in structural rearrangements were 18q11 and 22q11, seen in two tumours each. It could be noted that while 5/6 cases from typical sites were diploid or hypodiploid, 4/5 tumours from atypical sites showed near-triploidy or near-tetraploidy.

Prognostic factors

ES is an aggressive sarcoma which tends to propagate along fascial planes, and tendon and nerve sheaths. The recurrence rate, which depends mainly on the adequacy of the initial excision, varies between 34% {876} and 77% {336, 1810}. Metastases develop in about 40% of the patients, usually following repeat-

ed recurrences, and primarily involve the lungs, but also, in descending order of frequency, regional lymph nodes, scalp, bone, and brain {336,625,1723,1810}. Five- and ten-year overall survival rates range between 50% {336, 625} and 80% {231, 292}, underlining the characteristic protracted and unpredictable clinical course of the lesion. The overall recurrence rate is about 80% at 10 years {335}.

Adverse prognostic factors in ES include male sex {336}, advanced age at diagnosis, large tumour size (>5 cm) {625}, deep location {231}, nuclear pleomorphism, high mitotic activity, presence of vascular and/or nerve invasion {1723}, multiple recurrences and presence or absence of regional lymph node metastases at diagnosis {292,1723}.

Proximal-type epithelioid sarcoma

Recently, attention has been drawn to a special type of aggressive malignant soft tissue neoplasm thought to represent a «proximal» variant of epithelioid sarcoma {855,897}. In this variant, the tumours develop predominantly (but not excusive-

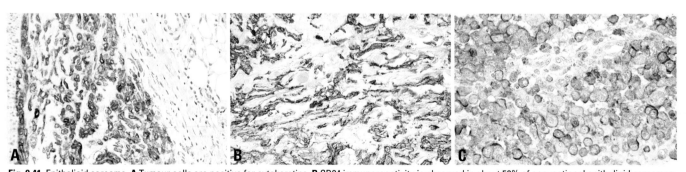

Fig. 9.41 Epithelioid sarcoma. **A** Tumour cells are positive for cytokeratins. **B** CD34 immunoreactivity is observed in about 50% of conventional epithelioid sarcomas. **C** Proximal-type epithelioid sarcoma: tumour cells displaying membranous positivity for EMA

ly) in the pelvis, perineum and genital tract (pubis, vulva, penis). Most of them are deep-seated and they tend to occur in older adults than in the «distal» conventional variant of ES.

Microscopically, «proximal-type» ES, which often shows a multinodular pattern of growth, consists of large epithelioid carcinoma-like cells with marked cytological atypia, vesicular nuclei and prominent nucleoli. Rhabdoid features are frequently observed and may even predominate in some lesions to the point that morphological distinction from an malignant extrarenal rhabdoid tumour (see page 219) may be almost impossible {334,1487,1692}. Rare cases show hybrid histologic features of the classical and proximal subtypes. Tumour necrosis, a common finding, seldom results in a granuloma-like pattern like that observed in the classical «distal» form of ES. Immunohistochemical and ultrastructural features are similar to «distal» ES {855, 897}.

Like malignant extrarenal rhabdoid tumours, «proximal-type» ES seems also to be associated with a more aggressive clinical course, multimodal therapy resistance, and earlier tumour-related deaths as compared with the more indolent behaviour of conventional ES {336, 855,897,1397}. It is not clear yet if this unfortunate behaviour is related to the prominent rhabdoid phenotype or merely to classical prognostic factors such as tumour size, depth, proximal / axial location, resectability, or vascular invasion.

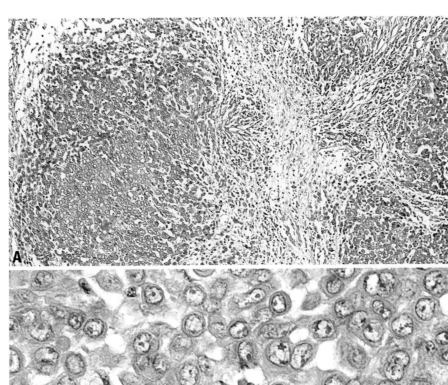
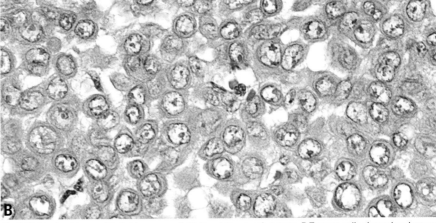

Fig. 9.42 Proximal-type epithelioid sarcoma. **A** Multinodular growth pattern. **B** Tumour cells show abundant and densely eosinophilic cytoplasm, enlarged vesicular nuclei and prominent nucleoli, resulting in a carcinoma-like appearance.

Alveolar soft part sarcoma

N. Ordóñez
M. Ladanyi

Definition

Alveolar soft part sarcoma (ASPS) is a rare tumour affecting mainly adolescents and young adults. It is composed of large, uniform, epithelioid cells having abundant eosinophilic, granular cytoplasm arranged in solid nests and / or alveolar structures, separated by thin, sinusoidal vessels.

ICD-O code   9581/3

Epidemiology

ASPS is a rare tumour with a reported frequency of 0.5% to 0.9% of all soft tissue sarcomas {901, 1227}. It can occur at any age, but is most common between 15 and 35 years. It is rare before 5 and after 50 years of age. There is a female predominance before age 30 and a slight male predominance over age 30 {1617,1719}.

Sites of involvement

In adults, the tumour most commonly occurs in the extremities, especially in the deep soft tissues of the thigh. In 41% of 176 cases from the two largest series, the tumour originated in the thigh or buttock {1258,1719}. In children and infants, the head and neck region, especially the orbit and tongue, is the most common site of origin. Isolated cases have been reported in a wide variety of unusual locations, including the female genital tract {1563,1742}, mediastinum {691}, lung {1991}, stomach {2321}, and bone {1661}.

Clinical features

ASPS usually presents as a slowly growing, painless mass that is easily overlooked due to its relative lack of symptoms. Early metastasis is a characteristic feature of this tumour and, in a good number of cases, metastasis to the lung or brain is the first manifestation of the disease. Orbital lesions present most commonly with proptosis and lid swelling. Because of the high vascularity of the tumour, on occasion, pulsation or a distinctly audible bruit can occur. Hypervascularity with prominent draining veins can be demonstrated by angiography or contrast-enhanced CT {1285}, and high signal intensity on T1- and T2-weighted images on MRI are highly suggestive of ASPS {2052}.

Macroscopy

Alveolar soft part sarcomas tend to be poorly circumscribed, pale grey or yellowish in colour, and present a soft consistency. Areas of necrosis and haemorrhage are common, especially in the larger tumours.

Histopathology

The most characteristic light microscopic feature is that of an organoid or nesting pattern which is best seen at low magnification. The nests tend to be uniform, but may vary in size and shape. They are separated by delicate partitions of connective tissue containing sinusoidal vascular channels lined by flattened endothelium. Loss of cellular cohesion and necrosis of the centrally located cells in the nests results in the commonly seen pseudo-alveolar pattern and is the source of the descriptive "alveolar" designation. In some instances, especially in infants and children, the tumour may grow as diffuse sheets of cells without an apparent nesting pattern. The individual tumour cells are large round or polygonal and exhibit little variation in size and shape. They contain one or two vesicular nuclei with prominent nucleoli, but on occasion as many as five nuclei can be seen in the same cell. Nuclear atypia is uncommon, but can occur. The cell borders are sharply defined conferring a distinctly epithelioid appearance. The cytoplasm is abundant, eosinophilic, and finely granular but, on occasion, may appear clear or vacuolated. Mitotic figures are uncommon. The cells frequently contain rhomboid or rod-shaped crystalline inclusions that may be faintly

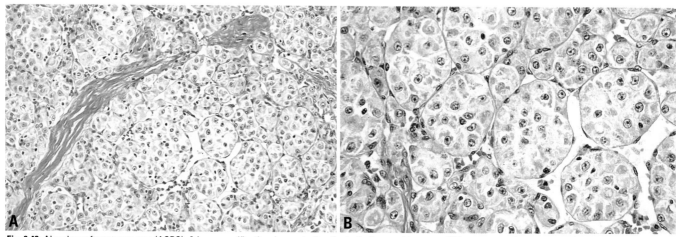

Fig. 9.43 Alveolar soft part sarcoma (ASPS). **A** Low magnification demonstrating the typical organoid pattern. **B** The tumour cell nests are outlined by sinusoidal vascular channels.

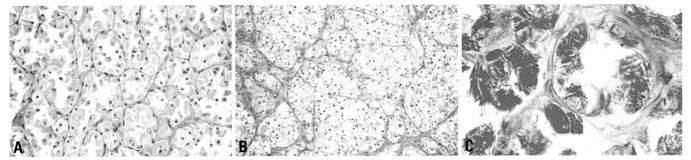

Fig. 9.44 Alveolar soft part sarcoma (ASPS). **A** Area showing the pseudoalveolar pattern. **B** Clearing of the cytoplasm, probably caused by degeneration, can mimic renal cell carcinoma. **C** PAS stain with diastase digestion demonstrates the presence of crystals.

apparent on haematoxylin-and-eosin stained histological preparations but can be better demonstrated with PAS stain after diastase digestion. These inclusions vary greatly in number from case to case. They can be seen in virtually every tumour cell in some cases, while they are rare or even absent in others. In addition to the crystals, variable amounts of glycogen and diastase-resistant granules, which probably represent precursors of the crystals, can also be found. Vascular invasion is an almost invariable feature.

Immunophenotype

ASPS has been extensively studied by immunohistochemical methods with no consistently positive findings {713,1617-1619,2213}. Among the muscle markers that have been investigated, desmin is sometimes positive, particularly in frozen sections, and there is often cytoplasmic (but not nuclear) reactivity for MyoD1. Immunostaining for myogenin has been consistently negative {1618, 2213}. Positivity for S100 protein or neuron-specific enolase has been demonstrated in about one-fourth of the cases, but the expression of these markers has no diagnostic value or significance in the histo-

genesis of this tumour {1617, 1619}. ASPS do not express synaptophysin, chromogranin, neurofilament proteins, cytokeratin, or epithelial membrane antigen.

The majority of cells show moderate to strong nuclear staining with the antibody to the carboxy-terminal portion of TFE3 retained in the fusion protein, in contrast to most normal cells which show only weak to absent nuclear staining with this type of TFE3 antibody {1203}. The PAS-diastase-resistant cytoplasmic granules associated with crystal formation are immunoreactive for MCT1 and CD147 {1202}. MCT1 is a monocarboxylate transporter and CD147 functions, in part, as its chaperon protein.

Ultrastructure

By electron microscopy, the nests of tumour cells are shown to be surrounded by a discontinuous basal lamina. The cell membranes are joined by scattered, poorly developed junctions, and the cytoplasm contains numerous mitochondria, abundant rough endoplasmic reticulum, and prominent Golgi complexes. The most characteristic ultrastructural feature is the presence of membrane-bound or free rhomboid crystals with a

periodicity of 10 nm (see above) {1258, 1619}. Secretory granules containing homogeneous secretory material that on occasion exhibits small foci of crystallization are often seen {1618}.

Genetics

Cytogenetic studies of ASPS have identified a specific alteration, der(17)t(X;17)(p11;q25) {927,1048}. Because the der(X) resulting from the t(X;17)(p11;q25) is almost always absent, the der(17)t(X;17) may be described in some cases as add(17)(q25) unless the quality of the banding allows for positive identification of the additional material as the short arm of X {1907}. This translocation has recently been shown to result in the fusion of the *TFE3* transcription factor gene (from Xp11) with *ASPL* (a.k.a. *ASPSCR1* or *RCC17*) at 17q25 {1207}. The ASPL/TFE3 fusion protein localizes to the nucleus and can function as an aberrant transcription factor. Although the presence of the *ASPL/TFE3* fusion appears highly specific and sensitive for ASPS among sarcomas {1207}, the same gene fusion is also found in a small but unique subset of renal adenocarcinomas arising in paediatric and young adult patients {77,928}.

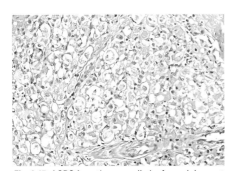

Fig. 9.45 ASPS from the upper limb of an adolescent male. Note the solid growth pattern.

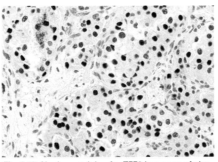

Fig. 9.46 Nuclear staining for TFE3 in a case of alveolar soft part sarcoma (ASPS).

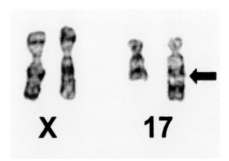

Fig. 9.47 Partial karyotype of ASPS showing the characteristic der(17)t(X;17)(p11.2;q25).

Prognostic factors

ASPS is characterized by relatively slow growth and seldom recurs locally after complete resection; however, it is highly metastatic. Metastasis can occur early in the course of the disease, sometimes prior to the detection of the primary lesion, or much later, even decades, after resection of the primary, despite the absence of local recurrence {95, 1258, 1261, 2191}. In a large study from the Memorial Sloan-Kettering Cancer Centre, the survival rate for patients with no evidence of metastasis at the time of diagnosis was 60% at 5 years, 38% at 10 years, and 15% at 20 years {1258}.

Factors that can influence prognosis are patient age at presentation, tumour size, and the presence of metastasis at diagnosis. Histological features have no prognostic significance. It has been reported that there is an increase in the risk of metastasis with increasing age

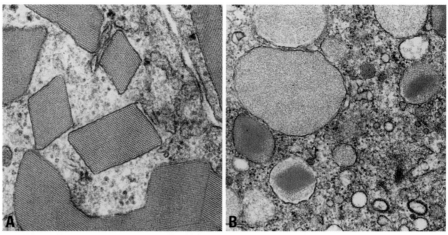

Fig. 9.48 Alveolar soft part sarcoma (ASPS). **A** Membrane-bound, fully developed crystals may adhere to one another, forming a variety of shapes. **B** Some of the large, membrane-bound secretory granules contain foci of crystallization.

{1258} and that patients who present with larger tumours are most likely to have metastasis at the time of diagnosis {618}. The most common sites of metas-tasis in decreasing order of frequency are lung, bone, and brain {1258,1719}. Metastasis to the lymph nodes is uncommon.

Clear cell sarcoma of soft tissue

R. Sciot
F. Speleman

Definition
A soft tissue sarcoma of young adults with melanocytic differentiation, typically involving tendons and aponeuroses. This tumour is unrelated to paediatric lesions currently known as clear cell sarcoma of the kidney.

ICD-O code   9044/3

Synonym
Malignant melanoma of soft parts.

Epidemiology
These rare tumours usually affect young adults, with a peak incidence in the third and fourth decade. Presentations under the age of 10 or above 50 years are rare. There is a slight female predominance {354,484,567,589,1291,1499}.

Sites of involvement
The extremities are the principal site of involvement (90-95%) with the foot/ankle region accounting for about 40% of cases. Clear cell sarcoma is usually deep seated and often attached to aponeuroses and tendons. The tumour may extend into the subcutis or lower dermis, but the epidermis is typically intact. The head and neck and the trunk region are rarely involved {354,484,567, 589,1291,1499}. The visceral organs, retroperitoneum, bone, penis and spinal nerve roots are exceptional locations {535,573,731,1347,1662,1817,1866, 2065,2324}.

Clinical features
The tumour usually presents as a slowly growing mass, being present for several weeks to several years. Pain and/or tenderness is present in up to 50% of cases. On MRI imaging, clear cell sarcoma usually has a benign looking appearance with a slightly increased intensity on T1-weighted images compared to muscle in about half the cases {465}.

Macrosocopy
Most tumours are relatively small (2-6 cm), although lesions as large as 15 cm

have been described. The cut surface usually shows a lobulated grey-white mass. Pigmented areas are found in rare cases. Necrosis or cystic degeneration is occasionally seen.

Histopathology
Clear cell sarcoma shows a typical uniform, nested to fascicular growth pattern. Tumour cells are polygonal or spindle-shaped with abundant eosinophilic or clear cytoplasm. The nuclei are typically vesicular with a prominent nucleolus. Thin fibrous septa delineate the tumour cell nests. Scattered wreath-like multinucleated giant cells are present in about 50% of cases. The mitotic activity is usually relatively low as also is the degree of pleomorphism. Melanin is rarely seen on H&E stains, but can be detected by melanin stains in +/-50% of cases {354, 484,567,589,1291,1499}. Less common morphological variations on the typical appearance, are: spindle cell arrangement, marked pleomorphism and mitotic activity (especially in recurrent and

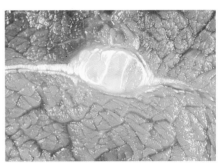

Fig. 9.49 Clear cell sarcoma. This well circumscribed tumour arose in the plantaris tendon of an 18-year-old woman. Despite the small size of the tumour, she died from disseminated metastases four years later.

metastatic lesions), solid round cell aspect, microcystic aspect, and the presence of myxoid stroma {354,416, 484,567,589,1291,1499}.

Immunophenotype
Positivity for S100 protein, HMB45 and other melanoma antigens is seen in almost all cases {829,1115,1291,1499,

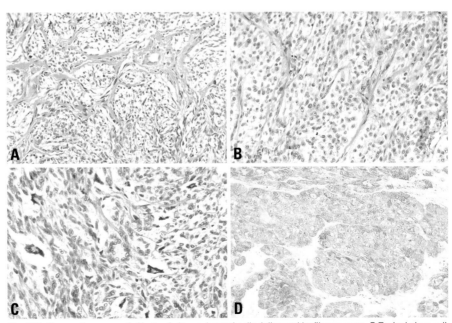

Fig. 9.50 Clear cell sarcoma. **A** Nests of clear polygonal cells delineated by fibrous septa. **B** Typical clear cell sarcoma with more eosinophilic cytoplasm. Note the prominent vesicular nuclei and nucleoli. **C** Area showing wreath-like giant cells. **D** Strong S100 staining is a consistent feature.

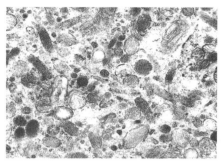

Fig. 9.51 Ultrastructural appearance of clear cell sarcoma from a 23 year-old male, showing a mixture of stage II and III melanosomes.

2065}. Positivity for HMB45 is often stronger and more diffuse than for S100 protein. Expression of neuron-specific enolase, synaptophysin, CD57 (Leu-7), and even cytokeratin and actin have been noted {416,1291,1499,1501,2065}.

Ultrastructure

Melanosomes in varying stages of development are present in the majority of cases. Variably abundant cytoplasmic glycogen, swollen mitochondria and a basal lamina complete the picture {1115, 1453, 1517}.

Genetics

The cytogenetic hallmark of clear cell sarcoma is the presence of a reciprocal translocation, t(12;22)(q13;q12). This translocation has been detected in the majority of clear cell sarcoma cases reported in the literature but not in other malignancies {1477}. The t(12;22)(q13;q12) results in fusion of the EWS (22q12) and ATF1 (12q13) genes {74, 2350}.

The t(12;22) has been reported as the sole chromosomal aberration in clear cell sarcoma, however, most cases also display additional chromosomal aberrations, often complex in nature. These additional cytogenetic changes include +8, structural and numerical aberrations involving chromosome 22 (other than the t(12;22)) and +7 {1262, 2007, 2128}. No variant or cryptic translocations, resulting in an EWS/ATF1 fusion transcript have been reported.

The EWS/ATF1 fusion protein invariably contains the N-terminal domain of EWS and the ATF1 bZIP domain. An EWS/ATF1 fusion transcript is detectable with RT-PCR in more than 90% of the cases {74}. The type 1 fusion transcript (EWS exon 8-ATF1 codon 65) is by far the most common, but other variants account for approximately 10% of the cases. The reciprocal ATF1/EWS transcript probably does not contribute to malignant conversion, since it is out of frame. ATF1 is a member of the CREB/ATF basic leucine-zipper type of transcription factor family and binds to cAMP inducible promoters. It was shown that the EWS/ATF1 fusion converts ATF1 to a constitutive transcriptional activator that represses TP53/CBP-mediated transactivation {728,729}.

By RT-PCR analysis it was shown that 4/4 cases expressed the melanocyte-specific splice form of the microphthalmia transcription factor (MITF) transcript {74}.

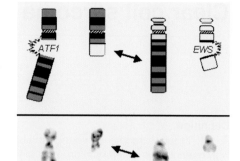

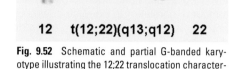

12   t(12;22)(q13;q12)   22

Fig. 9.52 Schematic and partial G-banded karyotype illustrating the 12;22 translocation characteristic of clear cell sarcoma.

Prognostic factors

The prognosis is poor with a mortality rate ranging from 37% to 59% in the largest series {354,484,567,589,1291, 1499}. Many patients develop recurrences and metastases, albeit sometimes more than 10 years after diagnosis. Five-year survival figures thus overestimate the long term survival. In the Mayo Clinic series, the survival at 5, 10 and 20 years was 67%, 33% and 10%, respectively {1291}. Nodal metastasis develops in up to 50% of patients. There is as yet no answer to the question of prophylactic regional lymph node dissection. The lung and bone are other frequent sites of metastasis. Tumour size (greater than 5 cm), necrosis and local recurrence are unfavourable prognostic factors {1291, 1499,1862}.

Extraskeletal myxoid chondrosarcoma

D.R. Lucas
S. Heim

Definition

Extraskeletal myxoid chondrosarcoma (EMC) is a malignant soft tissue tumour characterized by a multinodular architecture, abundant myxoid matrix, and malignant chondroblast-like cells arranged in cords, clusters, or delicate networks. Despite the name, there is no convincing evidence of cartilaginous differentiation.

ICD-O code   9231/3

Synonym

Chordoid sarcoma.

Epidemiology

EMC is a rare tumour, accounting for less than 3% of soft tissue sarcomas {2143}. It is primarily a tumour of adulthood with the median age in the sixth decade and a male:female ratio of 2:1. Only rare cases in childhood or adolescence have been reported {864}.

Sites of involvement

Most EMCs arise in the deep soft tissues of the proximal extremities and limb girdles {597,1385}. Thigh is the most common location. Less common sites include trunk, paraspinal region, foot, and head and neck region. Rare tumours have also been reported in the finger {1603}, intracranial location {1864}, retroperitoneum {730}, pleura {801}, and bone {1105}.

Clinical features

Patients typically present with an enlarging soft tissue mass. Pain and tenderness characterize some cases, and tumours around joints may restrict range of motion. Large or superficial tumours may ulcerate the skin. Although imaging characteristics are nonspecific, most tumours appear lobulated, and highly myxoid tumours have a homogeneous high signal on T2 weighted MRI image. Tumours with necrosis or hemorrhage have a more heterogeneous signal.

Macroscopy

Most EMCs form large, well demarcated tumours contained by a pseudocapsule.

The median size is 7 cm {1385}. However, tumour size is quite variable, including very large masses (20-25 cm) in some cases. On cut section, the tumour has a well defined multinodular architecture comprised by gelatinous nodules separated by fibrous septa. Intratumoural cysts and haemorrhage, both recent and remote, and geographic areas of necrosis may be present. Highly cellular tumours have a fleshy consistency.

Histopathology

Conventional 'well differentiated' EMC has a multinodular architecture defined by fibrous septa that divide the tumour into circumscribed areas filled with pale blue myxoid or chondromyxoid stroma that is rich in sulfated proteoglycans. Lobules often show higher cellularity at the periphery. Well formed hyaline cartilage is rarely, if ever seen. The stroma is strikingly hypovascular.

The neoplastic cells usually have a modest amount of deeply eosinophilic, finely granular to vacuolated cytoplasm and uniform round to oval nuclei. The chromatin is usually evenly distributed often with a small, inconspicuous nucleolus. The cells characteristically interconnect with one another to form cords or clus-

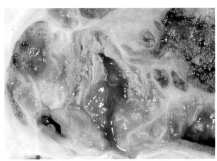

Fig. 9.53 Extraskeletal myxoid chondrosarcoma typically forms a demarcated tumour encased by a pseudocapsule, and divided into multiple gelatinous nodules by fibrous septa. Intratumoral cysts and hemorrhage are common.

ters. In some tumours they form complex, filigree or cribriform arrays, while others show spindle cell patterns. Epithelioid cells with abundant eosinophilic cytoplasm and vesicular nuclei with prominent nucleoli, or rhabdoid cells with hyalinized cytoplasmic globules, are found in some EMCs. Mitotic activity is usually low (<2 mitotic figures per 10 high power field) in most cases. Areas of recent and remote intratumoural haemorrhage are common.

EMC may have more cellular areas, characterized by closely spaced cells with

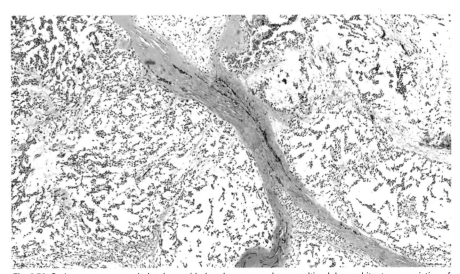

Fig. 9.54 On low power, extraskeletal myxoid chondrosarcoma has a multinodular architecture consisting of myxoid areas demarcated by fibrous septa.

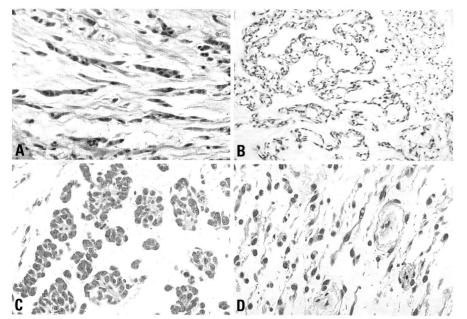

Fig. 9.55 Extraskeletal myxoid chondrosarcoma (EMC). Tumour cells typically have low grade cytologic features and interconnect with one another to form **(A)** cords, **(B)** delicate networks, **(C)** clusters, or **(D)** spindle cell patterns.

Fig. 9.56 A,B EM features of EMC include granular extracellular matrix, cytoplasm rich in mitochondria and RER, and intracysternal microtubules.

minimal myxoid stroma. Diffusely cellular tumours are referred to as "cellular variants". The cells in these tumours frequently have epithelioid morphology and greater mitotic activity. Some EMCs display sheets of anaplastic epithelioid cells devoid of matrix, fibrosarcomatous areas, brisk mitotic activity with abnormal division figures, and large geographic areas of necrosis. In such high grade tumours, one may need to search for areas of conventional EMC morphology in order to make the diagnosis. Finally, small cells with scant cytoplasm may comprise some EMCs {864, 1385}.

Immunophenotype
Vimentin is the only marker consistently expressed in EMC {494,1385}. S100 protein, cytokeratin, and epithelial mem-

brane antigen are expressed in a minority of tumours and usually only focally. Synaptophysin or neuron-specific enolase expression has been demonstrated in some tumours {889,1603,1611}.

Ultrastructure
Interconnecting, rounded mesenchymal cells surrounded by abundant granular amorphous extracellular stroma characterize its fine structure. The cytoplasm is rich in organelles, especially mitochondria, rough endoplasmic reticulum (RER), and intermediate filaments, which are sometimes arranged in perinuclear whorls. Dilations within the RER filled with granular amorphous material identical to the extracellular stroma, and ruffled cytoplasmic borders are common findings. Intracisternal microtubules are very char-

acteristic of EMC. However, they are present in less than half the cases {65, 1385, 1672}. Dense core neurosecretory granules have also been report in some cases {889}.

Genetics
Myxoid chondrosarcoma has been examined both at the cytogenetic and molecular genetic levels. Of the more than 20 such tumours that have been reported to carry clonal chromosomal aberrations {205,253,266,459,949,950, 1332,1633,2028,2144}, the reciprocal translocation t(9;22)(q22;q12) was seen in around half of all cases. Sometimes three-way variant translocations were observed, and more often than not there are additional, secondary chromosomal aberrations. The t(9;22) (q22;q12) has

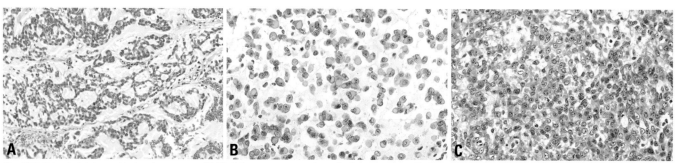

Fig. 9.57 Extraskeletal myxoid chondrosarcoma (EMC). **A** In some tumours the cells form complex cribriform arrays. **B** Rhabdoid cells with eccentric hyaline globules, are occasionally seen in EMC. **C** 19 Densely cellular areas with minimal matrix characterize the cellular higher grade variant of EMC.

not been associated with other diagnostic entities. A second cytogenetic subgroup of extraskeletal myxoid chondrosarcoma characterized by the presence of a t(9;17)(q22;q11) was also identified {205}; this translocation is equally specific but less common than the t(9;22).

The molecular genetic consequences of both the t(9;22)(q22;q12) and the t(9;17)(q22;q11) have been unravelled {359,1201,1643,1963}. In the former translocation, the genes *NR4A3* (a.k.a. *CHN*, *TEC*, from 9q22) and *EWS* (from 22q12) are fused. It seems that two main *EWS/NR4A3* transcripts exist, joining *EWS* exons 12 and 7, respectively, to *NR4A3*. In the t(9;17)(q22;q11), *NR4A3* is recombined instead with the *RBP56* gene from 17q11 to generate a chimeric *RBP56/NR4A3*. RBP56 encodes a putative RNA-binding protein similar to the EWS and FUS proteins. It appears that the N-terminal parts of EWS and RBP56 have similar oncogenic potential making them pathogenetically equivalent in oncoproteins arising from fusions with certain transcription factors. A third chromosomal variant, t(9;15)(q22;q21), which has been described in a single case, leads to the fusion of the *TCF12* and *NR4A3* genes {1964}.

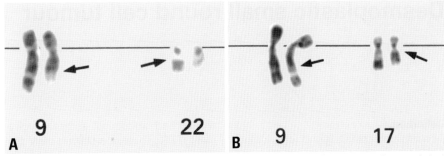

Fig. 9.58 A The translocation t(9;22)(q22;q12) (arrows indicate breakpoints) is pathognomonic for extraskeletal myxoid chrondrosarcoma and is found in half of all such tumours. It recombines the two genes *NR4A3* (from 9q22) and *EWS* (from 22q12). **B** The translocation t(9;17)(q22;q11) (arrows indicate breakpoints) is also typical for extraskeletal myxoid chrondrosarcoma but is found only in a minority of lesions. It recombines the genes *NR4A3* (from 9q22) and *RBP56* (from 17q11).

Prognostic factors

EMC is a tumour with long survival but is known, with prolonged follow-up, to have high potential for local recurrence and metastasis, and a high disease-associated death rate {1385,1847}. Local recurrences and metastases each occur in approximately half of cases. Metastases are usually pulmonary. However, extrapulmonary and disseminated metastases also occur {1847}. Interestingly, prolonged survivals even in the face of metastatic disease are not uncommon in EMC. In a recent large study of 99 patients, Meis-Kindblom et al. {1385} report 5, 10, and 15 year survivals of 90, 70, and 60%, respectively.

Large tumour size, especially greater than 10 cm, appears to be a significant negative prognostic factor in EMC {1385, 1611}. Although a number of studies deny the significance of histologic variables such as grade, cellularity, and mitotic rate on clinical behaviour {1028, 1385,1847}, others suggest that examples showing increased cellularity and atypia are more aggressive {65, 1289, 1611}. A few studies have also suggested that the presence of rhabdoid cells may be an adverse histologic variable {1611,1622}.

Malignant mesenchymoma

H.L. Evans

The term "malignant mesenchymoma" has been applied to sarcomas that exhibit two or more lines of specialized differentiation. However, it has become apparent that this group does not form a clinicopathological entity, and that potential candidates for the designation can be more appropriately classified in other ways. Among those with a fatty component are myxoid liposarcomas with carti-lagenous metaplasia, atypical lipomatous tumours (well differentiated liposarcomas) with osseous, cartilagenous, smooth muscle, or skeletal muscle elements, dedifferentiated liposarcomas with the same elements in the dedifferentiated component, and pleomorphic liposarcomas with osteogenic areas. Nonfatty neoplasms meeting the definition include the rare leiomyosarcomas that have osteosarcomalike or rhabdomyosarcomatous zones and the occasional embryonal rhabromyosarcomas that demonstrate focal cartilage. Obviously all of these are different neoplasms, and "lumping" them together under one heading is misleading.

ICD-O code   8990/3

Desmoplastic small round cell tumour

C.R. Antonescu
W. Gerald

Definition
Desmoplastic small round cell tumour (DSRCT) is composed of small round tumour cells of uncertain histogenesis, associated with prominent stromal desmoplasia and polyphenotypic differentiation. The presence of the t(11;22)(p13;q12) translocation is a consistent cytogenetic feature.

ICD-O code   8806/3

Synonyms
Intraabdominal desmoplastic small round cell tumour, intrabdominal desmoplastic small cell tumour with divergent differentiation, polyphenotypic small round cell tumour.

Epidemiology
DSRCT primarily affects children and young adults, who usually present with widespread abdominal serosal involvement {777}. There is a striking male predominance, with a peak incidence in the third decade of life (with a wide range from 1st to 5th decade).

Sites of involvement
The vast majority of patients develop tumour in the abdominal cavity, frequently located in the retroperitoneum, pelvis, omentum, and mesentery. Multiple serosal implants are common. Clinical presentation outside the abdominal cavity is very rare, and is mainly restricted to the thoracic cavity and paratesticular locations {412}. Isolated cases occur in limbs, head and neck and brain.

Clinical features
Presenting symptoms are usually related to the primary site, such as pain, abdominal distension, palpable mass, acute abdomen, ascites, and organ obstruction. Presentation at an exceptional site (see above) should prompt a careful search for an intra-abdominal primary.

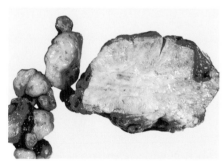

Fig. 9.59 Desmoplastic small round cell tumour presenting as one dominant tumour mass and multiple smaller tumour nodules. The cross section shows a solid white-tan cut surface, with foci of necrosis.

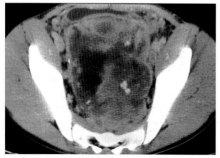

Fig. 9.60 CT image of a large pelvic desmoplastic small round cell tumour.

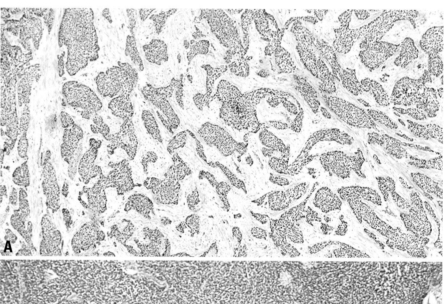

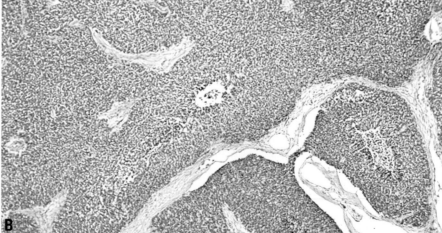

Fig. 9.61 Histological spectrum of desmoplastic small round cell tumour. **A** Characteristic morphology with variably sized nests in a desmoplastic stroma. **B** Solid growth pattern with large confluent nests.

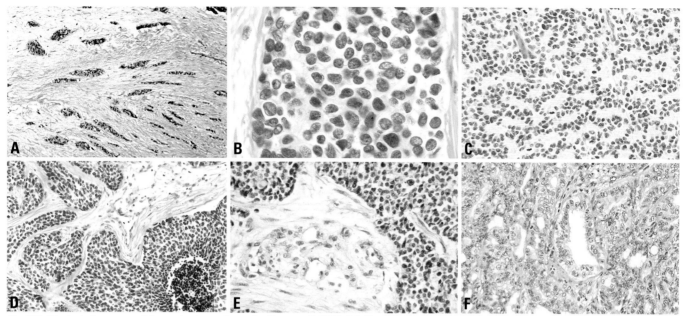

Fig. 9.62 Histological spectrum of desmoplastic small round cell tumour (DSRCT). **A** Infiltrative growth pattern and "indian-file" appearance. **B** Small round cells with minimal nuclear pleomorphism. **C** Rosette formation. **D** Focal necrosis. **E** "Glomeruloid" vascular proliferation. **F** Epithelial features with gland formation.

Macroscopy

The typical gross appearance consists of multiple tumour nodules studding the peritoneal surface. Often there is a dominant tumour mass accompanied by smaller nodules. The cut surface is firm, grey-white, with foci of haemorrhage and necrosis.

Histopathology

Histologically, DSRCT is characterized by variably sized and shaped, sharply outlined nests of small neoplastic cells surrounded by a prominent desmoplastic stroma. The size of the nests varies considerably, from minute clusters to large irregular confluent sheets. Central necrosis is common and cystic degeneration can also be seen. Some tumours focally exhibit epithelial differentiation, with glands or rosette growth pattern. The tumour cells are typically uniform with small hyperchromatic nuclei, scant cytoplasm and indistinct cytoplasmic borders. In about half of cases a small component of tumour cells show intracytoplasmic eosinophilic rhabdoid inclusions. Some tumours have larger cells and greater pleomorphism. The chromatin is typically dispersed, with inconspicuous nucleoli. Mitoses are frequent and individual tumour cell necrosis is common. The desmoplastic stroma is composed of fibroblasts or myofibroblasts embedded in a loose extracellular material or collagen. Prominent stromal vascularity is also present, suggestive of a hyperplastic response to the tumour. The hyperplastic vessels vary from complex capillary tufts to larger vessels with eccentric thickened walls and prominent endothelial and pericytic cells.

Immunophenotype

The immunoprofile of DSRCT is consistent and distinctive, showing a complex pattern of simultaneous multi-phenotypic differentiation, expressing proteins associated with epithelial, muscular, and neural differentiation {778, 779}. The majority of cases are immunoreactive for cytokeratins, epithelial membrane antigen, vimentin, desmin, and NSE. A distinctive dot-like intracytoplasmic localization is seen with desmin and occasionally with other intermediate filaments. Myogenin and myoD1 are consistently negative. Nuclear expression of WT1 (using antibodies to the carboxy terminus) is usually seen {124, 947}. The stromal component is positive for vimentin and common or smooth muscle actin, suggesting myofibroblastic origin.

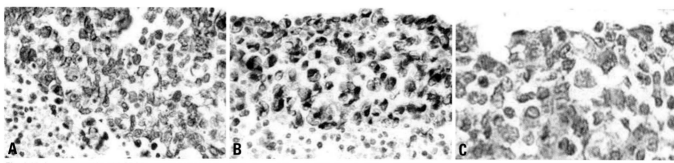

Fig. 9.63 Immunoprofile of DSRCT: strong immunoreactivity for cytokeratin (**A**), desmin (**B**), and NSE (**C**).

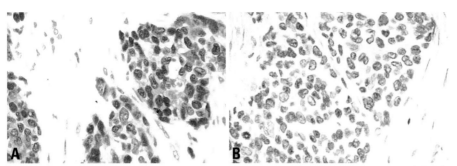

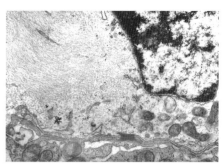

Fig. 9.64 Immunodetection of EWS/WT1 chimeric protein in desmoplastic small round cell tumour (DSRCT). **A** Strong nuclear reactivity with the WT1 (C19) antibody directed to the carboxy terminus of WT1. **B** No reactivity with the WT1 antibody directed to the amino terminus of WT1.

Fig. 9.65 EM of DSRCT: neoplastic cells with typical whorls of intermediate filaments and well formed desmosome junctional structures.

Ultrastructure

Most cells have a primitive / undifferenti-ated appearance with small amounts of cytoplasm and scant organelles. A notable feature is the presence of paranuclear aggregates and whorls of intermediate filaments. Rare dense core granules can be also seen in some cases. Few cells are connected by cell junction complexes, including well formed desmosomes.

Genetics

DSRCT is characterized by a specific chromosomal abnormality, t(11;22) (p13;q12) {190,1801,1871}, unique to this tumour, involving two chromosomal regions previously implicated in other malignant tumours. The translocation results in the fusion of the Ewing sarcoma gene, *EWS*, on 22q12 and the Wilms tumour gene, *WT1*, on 11p13 {461, 780, 1206}. Interestingly, the most common primary site of DSRCT, the serosal lining of body cavities, has high transient fetal expression of *WT1* gene. WT1 is expressed in tissues derived from the intermediate mesoderm, primarily those undergoing transition from mesenchyme to epithelium, in a specific period of development {1729,1751}. This stage of differentiation is reminiscent of DSRCT with early features of epithelial differenti-ation.

The most commonly identified *EWS/WT1* chimeric transcript is composed of an in-frame fusion of the first seven exons of *EWS*, encoding the potential transcrip-tion modulating domain, and exons 8 through 10 of *WT1*, encoding the last three zinc-fingers of the DNA-binding domain. Rare variants including addition-al exons of *EWS* occur {70}. Intranuclear chimeric protein can be detected and shown to contain the carboxy terminus of WT1 {776}. Detection of the *EWS/WT1* gene fusion and chimeric transcript serves as a sensitive and specific mark-er for DSRCT {776}.

Prognostic factors

The overall progression-free survival remains very poor, despite multimodal therapy {776,1189}.

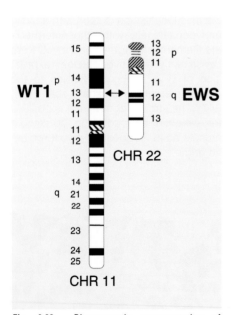

Fig. 9.66 Diagrammatic representation of chromosomal breakpoints in DSRCT with t(11;22)(p13;q12) translocation.

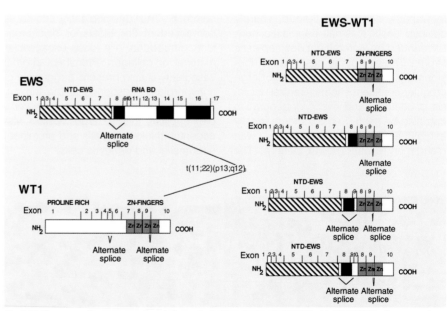

Fig. 9.67 Diagrammatic representation of chromosomal breakpoints in DSRCT with *EWS/WT1* fusion transcripts. All chromosome 11 breakpoints involve intron 7 of *WT1*, suggesting that the preservation of the last three zinc-finger motifs of WT1 is crucial to sarcomagenesis. The majority of chromosome 22 breakpoints involve intron 7 of *EWS* and, infrequently, introns 8 and 9.

Extrarenal rhabdoid tumour

D. Schofield

Definition

Soft tissue rhabdoid tumour is a malignant tumour of infants and children, characterized by neoplastic cells with large nuclei, prominent nucleoli, and abundant, eccentric cytoplasm with variably prominent eosinophilic, cytoplasmic "inclusions". These inclusions are ultrastructurally composed of whorls of intermediate filaments. Since a rhabdoid phenotype may be present in a wide spectrum of tumours, particularly those occurring in adults, the diagnosis of rhabdoid tumour requires exclusion of an underlying alternative line of differentiation.

ICD-O code 8963/3

Epidemiology

Malignant rhabdoid tumours are well defined and characterized entities in both the kidney and central nervous system. Due to histological overlap with other neoplasms, rhabdoid tumour as a distinct entity arising in soft tissue has taken longer to define. However, it has become apparent that these tumours, if carefully defined, are confined almost exclusively infants and children. Congenital and even fetal cases, some with disseminated disease at the time of diagnosis, are well documented {972, 980, 2259}. An increasing number of familial cases are recognized {406, 1733}.

Sites of involvement

The tumours may arise at a variety of topographic locations, including liver, heart and gastrointestinal system. Soft tissue lesions seem to arise most frequently in deep, axial locations, including the neck and paraspinal regions. Cutaneous lesions are well described.

Imaging studies are not felt to be particularly helpful in the diagnosis of soft tissue rhabdoid tumours, other than to delineate the extent of tumour as the features are non-specific {1802}.

Macroscopy

Rhabdoid tumours have been described as primarily unencapsulated masses, generally less than 5 cm in greatest dimension. The cut surface is soft and grey to tan in colour. Foci of both haemorrhage and necrosis are frequently observed {1150}.

Histopathology

Rhabdoid tumours are densely cellular, comprised of sheets or solid trabeculae of neoplastic cells with large, vesicular, round to bean-shaped nuclei, prominent centrally located nucleoli, and abundant eccentric cytoplasm. Less common features include scattered non-neoplastic, osteoclast-like giant cells, a myxoid background, a lack of cellular cohesiveness, and increased collagen deposition between trabeculae of tumour cells. Mitoses are frequent, averaging approximately one per high power field, and necrosis is common.

The diagnostic hallmark of this tumour by routine haematoxylin and eosin staining is a distinctive, globoid, hyaline, eosinophilic, cytoplasmic inclusion. While these distinctive cells are numerous in most tumours, occasional tumours may consist primarily of primitive, undifferentiated "small round blue cells" with only a minority of cells having a rhabdoid phenotype. In these cases, the rhabdoid cells may occur in clusters or scattered singly throughout the tumour, highlighting a potential diagnostic challenge in a small biopsy sample.

A wide variety of tumours, including some carcinomas, sarcomas, meningiomas, melanomas, lymphomas, and mesotheliomas, may display rhabdoid features, either focally or diffusely, fuelling much of the "entity vs phenotype" debate that has surrounded these tumours in the past. When present in a tumour with an otherwise documentable line of differentiation, the rhabdoid phenotype should be reflected in the diagnosis, either as a composite extrarenal rhabdoid tumour (particularly if the phenotypic appearance is mixed) or as a modifier (if the phenotype is diffuse). In addition, there are rare cases of rhabdoid tumours apparently arising in proximity to cutaneous, benign, mesenchymal lesions in neonates {764,1686}.

Immunophenotype

As a variety of tumours may express the rhabdoid phenotype, immunohistochemical stains are frequently an invaluable adjunct. The majority of rhabdoid tumours coexpress vimentin and an epithelial antigen, such as keratin, epithelial mem-

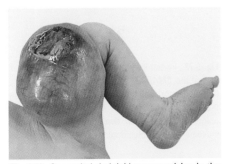

Fig. 9.68 Congenital rhabdoid tumour arising in the soft tissue of the thigh of a neonate.

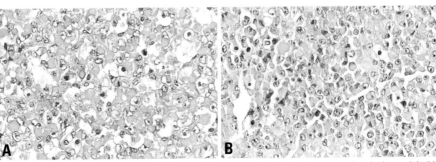

Fig. 9.69 Extrarenal rhabdoid tumour. **A** Cells contain abundant eosinophilic cytoplasm and vesicular nuclei with prominent nucleoli. **B** Note prominent pale-pink inclusions.

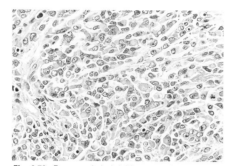

Fig. 9.70 Extrarenal rhabdoid tumour. Note diffuse, discohesive growth pattern and prominent cytoplasmic inclusions.

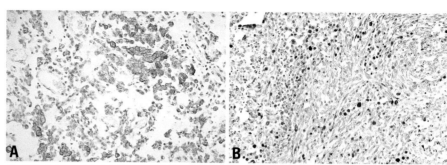

Fig. 9.71 Extrarenal rhabdoid tumour. **A** Focal positivity for epithelial membrane antigen is a frequent finding. **B** Positivity for cytokeratin AE-1/AE-3 in the cytoplasm, with accentuation of the filamentous inclusions, is commonly seen.

brane antigen and/or CAM5.2. In addition, a significant percentage of tumours frequently express neuroectodermal antigens such as CD99, synaptophysin, and/or NSE. Expression of muscle specific actin and focal S-100 positivity are also not uncommon. However, despite the frequent polyphenotypic appearance, desmin, myoglobin and CD34 are not expressed {634,1150,2141}.

Ultrastructure

The classic rhabdoid tumour cell is ultrastructurally characterized by cytoplasmic whorls of intermediate filaments measuring 8-10 mn in diameter. These filamentous whorls may incorporate mitochondria, lipid droplets or fragments of endoplasmic reticulum. A double immunofluorescence and three dimensional imaging study suggests that these whorls represent cytokeratin, while vimentin forms a filamentous network throughout the cytoplasm. In addition to the distinctive whorls, rhabdoid tumour cells, contain the usual, non-specific cadre of cytoplasmic organelles, including few mitochondria, lysosomes, free ribosomes and dilated rough endoplasmic reticulum, along with scattered lipid droplets. Variably developed intercellular attachments may be seen, but true desmosomes are not present {2137}.

Due to sampling, typical rhabdoid cells may or may not be identified in tumours with a rhabdoid phenotype, regardless of whether the lesion is a true rhabdoid tumour or otherwise. Ultrastructural examination of these tumours is probably most helpful in excluding rhabdoid tumour histology as an uncommon phenotypic presentation of an otherwise typical sarcoma or carcinoma of known histogenesis.

Genetics

The identification of deletions and occasional translocations (the latter involving partner chromosome regions 1p36, 6p12, 11p15 and 18q21) {881, 1548, 1689, 1813} of chromosome 22 band q11.2 in a number of soft tissue rhabdoid tumours provided the first and most convincing evidence that at least a subgroup of these tumours represented a distinct clinicopathological entity. Conversely, chromosome 22 deletions were distinctly uncommon in a limited number of composite extrarenal rhaboid tumours studied, supporting the hypothesis that the rhabdoid phenotype was a manifestation of anaplastic progression modulated by a separate genetic mechanism {743}. Subsequent identification of mutations and homozygous deletions of the SMARCB1 (a.k.a. hSNF5 or INI1) gene in the majority of rhabdoid tumours has confirmed the initial karyotypic and molecular cytogenetic observations {192, 1921, 2201}. SMARCB1 mutations and deletions are also characteristic of rhabdoid tumours originating in the kidney and central nervous system and have been identified in a subset of choroid plexus carcinomas, medulloblastomas, central PNETs, along with a rare glioblastoma multiforme and rhabdomyosarcoma {483, 1922}.

Although SMARCB1 functions as a tumour suppressor gene, the mechanism of its inactivation is usually not the classic "mutation and subsequent deletion of the second normal allele." Most malignant rhabdoid tumours are characterized by either a homozygous deletion or partial / complete isodisomy of chromosome 22. Homozygous deletions seem to be present in the majority of cases in which a translocation is documented {1813}.

In addition to chromosome 22 rearrangements and SMARCB1 inactivation, other chromosomal abnormalities and TP53 mutation / overexpression have been reported in isolated soft tissue rhabdoid tumours {394,546,1052,1122,2021}.

Prognostic factors

Extrarenal rhabdoid tumours, like their renal and central nervous system counterparts, are characterized by aggressive biological behaviour. Regardless of therapy and current identifiable tumour or patient-specific features, survival rates are dismal.

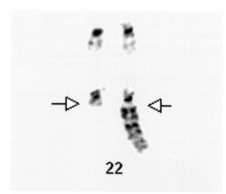

Fig. 9.72 Partial karyotype illustrating homozygous loss of the SMARCB1 locus on 22q. One homologue (left) is deleted, and the other (right) is involved in an unbalanced translocation. Arrows indicate breakpoints. For comparison, two normal copies of chromosome 22 are shown (top).

Neoplasms with perivascular epithelioid cell differentiation (PEComas)

A.L. Folpe

Definition

Neoplasms with perivascular epithelioid cell differentiation (PEComas) are mesenchymal tumours composed of histologically and immunohistochemically distinctive perivascular epithelioid cells. The PEComa family of tumours includes angiomyolipoma (AML), clear cell "sugar" tumour of the lung (CCST), lymphangioleiomyomatosis (LAM), clear cell myomelanocytic tumour of the falciform ligament / ligamentum teres (CCMMT) and unusual clear cell tumours of the pancreas, rectum, abdominal serosa, uterus, vulva, thigh, and heart. Some of these lesions are discussed in the WHO Classification of renal (AML), hepatic (AML) and pulmonary (CCST, LAM) tumours.

Synonyms

Extrapulmonary sugar tumour, perivascular epithelioid cell tumour (PECT), monotypic epithelioid angiomyolipoma.

Epidemiology

PEComas other than AML, CCST or LAM are exceedingly rare. Approximately 31 PEComas other than AML, LAM or CCST have been reported {225,417,698,701,802,1441,1676,2084, 2100,2186, 2335}.
CCMMT usually occurs in young girls, with a mean age at diagnosis of 11 years {698,2084}. Uterine PEComas have a mean age at diagnosis of 54 years {417, 1441,1821,2186}. Almost all other reported PEComas have been in women, with a wide age range {225,802,2100}.

Sites of involvement

PEComas have been reported in the uterus (13 cases), falciform ligament (8 cases), large and small bowel (3 cases), pancreas (1 case), pelvic sidewall (1 case), vulva (1 case), thigh (1 case) and heart (1 case) {225,417,698,701,802,1441,1676,2084, 2100,2186,2335}.

Clinical features

CCMMT presents as a painful abdominal mass. Uterine PEComas may present with vaginal bleeding. Other PEComas typically present as a painless mass. No association with tuberous sclerosis complex has been demonstrated in non-AML, CCST or LAM PEComas.

Histopathology

Perivascular epithelioid cells (PECs) are characterized by perivascular location, often with a radial arrangement of cells around the vascular lumen {227,1675}. Typically, PECs in an immediate perivascular location are most epithelioid and spindled cells resembling smooth muscle are seen away from vessels. Great variation is seen in the relative proportion of epithelioid and spindled cells. PECs have clear to granular, lightly eosinophilic cytoplasm, rather than the dense eosin- ophilia of true smooth muscle cells. They typically display small, centrally placed, normochromatic, round to oval nuclei with small nucleoli, although striking hyperchromasia and nuclear irregularity may be present.

The majority of PEComas resemble CCST, with PEC arrayed around thin-walled blood vessels {2100,2186,2335}. However, a significant percentage of reported PEComas display striking nuclear atypia, elevated mitotic activity and necrosis {225,1786,2100}. Uterine PEComas may show an infiltrative growth pattern similar to that of low grade endometrial stromal sarcoma {2186}. CCMMT differs somewhat from other PEComas in that it is almost exclusively a spindle cell lesion, with uniform moderately sized cells arranged in fascicles and nests {698,701,2084}. A striking feature is the elaborate vasculature, with small arcing vessels that subdivide the tumour into coarse packets, reminiscent of renal cell carcinoma. Mitotic activity, angiolymphatic invasion and necrosis have not been reported.

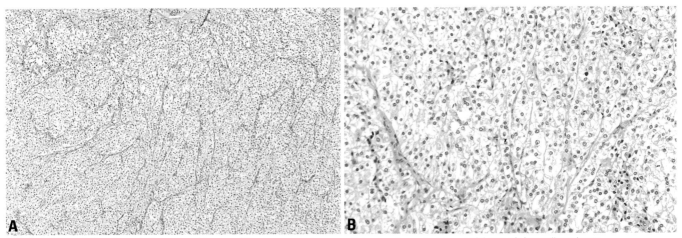

Fig. 9.73 PEComa. **A** Note the typical nested architecture. **B** In many cases, tumour cells have a clear cytoplasm, reminiscent of clear cell carcinoma.

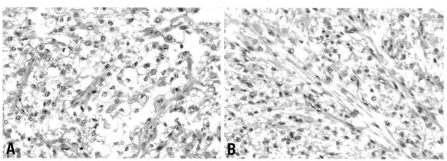

Fig. 9.74 A Epithelioid cytomorphology in a PEComa. **B** PEComa consisting of clear to lightly eosinophilic spindle cells.

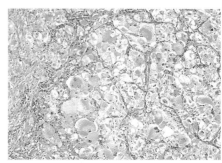

Fig. 9.76 Some PEComa cases show marked cytological pleomorphism.

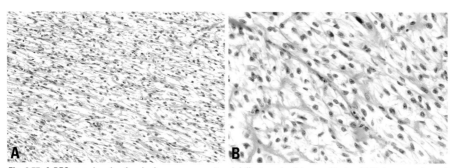

Fig. 9.75 A PEComa showing fascicular arrangement and delicate, arborizing capillaries. **B** High power view of a PEComa with round nuclei with small nucleoli.

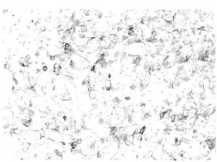

Fig. 9.77 PEComas are consistently immunoreactive for HMB45.

Immunohistochemistry

The PEC is characterized by positivity with melanocytic markers, such as HMB-45, Melan-A, tyrosinase, microphthalmia transcription factor, and NKI/C3 and muscle markers, such as smooth muscle actin, pan-muscle actin, muscle myosin and calponin {225, 226, 288, 329, 698, 1199, 1674, 2034, 2100, 2224, 2339}. Desmin is less often positive and cytokeratin and S100 protein are usually absent. In PEComas, the most sensitive melanocytic markers are HMB-45, Melan-A and microphthalmia transcription factor {2034, 2339}.

Ultrastructure

Ultrastructural studies have documented abundant cytoplasmic glycogen, pre-melanosomes, thin filaments with occasional dense bodies, hemidesmosomes and poorly formed intercellular junctions {698, 2084, 2100}.

Genetics

The presence of a t(3;10)(?p13;?q23) has been reported in one CCMMT {698}. Other PEComas have not been studied by cytogenetic or molecular genetic methods. A small number of CCMMT have also been shown to lack expression of the tuberous sclerosis-associated *TSC2* gene product tuberin {698}.

Prognostic factors

Clear criteria for malignancy in PEComas have not been elaborated, owing to their rarity. Development of such criteria has also been complicated by the relatively frequent presence of pseudomalignant changes in the most common PEComa, AML. However, clinically malignant (i.e., metastatic) AML, usually of the epithelioid type, have been convincingly documented, and these tumours closely resemble many

reported PEComas of non-AML, LAM or CCST type {1199, 1339, 1673, 1744, 1786, 2323}. Sarcomas arising in pre-existing benign AML have also been reported {356, 655}. Furthermore, clinically malignant pulmonary CCST have been reported {752}. Clinically malignant PEComas of the bowel, uterus, and heart have been reported {225, 2100}. On the basis of these prior reports, it appears that PEComas displaying any combination of infiltrative growth, marked hypercellularity, nuclear enlargement and hyperchromasia, high mitotic activity, atypical mitotic figures, and coagulative necrosis should be regarded as malignant. Malignant PEComas are aggressive sarcomas that frequently result in the death of affected patients. In contrast to other forms of PEComa, CCMMT to date appears relatively benign.

Intimal sarcoma

B. Bode-Lesniewska
P. Komminoth

Definition
Intimal sarcomas are malignant mesenchymal tumours arising in large arterial blood vessels of the systemic and pulmonary circulation. The defining feature is the predominant intraluminal growth with obstruction of the lumen of the vessel of origin and the seeding of emboli to peripheral organs.

ICD-O code   8800/3

Epidemiology
Intimal sarcomas are very rare tumours {219, 286}. According to the published case reports pulmonary intimal sarcomas are almost twice as common as tumours of aortic origin (165 versus 100 reported patients) {219, 286, 772, 1916}. Pulmonary intimal sarcomas show a slight female predominance (female to male ratio of about 1.3), while no sex predilection could be observed for aortic tumours. Intimal sarcomas are tumours of adulthood with a broad age range. The mean age at the time of diagnosis is 48 years for pulmonary and 62 years for aortic intimal sarcoma {286}.

Sites of involvement
Intimal sarcomas of the pulmonary circulation mainly involve the proximal vessels and are frequently located in the pulmonary trunk (80%), the right or left main pulmonary arteries (50-70%), or both (40%) {286, 287, 1577}. Some tumours also involve the pulmonary valve or extend into the right ventricular outflow tract. Direct infiltration or lung metastases are observed in 40% of affected patients while extrathoracic spread occurs in about 20% of cases, involving the lungs, kidneys, lymph nodes, the brain and skin {286, 1577}.

Aortic intimal sarcomas mostly arise in the abdominal aorta between the celiac artery and the iliac bifurcation and approximately 30% of tumours are located in the descending thoracic aorta. Arterial embolic tumour dissemination in these patients is frequent and results in distant metastases involving bone, peritoneum, liver and mesenteric lymph nodes {286, 1861}.

Clinical features
The clinical presentation of intimal sarcomas is often unspecific and related to tumour emboli. Due to rarity of this tumour, proper diagnosis is often delayed or made post mortem. In pulmonary intimal sarcomas recurrent pulmonary embolic disease is the most common primary diagnosis. Intimal sarcomas of the aorta most commonly present with consequences of embolic incidents such as claudication and absent pulses of lower extremities, back pain and abdominal angina resulting from mesenteric artery occlusion, malignant hypertension or rupture of aneurysm formed by the tumour {1572}.

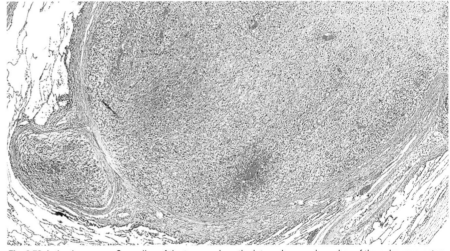

Fig. 9.79 Intimal sarcoma. Spreading of the tumour along the intrapulmonary branches of the pulmonary artery (from B. Bode-Lesniewska et al. {219}).

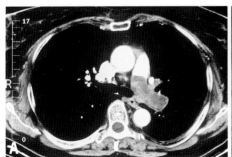 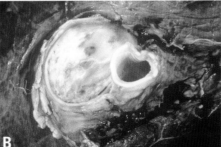 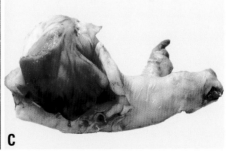

Fig. 9.78 Intimal sarcoma. **A** Chest CT of a patient with an intimal sarcoma of the left pulmonary artery. **B** View of the hilum of the resected lung of this patient with obstruction of the lumen of the pulmonary artery by tumour tissue. **C** Endarterectomy specimen of another patient with intimal sarcoma of the pulmonary artery (from B. Bode-Lesniewska et al. {219}).

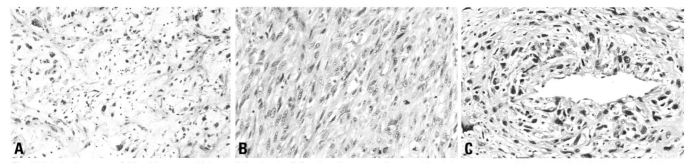

Fig. 9.80 Intimal sarcoma. **A** Myxoid tumour with low cellular density. **B** Bundles of tumour cells resembling leiomyosarcoma. **C** An endothelially lined vascular cleft surrounded by pleomorphic tumour cells (from B. Bode-Lesniewska et al. {219}).

The conventional imaging methods are often disappointingly non-specific, but the neoplastic nature of the tissue occluding the lumen can be suspected in modern diagnostic procedures (CT, MRI, PET) {1745, 2112}.

Macroscopy

Intimal sarcomas are by definition mostly intravascular polypoid masses attached to the vessel wall and grossly resembling thrombi. They may extend distally along the branches of the involved vessels. Occasionally a mucoid lumen cast can be recovered intraoperatively. Some of the aortic tumours may cause thinning and aneurysmal dilatation of the vessel wall with adherent thrombotic material suggesting atherosclerotic changes, particularly in the abdominal aorta. Some of these lesions of the pulmonary arteries may have harder, bony areas corresponding to osteosarcomatous differentiation.

Histopathology

Intimal sarcomas are usually poorly differentiated mesenchymal malignant tumours of fibroblastic or myofibroblastic differentiation, consisting of mildly to severely atypical spindle cells with varying degrees of atypia, mitotic activity, necrosis and nuclear polymorphism. Some tumours show large myxoid areas or epithelioid appearance of tumour cells {804, 974}. Prominent spindling and bundling of the tumour cells may resemble leiomyosarcoma. Rare cases may contain areas of rhabdomyo-, angio- or osteosarcomatous differentiation {286, 287, 804, 974, 1577}. Aortic intimal sarcomas – unlike pulmonary ones – uncommonly contain areas of specific differentiation other than a myofibroblastic one, although some tumours with angio- and rhabdomyosarcomatous appearance have been described in case reports {1466, 1861}.

Immunophenotype

The undifferentiated tumour cells of intimal sarcomas usually exhibit immunoreactivity for vimentin and osteopontin {771}. Variable positivity for smooth muscle actin has been observed and few tumours exhibit some positive staining with antibodies against desmin. In a typical case of intimal sarcoma the vascular markers (CD31, CD34 and FVIII) are negative, but may be positive in areas with angiosarcomatous differentiation.

Ultrastructure

Ultrastructurally, microfilaments, dense bodies, as well as a discontinuous external lamina can be found in intimal sarcomas as features compatible with myofibroblastic differentiation {286, 1039}. In tumours with rhabdomyosarcomatous differentiation some rudimentary sarcomeric structures may be observed {1466}.

Genetics

In a recent study using comparative genomic hybridization (CGH), gains and amplifications of the 12q13-14 region were identified in 6/8 tumours. Other, less consistent alterations were losses on 3p, 3q, 4q, 9p, 11q, 13q, Xp and Xq, gains on 7p, 17p and 17q as well as amplifications on 4q, 5p, 6p and 11q {219}.

Prognostic factors

The prognosis of intimal sarcomas originating both in the aorta and in pulmonary arteries is poor with mean survival times of about 5-9 months in patients with aortic tumours and of 13-18 months in patients with pulmonary sarcomas {1916}. Surgical and adjuvant therapy may prolong survival without influencing the generally poor outcome {219, 286, 1577}.

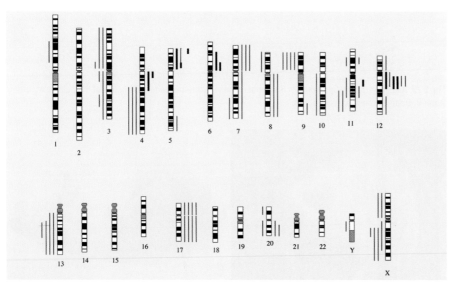

Fig. 9.81 CGH analysis of 8 intimal pulmonary artery sarcomas. Bars to the left of the chromosomes correspond to losses, bars to the right, to gains; thick bars correspond to amplifications of genetic material (from B. Bode-Lesniewska et al. {219}).

WHO Classification
of Bone Tumours

Primary neoplasms of the skeleton are rare, amounting to only 0.2% of the overall human tumour burden. However, children are frequently affected and the aetiology is largely unknown.

Significant progress has been made in the histological and genetic typing of bone tumours. Furthermore, advances in combined surgical and chemotherapy havelead to a significant increase in survival rates even for highly malignant neoplasms, including osteosarcoma and Ewing sarcoma.

Several bone tumours occur in the setting of inherited tumour syndromes, but their histology differs little from the respective sporadic counterparts.

WHO classification of bone tumours

CARTILAGE TUMOURS
Osteochondroma	9210/0*
Chondroma	9220/0
Enchondroma	9220/0
Periosteal chondroma	9221/0
Multiple chondromatosis	9220/1
Chondroblastoma	9230/0
Chondromyxoid fibroma	9241/0
Chondrosarcoma	9220/3
Central, primary, and secondary	9220/3
Peripheral	9221/3
Dedifferentiated	9243/3
Mesenchymal	9240/3
Clear cell	9242/3

OSTEOGENIC TUMOURS
Osteoid osteoma	9191/0
Osteoblastoma	9200/0
Osteosarcoma	9180/3
Conventional	9180/3
chondroblastic	9181/3
fibroblastic	9182/3
osteoblastic	9180/3
Telangiectatic	9183/3
Small cell	9185/3
Low grade central	9187/3
Secondary	9180/3
Parosteal	9192/3
Periosteal	9193/3
High grade surface	9194/3

FIBROGENIC TUMOURS
Desmoplastic fibroma	8823/0
Fibrosarcoma	8810/3

FIBROHISTIOCYTIC TUMOURS
Benign fibrous histiocytoma	8830/0
Malignant fibrous histiocytoma	8830/3

EWING SARCOMA/PRIMITIVE NEUROECTODERMAL TUMOUR
Ewing sarcoma	9260/3

HAEMATOPOIETIC TUMOURS
Plasma cell myeloma	9732/3
Malignant lymphoma, NOS	9590/3

GIANT CELL TUMOUR
Giant cell tumour	9250/1
Malignancy in giant cell tumour	9250/3

NOTOCHORDAL TUMOURS
Chordoma	9370/3

VASCULAR TUMOURS
Haemangioma	9120/0
Angiosarcoma	9120/3

SMOOTH MUSCLE TUMOURS
Leiomyoma	8890/0
Leiomyosarcoma	8890/3

LIPOGENIC TUMOURS
Lipoma	8850/0
Liposarcoma	8850/3

NEURAL TUMOURS
Neurilemmoma	9560/0

MISCELLANEOUS TUMOURS
Adamantinoma	9261/3
Metastatic malignancy	

MISCELLANEOUS LESIONS
Aneurysmal bone cyst	
Simple cyst	
Fibrous dysplasia	
Osteofibrous dysplasia	
Langerhans cell histiocytosis	9751/1
Erdheim-Chester disease	
Chest wall hamartoma	

JOINT LESIONS
Synovial chondromatosis	9220/0

_____

* Morphology code of the International Classification of Diseases for Oncology (ICD-O) {726} and the Systematized Nomenclature of Medicine (http://snomed.org). Behaviour is coded /0 for benign tumours, /1 for unspecified, borderline or uncertain behaviour, /2 for in situ carcinomas and grade III intraepithelial neoplasia, and /3 for malignant tumours.

WHO classification of tumours of bone: Introduction

H.D. Dorfman   D. Vanel
B. Czerniak   Y.K. Park
R. Kotz   K.K. Unni

Among the wide array of human neoplasms, primary tumours of bone are relatively uncommon. Not only has this contributed to the paucity of meaningful and useful data about the relative frequency and incidence rates of the various subtypes of bone tumours, but it also explains our rudimentary understanding of risk factors.

Little information is available concerning the aetiology and epidemiologic features of benign bone tumours since most published statistical studies have dealt with bone sarcomas. The benign lesions will be considered from the epidemiologic and aetiologic standpoint under the individual chapter headings, where they are known.

Incidence

In general, bone sarcomas account for only 0.2% of all neoplasms for which data were obtained in one large series (SEER) {1789}. Comparison of the incidence rate of bone sarcomas with that of the closely related group of soft tissue sarcomas indicates that osseous neoplasms occur at a rate approximately one tenth that of their soft tissue counterparts {537,946,1304}.

In North America and Europe, the incidence rate for bone sarcomas in males is approximately 0.8 new cases per 100,000 population and year. Somewhat higher incidence rates have been observed for males in Argentina and Brazil (1.5-2) and Israel (1.4) {1665}. Cancer registry data with histological stratification indicate that osteosarcoma is the most common primary malignant tumour of bone, accounting for approximately 35 percent of cases, followed by chondrosarcoma (25%), and Ewing sarcoma (16%). In countries and regions with higher incidence rates, the relative fraction of osteosarcomas appears to be larger. Chordomas and malignant fibrous histiocytoma are much less frequent, constituting approximately 8 and 5% of bone tumours, respectively. In recent years, the diagnosis of fibrosarcoma primary in bone has largely been replaced by that of malignant fibrous histiocytoma, accounting for a marked decline in the frequency of the former diagnostic category.

Age and site distribution

The age-specific frequencies and incidence rates of bone sarcomas as a group are clearly bimodal. The first well defined peak occurs during the second decade of life, while the second occurs in patients older than sixty. The risk of development of bone sarcomas during the second decade of life is close to that of the older than 60 population, but there are more cases in the second decade. The bimodal age-specific incidence rate pattern of bone sarcomas is clearly different from that of soft tissue sarcomas, which shows a gradual increase of incidence with age.

Osteosarcoma occurs predominantly in patients younger than age twenty, and in this group 80% occur in long bones of the extremities. In this age group, a small proportion of cases involve other parts of the skeleton, such as craniofacial bones, the spine, and pelvis. The clear predilection of osteosarcoma for the appendicular skeleton has a tendency to decrease with age. In patients older than fifty, osteosarcoma of the extremity bones makes up only 50 % of cases. In this group, the pelvis and craniofacial bones each account for about 20 % of the cases. The incidence rate of extremity bone involvement for patients older than 50 is approximately one third of that for persons in the younger age groups.

Chondrosarcomas have age-specific incidence rates showing a gradual increase up to age 75. The age adjusted rates show little difference by sex and race. More than 50 % of chondrosarcomas occur in the long bones of the extremities. The other major sites of involvement are the pelvis and ribs. The latter site and the sternum are high risk sites for malignant cartilage tumours.

Ewing sarcoma has epidemiological features similar to those of osteosarcoma, but while osteosarcomas tend to occur in the metaphyseal areas of long bones of skeletally immature patients, particularly in the knee region, Ewing sarcoma tends to arise in the diaphysis. The age-specific relative frequency and incidence mir-

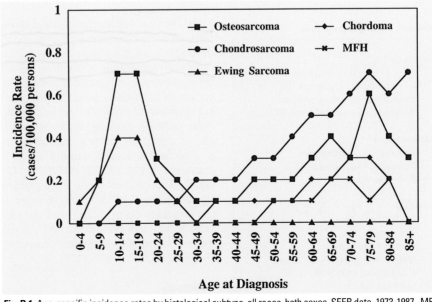

Fig. B.1 Age-specific incidence rates by histological subtype, all races, both sexes, SEER data, 1973-1987. MFH, malignant fibrous histiocytoma and fibrosarcoma.

Relative frequencies of bone sarcomas by histological type, sex, and race: SEER data 1973-1987

Histological type	Total No.	Total %	White No.	White %	Black No.	Black %
Osteosarcoma	922	35.1	743	32.6	106	57.9
Chondrosarcoma	677	25.8	615	27.0	35	19.1
Ewing sarcoma	420	16.0	392	17.3	7	3.8
Chordoma	221	8.4	200	8.8	4	2.2
Malignant fibrous histiocytoma	149	5.7	125	5.5	13	7.1
Angiosarcoma	36	1.4	35	1.5	1	0.5
Unspecified	32	1.2	27	1.2	3	1.6
Other	170	6.4	139	6.1	14	7.8
Total	2627	100.0	2276	100.0	183	100.0

From H. Dorfman & B. Czerniak {537}.

ror those of osteosarcoma with the major peak occurring during the second decade of life. Although there is a rapid decrease in incidence after age 20, cases are seen in all age groups. Unlike osteosarcoma, Ewing sarcoma is reported to occur almost exclusively in the white population.

Precursor lesions

Although the majority of primary bone malignancies arise do novo, it is increasingly apparent that some develop in association with recognizable precursors. Some of these represent non-neoplastic

Precursors of malignancy in bone

High Risk
Ollier disease (Enchondromatosis) and Maffucci syndrome
Familial retinoblastoma syndrome
Rothmund-Thomson syndrome (RTS)

Moderate Risk
Multiple osteochondromas
Polyostotic Paget disease
Radiation osteitis

Low Risk
Fibrous dysplasia
Bone infarct
Chronic osteomyelitis
Metallic and polyethylene implants
Osteogenesis imperfecta
Giant cell tumour
Osteoblastoma and chondroblastoma

lesions that predispose to malignant transformation. Others are benign neoplasms that can be the source of a malignant neoplastic process. The likelihood of discovering such associated lesions can be facilitated by attention to clinicopathological correlation of all available data before arriving at a diagnosis. In bone, the inclusion of radiographic imaging data in the diagnostic process offers a unique opportunity to discover clues to causal relationships that may not be reflected in histological patterns or in other laboratory data. This is especially true when serial radiographs are available for review.

Paget disease, radiation injury, and some of the more common benign cartilaginous dysplasias are the most clearly established precancerous conditions. Both osteosarcoma and malignant fibrous histiocytoma have been linked to pre-existing condition of bone such as Paget disease, radiation damage, bone infarction, fibrous dysplasia, chronic osteomyelitis, and some genetically determined syndromes {25,132,390,797,867,989,1042, 2263}. The relative rarity of malignant transformation in fibrous dysplasia, osteomyelitis, bone cysts, osteogenesis imperfecta, and bone infarction places these conditions in a separate category {540,725,760, 892,1471,2122}.

Aetiology

While radiation and chronic inflammatory states are established, though rare caus-

es of bone malignancies, other exposures and conditions have been suspected (e.g. chromium, nickel, cobalt, aluminum, titanium, methyl-methacrylate, and polyethyelene) but not unequivocally confirmed. Recently attention has been focused on a small number of reported cases of bone sarcomas arising in association with implanted metallic hardware and joint prostheses {788, 879, 1083,1683,2225}. However, the epidemiological evidence for a causitive role is still limited or inconclusive {6}. Future molecular epidemiological studies in patients who have undergone orthopaedic implantation of metallic and other foreign materials may provide clues to the pathogenetic mechanisms underlying malignant transformation in bone.

Clinical features

The clinical features of bone tumours are non-specific, therefore a long period of time may elapse until the tumour is diagnosed. Pain, swelling and general discomfort are the cardinal symptoms that lead to the diagnosis of bone tumours. However, limited mobility and spontaneous fracture may also be important features.

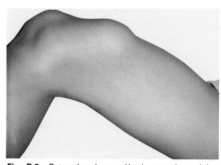

Fig. B.2 Osteochondroma. Hard, smooth, nodular swelling of the distal femur, skin and soft tissues are easily movable and the knee joint is freely mobile.

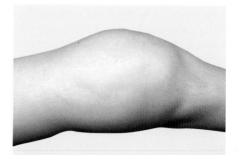

Fig. B.3 Osteosarcoma, causing swelling in the distal femur. Soft tissues poorly movable, consistency ranging from tough to hard, hyperthermia of the skin and marked veins.

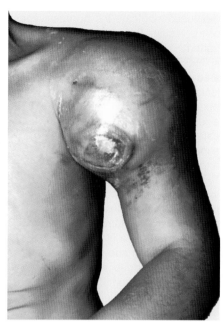

Fig. B.4 Ewing sarcoma of the proximal humerus, presenting as tightly elastic, tense, ulcerated lesion with shining skin, on a grey-white background. Note the marked veins and skin striation.

Pain

Pain is the first and most common symptom in nearly all malignant bone tumours {388,429,1025,1159,1254}. If a spontaneous fracture does not occur, the symptoms usually commence slowly. Initially the patient has tearing neuralgia-like pain, which may also be interpreted as "rheumatic pain". Although the symptoms may initially occur intermittently and only at rest, the pain might subsequently become more intense, disturb sleep at night, spread into the adjacent joint and is frequently misinterpreted as arthritis or as a post-traumatic phenomenon.

A further intensification of pain is experienced as a persistent and piercing pain. During disease progression, the pain becomes excruciating and intolerable, requiring opiate treatment.

In case of pressure on nerve trunks or nerve plexuses, the patient may experience radiating pain. A specific kind of pain occurs when the tumour is located in the spine and causes radicular or spinal compression symptoms with paralysis.

Swelling

The second most important symptom in bone tumours is swelling, which may frequently be of very long duration, especially in benign neoplasms, and cause no additional complaints. Swelling is only observed if there is an extraosseous part of the tumour or the bone is expanded by the tumourous process. In malignant tumours, swelling develops more rapidly. A description of consistency is important e.g. hard, coarse, tightly elastic or soft. Metric data concerning swelling (in centimeters) should be given; ultrasonic examination may be helpful to establish objective sizes. In advanced stages, tumour swelling may also cause skin changes, including tensed shining skin with prominent veins, livid colouring, hyperthermia, as well as striation of the skin and eventually, ulceration. The mobility of the skin, subcutis and musculature above the tumour should also be assessed. The less the mobility, the more likely is this factor a criterion of malignancy.

Limitation of movement

Mobility may be limited in cases of lesions close to the joint, in tumours such as osteoblastoma, chrondroblastoma, giant cell tumours and all types of sarcomas. Occasionally it is not the tumour but reactive synovitis in the joint, especially in chondroblastoma, that causes limitation of movement and masks the true diagnosis.

Pathologic fracture

Fracture is diagnosed early, as it causes the patient to seek attention immediately. It may occur with no prior symptoms at all, as is frequently the case in juvenile cysts and in some non-ossifying bone fibromas. In cases of malignant bone tumours, fracture is a rather rare primary event, as it usually occurs in advanced stages of osteolytic malignant tumours and the patient will have experienced pain and tumour growth prior to it.

General symptoms

These mainly consist of fever, exhaustion and loss of weight. They are late signs in malignant tumours, and will be absent in nearly all cases of benign bone lesions.

Imaging of bone tumours
Diagnosis

Combining both radiological and histological criteria is most appropriate.

Based on clinical and radiological signs, one should first diagnose benign lesions for which a subsequent biopsy may not be necessary:
> Metaphyseal fibrous defect
> Fibrous dysplasia
> Osteochondroma
> Enchondroma
> Simple bone cyst
> Vertebral haemangioma

Age is useful information: before age of 5, a malignant tumour is often metastatic neuroblastoma; between 5 and 15 years old, osteosarcoma or Ewing sarcoma; and after 40 years, metastasis or myeloma.

The first step is to determine tumour aggressiveness by conventional radiology. Important parameters include tumour

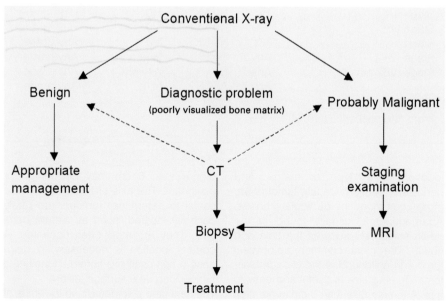

Fig. B.5 The choice of the imaging technique.

Primary tumour (T)	TX:	primary tumour cannot be assessed
	T0:	no evidence of primary tumour
	T1:	tumour ≤ 8 cm in greatest dimension
	T2:	tumour > 8 cm in greatest dimension
	T3:	discontinuous tumours in the primary bone site

Regional lymph nodes (N)	NX:	regional lymph nodes cannot be assessed
	N0:	no regional lymph node metastasis
	N1:	regional lymph node metastasis

Note: Regional node involvement is rare and cases in which nodal status is not assessed either clinically or pathologically could be considered N0 instead of NX or pNX.

Distant metastasis (M)	MX:	distant metastasis cannot be assessed
	M0:	no distant metastasis
	M1:	distant metastasis
	M1a:	lung
	M1b:	other distant sites

G Histopathological Grading

Translation table for 'three' and 'four grade' to 'two grade' (low vs. high grade) system

TNM two grade system	Three grade systems	Four grade systems
Low grade	Grade 1	Grade 1
		Grade 2
High grade	Grade 2	Grade 3
	Grade 3	Grade 4

Note: Ewing sarcoma is classified as high grade.

Stage IA	T1	N0,NX	M0	Low grade
Stage IB	T2	N0,NX	M0	Low grade
Stage IIA	T1	N0,NX	M0	High grade
Stage IIB	T2	N0,NX	M0	High grade
Stage III	T3	N0,NX	M0	Any grade
Stage IVA	Any T	N0,NX	M1a	Any grade
Stage IVB	Any T	N1	Any M	Any grade
	Any T	Any N	M1b	Any grade

From references {831,1979}.

destruction indicate the aggressiveness of the lesion. Type 1 is the geographic pattern. 1A is characterized by a rim of sclerosis between the normal and lytic area. 1B indicates a very well limited lesion, with sharp separation with normal bone, but no sclerosis. 1C characterizes a less sharp limit. Type 2 is the moth-eaten pattern. It is made of multiple holes separated by not yet destroyed bone and indicates a more aggressive growth. Type 3 is the permeative pattern. Indistinct transition indicates a very rapid progression of the lesion. The pattern of the margins of the tumour only means the rate of progression of the lesion and not directly its malignancy.

Most lesions appear radiolucent on the radiographs but some are sclerotic. The typical arciform calcifications suggest cartilaginous tumours.

The pattern of periosteal new bone formation reacting to the tumour crossing the cortex depends upon the rate of progression of the tumour. When the tumour grows slowly, the periosteum has enough time to build a thick layer of bone. When multiple layers of periosteal formation are present, there is probably a succession of fast and slow growth phases of progression. Perpendicular periosteal formations are a very useful radiological sign, strongly suggesting malignancy.

The Codman's triangle indicates an elevated periosteal reaction, broken by the growth of the tumour. It can be seen in both benign and malignant processes.

Cortical disruption, and soft tissues involvement usually indicate aggressiveness. A thin layer of new bone formation ossified around the tumour suggests a slow evolution and therefore a benign process, even if the cortex is destroyed. On the contrary, tumour on both sides of a not yet destroyed cortex indicates a very aggressive lesion.

Multiple lesions are seen in chondromas, osteochondromas, Langerhans cell histiocytosis, metastases, and more rarely in multifocal osteosarcomas and metastatic Ewing sarcoma.

A flow chart of diagnostic procedures is shown in Fig. B.05. In general, conventional X-ray radiography is the starting point. CT is the examination of choice in the diagnosis of the nidus of osteoid osteoma in dense bone {798}. Small lucency of the cortex, localized involvement of the soft tissues, and thin peripheral periosteal reaction can be seen

location, size, type of matrix, and periosteal reaction. Certain tumours are more common in particular bones. Adamantinoma, usually found in the adult, selectively involves the tibia and fibula. The most common epiphyseal tumour in childhood is the chondroblastoma. Tumour size is useful and easy to use. A tumour less than 6 cm in greatest dimension is likely benign whereas one bigger than 6 cm may be benign or malignant. The axis of the lesion is also useful to determine. Tumours are rarely centrally located, such as simple bone cyst. They are most often eccentric. A cortical location is necessary to diagnose a non-ossifying fibroma. Finally the tumour can be a surface lesion.

The next step is to determine the limits of the tumour. The patterns of bone

Musculoskeletal Tumour Society staging of malignant bone lesions

Stage:	Definition:
IA	Low grade, intracompartmental
IB	Low grade, extracompartmental
IIA	High grade, intracompartmental
IIB	High grade, extracompartmental
III	Any grade, metastatic

Musculoskeletal Tumour Society staging. Surgical margins

Type:	Plane of Dissection:
Intralesional	Within lesion
Marginal	Within reactive zone-extracapsular
Wide	Beyond reactive zone through normal tissue within compartment
Radical	Normal tissue extracompartmental

{279}. CT also allows measurement of the thickness of a non-calcified cuff of a cartilaginous tumour: the cuff is thin in benign lesions and thick (more than 3 cm) in chondrosarcomas {1092}. MRI is rarely useful in the diagnosis, but can display better than CT fluid levels in blood filled cavities, especially aneurysmal bone cysts.

Staging
Focal extent and staging is based on MRI {24,216,222}. The main advantages are high contrast and the possibility of choosing the plane of examination without moving the patient.
Bone metastases are best detected on radionuclide bone scans. Pulmonary metastases are evaluated on conventional chest radiographs and chest CT {2185}. Positron emission tomography (PET) is still under evaluation.
Effectiveness and follow-up of treatment
Most primary malignant tumours are treated with preoperative chemotherapy before removal. Plain films and CT can provide information on the size, margins and ossifications of the tumour. MRI, however, provides a more accurate study of the tumour volume. Signal decrease on T2-weighted sequences suggests in-

creased ossification or more fibrous tissue in the tumour {964}. Lack of increase in signal intensity of the lesion after injection of the contrast agent suggests necrosis. MR imaging with dynamic contrast-enhancement may be useful for differentiating post-chemotherapeutic change from viable tumour, because viable tumour enhances rapidly, and the post-chemotherapeutic changes enhance slowly {463,2175,2202}.

Grading and staging of bone sarcomas
Grading
Histological grading is an attempt to predict the biological behaviour of a malignant tumour based on histological features. The principles used for grading sarcomas are similar to those proposed by Broders for grading of squamous cell carcinoma {272}. In bone tumours, cellularity, i.e., the relative amount of cells compared to matrix, and nuclear features of the tumour cells are the most important criteria used for grading. Generally, the higher the grade, the more cellular the tumour. Irregularity of the nuclear contours, enlargement and hyperchromasia of the nuclei are correlated with grade. Mitotic figures and necrosis are addition-

al features useful in grading {624}.
Spindle cell sarcomas such as osteosarcoma and fibrosarcoma need to be graded. Many studies have shown that histological grading correlates with prognosis in chondrosarcoma and malignant vascular tumours {624,1006,1858}. Tumours which are monomorphic, such as small cell malignancies (Ewing sarcoma, malignant lymphoma and myeloma), do not lend themselves to histological grading. Mesenchymal chondrosarcomas and dedifferentiated chondrosarcomas are always high grade, whereas clear cell chondrosarcomas are low grade. Clinicopathological studies have shown that grading is not useful in predicting prognosis in adamantinoma and chordoma.
The significance of histological grading is limited by inter-observer variability and the fact that the majority of tumours fall into the intermediate range.

Staging
In bone tumours, staging incorporates the degree of differentiation as well as local and distant spread, in order to estimate the prognosis of the patient.
The universal TNM staging system used for most carcinomas is not commonly used for sarcomas because of their rarity with which sarcomas metastasize to lymph nodes. Hence the special staging system adopted by the musculoskeletal society first described by Enneking and co-authors have gained acceptance {2291}. Although staging systems have been described for both benign and malignant bone tumours, the usefulness is primarily in description of malignant bone tumours. Benign lesions are classified using Arabic numerals and malignant ones with Roman numerals. Stage 1 benign lesions are latent lesions having negligible recurrence rate following intracapsular excision. Stage 2 benign lesions are actively growing with a significant recurrence rate after intracapsular procedures but a negligible recurrence rate after marginal en bloc excision. Stage 3 benign lesions are locally aggressive with extracapsular extension having a high recurrence rate after either intracapsular or marginal procedures.
A surgical staging system for malignant lesions is most logically accomplished with the assessment of the surgical grade (G), the local extent (T), and the presence or absence of regional or dis-

tant metastases (M). Any neoplasm can be divided into two grades; low (G1) and high (G2). In general, low grade lesions correspond to Broders grade 1 and 2 and have less than 25% risk of metastasis. High grade lesions (Broders grade 3 and grade 4) have a great risk of local recurrence and greater than 25% risk of distant spread. The anatomic extent (T) is subdivided according to whether the lesion is intracompartmental (A) or extracompartmental (B) {55, 1677}. The presence or absence of metastasis (M) is the third major factor related to both prognosis and surgical planning.

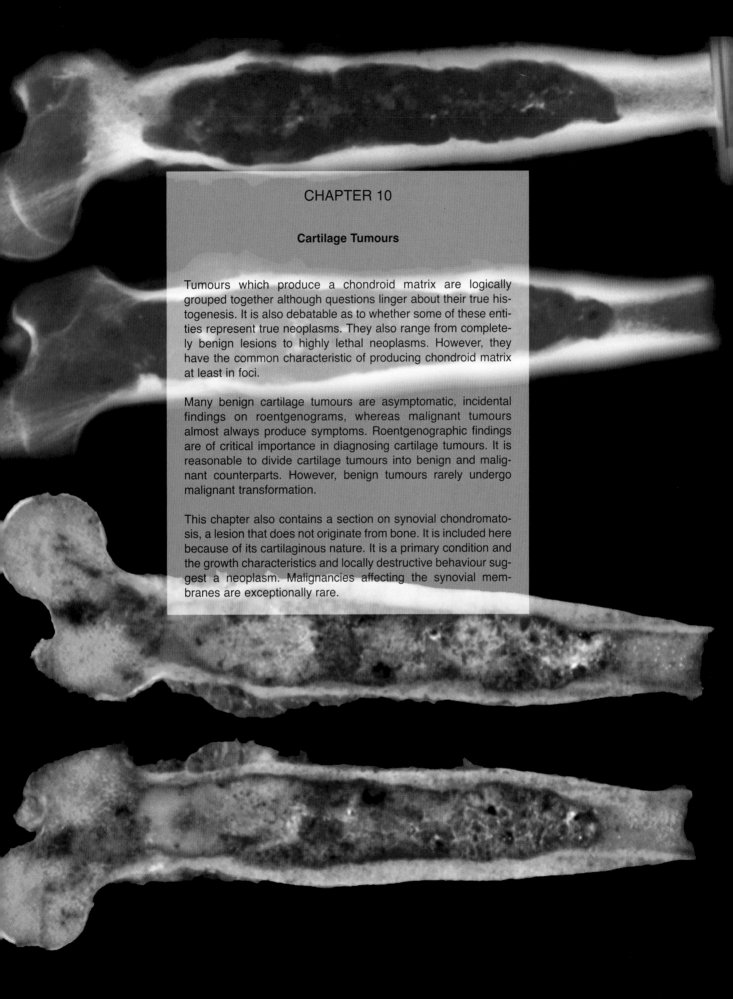

CHAPTER 10

Cartilage Tumours

Tumours which produce a chondroid matrix are logically grouped together although questions linger about their true histogenesis. It is also debatable as to whether some of these entities represent true neoplasms. They also range from completely benign lesions to highly lethal neoplasms. However, they have the common characteristic of producing chondroid matrix at least in foci.

Many benign cartilage tumours are asymptomatic, incidental findings on roentgenograms, whereas malignant tumours almost always produce symptoms. Roentgenographic findings are of critical importance in diagnosing cartilage tumours. It is reasonable to divide cartilage tumours into benign and malignant counterparts. However, benign tumours rarely undergo malignant transformation.

This chapter also contains a section on synovial chondromatosis, a lesion that does not originate from bone. It is included here because of its cartilaginous nature. It is a primary condition and the growth characteristics and locally destructive behaviour suggest a neoplasm. Malignancies affecting the synovial membranes are exceptionally rare.

Osteochondroma

J. Khurana
F. Abdul-Karim
J.V.M.G. Bovée

Definition
Osteochondroma is a cartilage capped bony projection arising on the external surface of bone containing a marrow cavity that is continuous with that of the underlying bone.

ICD-O codes
Osteochondroma   9210/0
Osteochondromatosis NOS   9210/1

Synonyms
Osteochondroma:
Osteochondromatous exostosis, solitary osteochondroma.

Multiple osteochondromas:
Hereditary osteochondromatosis, hereditary deforming osteochondromatosis, hereditary chondrodysplasia, diaphyseal aclasis, metaphyseal aclasis, hereditary multiple exostoses.

Epidemiology
Solitary osteochondroma
Osteochondroma may be the most common bone tumour {988,1875,2155}. The reported incidence, 35% of benign and 8% of all bone tumours, probably is an underestimate as the majority are asymptomatic and not clinically apparent {2155}. Most reported cases have been in the first 3 decades with no known sex predilection.

Multiple osteochondromas
Approximately 15% of patients (of all osteochondromas) have multiple lesions {2155}, with an incidence up to 1:50,000 in some series {1887}. The age of patients with multiple lesions is similar to those with solitary osteochondromas and there is also no sex predilection. Inheri-tance is autosomal dominant.

Sites of involvement
Osteochondromas generally arise in bones preformed by cartilage. The most common site of involvement is the metaphyseal region of distal femur, upper humerus, upper tibia and fibula {2155}.

Involvement of flat bones is less common with the ilium and scapula accounting for most of the cases.

Clinical features
Signs and symptoms
Many, if not most lesions, are asymptomatic and found incidentally. In symptomatic cases, the symptoms are often related to the size and location of the lesion. The most common presentation is that of a hard mass of long-standing duration. Some cases present with symptoms related to secondary complications such as mechanical obstruction, nerve impingement, bursa forming over the osteochondroma, pseudoaneurysm of an overlying vessel, infarction of the osteochondroma or fracture of the stalk of the lesion {131,188,470,988,1072, 1468,1681,1875,2119,2152,2155}.
Increasing pain and/or growing mass may be a manifestation of malignant transformation of osteochondromas. It is estimated to be less than 1% in patients with solitary and approximately 1-3% in patients with multiple osteochondromas. Higher incidences, some up to 20% of malignant transformation in multiple osteochondromas have been reported because of case selection and variable criteria used {211,1131,1875,2155, 2206}.

Imaging
Solitary osteochondromas may be pedunculated or sessile lesions. The characteristic feature is a projection of the cortex in continuity with the underlying bone. Irregular calcification is often seen. Excessive cartilage type flocculent calcification should raise the suspicion of malignant transformation. CT scan or MRI images typically show continuity of the marrow space into the lesion. These modalities may also predict the thickness of the cartilage cap {464,775, 2285}. A thick cap raises the suspicion of malignant transformation. Osteochondromas grow away from the site of active growth, most likely due to forces from adjacent tendons and muscles.

Multiple osteochondromas are similar to the solitary ones but are generally associated with remodeling defects of bone. Many are flat and cauliflower shaped.

Aetiology
The aetiology is not known. Based on the resemblance of the cartilage cap to the growth plate, several hypotheses have been offered. These include the possibility of breakage, rotation and aberrant growth of the physeal plate or herniation of the plate in the metaphysis {415,988, 1457,1464,1718}.

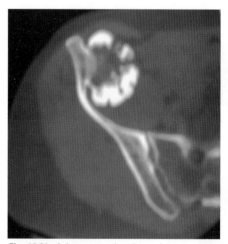

Fig. 10.01 A large ostechondroma is seen at the upper ilium extending into the false pelvis.

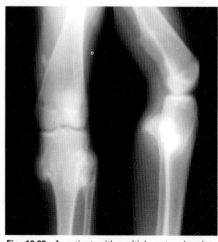

Fig. 10.02 A patient with multiple osteochondromas. The limb shows shape and modeling defects.

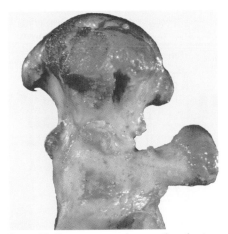

Fig. 10.03 Outer aspect and cut section of osteo-chondroma of the upper fibula demonstrating the continuity of the cortex and marrow cavity of the osteochondroma with that of the underlying bone.

Macroscopy

An osteochondroma may be sessile or pedunculated. The cortex and medullary cavity extend into the lesion. The cartilage cap is usually thin (and decreases in thickness with age). A thick and irregular cap (greater than 2 cm) may be indicative of malignant transformation.

Histopathology

The lesion has three layers – perichondrium, cartilage and bone. The outer layer is a fibrous perichondrium that is continuous with the periosteum of the underlying bone. Below this is a cartilage cap that is usually less than 2 cm thick (and decreases with age). Within the cartilage cap the superficial chondrocytes are clustered, whereas the ones close to the transition to bone resemble a growth plate. They are organised into chords and undergo endochondral ossification similar to the zone of provisional mineralization. Loss of the architecture of cartilage, wide fibrous bands, myxoid change, increased chondrocyte cellularity, mitotic activity, significant chondrocyte atypia and necrosis are all features that may indicate secondary malignant transformation. Fractures within a stalk may elicit a focal fibroblastic response.

Surface chondrosarcomas differ from osteochondromas by the absence of a stalk and the presence of lobular masses of cartilage that permeate and infiltrate the soft-tissues {1366}. Parosteal osteosarcoma may have a zone of typical cartilage simulating a "cap". They are, however, radiographically and

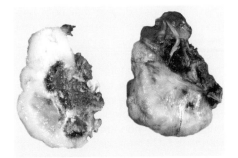

Fig. 10.04 Osteochondroma cut surface and outer surface showing the bony stalk and the overlying cartilage cap.

microscopically different from an osteochondroma. The characteristic fibroblastic proliferation and cytological atypia is not observed in an osteochondroma.

Bunions and osteophytes are bony growths (often without a cartilage cap) that have no marrow cavity or sometimes a poorly developed one that is not continuous with the medullary canal of the underlying bone. Exostoses that arise in the cranio-facial and jaw bones are sometimes called tori (sing. torus). These are usually osseous proliferations that are reactive to an irritant. A similar traumatic aetiology is most likely responsible for the subungual exostosis and the so-called aural meatal exostosis. Bizarre parosteal osteochondromatous proliferation (Nora's lesion) is a disorganized mass of bone, cartilage and fibrous tissue. Trevor disease (Dysplasia Epiphysealis Hemimelica) is a non-hereditary skeletal dysplasia that resembles an epiphyseal osteochondroma.

Genetics

It was long debated whether osteochondroma was a developmental disorder or a true neoplasm. Cytogenetic aberrations involving 8q22-24.1, where the *EXT1* gene is located, have been found in ten out of 30 sporadic and in 1 out of 13 hereditary osteochondromas {264, 1430}. Moreover, DNA flow cytometry of the cartilaginous cap demonstrated aneuploidy (DNA index range 0.88-1.17) in four of 10 osteochondromas {238}. LOH detected by microsatellite analysis using DNA isolated from the cartilaginous cap was found almost exclusively at the *EXT1* locus in 3 of 8 sporadic and 2 of six hereditary osteochondromas {238}. Fluorescence in situ hybridization revealed loss of the 8q24.1 locus in 27 of 34 (79%) osteochondromas {645}.

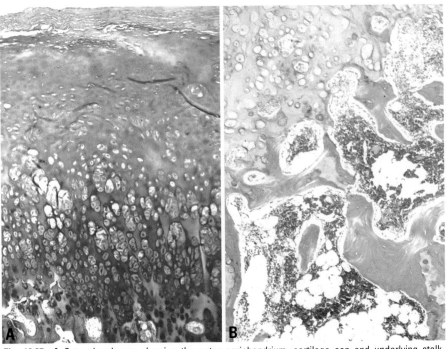

Fig. 10.05 A Osteochondroma, showing the outer perichondrium, cartilage cap and underlying stalk. Variable amount of endochondral ossification occurs at the bone/cartilage interface. **B** Endochondral ossification is often seen at the base of the osteochondroma. This is a normal feature and should not be interpreted as a malignancy invading into the stalk.

These findings suggest that both sporadic and hereditary osteochondromas are true neoplasms.

The *EXT* genes, involved in hereditary multiple osteochondromas (HMO), are hypothesised to be tumour suppressor genes. Most of the mutations found in HMO patients are predicted to result in a truncated or non-functional protein. Germline *EXT1* mutations combined with loss of the remaining wild type allele was demonstrated in three osteochondromas of two HMO patients {238}. One sporadic osteochondroma was described to harbour a deletion of one *EXT1* gene combined with an inactivating mutation in the other *EXT1* gene {168}. Although second mutations have been demonstrated in the minority of cases so far, these findings strongly suggest that inactivation of both copies of an *EXT* gene in a cartilaginous cell of the growth plate is required for osteochondroma formation in both hereditary and sporadic cases. Indeed, diminished levels of the EXT1 and EXT2 proteins {168} and of their putative downstream effectors (IHh/PTHrP and FGF signalling pathway, see chapter 21) {241} were

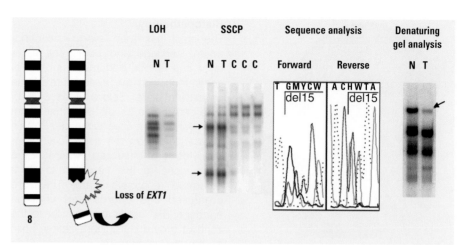

Fig. 10.06 Chromosomal band 8q24 rearrangement in sporadic osteochondroma (on the left). LOH at 8q24 in a patient with multiple exostoses is demonstrated by microsatellite analysis (D8S198). SSCP mutation analysis reveals aberrant bands (indicated by arrows) in both normal (N) and osteochondroma (T) DNA. Sequence analysis reveals a constitutional 15 bp deletion. The PCR fragment containing the mutation is run on a denaturing gel, illustrating loss of the wild-type allele (arrow).

demonstrated in both sporadic and hereditary osteochondroma chondrocytes {168}. Moreover, *EXT* mutations were described to induce cytoskeletal abnormalities (altered actin distribution) in osteochondroma chondrocytes {168, 169,1237}.

Prognostic factors

Excision of the osteochondroma is usually curative. Recurrence is seen with incomplete removal, however, multiple recurrences or recurrence in a well excised lesion should raise the suspicion of malignancy.

Chondromas: enchondroma, periosteal chondroma, and enchondromatosis

D.R. Lucas
J.A. Bridge

This group of generally benign tumours of hyaline cartilage share many histological features. However, they differ with respect to location and clinical features. Enchondroma and periosteal chondroma are sporadic while enchondromatosis usually manifests as a congenital tumour syndrome (see Chapter 21, page 356).

Enchondroma

Definition
Enchondroma is a benign hyaline cartilage neoplasm of medullary bone. Most tumours are solitary, however, they occasionally involve more than one bone or site in a single bone.

ICD-O codes
Chondroma   9220/0
Enchondroma   9220/0

Synonyms
Solitary enchondroma, central chondroma.

Epidemiology
Enchondromas are relatively common, accounting for 10-25% of all benign bone tumours {1874,2155}. The true incidence is actually much higher since many tumours are detected incidentally and never biopsied. The age distribution is wide, ranging from 5-80 years. However, the majority of patients present within the second through fourth decades of life. The sexes are equally affected.

Sites of involvement
Half of all enchondromas in surgical pathology series occur in the hands and feet {1469,1874,2155}. It is the most common bone tumour of the hand, where it most often affects the small tubular bones. The long tubular bones, especially proximal humerus and proximal and distal femur, are next in frequency.

Enchondromas are uncommon in the flat bones such as pelvis, ribs, scapula, sternum or vertebrae, and are exceedingly rare in the craniofacial bones.

Clinical features / Imaging
Enchondromas in the small bones of the hands and feet typically present as palpable swellings, with or without pain. Because they often expand these small bones and attenuate the cortex, they frequently present with pathological fractures. Long bone tumours are more often asymptomatic, and many are detected incidentally in radiographs or bone scans taken for other reasons. Tumours other than those located in small bones are usually painless unless aggravated by stress. Enchondromas are usually "hot" on bone scan.

Radiographically, enchondromas form well marginated tumours that vary from radiolucent to heavily mineralized. When present, the mineralization pattern is high-

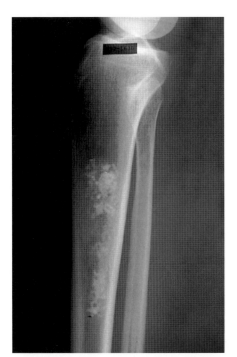

Fig. 10.07 Enchondromas can be heavily mineralized. Flocculent, punctate, and ring and arc patterns of mineralization, as seen in this tibial diaphyseal tumor, are highly characteristic of hyaline cartilage tumors.

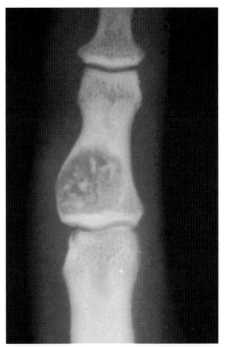

Fig. 10.08 Enchondromas are most commonly located in the small bones of the hands and feet. This radiograph depicts a slightly expansile enchondroma of the finger with punctate mineralization.

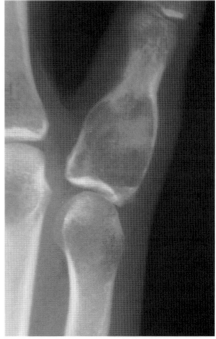

Fig. 10.09 In small bones, enchondromas can be very expansile, as seen in this radiolucent finger tumour.

ly characteristic, consisting of punctate, flocculent, or ring and arc patterns. Long bone tumours are usually centrally located within the metaphysis. Diaphyseal long bone tumours are less common, and epiphyseal tumours are rare. Enchondromas in the small tubular bones can be centrally or eccentrically located, and larger tumours can completely replace the medullary cavity {2081}. In small and medium-sized tubular bones and in thin flat bones, enchondromas are frequently expansile. By contrast, in the large long bones, such as the femur, tibia or humerus, only minimal degrees of bony expansion and endosteal erosion (or "scalloping") are acceptable. More extensive endosteal erosion is considered suspicious for low grade chondrosarcoma. Cortical destruction and soft tissue invasion should never be seen in enchondomas.

Macroscopy

Most enchondromas measure less than 3 cm and tumours larger that 5 cm are uncommon. Because most tumours are treated by curettage, the specimen is usually received in fragments. The tissue is white-grey and opalescent. Gritty yellow or red foci represent areas of calcification or ossification. In the intact state, enchodromas are well marginated. They frequently have a multinodular architecture, comprised by nodules of cartilage separated by bone marrow. This multinodular pattern appears to be more common in long

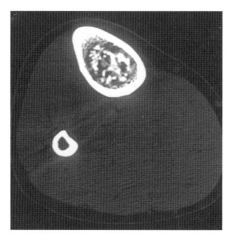

Fig. 10.10 This CT scan highlights punctate and solid patterns of mineralization in a tibial enchondroma.

bones compared to small tubular bones, where enchondromas usually have a confluent growth pattern.

Histopathology

In general, chondromas are hypocellular, avascular tumours with abundant hyaline cartilage matrix. They typically stain pale blue with haematoxylin and eosin due to high content of matrix proteoglycans. The chondrocytes are situated within sharp-edged lacunar spaces, and have finely granular eosinophilic cytoplasm that is often vacuolated. The nuclei are typically small and round with condensed chromatin. Slightly larger nuclei with open chromatin and small nucleoli are not

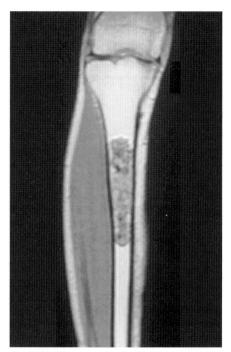

Fig. 10.11 This coronal MRI of a tibial enchondroma highlights its sharp margination, multinodular architecture, and lack of endosteal erosion.

uncommon. The cells can be evenly distributed or arranged in small clusters. More than one cell per lacuna, as well as occasional binucleated cells, can be present. Mitotic activity is very low, and usually not detectable. Focally, in some tumours, the matrix can be myxoid. Here, the chondrocytes, which are no longer confined to lacunae, assume bipolar or stellate shapes. Myxoid matrix rarely accounts for more than a minor component of a tumour. The architecture of enchondroma varies from confluent to multinodular. Delicate fibrous septa or thin mantles of lamellar bone surround the nodules. Normal marrow elements are often present between nodules. Although endosteal erosion is present in some cases, enchondromas do not invade into the Haversian system. The degree of mineralization is variable. Both basophilic stippled calcification and endochondral ossification account for it. Areas of ischaemic necrosis are common, especially in heavily calcified tumours. Here, the chondrocytes are reduced to eosinophilic bodies.

Enchondromas in the small bones of the hands and feet can be more cellular and cytologically atypical than long bone tumours. Without proper radiological correlation, such lesions can be mistaken for low grade chondrosarcomas.

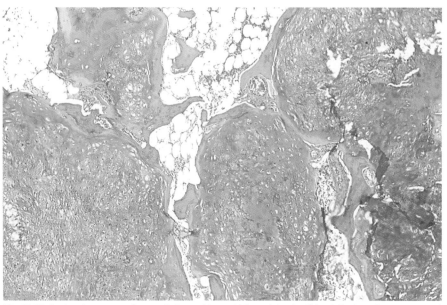

Fig. 10.12 Enchondromas are frequently formed by multiple nodules (or "islands") of cartilage separated from one another by bone marrow.

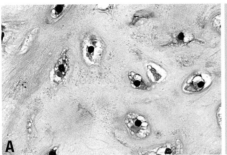
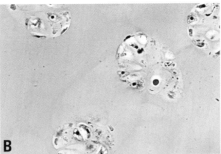

Fig. 10.13 A Enchondromas are typically hypocellular tumors with abundant hyaline cartilage matrix. The chondrocytes are situated within lacunar spaces, have uniform small round nuclei, and finely granular, often vacuolated, eosinophilic cytoplasm. **B** The lesions of enchondromatosis consist of mature hyaline cartilage. The chondrocytes are frequently arranged in clusters, as depicted.

Genetics

A diploid pattern with low cell proliferative activity is with rare exception typical of chondromas, as assessed by DNA flow cytometric / cytofluorometric studies and comparative genomic hybridization {36,1190}. Diploid or near-diploid complements with simple structural abnormalities, particularly involving chromosomes 6 and 12, have been detected by conventional cytogenetic analysis {265,856,1870, 2105}.

Prognostic factors

Enchondromas are successfully treated by intralesional curettage in most cases, and local recurrences are uncommon. Occasionally, an enchondroma will recur many years later, and rarely recur as a low grade chondrosarcoma {411}.

Periosteal chondroma

Definition

Periosteal chondroma is a benign hyaline cartilage neoplasm of bone surface that arises from the periosteum.

ICD-O code   9221/0

Synonyms

Juxtacortical chondroma, parosteal chondroma.

Epidemiology

Periosteal chondromas are much less common, accounting for less than 2% of chondromas {270,1874,2155}. They occur both in children and adults with equal sex distribution {144,1248,1256}.

Sites of involvement

Periosteal chondromas occur most commonly in the long bones. Proximal humerus is a characteristic location. The small tubular bones are also common sites {144,270,1248,1256,2155}.

Clinical features / Imaging

Periosteal chondromas present as palpable, often painful, masses {144,1248}. Radiographically, they appear as radiolucent or mineralized bone surface tumours that form sharply marginated erosions (or "saucerization") of the cortex. Typically, the underlying cortex is thickened, and the tumour is bordered by solid periosteal buttressing.

Macroscopy

Periosteal chondromas form well-marginated bone surface tumours. The cortex underlying the tumour is usually indented and thickened. Solid periosteal buttressing encloses the tumour on its sides. Tumours are usually less than 6 cm in greatest dimension {144,1248, 2155}.

Histopathology

Periosteal chondromas have a sharp margin with the underlying thickened cortex. They do not penetrate into cancellous bone. Although the degree of cellularity and the cytological features are similar to other chondromas, occasionally periosteal chondromas can be more cellular and show greater nuclear pleomorphism and more binucleation.

Genetics

One case of periosteal chondroma exhibited structural changes of the same band on both chromosome 12 homologues {1323}.

Prognostic factors

Periosteal chondromas have been treated with intralesional, marginal, and en bloc excisions, and the recurrence rate is low regardless of type of surgery {144,1248}.

Enchondromatosis

Definition

Ollier disease is a developmental disorder caused by failure of normal enchondral ossification. There is failure of normal enchondral ossification. Furthermore, there is production of cartilaginous masses (enchondromas) in the metaphysis and adjacent regions of the shafts and flat bones, with varying degrees of bone deformity. There is predominant unilateral involvement. The multiple enchondromas appear in childhood and there is a wide spread skeletal involvement.
Maffucci syndrome combines the features of Ollier disease associated with angioma of the soft tissue (rarely viscera).

ICD-O code   9220/1

Synonyms

Multiple chondromatosis, multiple enchondromatosis, chondrodysplasia, Ollier disease, Maffucci syndrome.

Epidemiology

Enchondromatosis is rare. On average, patients are younger than those with solitary tumours, the majority presenting during the first two decades of life {2155}. It has been estimated that chondrosarcomas develop by age 40 in approximately 25% of patients with Ollier disease. In Maffucci syndrome the risk of secondary malignancy is even higher. Age at presentation is inversely proportional to severity of disease. Severe cases present in early childhood. The sexes are equally affected.

Sites of involvement

The localization and extent of skeletal involvement in enchondromatosis varies greatly among individuals, ranging from cases limited to multifocal involvement of a single bone to cases with widespread lesions and crippling deformation. The hand is the most common site. Other common sites are foot, femur, humerus, and forearm bones. In severe cases, the flat bones are also affected. Frequently, the disease is limited to a single extremity or to one side of the body. Many cases, however, have bilateral involvement. In bilateral disease, one side of the body is usually more affected than the other.

Clinical features / Imaging

The clinical presentation of enchondromatosis depends on the extent of disease. For example, it can range from a few small lesions in the hand or foot to multiple, widely distributed, sizeable lesions and marked skeletal deformation. Pathological fractures, limb length discrepancies, and bowing deformities are common in severe cases. Change in symptoms and extension beyond the bony cortex into the adjacent soft tissue herald the development of chondrosarcomas in both Ollier disease and Maffucci syndrome. Malignant transformation occurs in approximately 25-30% of cases {269,1274,1901}.

Radiographically, the lesions of enchondromatosis can be radiolucent or mineralized, and can be intramedullary or periosteal in location. Bony expansion is common. Any part of a tubular bone can be affected, including the articular cartilage and the epiphysis {1469}. However, the metaphysis is most common. Radiolucent columns that extend from the growth plate into the metaphysis are highly characteristic. In severe cases, the flat bones, particularly the iliac crest, can be affected. In Maffucci syndrome, soft tissue calcifications due to pleboliths within the haemagiomas can be visualised in radiographs.

Macroscopy

The gross extent of disease in enchondromatosis is variable. In severe cases, marked expansion and cortical attenuation can be seen even in large bones.

Histopathology

The microscopic appearance of lesions in enchondromatosis resembles that described above. However, they can be more cellular and cytologically atypical than typical solitary enchondromas of the long bones.

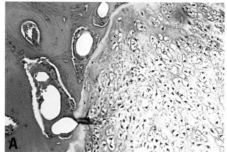

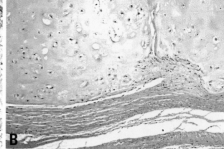

Fig. 10.14 A Although enchondromas can erode the endosteal surface of the cortex, the bone-tumor interface is typically broad without evidence of destructive invasion. **B** Periosteal chondromas are covered by a periosteal fibrous membrane.

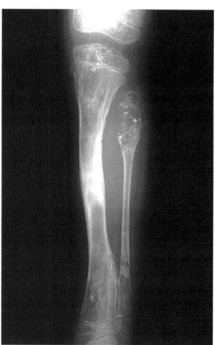

Fig. 10.15 This X-ray is from a 6-year-old boy with enchondromatosis. Note the following features: 1) extensive involvement of multiple bones; 2) localization of lesions primarily to the metaphyses, but also with diaphyseal and epiphyseal involvement; 3) radiolucent columns of dysplastic cartilage that extend from the growth plate into the metaphysis to create a fluted pattern, a highly characteristic finding in this disease; 4) bony expansion; 5) punctate mineralization; 6) bowing deformation; 7) and fracture callus in tibial diaphysis.

Genetics

A description of molecular alterations identified in enchondromatosis is included within the section on congenital tumour syndromes (see chapter 21).

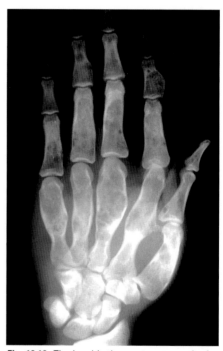

Fig. 10.16 The hand is the most common site for enchondromatosis (Ollier disease). Expansile, radiolucent and mineralized lesions involve multiple metacarpal and phalangeal bones in this case.

Prognostic factors

The prognosis of enchondromatosis depends upon the extent and severity of disease. Malignant transformation occurs in 25-30% of cases, usually as low grade chondrosarcoma {1274, 1901}. However, high grade sarcomas, such as osteosarcoma or dedifferentiated chondrosarcoma {270,1274}, can also occur.

Chondroblastoma

S.E. Kilpatrick
M. Parisien
J.A. Bridge

Definition
Chondroblastoma is a benign, cartilage-producing neoplasm usually arising in the epiphyses of skeletally immature patients.

ICD-O code   9230/0

Synonyms
Calcifying giant cell tumour, epiphyseal chondromatous giant cell tumour.

Epidemiology
Chondroblastoma accounts for less than 1% of all bone tumours. Most patients are between 10 and 25 years of age at diagnosis and there is a male predominance. Patients with skull and temporal bone involvement tend to present at an older age (40-50 years) {2147}.

Sites of involvement
Greater than 75% involve the long bones; the most common anatomic sites are the epiphyseal and epimetaphyseal regions of the distal and proximal femur, proximal tibia, and proximal humerus {215,2147}. Equivalent sites within flat bones such as the acetabulum and ilium are not uncommon. Other unusual but classic sites of involvement include the talus, calcaneus, and patella. Within the craniofacial region, the temporal bone is most frequently affected. Chondroblastomas almost invariably involve a single bone but multifocal lesions arising in 2 separate bones have been reported {1795}.

Clinical features
The vast majority of patients complain of localized pain, often mild, but sometimes of many years duration. Soft tissue swelling, joint stiffness and limitation, and limp are reported less commonly. A minority of patients may develop joint effusion, especially around the knee. Temporal bone involvement may be associated with hearing loss, tinnitus, and/or vertigo {186,2147}. Radiologically, chondroblastomas are typically lytic, centrally or eccentrically placed, relatively small lesions (3 to 6 cm), occupying less than one half of the epiphysis and are sharply demarcated, with or without a thin sclerotic border. The presence of sclerotic rim, along with the younger age of the patient, helps to differentiate chondroblastoma from giant cell tumour of bone, which generally lacks a sclerotic border and occurs in patients older than 20 years. There generally is no expansion of the bone or periosteal reaction. However, larger lesions involving flat bones or small tubular bones may exhibit a periosteal reaction. Concomitant involvement of the metaphysis is commonly observed {215, 2147}. Although often helpful, matrix calcifications are only visible in about 1/3 of patients {2147}.

Macroscopy
Curetted fragments are tan with areas of white colourations. The lesions may be partly cystic.

Histopathology
Histologically, the characteristic cell is a remarkably uniform, round to polygonal cell with well defined cytoplasmic borders, clear to slightly eosinophilic cytoplasm and a round to ovoid nucleus (chondroblasts). The nucleus often displays clefts or longitudinal grooves and contains one or more small to inconspicuous nucleoli. Chondroblasts are packed in pseudo-lobulated sheets often showing a pavement-like pattern. Randomly distributed osteoclast-type giant cells are almost always present. Variably-sized nodules of light-staining, amorphous, bluish to eosinophilic material (chondroid) accompany the chondroblasts {993,2147}. Mature, basophilic-staining, hyaline cartilage is relatively uncommon. A fine network of pericellular calcification defines the so called "chicken wire calcification" seen in many of cases. Individual chondroblasts may exhibit cytological atypia most often represented by large, hyperchromatic nuclei; nevertheless, such features do not adversely affect prognosis {1878, 2015}. Mitoses are observed but atypical forms are never seen. Aneurysmal bone cyst-like changes may be found in up to 1/3 of cases {2147}. Ultrastructural studies reveal deep indentations of the nuclear membrane and features, such as abundant rough endoplasmic reticulum and long cytoplasmic processes, typical of fetal chondroblasts {2025}.

Immunophenotype
The chondroblasts generally express S100 protein and vimentin {1493}. The expression of other antigens has been reported with cytokeratin being among the most commonly observed {569,918}.

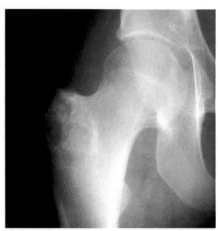

Fig. 10.17 Plain X-ray showing a multiloculated, circumscribed lytic defect with a sclerotic rim involving the greater trochanter. Involvement of the apophysis, such as the greater trochanter, is considered analogous to epiphyseal involvement of a long bone and not uncommon in chondroblastoma.

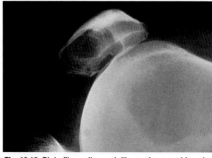

Fig. 10.18 Plain film radiograph illustrating a multicystic, well-circumscribed lesion involving the patella.

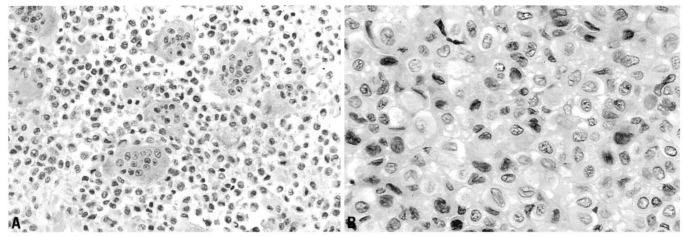

Fig. 10.19 **A** Chondroblastoma with sheets of mostly uniform-appearing chondroblasts and numerous randomly-distributed osteoclast type giant cells. **B** Cytologically, the individual chondroblasts are round to polygonal with sharply defined cytoplasmic borders, round to ovoid nuclei, and occasional small nucleoli. Nuclear grooves and indentations are frequently seen.

Genetics

Flow cytometric studies have revealed that most chondroblastomas are diploid with low proliferative fractions, however, near-diploid aneuploid populations have been detected in a subset of cases {414, 576,1798,2092}. Clonal abnormalities have been described in six benign and one 'malignant' chondroblastoma {253, 1333,2068,2184}. The observation of recurrent structural anomalies involving chromosomes 5 and 8 suggests that there may be preferential involvement of these chromosomes {2068}. Rearrangements of chromosome band 8q21 were detected exclusively in aggressive chondroblastomas {253,2068}. Multiple DNA aneuploid populations, and immunohistochemical evidence of *TP53* mutation and extensive proliferative activity, were detected in a malignant chondroblastoma {1624}.

Prognostic factors

Between 80-90% of chondroblastomas are successfully treated by simple curettage with bone grafting. Local recurrence rates range between 14-18% and occur usually within two years {215,1878, 2015,2147}. Likely the result of anatomic localization and difficulties of surgical extirpation, temporal bone lesions may recur in up to 50% of cases {186}. Huvos et al. {993} documented a higher recurrence rate among chondroblastomas with a concomitant aneurysmal bone cyst component; however, others have not observed this association {2015, 2147}. The rare development of pulmonary metastases in histologically benign chondroblastoma is well documented {833,1788,2282}. However, these metastases are clinically non-progressive and can often be satisfactorily treated by surgical resection and/or simple observation {1788}. Unfortunately, there are no reliable histological parameters capable of predicting more aggressive behaviour. The existence of a true "malignant" variant of chondroblastoma is controversial and many investigators propose that most such tumours represent postradiation sarcomas or simply misdiagnoses {2147}.

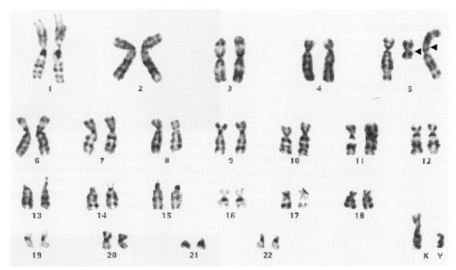

Fig. 10.20 G-banded karyotype of a chondroblastoma with the karyotype: 47,XY,+5,t(5;5)(p10;p10).

Chondromyxoid fibroma

M.L. Ostrowski
H.J. Spjut
J.A. Bridge

Definition

Chondromyxoid fibroma is a benign tumour characterized by lobules of spindle shaped or stellate cells with abundant myxoid or chondroid intercellular material.

ICD-O code   9241/0

Epidemiology

Chondromyxoid fibroma is one of the least common tumours of bone, comprising less than 1% of bone tumours and less than 2% of benign bone tumours {2155}. It comprises 2.3% and 2.4% of cartilaginous tumours in children and adults, respectively {1625}, and occurs in males more often than females {781, 2300}. This tumour presents most frequently in the second and third decades of life {644,2300}.

Sites of involvement

Chondromyxoid fibroma occurs in almost any osseous site. It is most frequent in the long bones, most often the proximal tibia (the most common site) and the distal femur. Approximately 25% of cases occur in the flat bones, mainly the ilium. The bones of the feet are also involved, especially the metatarsals. Other sites of involvement include the ribs, vertebrae, skull and facial bones, and tubular bones of the hand.

Clinical features / Imaging

Pain is the most common symptom, usually mild and sometimes present for several years {644,1748}. Swelling is noted infrequently, more often in tumours of the bones of the hands and feet. Lesions of the rib or ilium may be discovered as incidental radiological findings {2345}. Chondromyxoid fibroma in a long bone is typically a metaphyseal, eccentric, sharply marginated oval zone of rarefaction with attenuation and expansion of one cortex. The longtitudinal axis of the lesion corresponds to that of the involved bone, and the size ranges from 1 to 10 cm with an average of 3 cm {988}. In the small bones, fusiform expansion of the

entire bone is typical. Trabeculations, scalloped borders, and sclerotic rims are common. Most lesions are entirely lucent; approximately 10% may show focal calcified matrix, more often detectable with computed tomography scans. There may be cortical destruction and extension into

soft tissues, but the adjacent periosteum is typically intact {1748}. Rarely, contiguous bones are affected {282} or the tumour is juxtacortical {1329}. Soft tissue extension is best demonstrated with magnetic resonance image studies {1301}.

Macroscopy

Gross features of chondrodromyxoid fibroma include an expansile bluish, grey, or white tumour, without necrosis, cystic change, or liquefaction. Typical hyaline cartilage is not present. In flat

bones, the tumour is multilobulated and well demarcated from the surrounding bone. The scalloped margins correspond to the trabeculations or septations noted with radiological studies. In rare soft tissue implants, the gross features are identical to the intraosseous tumours.

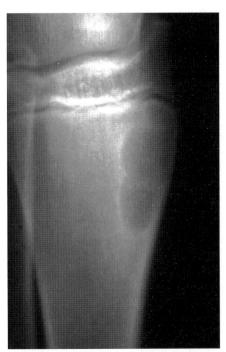

Fig. 10.21 Proximal tibial chondromyxoid fibroma in a 14-year-old boy. This lytic lesion exhibits sharply circumscribed and sclerotic borders with scalloping.

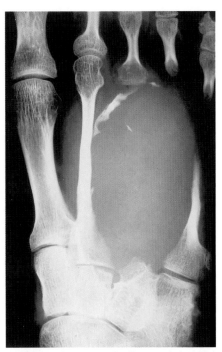

Fig. 10.22 Chondromyxoid fibroma of the third metacarpal. The lytic and fusiform tumour has greatly expanded the bone, typical for location in the small tubular bones of the foot.

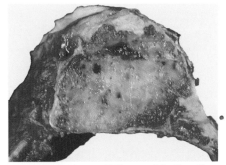

Fig. 10.23 Chondromyxoid fibroma of the ilium. Note the yellow-grey relatively uniform lesion, with sharply demarcated borders and expansion of the bone.

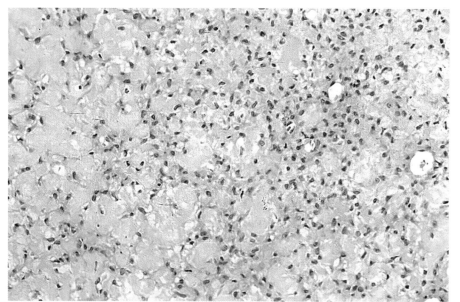

Fig. 10.24 Chondromyxoid fibroma. Subtle microlobular pattern. Note the myxoid regions among which cells are situated in a sieve-like pattern. The spindle cells show eosinophillic cytoplasm.

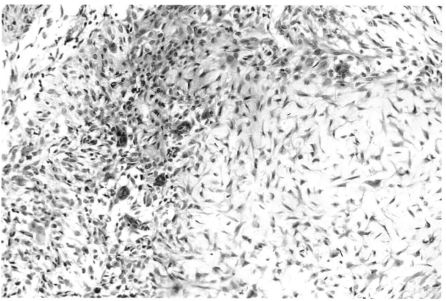

Fig. 10.25 Chondromyxoid fibroma. Cellular regions with giant cells are present peripheral to the lobules.

Histopathology

Chondromyxoid fibroma shows a variety of histological features that are nonetheless quite distinct. The tumour is typically sharply demarcated from the surrounding bone. Rarely there is entrapment of surrounding bone trabeculae by tumour, or lobules of tumour may be separate from the main lesion.

The classic features include a lobular pattern with stellate or spindle-shaped cells in a myxoid background {1876}. Occasionally, a more vague lobular pattern is present. Lobules demonstrate hypocellular centres and hypercellular peripheries.

Individual cells within lobules have oval to spindled nuclei and indistinct to densely eosinophillic cytoplasm. Cytoplasmic extensions, often bipolar or multipolar, are frequent. Enlarged, hyperchromatic and pleomorphic nuclei are noted in 20-30% of cases. These features may suggest malignancy, but they are usually focal and associated with voluminous cytoplasm as well, sometimes with smudgy or degenerative features, similar to ancient schwannoma {109,2155}. Microscopic cystic or liquefactive change is uncommon and usually focal when present. Hyaline cartilage is present in 19% of cases {2300}. Calcification when present is usually coarse and occurs more frequently in tumours from patients over 40 years of age and in flat bone tumours {2315}. Mitoses are uncommon {644,2300}; atypical mitoses have not been noted. Osteoclast like giant cells are often present at the lobular peripheries. There may be haemosiderin deposition in these regions as well, and inflammatory cells, usually lymphocytes. Aneurysmal bone cyst areas are noted in approximately 10% of long and flat bone lesions {2300}.

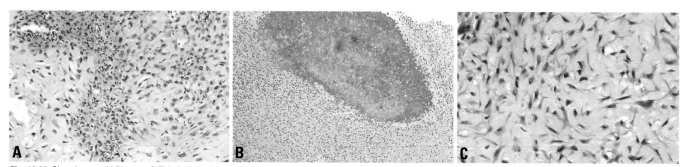

Fig. 10.26 Chondromyxoid fibroma. **A** This lesion shows more nuclear atypia than the typical case, with densely cellular areas at the periphery of the lobules. **B** Focal coarse calcification. Note that these elements surround hyaline cartilage. **C** Moderate nuclear enlargement is present in these cells, and the eosinophillic cytoplasmic processes are prominent.

Immunophenotype

S100 protein has been reported in chondromyxoid fibroma {213,2345}. Immuno-reactivity for smooth muscle actin, muscle actin and CD34 has been noted in regions peripheral to the lobules, but not elsewhere in these tumours {1558}.

Ultrastucture

Ultrastructurally, the stellate cells have irregular cell processes, scalloped cell membranes, cytoplasmic fibrils and glycogen, features of both chondroblastic and fibroblastic differentiation {1930, 2162}. Cells with classic features of chondrocytes, those with myofibroblastic features, and intermediate forms have been described in chondromyxoid fibroma {1558}.

Genetics

Cytogenetic studies are limited; however, clonal abnormalities of chromosome 6 appear to be non-random {828,870, 1836,1870,2082}. In particular, rearran-

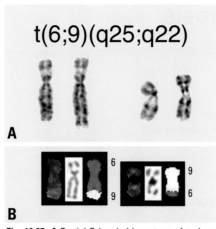

t(6;9)(q25;q22)

A

B

Fig. 10.27 A Partial G-banded karyotype of a chondromyxoid fibroma exhibiting structural rearrangement of 6q, a nonrandom finding in this neoplasm. **B** Spectral karyotypic image of the derivative chromosomes in the translocation presented in part A.

gements of the long arm of chromosome 6 at bands q13 and q25 are recurrent. Expression analysis of matrix components, particularly of collagens,

can serve as marker systems for cell differentiation patterns in mesenchymal neoplasms {22,2174}. An examination of the matrix composition and gene expression pattern in chondromyxoid fibroma has shown pronounced expression of hydrated proteoglycans (major constituent of the myxoid matrix) and focal expression of collagen type II (a marker of chondrocytic cell differentiation) as well as collagen types I, III, and VI {1980}. Importantly, this unique biochemical composition and gene expression pattern in chondromyxoid fibroma has not been detected in other mesenchymal neoplasms, including chondroblastoma, osteochondroma, enchondroma and chondrosarcoma {1980}.

Prognostic factors

The prognosis for this tumour is excellent, even with recurrence, including soft tissues which occurs in approximately 15% of cases treated with curettage and bone grafting.

Synovial chondromatosis

M.V. Miller
A. King
F. Mertens

Definition
Synovial chondromatosis is a benign nodular cartilaginous proliferation arising in the synovium of joints, bursae or tendon sheaths.

Synonyms
Synovial osteochondromatosis, primary synovial chondromatosis, synovial chondrometaplasia.

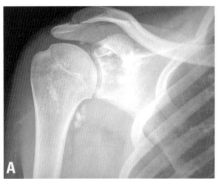
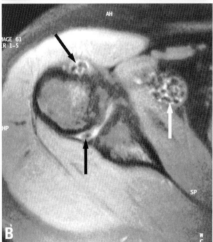

Fig. 10.28 Synovial chondromatosis. **A** Plain radiograph showing small ossific loose bodies in the axillary recess, biceps sheath and subscapularis recess of the shoulder joint. **B** Fat suppressed T2 weighted axial MRI of the same patient showing low signal ossific nodules (arrows) in shoulder joint, biceps sheath and subscapsularis recess, surrounded by bright fluid.

Epidemiology
Synovial chondromatosis is an uncommon condition, usually occurring in adults, twice as commonly in males {643}.

Sites of involvement
Usually only one joint is involved, most often the knee, less commonly the hip, elbow, wrist, ankle, shoulder or temporomandibular joint.

Clinical features / Imaging
Symptoms, where present, are non-specific including recurrent pain, swelling, stiffness or joint locking. Rarely the lesion presents as a painless soft tissue mass adjacent to a joint. Radiography may be negative except for effusion, unless there is calcification or ossification of the nodules. Magnetic resonance imaging demonstrates the cartilaginous or ossific nodules within the joint.

Macroscopy
Lesional tissue consists of multiple glistening blue/white ovoid bodies or nodules within synovial tissue, from less than a millimeter to several centimeters.

Histopathology
The nodules are of variably cellular hyaline cartilage covered by a fine fibrous layer, and sometimes by synovial lining cells. The chondrocytes are clustered, may have plump nuclei with moderate nuclear pleomorphism and binucleate cells are common. Mitoses are uncommon. There may be ossification, sometimes with fatty marrow in intertrabecular spaces.

Genetics
Cytogenetic analyses have disclosed clonal chromosome aberrations in six tumours, all affecting the knee {1426, 1906,2082}. All cases had near-diploid or pseudo-diploid karyotypes, with three showing only simple numerical changes (-X, -Y, and +5, respectively). Among the three cases with structural aberrations, all displayed rearrangement of the bands 1p13-p22.

Prognostic factors
Synovial chondromatosis is self-limiting but may recur locally after excision or incomplete synovectomy, especially in the early phase of the disease.
Damage to the joint surfaces may result in secondary degenerative joint disease. Bone erosion with cranial extension from a temporomandibular joint lesion has been reported {1069}.
Chondrosarcoma may uncommonly develop from synovial chondromatosis {454}. A long clinical history of joint symptoms leading to intractable pain may indicate malignant transformation.

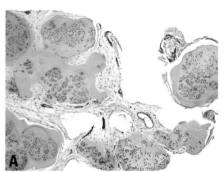
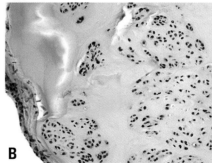

Fig. 10.29 Synovial chondromatosis. **A** Nodules of cartilage with clustered chondrocytes. **B** Cartilaginous nodule covered by synovial lining cells.

Chondrosarcoma

F. Bertoni
P. Bacchini
P.C.W. Hogendoorn

Definition
Chondrosarcoma (CHS) is a malignant tumour with pure hyaline cartilage differentiation. Myxoid changes, calcification or ossification may be present. The term CHS is used to describe a heterogeneous group of lesions with diverse morphologic features and clinical behaviour. This section will deal with primary, secondary and periosteal CHS.

ICD-O codes
Chondrosarcoma　　　　　　9220/3
Periosteal chondrosarcoma　　9221/3

Primary Chondrosarcoma

Primary CHS (or conventional CHS) arises centrally in a previously normal bone and the previous definition is pertinent to all primary CHS.

Epidemiology
Primary CHS accounts for approximately 20% of malignant bone tumours in one large series {2155}. It is the third most common primary malignancy of bone after myeloma and osteosarcoma. In the total group of CHS more than 90% are primary (conventional) type.

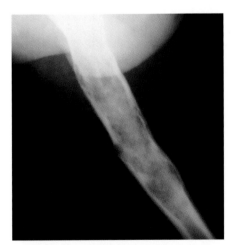

Fig. 10.30 A 56-year-old male with left thigh pain of 2 years duration and swelling for 2 months. Plain X-ray: extensive osteolysis of the left proximal femur.

Age and sex
Primary CHS is a tumour of adulthood and old age. The majority of patients are older than 50 years. The peak incidence is in the fifth to seventh decades of life.
There is a slight preference for male patients.

Sites of involvement
The most common skeletal sites are the bones of the pelvis (the ilium is the most frequently involved bone) followed by the proximal femur, proximal humerus, distal femur and ribs. Approximately three-fourths of the tumours occur in the trunk and upper ends of the femur and humerus. The small bones of the hands and feet are rarely involved by primary CHS (1% of all CHS). Chondrosarcoma is extremely rare in the spine and craniofacial bones.

Clinical features / Imaging
Local swelling and pain, alone or in combination, are significant presenting symptoms. The symptoms are usually of long duration (several months or years).
Radiographic findings are very important in the diagnosis of cartilaginous tumours. In the long bones primary CHS occur in the metaphysis or diaphysis were they produce fusiform expansion with cortical thickening of the bone. They present as an area of radiolucency with variably distributed punctate or ring-like opacities (mineralization). Cortical erosion or destruction is usually present. The cortex is often thickened but periosteal reaction is scant or absent.
MRI can be helpful in delineating the extent of the tumour and establishing the presence of soft tissue extension.
CT scans aid in demonstrating matrix calcification.

Macroscopy
The cut surfaces of CHS tend to have a translucent, blue-grey or white colour corresponding to the presence of hyaline cartilage. A lobular growth pattern is a consistent finding. There may be zones containing myxoid or mucoid material and cystic areas. Yellow-white, chalky areas of calcium deposit are commonly present (mineralization). Erosion and destruction of the cortex with extension into soft tissue may be present expecially in CHS of the flat bones (pelvis, scapula and sternum).

Histopathology
At low magnification CHS shows abundant blue-grey cartilage matrix production. Irregularly shaped lobules of cartilage varying in size and shape are present. These lobules may be separated by fibrous bands or permeate bony trabeculae.

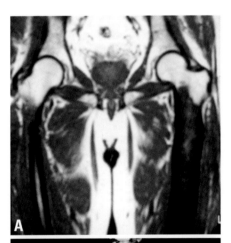

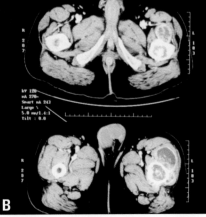

Fig. 10.31 Expansion of the cortical contour and endosteal involvement is detected. **A** MRI and **(B)** CT: the lesion is extensively involving the femoral shaft. Cartilage matrix calcification is present on CT along with cortical destruction and soft tissue extension.

Chondrosarcomas are hypercellular when compared to an enchondroma. It may vary from field to field, however, the overall picture should be one of increased cellularity. The chondrocytes are atypical varying in size and shape and contain enlarged, hyperchromatic nuclei. The extent of atypia is usually mild to moderate. Binucleation is frequently seen. Permeation of cortical and/or medullary bone is an important characteristic of CHS that can be used to separate it from enchondroma. In some enchondromas, nodules of cartilage may be found in the marrow cavity separate from the main tumour mass. This differs from true permeation of host bone where the tumour fills up the marrow cavity entrapping pre-existing bony trabeculae or invades through cortical bone into soft tissue. Myxoid changes or chondroid matrix liquefaction is a common feature of chondrosarcomas. Necrosis and mitoses can be seen in chondrosarcoma, particularly in high grade lesions.

It is important to stress that the histological guidelines used for a diagnosis of CHS in a small bone of the hand and foot are different. Increased cellularity, binucleated cells, hyperchromasia and myxoid change may all be present in enchondroma in this location. The most significant histological feature of CHS involving the small bones is permeation through the cortex into soft tissue and a permeative pattern in the cancellous bone.

Grading is important in CHS. Several studies have confirmed its usefulness in predicting histological behaviour and prognosis: there are several grading systems. Chondrosarcomas are graded on a scale of 1-3. The grading is based primarily on nuclear size, nuclear staining (hyperchromasia) and cellularity {624}.

Grade 1: Tumours are moderately cellular and contain hyperchromatic plump nuclei of uniform size. Occasionally binucleated cells are present. The cytology is very similar to enchondroma.

Grade 2: Tumours are more cellular and contain a greater degree of nuclear atypia, hyperchromasia and nuclear size.

Grade 3 lesions are more cellular and pleomorphic and atypical than grade 2. Mitoses are easily detected.

The vast majority of primary CHS are grade 1 or 2. Rarely grade 3 CHS are

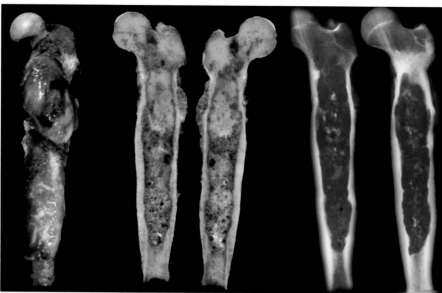

Fig. 10.32 Chondrosarcoma. The surgical specimen. The proximal femur and the femoral shaft with bulging in the proximal shaft. Side by side: bisected tumour and X-ray of surgical specimen. The lesion has thickened the cortex or irregularly eroded it. Discrete punctate opacities predominate.

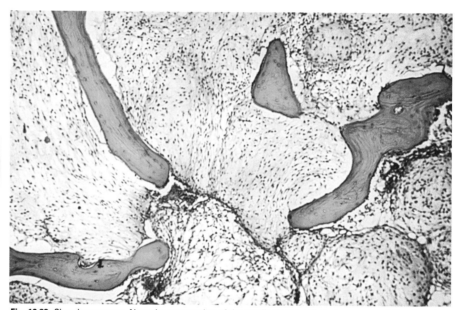

Fig. 10.33 Chondrosarcoma. Note the permeation of the cartilaginous cells between preexisting bony trabeculae. The lesion is very cellular and has pleomorphic appearance of grade 2 central chondrosarcoma.

reported. Bjornsson et al. {208} reviewing 338 patients with CHS of pelvis, shoulder and tubular bones found that 61% were grade 1, 36% were grade 2, and 3% were grade 3.

Prognostic factors

Several histological parameters are associated with increased risk of recurrence and metastasis including grade, tumour necrosis, mitotic count and myxoid tumour matrix. Analysed in a multi-variate fashion, histological grade is the single most important predictor of local recurrence and metastasis {208}. The five-year survival is 89% for patients with grade 1, the combined group of patients with grade 2 and 3 have a five-year survival of 53%. Approximately 10% of tumours that recur have an increase in the degree of malignancy. Occasionally in chondrosarcomas there is the coexistence of various histological grades in the same tumour.

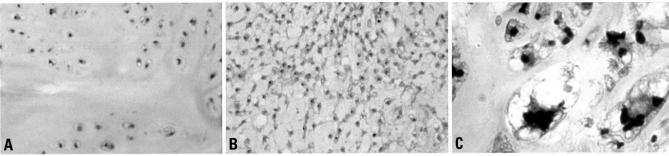

Fig. 10.34 A Grade 1 chondrosarcoma: Few cells with no variation in size and shape (the cytology is indistinguishable from that of enchondroma). B Grade 2 chondrosarcoma is characterized by hypercellularity. The cells show variation in size and shape. Extensive myxoid component. C Grade 3 chondrosarcoma: High cellularity, with prominent pleomorphic appearance and atypia. Mitotic figures are present.

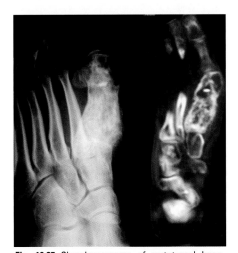

Fig. 10.35 Chondrosarcoma of metatarsal bone. Plain X-ray and CT show alteration of the bone contour and calcification.

the cortex with indistinct margins. It is generally larger than periosteal chondroma (more than 5 cm) It is a radiolucent lesion with punctate radiodensity (calcification) It is covered by elevated periosteum and it is pasted on the cortical bone showing variable erosion of it.

Macroscopy
A large (more than 5 cm) lobulated mass is attached to bone surface. On the cut section a lucent glistening appearance is often associated with gritty white areas of enchondral ossification and calcification.

Histopathology
Histological features are similar to that of conventional chondrosarcoma. Nodules of tumour invade surrounding soft tissues.

Secondary chondrosarcoma

Definition
Secondary chondrosarcoma is a chondrosarcoma arising in a benign precursor, either an osteochondroma or enchondroma

ICD-O code   9220/3

Epidemiology
There are no reliable figures about risk of developing chondrosarcoma in the benign precursors which are frequently asymptomatic. Information available is from surgical series which introduces a selection bias. The risk for chondrosarcoma in solitary osteochondroma

Periosteal chondrosarcoma

Definition
Periosteal chondrosarcoma is a malignant hyaline cartilage tumour, which occurs on the surface of bone.

Synonym
Juxtacortical chondrosarcoma.

Epidemiology
In the SEER data, only 3 of 667 chondrosarcoma were classified as periosteal {538}. The tumour occurs in adults.

Sites of involvement
The metaphyses of long bones are involved, especially the distal femur.

Clinical features / Imaging
Patients present with pain with or without swelling. The lesion appears to involve

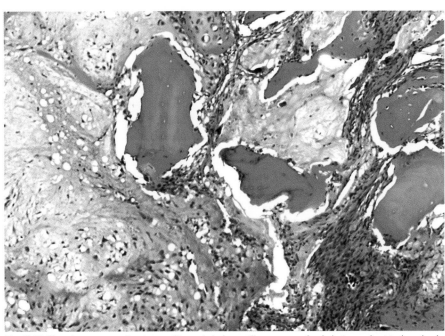

Fig. 10.36 Chondrosarcoma of metatarsal bone. Lobular cartilage permeating in between host trabeculae is present (Grade 2 central chondrosarcoma).

has been reported to be 2% and that for osteochondromatosis 5-25% {538}. It is difficult to prove malignant transformation in enchondromas. Patients with Ollier disease and Maffucci syndrome have a 25-30% risk of developing chondrosarcoma {269, 1274, 1901}. Patients are generally younger than patients with primary chondrosarcoma.

Sites of involvement
Any portion of the skeleton may be involved. However, the pelvic and shoulder girdle bones are more frequently affected.

Clinical features / Imaging
A change in clinical symptoms in a patient with a known precursor lesion heralds the development of chondrosarcoma. Sudden pain or increase in swelling are frequent complaints.
In osteochondromas, plain roentgenograms show irregular mineralization and increased thickness of the cartilage cap. In preexisting chondromas, destructive permeation of bone and development of a soft tissue mass are seen. CT and MRI are helpful in delineating the thickness of the cartilage cap and presence of cortical destruction and soft tissue mass.

Macroscopy
Chondrosarcomas secondary to osteochondroma show a thick (more than 2 cm) lobulated cartilage cap. The cartilage usually shows cystic cavities. Chondrosarcoma arising in chondromatosis is usually very myxoid and hence appears mucoid. The tissue "runs" when sectioned leaving behind cystic cavities. This contrasts with the solid blue matrix of the areas of chondromatosis.

Histopathology
Secondary chondrosarcomas are generally low grade tumors. Invasion of surrounding tissues and marked myxoid change in the matrix are helpful features.

Prognostic factors
Patients with chondrosarcoma and osteochondromas have excellent prognosis. Chondrosarcoma in enchondromatosis has the same prognosis as conventional chondrosarcoma and depends on the site and grade of the tumour.

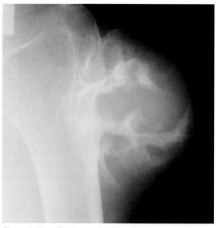

Fig. 10.37 Periosteal chondrosarcoma. X-ray shows the lesion arising on the bone surface with multilobular appearance.

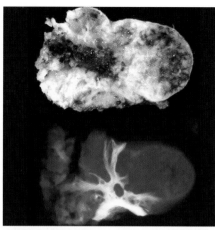

Fig. 10.38 Periosteal chondrosarcoma. Gross features and the X-ray of the surgical specimen from the partial cortex resection of the lesion.

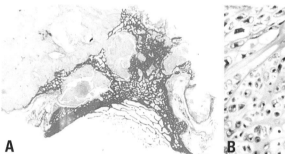

Fig. 10.39 A Periosteal chondrosarcoma. On low power the cartilage lesion is pasted on the cortex. B High power view: highly cellular and pleomorphic cartilaginous cells with the cytologic features of grade 2 chondrosarcoma.

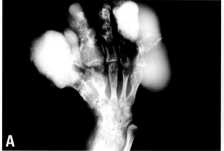
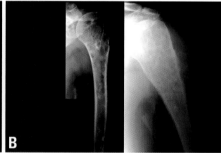

Fig.10.40 A,B Secondary chondrosarcoma in Maffucci syndrome. Multiple cartilaginous masses involve bones of the hand and are associated with soft tissue angioma. In the proximal humerus the enchondroma enlarged in size and had the radiographic features of chondrosarcoma.

Secondary chondrosarcoma in Ollier disease and Maffucci syndrome

The secondary chondrosarcoma in these conditions is characterized histologically by increased cellularity and nuclear atypia in comparison to the enchondroma of Ollier and Maffucci diseases. In these two conditions the histology of enchondromas is characterized by hypercellularity and nuclear atypia. So the differential diagnosis between enchondroma and grade 1 CHS on cytology is difficult. The diagnosis needs to be supported by the radiographic and clinical background.

Genetics
The cytogenetic data on chondrosarcomas are heterogeneous with karyotypic

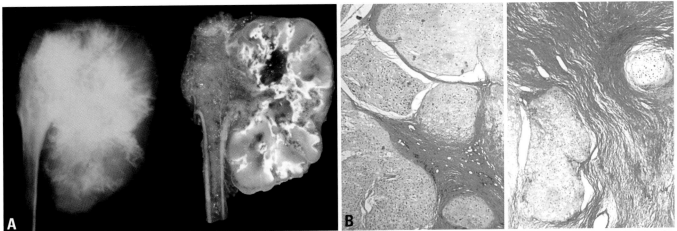

Fig. 10.41 Chondrosarcoma in a patient with multiple osteochondromas. **A** Plain X-radiograph and surgical specimen of the tumour of right proximal fibula: Note the thickness of the cartilaginous cap and flaring of the cortex (macro) and the fuzzy indistinct margins with irregular mineralization visible on X-ray. **B** Discrete peripheral nodules of cartilage are embedded in the soft tissue at the periphery of the lesion. These features explain the irregular margins and the possibility of local recurrence when the lesion is resected with inadequate surgical margins.

complexity ranging from single numerical or structural chromosomal aberrations to heavily rearranged karyotypes. In most cytogenetic reports in the literature, however, no strict distinction between primary conventional, secondary peripheral and periosteal chondrosarcomas is made, resulting in the description of many non-specific structural or numerical aberrations. Although no recurrent structural aberrations are described in these studies, the pattern of changes tends to be nonrandom {253,1315, 2082}. Total or partial gains and losses predominate, and the most common imbalances are loss of chromosomes/chromosome segments 1p36, 1p13-22, 4, 5q13-31, 6q22-qter, 9p22-pter, 10p, 10q24-qter, 11p13-pter, 11q25, 13q21-qter, 14q24-qter, 18p, 18q22-qter, and 22q13, and gain of 7p13-pter, 12q15-qter, 19, 20pter-q11, 21q {1315}. Loss of material from 13q was found to be an independent predictor of metastasis development, regardless of tumour grade or size {1315}.

Recent studies have indicated that primary conventional and secondary peripheral (arising within the cartilaginous cap of a preexisting osteochondroma) chondrosarcomas may differ in their genetic make up, as reflected by a clear difference in the loss of heterozygosity (LOH) pattern, LOH incidence, DNA ploidy status and cytogenetic aberrations {236,240}. Primary conventional chondrosarcomas are characterized by peridiploidy with limited LOH, often affecting the 9p12-22 region, whereas

secondary peripheral chondrosarcomas are characterized by genetic instability, a high percentage of LOH and a broad range of DNA ploidy. Trisomy 22 was only detected in primary conventional chondrosarcomas {240}.

Also comparative genomic hybridization studies point to deletions of 9p {1220}. The *CDKN2A* tumour suppressor gene (P16) is a potential target for the deletions in this region. Mutations have not been documented so far {91,236}, but *CDKN2A* methylation has been detected in a substantial number of chondrosarcomas {91}.

Primary conventional chondrosarcomas and enchondromas have been found to occur in high association with the development of breast cancer at early age, not associated with previously recognized breast cancer syndromes {1595}. Recently, one somatic and one germline mutation in the gene encoding the PTH/PTHrP type I receptor were identified in a subset of patients with Ollier disease {968}.

Cytogenetic data on periosteal chondrosarcoma are limited to two cases. No shared breakpoints were found {240}.

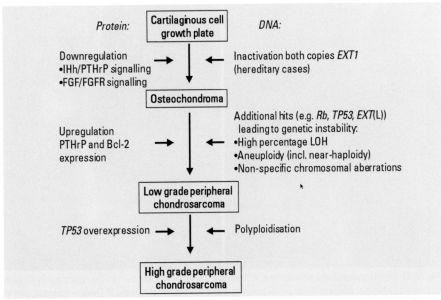

Fig. 10.42 Multistep molecular genetic model for peripheral secondary chondrosarcoma tumourigenesis.

Dedifferentiated chondrosarcoma

S. Milchgrub
P.C.W. Hogendoorn

Definition

Dedifferentiated chondrosarcoma is a distinct variety of chondrosarcoma containing two clearly defined components, a well differentiated cartilage tumour, either an enchodroma or a low grade chondrosarcoma, juxtaposed to a high grade noncartilaginous sarcoma. There is a histologically abrupt transition between the two components.

ICD-O code   9243/0

Synonym

Chondrosarcoma with additional mesenchymal component.

Epidemiology

Dedifferentiated chondrosarcoma makes up 10% of all reported chondrosarcomas. The average age of presentation is between 50 and 60 years, and the age range 29 to 85 years.

Sites of involvement

The most common sites of involvement are pelvis, femur and humerus.

Clinical features / Imaging

The most common presenting symptom is pain, however, swelling, paresthesia and pathological fractures are also common. The tumour usually produces an ill defined, lytic, intraosseous lesion often associated with cortical perforation and extraosseous extension. The pre-existing cartilaginous portion, which may show the ring-like densities seen in enchondromas or other radiologic findings of cartilaginous matrix, is sharply distinct from the lytic permeable and destructive component.

Macroscopy

Typically, both tumour components, cartilaginous and noncartilaginous, are grossly evident in varying proportions.

The blue-grey lobulated low grade cartilaginous component is usually located centrally, while the overgrowth and expanded fleshy or haemorrhagic higher grade component is predominantly extraosseous.

Histopathology

The cartilaginous component is usually a low grade chondrosarcoma. Malignant fibrous histiocytoma is the most frequent pattern reported in the high grade sarcoma component; however, osteosarcoma, fibrosarcoma and rhabdomyosarcoma are also encountered. There is abrupt demarcation between the two components.

Genetics

Cytogenetic data available at present justify a conclusion that no specific aberrations seem to be associated with dedifferentiated chondrosarcoma {240,254,1315,1592,1631,1870,2067, 2093,2334} Structural and numerical aberrations are most frequently reported for chromosomes 1 and 9. The non-uniform karyotype is reflecting the wide variety of histology of the "dedifferentiated" part. Based upon mutation analysis of *TP53*, it was

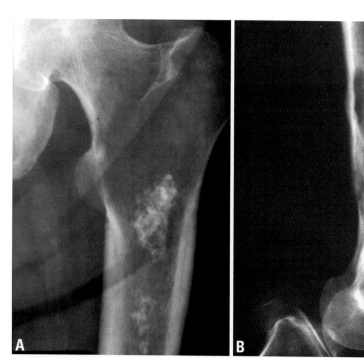

Fig. 10.43 Dedifferentiated chondrosarcoma. **A** The distal portion of the tumour has the typical mineralization of a cartilage tumour, whereas the proximal part is lytic and destructive appearing. **B** There is a central area of calcification associated with large areas of lysis.

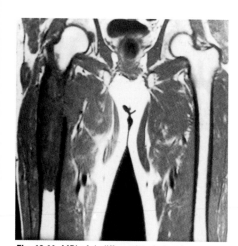

Fig. 10.44 MRI of dedifferentiated chondrosarcoma of proximal femur. In addition to large areas of destruction in the medullary cavity, there is a large soft tissue mass medially.

shown that both components – sharing identical and uncommon *TP53* mutations – have a common origin, though the apparent numerous additional genetic differences suggest an early division of the two cell clones {237}. Support for this concept comes from combined cytogenetic and immunophenotypic analyses, showing numerical aberrations of chromosome 7 in both components {254}. When considering two subtypes of dedifferentiated chondrosarcoma, i.e., the classical type with a low grade chondroid component and a second type with a more high grade chondrosarcomatous component next to the "dedifferentiated component", the model presented might not be entirely satisfying for both subtypes {23}. This view is supported by studies on the immunohistochemical and ultrastructural levels, as well as based on growth rates of both components. As molecular data

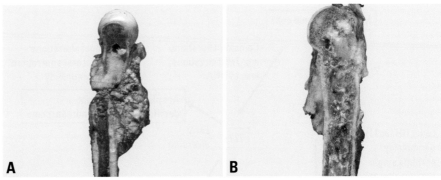

Fig. 10.45 A Dedifferentiated chondrosarcoma of proximal femur. The medullary part has the appearance of cartilage tumour, whereas a soft tissue mass is fleshy. **B** Dedifferentiated chondrosarcoma of proximal humerus with cartilaginous areas juxtaposed to fleshy, sarcomatous areas.

on these subtypes separately and more specifically the first mentioned subtype are lacking, the suggestion of two subtypes of dedifferentiated chondrosarcoma with two different genetic routes for tumourigenesis remains speculative.

Prognostic factors

Dedifferentiated chondrosarcomas are aggressive neoplasms and have a dismal prognosis. Despite aggressive therapy, approximately 90% of patients are dead, with distant metastasis within two years.

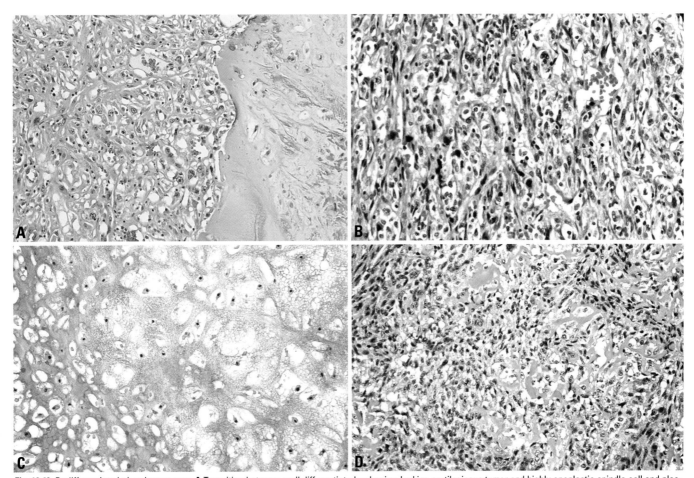

Fig. 10.46 Dedifferentiated chondrosarcoma. **A** Transition between well differentiated or benign-looking cartilaginous tumor and highly anaplastic spindle cell and pleomorphic sarcoma is abrupt without morphologic continuity. **B** In this lesion, the high grade component has a slightly epithelioid appearance. **C** Cartilaginous portion of dedifferentiated chondrosarcoma. There is minimal cytological atypia. **D** Dedifferentiated portion presents as markedly atypical spindle cells with matrix formation.

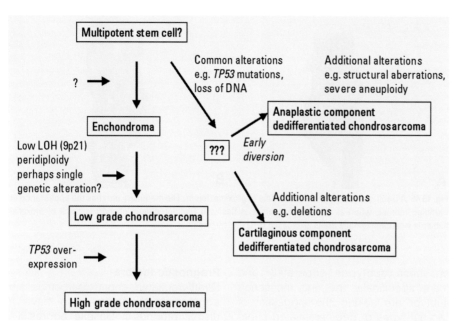

Common alterations
e.g. *TP53* mutations,
loss of DNA

Additional alterations
e.g. structural aberrations,
severe aneuploidy

Fig. 10.47 Multistep model of tumourigenesis of dedifferentiated chondrosarcoma (adapted from J.V Bovee et al. {237}). Genetic analysis provides evidence for a monoclonal origin of both parts, sharing identical genetic alterations. The presence of multiple additional alterations suggest early separation of the cartilaginous and "dedifferentiated" clone.

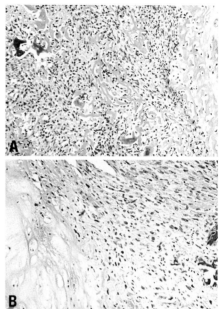

Fig. 10.48 Dedifferentiated chondrosarcoma. **A** Typical example with low grade chondrosarcoma juxtaposed to a high grade spindle cell sarcoma. **B** The low grade chondrosarcoma (left) is juxtaposed to a spindle cell sarcoma with bone formation.

Mesenchymal chondrosarcoma

Y. Nakashima
Y.K. Park
O. Sugano

Definition

Mesenchymal chondrosarcoma is a rare malignant tumour characterized by a bimorphic pattern that is composed of highly undifferentiated small round cells and islands of well differentiated hyaline cartilage.

ICD-O code   9240/3

Epidemiology

Mesenchymal chondrosarcoma makes up less than 3 to 10 percent of all primary chondrosarcomas. Although occurring at any age, the peak incidence is in the second and the third decades. Males and females are affected equally {310, 421,994,1533,1881}.

Sites of involvement

The skeletal tumours show a widespread distribution. The craniofacial bones (especially the jawbones) {1276,2197}, the ribs, the ilium, and the vertebrae are the most common sites {182,891,1364}.

Patients with involvement of multiple bones are reported {1533}. Approximately one-fifth to one-third of the lesions primarily affect the somatic soft tissues {182,891,1023,1364,2061} and the meninges are one of the most common sites of extraskeletal involvement {1824, 1881}.

Clinical features / Imaging

The cardinal symptoms are pain and swelling ranging from few days to several years, frequently more than one year in duration {182,849,891,1364}. Oncogenic osteomalacia secondary to mesenchymal chondrosarcoma has been reported {2353}.

Radiologically, skeletal lesions are primarily lytic and destructive with poor margins, not significantly differing from ordinary chondrosarcoma in most cases. Mottled calcification is sometimes prominent. Some have well defined margins with a sclerotic rim. Expansion of the bone is frequent, and cortical destruction or cortical breakthrough with extraosseous extension of soft tissue is common. Bony sclerosis, cortical thickening, and superficial involvement of the bone surface are also seen. Imaging features of extraskeletal tumours are also nonspecific, showing chondroid-type calcifications and foci of low signal intensity within enhancing lobules {1927}.

Macroscopy

The tumours are grey-white to grey-pink, firm to soft, and usually well defined, circumscribed masses varying from 3 to 30 cm in maximum diameter {994,1533}. Lobulation is rare. Most lesions contain hard mineralized deposits that vary from dispersed foci to prominent areas. Some tumours show a clearly cartilaginous appearance, even in a small section. Foci of necrosis and haemorrhage may be prominent. As evidenced on X-rays, bony expansion with cortical thinning or, more commonly, bone destruction and invasion of soft tissue is frequent.

Histopathology

The typical biphasic pattern is composed of undifferentiated small round cells admixed with islands of hyaline cartilage. The amount of cartilage is highly variable. The cartilage may be distinct

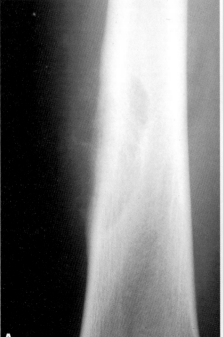
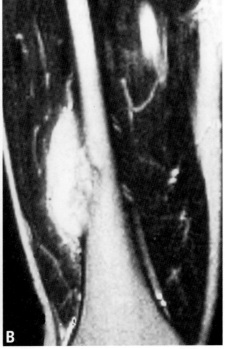

Fig. 10.49 Mesenchymal chondrosarcoma of the surface of the femur. There is a calcifying neoplasm involving predominantly the cortex and soft tissue. **A** Plain X-ray. **B** CT.

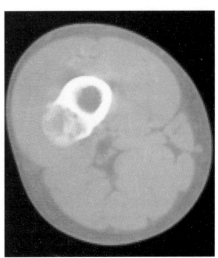

Fig. 10.50 MRI shows a fairly extensive soft tissue mass attached to the cortex.

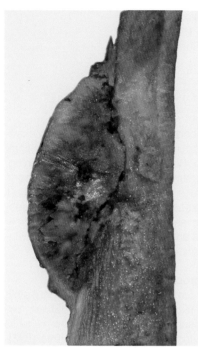

Fig. 10.51 Gross specimen of mesenchymal chondrosarcoma of the surface of the femur, showing a reasonably well-demarcated lesion involving the cortex and soft tissues.

from the undifferentiated component or blend gradually with it. In the undifferentiated areas, the small round cells typically simulate Ewing sarcoma, and a haemangiopericytomatous vascular pattern is common. The small cells may be spindle-shaped to some extent. Osteoclast-like multinucleated giant cells may occasionally be seen, and osteoid and even bone may be present.

Immunophenotype

Immunohistological studies {508, 513, 827, 958, 1844, 2064} of mesenchymal chondrosarcoma are not specifically helpful in the differential diagnosis among small round cell lesions. The small cell component of mesenchymal chondrosarcomas are positive for vimentin, Leu7 {508,2064}, and CD99 {827,958} making differentiation from Ewing sarcoma difficult, whereas cells in the chondroid areas are positive for S100 protein {508, 958, 2064}.

Ultrastructure

The biphasic nature of neoplastic cells was demonstrated electron microscopically {182,529,727,1342,1358,2026}. In cartilaginous foci, the cells show a chondrocyte-like appearance, as is seen in conventional chondrosarcoma, and in the undifferentiated small cell areas, uniform sheets of round to oval cells with little intercellular matrix are similar to primitive mesenchymal cells.

Genetics

Only few cases of mesenchymal chondrosarcoma with chromosome aberrations have been reported {1477}. The observed changes have varied from a pseudodiploid karyotype with a balanced translocations as the sole aberration {1787} to highly complex karyotypes with more than 150 chromosomes and multiple numerical and structural rearrangements {529}. In two cases, a Robertsonian 13;21 translocation was detected {1542}. The 11;22 translocation of the Ewing family of tumours is not seen in mesenchymal chondrosarcoma.

In an immunohistochemical study, nuclear positivity for the TP53 protein was observed in 22-64% of the tumour cells, with positive staining in mesenchymal as well as chondroid components {1659}. PCR analysis revealed that approximately one-fifth of the cases had significantly reduced expression of TP53. However, no mutations resulting in amino acid substitution were found within exons 5-9 of the gene {1659}. Molecular analysis of the *CDKN2A* tumour suppressor gene revealed low expression levels in 7/33 cases, but single strand conformation polymorphism analysis of the entire coding region did not disclose any mutations {108}.

Prognostic factors

Mesenchymal chondrosarcoma is a highly malignant tumour with a strong tendency toward local recurrence and distant metastasis which are observed even after a delay of more than 20 years {1533}. The clinical course is frequently protracted and relentless, making long-term follow up mandatory. Mesenchymal chondrosarcoma of the jaw bones appears to have a more indolent course than those in other anatomic sites {2197}.

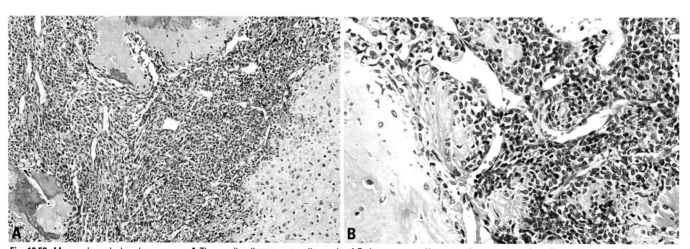

Fig. 10.52 Mesenchymal chondrosarcoma. **A** The small cells suggest a diagnosis of Ewing sarcoma. However, the presence of cartilage rules it out. **B** High power appearance of the small cell malignancy with a haemangiopericytomatous pattern.

Clear cell chondrosarcoma

E.F. McCarthy
A. Freemont
P.C.W. Hogendoorn

Definition
Clear cell chondrosarcoma is a rare, low grade variant of chondrosarcoma, which predilects the epiphyseal ends of long bones. It is characterized histologically by bland clear cells in addition to hyaline cartilage.

ICD-O code   9242/3

Epidemiology
Clear cell chondrosarcoma comprises approximately 2% of all chondrosarcomas {1724}.

Men are almost three times more likely to develop clear cell chondrosarcoma than women. The reported age range is 12 to 84 {209,1014}. However, most patients are between ages 25 and 50.

Sites of involvement
Most bones in the skeleton have been reported to be involved by clear cell chondrosarcoma, including skull, spine, hands, and feet. However, approximately two thirds of lesions occur in the humeral head or femoral head.

Clinical features / Imaging
Pain is the most common presenting symptom. Fifty five percent of patients had pain for longer than a year. In some patients (18%) symptoms were present longer than 5 years {209}. On occasion, the patient may have an elevated alkaline phosphatase {268}.

Radiographically, clear cell chondrosarcoma usually presents as a well defined lytic lesion in the epiphysis of a long bone. Occasionally, a sclerotic rim may be present. Some lesions may contain stippled radiodensities characteristic of cartilage. This radiographic appearance overlaps with that of chondroblastoma.

Macroscopy
Lesions range from 2 to 13 cm in maximum diameter. They contain soft but gritty material, sometimes with cystic areas. Gross features characteristic of cartilage are not usually present.

Histopathology
The neoplasm consists primarily of lobular groups of cells with round, large, centrally located nuclei with clear cytoplasms and distinct cytoplasmic membranes. Some cells have a pale pink cytoplasm and resemble the chondroblasts of chondroblastoma. Multinucleated osteoclast-like giant cells may also be present. Mitotic figures are rare. Many lesions also contain zones of conventional low grade chondrosarcoma with hyaline cartilage and minimally atypical nuclei. This cartilage may be focally calcified or ossified. Woven bone may form directly in the stroma, and areas of aneurysmal bone cyst are often present.

Immunophenotype
The clear cells and chondroblastoma-like cells are strongly positive for S100 protein and type II collagen.

Genetics
Only an isolated case report on the karyotype is available {2019}. *CDKN2A* alterations appear to be infrequent {1657}.

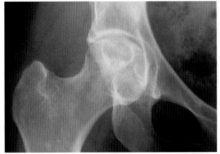

Fig. 10.53 Clear cell chondrosarcoma. X-ray showing a well defined lytic lesion in the femoral head. There is a thin sclerotic rim. The radiographic image is strongly suggestive of chondroblastoma.

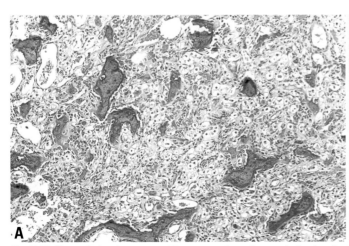
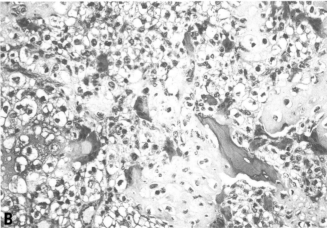

Fig. 10.54 Clear cell chondrosarcoma. **A** Low power photomicrograph showing sheets of clear cell admixed with seams of woven bone. **B** 1557 Sheets of clear cells with areas of mature hyaline cartilage.

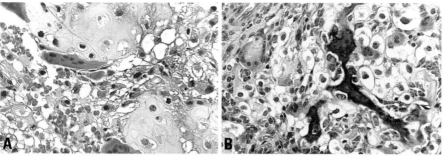

10.55 Clear cell chondrosarcoma. **A** Photomicrograph showing multinucleated giant cells associated with chondroid nodules. **B** High power photomicrograph of typical clear cells. A few osteoclast-like giant cells are present.

Prognostic factors
En bloc excision with clear margins usually results in cure. However, marginal excision or curettage provides unacceptable results with an 86% recurrence rate. In these incompletely excised cases, metastases, usually to the lungs and other skeletal sites, may develop, and the overall mortality rate in these cases is 15%. Dedifferentiation to high grade sarcoma has been reported in three cases {1054}.

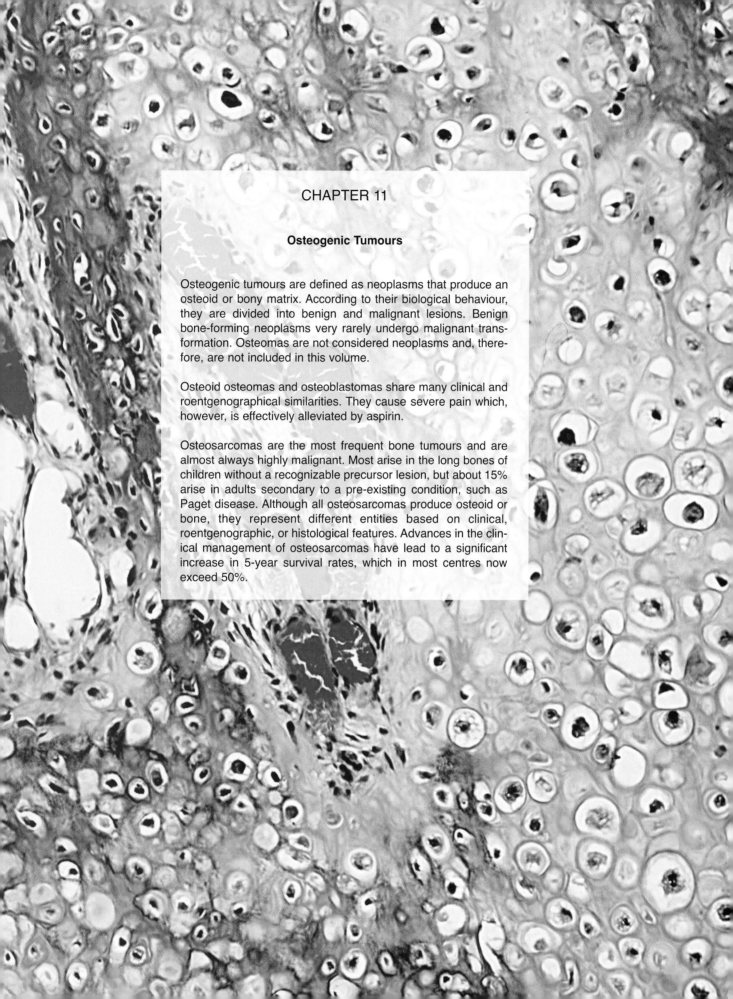

CHAPTER 11

Osteogenic Tumours

Osteogenic tumours are defined as neoplasms that produce an osteoid or bony matrix. According to their biological behaviour, they are divided into benign and malignant lesions. Benign bone-forming neoplasms very rarely undergo malignant transformation. Osteomas are not considered neoplasms and, therefore, are not included in this volume.

Osteoid osteomas and osteoblastomas share many clinical and roentgenographical similarities. They cause severe pain which, however, is effectively alleviated by aspirin.

Osteosarcomas are the most frequent bone tumours and are almost always highly malignant. Most arise in the long bones of children without a recognizable precursor lesion, but about 15% arise in adults secondary to a pre-existing condition, such as Paget disease. Although all osteosarcomas produce osteoid or bone, they represent different entities based on clinical, roentgenographic, or histological features. Advances in the clinical management of osteosarcomas have lead to a significant increase in 5-year survival rates, which in most centres now exceed 50%.

Osteoid osteoma

M.J. Klein
M.V. Parisien
R. Schneider-Stock

Definition
Osteoid osteoma is a benign bone-forming tumour characterized by small size, limited growth potential and disproportionate pain.

ICD-O code   9191/0

Epidemiology
Osteoid osteoma usually affects children and adolescents, although it is occasionally seen in older individuals. It is more common in males.

Sites of involvement
Osteiod osteoma has been reported in virtually every bone except for the sternum, but it is most common in the long bones, particularly in the proximal femur.

Clinical features / Imaging
The usual presenting complaint is pain. The pain, at first intermittent and mild with nocturnal exacerbation, eventually becomes relentless to the point of interfering with sleep. On the other hand, it is characteristic for salicylates and non-steroidal anti-inflammatory drugs to completely relieve the pain for hours at a time. Patients usually have become aware of this prior to seeking treatment, and about 80% report this characteristic feature {922}.

On physical examination, there is often an area of exquisite, very localized tenderness associated with the lesion, and there may be redness and localized swelling. There are sometimes unusual clinical manifestations that are site dependent. When lesions are located at the very end of a long bone, patients may present with swelling and effusion of the nearest joint. When osteoid osteoma arises in the spine, it usually affects the neural arch, and patients may present with painful scoliosis due to spasm of the spinal muscles {1126}. When the tumour occurs in the fingers, the persistent soft tissue swelling and periosteal reactions may result in functional loss that leads to numerous surgeries, large en-bloc excisions {1983} and even ray amputations.

Osteoid osteoma near or within joints may cause a reactive and inflammatory arthritis that can result in secondary osteoarthritis and in ectopic ossification {1579,2078}.

On plain films, the lesion is characterized by dense cortical sclerosis surrounding a radiolucent nidus. The cortical sclerosis may be so pronounced that the dense bone obscures the lesion. In those uncommon cases in which the centre of the lesion has ossified, the lesion can appear like a target, demonstrating central sclerosis within an area of circumscribed radiolucency. When plain x-rays demonstrate dense cortical sclerosis, particularly if it is eccentric and fusiform, osteoid osteoma should be suspected. The area containing the actual tumour may be visualised with a Technetium-99 bone scan if it can not be seen on a plain radiograph. Atypical and even misleading radiographic findings may be associated with osteoid osteomas in certain locations. Subperiosteal osteoid osteoma may produce a misleading degree of periostitis, while surface osteoid osteomas arising within joints may be virtually invisible on plain radiographs {1923}. The best imaging study to demonstrate osteoid osteoma is a CT scan {93}. The CT scan must be performed using bone windows, and it is essential to prepare the actual slices at 1 mm intervals rather than at conventional 5 mm or 1 cm intervals. The reason is that the standard CT slices may very easily cut above and below a small lesion. MRI may be useful in demonstrating medullary or periarticular lesions and peritumoural oedema {2014}.

Macroscopy
Osteoid osteoma is a small cortically based, red, gritty or granular round lesion surrounded by (and sharply circumscribed from) ivory white sclerotic bone.

Histopathology
Osteoid osteoma has a limited growth potential. Even though it may be present in a patient for several years, the lesion seldom exceeds 1 cm in greatest diameter. In fact, the term osteoblastoma is usually applied if a lesion of identical histology exceeds 2 cm in diameter; the implication is that lesions of this size are not limited in growth potential.

The tumour consists of a central area of vascularised connective tissue within which differentiating osteoblasts are

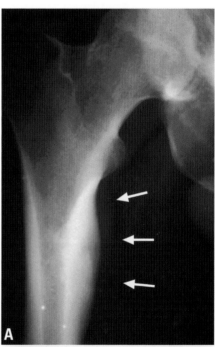

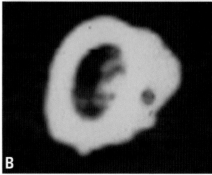

Fig. 11.01 **A** Osteoid osteoma of proximal femoral diaphysis, presenting on X-ray as dense, continuous fusiform sclerosis of the medial femoral cortex (arrows). **B** CT of the same lesion shows a circular radiolucency (nidus) in the outer portion of the thickened medial cortex.

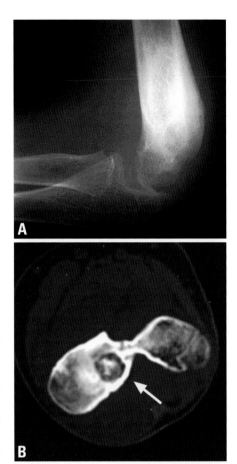

Fig. 11.02 Osteoid osteoma. **A** The lateral X-ray shows a radiolucent nidus with an unusual radiodense centre just medial to the olecranon fossa of the humerus. The surrounding bone demonstrates very dense reactive sclerosis. **B** On the CT scan, the target-shaped centrally dense nidus is very clear.

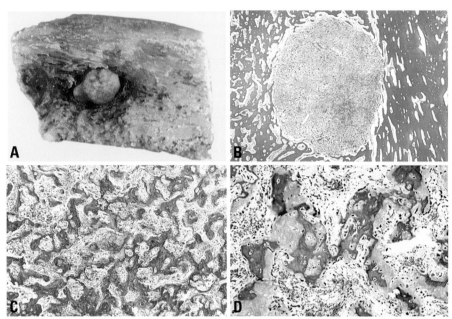

Fig. 11.03 Osteoid osteoma. **A** Grossly, the nidus is 5mm in diameter and has a hypervascular zone within the surrounding sclerotic cortex. **B** Very sharp circumscription of nidus near cortical surface showing dense cortex to the right and reactive neocortex above, below, and to the left of the lesion. **C** The histology of an undecalcified section from the centrally dense nidus shows interconnected, ossified bone trabeculae. **D** Clear ossification of osteoid trabeculae is seen (dark blue) as well as appositional osteoblast activity.

engaged in the production of osteoid and sometimes of bone. If actual bone is present, osteoclasts may also be seen engaged in remodelling, but the essential feature in the central portion of the lesion, or nidus {1024}, is the presence of differentiated osteoblastic activity. The osteoid may be microscopically disposed in a sheet-like configuration, but very often it is organized into microtrabecular arrays that are lined by plump appositional osteoblasts. It is this latter feature that helps to distinguish its pattern of bone formation from osteosarcoma. Additionally, nuclear pleomorphism is absent in osteoid osteoma. Cartilage is usually absent in osteoid osteoma. Surrounding the tumour, there is almost always an area of hypervascular sclerotic bone. This osteosclerosis tends to be more pronounced as lesions become closer to the bone surface and less pronounced in medullary lesions. The interface between osteoid osteoma and the surrounding reactive bone is very abrupt and circumscribed. When it can be demonstrated histologically, this interface provides very strong histological evidence of indolent local behaviour.

Even when the interface between tumour and reactive bone is not demonstrable in sections, the diagnosis becomes apparent by correlating the histological findings with satisfactorily prepared imaging studies.

Genetics
Only three osteoid osteomas, all with near-diploid karyotypes, have been described. In two cases each, involvement of chromosome band 22q13 and loss of the distal part of chromosome arm 17q were detected {136}.

Prognostic factors
The prognosis of osteoid osteoma is excellent. Recurrences are rare. Some lesions have been reported to have disappeared despite the lack of surgical therapy.

Osteoblastoma

A.J. Malcolm
A.L. Schiller
R. Schneider-Stock

Definitions

Osteoblastoma is a rare benign bone forming neoplasm which produces woven bone spicules, which are bordered by prominent osteoblasts.

ICD-O code   9200/0

Synonyms

Ossifying giant cell tumour, giant osteoid osteoma {427}.

Epidemiology

Osteoblastoma is rare, accounting for about 1% of all bone tumours and is more common in males (2.5:1) and affects patients in the age range of 10-30 years, with extremes of 5–70 years old. It is a disease of male teenagers and young adults.

Sites of involvement

Osteoblastoma is one of the few neoplasms that predilects for the spine, particularly the posterior elements, and the sacrum (40–55% of cases). In the appendicular sites, the proximal femur, distal femur and proximal tibia are the most frequent. Osteoblastoma less commonly involves the tarsal bones (talus and calcaneous). The cementoblastoma of the jaws is considered an osteoblastoma and is attached to the root of a tooth, particularly the lower molars, and therefore the jaws are also common sites. The vast majority of cases are intra-osseous (medullary) but a small percentage can occur on the surface of the bone in a periosteal (peripheral) site.

Clinical features

Osteoblastoma of the spine has similar symptoms and signs to that of osteoid osteoma namely back pain, scoliosis and nerve root compression {1547}. Jaw lesions produce tooth pain and/or swelling. The appendicular tumours also produce pain and/or swelling but these symptoms may be vague enough to last for months before the patient will see a clinician. Aspirin does not relieve the pain after prolonged therapy.

Imaging

An osteoblastoma is generally a lytic well circumscribed oval or round defect almost always confined by a periosteal shell of reactive bone. In the spine such an X-ray pattern gives rise to an aneurysmal bone cyst-like (ABC) picture. Limb tumours are metaphysical lytic defects with a thin periosteal bone shell. Large tumours also produce ABC – like changes. Some tumours may arise in a subperiosteal location but are still confined by a thin reactive bone shell. Most osteoblastomas are totally lytic and less than 30% may have focal areas of calcification indicative of tumour bone mineralisation {1292}.

The size of osteoblastomas varies from small (2-3 cm) to enormous dimensions of 15 cm or more. Most are in the 3–10 cm range. In those cases with secondary ABC changes, the tumours are generally larger.

Macroscopy

Osteoblastoma has an extremely rich vascular supply and, therefore, it is red or red brown and often with a gritty or sandpaper consistency due to the tumour bone. The tumour is usually round to oval with a thinned cortex and always with a thin periosteal reactive bone shell if the cortex is destroyed. In cystic lesions, blood-filled spaces simulating an ABC are prominent. The border between the tumour and medullary cavity is sharp, often with some reactive bone. The tumour has a "pushing" border rather than a permeative or infiltrative border against the endosteal cortical surface and trabecular bone of the marrow.

Histopathology

Osteoblastoma has identical histological features to osteoid osteoma {720,1022}. The tumour is composed of woven bone spicules or trabeculae. These spicules are haphazardly or chaotically arranged and are lined by a single layer of osteoblasts. The vascularity is rich, often with extravagated red blood cells. Osteoblasts may have mitoses but they are not atypical. Diffusely scattered osteoclast-type multinucleated giant cells are often present which may mimic giant cell tumour. In very rare cases, hyaline cartilage may be present and may represent micro callus formation. In some cases, the tumour woven bone may be in aggregates or nodules and in such cases careful scrutiny must be done to exclude osteosarcoma.

In some cases the tumour may have foci of large blood filled spaces which are not lined by endothelial cells. The walls of such spaces are composed of fibrovas-

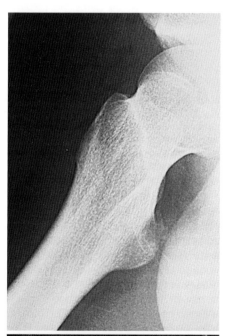

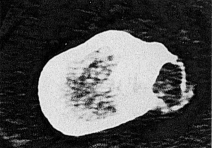

Fig. 11.04 A Osteoblastoma. Expanded radiolucent lesion of lesser trochanter in a 22 year-old male. **B** CT scan of same osteoblastoma showing a thin intact rim of encasing periosteal new bone.

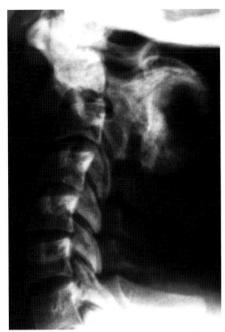

Fig. 11.05 Osteoblastoma. Plain X-ray of large expansile lesion of cervical vertebra.

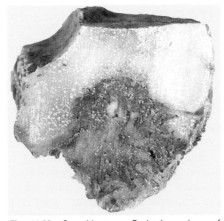

Fig. 11.06 Osteoblastoma. Excised specimen of femoral lesion showing a well-demarcated fleshy tumour.

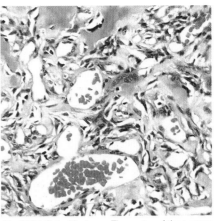

Fig. 11.07 Osteoblastoma. The centre of the tumour shows vascularity and irregular osteoid with osteoblasts and giant cells.

cular tissue with longer woven bone spicules usually in a parallel arrangement indicating reactive bone rather than tumour bone. Such foci are indistinguishable from an ABC and therefore more typical foci should be sought to confirm the diagnosis of osteoblastoma.

The pathologist, especially in large tumours, should definitely sample the border between pre-existing cortex or marrow trabeculae. Osteoblastomas do not infiltrate and isolate pre-existing lamellar bone structures as does osteosarcoma.

In some cases of osteoblastoma large, plump osteoblasts with a prominent nucleus and nucleoli, some with mitoses, may be present. The term epithelioid osteoblastoma has been used for this {541,1089}.

Genetics

Chromosomal rearrangements have been described in four cases, with chromosome numbers ranging from hypodiploid to hyperdiploid {443,1348, 1743}. No consistent aberration has been detected among them. In comparison with osteosarcomas, the total number of genetic alterations is rather low in osteoblastomas {1743}. Nevertheless, there are some hints that cell cycle dysregulation is correlated with the aggressive potential of these tumours. *MDM2* amplification was reported in one case {1743}, and *TP53* deletion at a splice region was demonstrated in an aggressive osteoblastoma {1184}. In accordance with the mostly benign character of osteoblastomas, they do not show telomerase activity {1100}, Overexpression of the hepatocyte growth factor receptor (MET/HGF receptor), a transmembrane tyrosine kinase encoded by the *MET* protooncogene, has been detected by PCR but not by Western blotting {653}. Serial analysis of the DNA content in one case of aggressive osteoblastoma showed that the appearance of aneuploidy could be demonstrated before malignancy was morphologically evident {824}.

Prognostic factors

Osteoblastoma should be treated by curettage. Large lesions may have to be excised. The prognosis is excellent and recurrences are unusual and more likely in those cases, which were curetted from a bone, which has difficult surgical access.

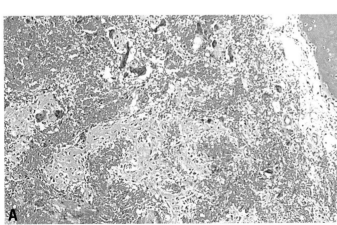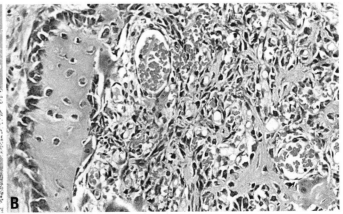

Fig. 11.08 Osteoblastoma. **A** Irregular osteoid, osteoblasts and giant cells, ectactic blood vessels and a reactive shell of periosteal new bone. **B** Classic osteoblastoma which is indistinguishable from an osteoid osteoma with small irregular islands of osteoid, osteoblasts and osteoclast-like giant cells and blood vessels.

Conventional osteosarcoma

A.K. Raymond
A.G. Ayala
S. Knuutila

Definition
Conventional osteosarcoma is a primary intramedullary high grade malignant tumour in which the neoplastic cells produce osteoid, even if only in small amounts.

ICD-O codes
Osteosarcoma,
  not otherwise specified   9180/3
Chondroblastic osteosarcoma   9181/3
Fibroblastic osteosarcoma,
  osteofibrosarcoma   9182/3
Central osteosarcoma,
  conventional central osteosarcoma,
  medullary osteosarcoma   9180/3
Intracortical osteosarcoma   9195/3

Synonyms
Conventional osteosarcoma, classical osteosarcoma, osteogenic sarcoma, osteosarcoma not otherwise specified, osteochondrosarcoma, osteoblastic sarcoma, chondroblastic osteosarcoma, fibroblastic osteosarcoma, osteofibrosarcoma, central osteosarcoma, central osteogenic sarcoma, conventional central osteosarcoma, medullary osteosarcoma, sclerosing osteosarcoma.

Epidemiology
Osteosarcoma is the most common, non-haemopoietic, primary malignant tumour of bone; estimated incidence of 4-5 per million population. There does not appear to be significant association with ethnic group or race. Conventional osteosarcoma is largely a disease of the young {537}. It most frequently occurs in the second decade with some 60% of patients under the age of 25 years. Although 30% of osteosarcomas occur in patients over 40 years of age, the possibility of a predisposing condition should always be considered in older patients (e.g., Paget disease of bone, post-radiation sarcoma) {986,988}. Conventional osteosarcoma affects males more frequently than females in a ratio of 3:2. This gender selection is even more pronounced in patients under 20 years of age and tends to become less dramatic with increasing age.

Sites of involvement
Conventional osteosarcoma shows a profound propensity for involvement of the long bones of the appendicular skeleton; in particular, the distal femur, proximal tibia, and proximal humerus. It tends to be a disease of the metaphysis (91%) or diaphysis (<9%). Primary involvement of the epiphyses is extraordinarily rare {1765}. Although the long bones remain the most frequent sites of primary conventional osteosarcoma, the relative incidence in non-long bone (i.e., jaws, pelvis, spine, and skull) involvement tends to increase with age. Osteosarcoma arising in bones distal to the wrists and ankles is extremely unusual {1472,1601}. Because of unusual clinical factors, imaging features, histological findings and/or unique treatment problems, tumours arising in certain sites (e.g., jaws, skull, spine, pelvis, intra-cortical, multicentric, and skip metastases) deserve special consideration {586,670, 857,995,1165,1196,1310,1578,1852, 1943,2113,2189}.

Clinical features / Imaging
Symptoms generally develop over a period of weeks to a few months. Early symptoms may wax and wane and thereby be difficult to interpret; eventually, they become unremitting. Although relatively non-specific, pain, with or without a palpable mass, is the cardinal symptom of conventional osteosarcoma. Pain is usually described as deep, boring and severe.
Findings on physical examination may be limited to a painful, tender mass. Other findings may include: decreased range of motion, limitation of normal function, oedema, localized warmth, telangectasias and bruit on auscultation. A sudden dramatic increase in tumour size is generally attributable to second-

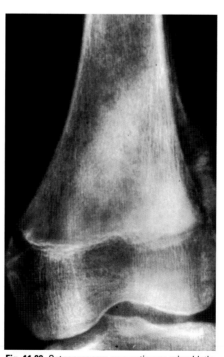

Fig. 11.09 Osteosarcoma presenting as mixed lytic / blastic lesion involving the distal femoral metaphysis of a skeletally immature patient. The radiodensity pattern is "cumulus cloud-like".

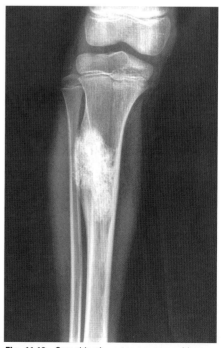

Fig. 11.10 Osteoblastic osteosarcoma with sunburst configuration involving the proximal tibial diaphysis. Such a location makes a patient a relatively ideal candidate for limb-sparing surgery.

ary changes such as intra-lesional haemorrhage. Pathological fracture occurs in 5-10% of patients. Laboratory findings are limited, although elevation of certain serum markers (e.g., alkaline phosphatase and lactic acid dehydrogenase) may be present and have been used to monitor disease status.

The overall radiographic appearance of conventional osteosarcoma is extremely variable. It may be purely osteoblastic or osteolytic {505}. In most cases, it is a mixed lytic/blastic lesion accompanied

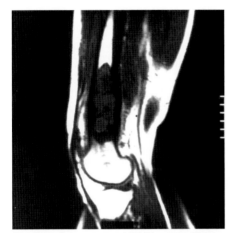

Fig. 11.11 Osteosarcoma. MRI, T1 weighted image. Decreased intramedullary signal intensity corresponds to area of pathology. Care must be taken not to over-interpret images; superimposed reactive changes (e.g., oedema, inflammation) may lead to an overestimation of the extent of tumour.

by cortical destruction and tumour extension into soft tissue. Tumours tend to be eccentric and the linear growth within the medullary cavity tends to stay ahead of its soft tissue counterpart. Rarely, non-contiguous intra-medullary growth within the parent bone or across adjacent joints may take place (i.e., "skip metastases") {586}. Soft tissue masses tend to be variably mineralized with the least calcification at the periphery. Tumour / periosteal interaction may lead to a variety of manifestations secondary to periosteal elevation (e.g., Codman's triangle) and periosteal reactive bone formation {538, 988}. Although involvement of true soft tissue eventually occurs, the radiographic soft tissue masses are frequently confined beneath the periosteum until late in disease evolution.

CT scan and MRI may be helpful in delineating the extent of the tumour preoperatively. {789,1378,1614,1768}. The latter studies are of paramount importance now that most patients have a potential for limb-salvage.

Tm99 radionuclide bone scan, may provide information regarding skip-metastases, multicentricity and systemic disease. Although not universally employed, the arteriogram can provide information pertaining to tumour response, or lack of response, to preoperative therapy. Osteosarcoma is a hypervascular lesion, with response to preoperative chemotherapy there is a decrease and elimination of tumour neovascularity {308,1183,1764}.

Aetiology

The precise aetiology of conventional osteosarcoma remains unknown. Although a history of trauma is frequently elicited, it is felt that trauma draws attention to the tumour rather than causing it. Paget disease of bone and radiation exposure have long been associated with an increased incidence of osteosarcoma {883,2263}. Although a wide variety of other tumours (e.g., osteoblastoma, osteochondroma, and fibrous dysplasia) and non-neoplastic conditions (e.g., osteomyelitis, and metal endoprosthesis implantation) have been linked with osteosarcoma, the extreme rarity of these associations suggests that any cause-and-effect relationship is tenuous {271,1164,1822}.

Macroscopy

Osteosarcoma is often a large (over 5 cm), metaphyseally centered, fleshy or hard tumour which may contain cartilage. It frequently transgresses the cortex and is associated with a soft tissue mass.

Some osteoblastic osteosarcomas may appear grey-tan and randomly granular (pumice-like), while others become denser, sclerotic and more yellow-white. Chondroblastic osteosarcomas tend to be white to tan, and variably calcified with a fish-flesh or rope-like cut surface.

Histopathology

As a sarcoma, conventional osteosarcoma is frequently referred to as a "spindle-cell" tumour; a reference which over-simplifies its cytological appearance. It tends to be a highly anaplastic, pleomorphic tumour in which the tumour cells may be: epithelioid, plasmacytoid, fusiform, ovoid, small round cells, clear cells, mono- or multinucleated giant cells, or, spindle cells. Most cases are complex mixtures of two or more of these cell types.

The diagnosis of osteosarcoma is predicated on the accurate identification of osteoid. Histologically, osteoid is a dense, pink, amorphous intercellular material, which may appear somewhat refractile. It must be distinguished from other eosinophilic extra-cellular materials such as fibrin and amyloid. Unequivocal discrimination between osteoid and non-osseous collagen may be difficult, and at times somewhat arbitrary. Non-osseous collagen tends to be linear, fibrillar, and compresses between neoplastic cells. In contrast, osteoid is curvilinear with small nubs, arborisation, and, what appears to be abortive, lacunae formation. The thickness of the osteoid is highly variable with the thinnest referred to as "filigree" osteoid. Osseous matrix also has a predisposition for appositional deposition upon previously existing normal bone trabeculae (i.e., "scaffolding"). When neoplastic cells are confined within large amounts of bone matrix, they frequently appear as small, pyknotic, minimally atypical cells, a feature referred to as "normalisaton." An under-appreciated architectural feature is the tendency for conventional osteosarcoma to grow in an angiocentric fashion which imparts an overall "basket-weave" or "cording" pattern to the tumour.

Conventional osteosarcoma can also produce varying amounts of cartilage and/or fibrous tissue. Many investigators further subdivide conventional osteosarcoma in terms of the predominant matrix {426,430,1764,1857,2155}. The algorithm is: identify the presence or absence of matrix and, if significant matrix is present, determine the matrix form. This system divides conventional osteosarcoma into three major subtypes: osteoblastic (50%), chondroblastic (25%), and fibroblastic (25%) osteosarcoma. Classification is a function of the primary tumour. There is a tendency for metastases to mimic the primary, but exceptions are frequent and there is a higher-than-expected incidence of fibroblastic differentiation in metastases.

Osteoblastic osteosarcoma

Bone and/or osteoid are the predominant matrix in osteoblastic osteosarcoma. The extremes of matrix production are thin, arborising osteoid (i.e., filigree) to dense, compact osteoid and bone (i.e., sclerotic).

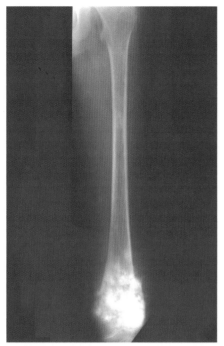

Fig. 11.12 Osteosarcoma. X-ray shows an ill defined radioopaque lesion involving the distal metaphysis and epiphysis with a hint of additional pathology in the more proximal femoral diaphysis.

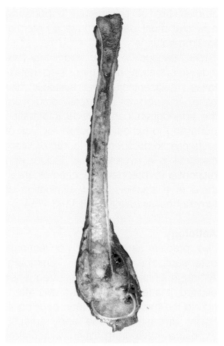

Fig. 11.13 Osteosarcoma. Surgical specimen demonstrating the presence of both primary tumour in the distal and skip metastases involving more proximal part of the femur.

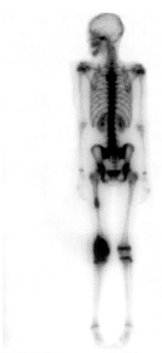

Fig. 11.14 Osteosarcoma. Tm99 bone scan. There is significant concentration of isotope at the primary lesion. Also, a second, discontinuous lesion is shown within the more proximal diaphysis.

Chondroblastic osteosarcoma

Chondroid matrix is predominant in chondroblastic osteosarcoma. It tends to be high grade hyaline cartilage, which is intimately associated, and randomly mixed, with non-chondroid elements. Myxoid and other forms of cartilage are uncommon, except in the jaws and pelvis. Grossly, an overt chondroid appearance is rare. This is probably secondary to the cartilage component being less well-formed, high grade, and mixing with non-chondroid elements resulting in a lack of large areas of pure chondroid differentiation and its attendant blue-grey lobulated appearance.

Fibroblastic osteosarcoma

A high grade spindle-cell malignancy with only minimal amounts of osseous matrix with or without cartilage is the hallmark of fibroblastic osteosarcoma. In general, the overall histological appearance is similar to fibrosarcoma or malignant fibrous histiocytoma. However, its loose definition (i.e., minimal matrix) makes fibroblastic osteosarcoma a de facto default classification.

There are many additional unusual morphological forms of osteosarcoma (Table 11.01), but lacking unique biological properties, they are merely considered forms or subtypes of the three major

groups {116,139,990,1166,1765, 1877, 2133}. In many cases the lack of significant amounts of osteoid, bone or cartilage relegates them to subtypes of fibroblastic osteosarcoma.

Historically, there has been little, if any, prognostic significance to such subtyping of conventional osteosarcoma. Rather, it has been an arguably artificial method of imparting some order to conventional osteosarcoma. However, recent data appear to indicate that there are some predictable survival differences between subtypes when contemporary multi-disciplinary therapy is employed {909}.

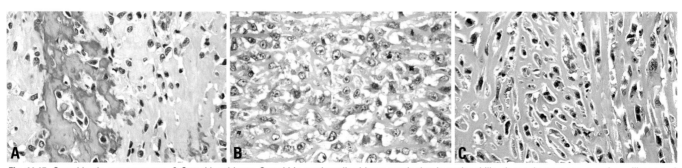

Fig. 11.15 Osteoblastic osteosarcoma. **A** Osteoid and bone. Osteoid is unmineralized bone matrix that is eosinophilic, dense, homogeneous and curvilinear and becomes bone as a result of mineralization (blue areas). **B** Filigree osteoid comprises thin, randomly arborizing lines of osteoid interweaving between neoplastic cells. **C** Osteoid seams may be flat and thick.

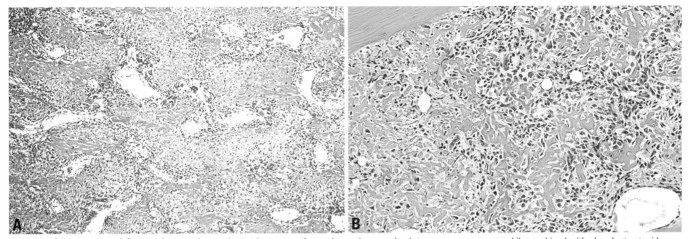

Fig. 11.16 Osteosarcoma. **A** Frequently occurring angiocentric pattern of growth may impart a basket-weave appearance while combined with abundant osteoid production. **B** Appositional osteoid/bone deposition of matrix onto previously existing normal bone trabeculum, a feature referred to as "scaffolding."

Management and interpretation of the post-chemotherapy, operative specimen is of critical importance since it yields an important prognostic determinant: response to pre-operative chemotherapy {1704,1763,1764}. The tumour-bearing bone is cut in the longitudinal axis in the plane that will demonstrate the greatest volume of tumour. The resulting cut-surface is sectioned and completely submitted (i.e., "mapped"). The orientation of these sections can be recorded by a number of techniques (i.e., specimen X-ray, and photocopy). Additional "non-mapped" sections from suspect areas should also be submitted for histological analysis. Response to therapy is recorded in terms of "tumour necrosis." The hallmark of osteosarcoma tumour necrosis is the absence of neoplastic cells (so-called "cell drop-out") in the face of residual tumour-produced matrix. Loose granulation tissue, fibrosis, and small numbers of inflammatory elements replace the cellular component of the tumour. The results of this analysis is generally reported in terms of percent tumour necrosis {988,1704,1764,2205,2292}.

Immunophenotype

The absence of reproducible evidence of specific findings minimises the use of both immunohistochemistry and electron microscopy in osteosarcoma {650,817, 893,1613,1666,2272}. In both cases their primary utility lies in their ability to exclude other diagnostic possibilities such as metastatic sarcomatoid carcinoma, and synovial sarcoma. Certain potential pitfalls exist. Osteosarcoma may be immunoreactive for cytokeratin and is frequently immunoreactive with antibodies to smooth muscle actin. Osteosarcoma usually has diffuse moderate to strong intra-cytoplasmic staining for CD99. Osteocalcin and osteonectin have sometimes been used to highlight osteoid.

Genetics

Cytogenetics

Most, if not all, osteosarcomas contain clonal chromosomal aberrations. The aberrations are complex, comprising an abundance of numerical and structural alterations {191,263,688,965,1428, 2090}. The modal chromosome number is highly variable. Multiple clones are common and may be related or unrelated. Diploid ploidy pattern by DNA cytofluorometry has been reported to be a poor prognostic sign {1191}.

Although no specific translocation or any other diagnostically consequential structural alteration has been assigned to

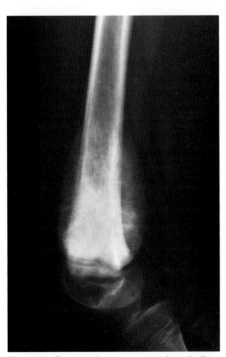

Fig. 11.17 Osteoblastic osteosarcoma is typically a radioopaque lesion, which may be purely blastic or mixed lytic / blastic. The tumour involves the metadiaphyseal region of the distal femur of a skeletally immature boy and has an overall "sunburst" configuration.

Fig. 11.18 Osteoblastic osteosarcoma presenting as dense, granular to sclerotic grossly bone-producing lesion. Note the deposition of tumour-produced bone on previously existing matrix and the well defined matrix within the soft tissues.

Table 11.01

Osteosarcoma: unusual histological forms*
- Osteoblastic osteosarcoma - sclerosing type
- Osteosarcoma resembling osteoblastoma
- Chondromyxoid fibroma-like osteosarcoma
- Chondroblastoma-like osteosarcoma
- Clear-cell osteosarcoma
- Malignant fibrous histiocytoma-like osteosarcoma
- Giant cell rich osteosarcoma
- Epithelioid osteosarcoma

*These forms are not associated with a specific biological behaviour that differs from conventional osteosarcoma. Therefore, these lesions are viewed as forms or subtypes of conventional osteosarcoma.

conventional osteosarcoma, involvement of certain chromosomal regions is recurrent. Chromosomal regions 1p11-13, 1q11-12, 1q21-22, 11p14-15, 14p11-13, 15p11-13, 17p and 19q13 are most frequently affected by structural changes, and the most common imbalances are +1, -6q, -9, -10, -13, and -17 {220,263}. Homogenously staining regions (hsr) and double minutes (dmin), cytogenetic manifestations of gene amplification, are frequently seen in conventional osteosarcomas {1404}.

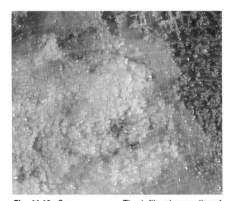

Fig. 11.19 Osteosarcoma. The infiltrative quality of the tumour becomes apparent on closer inspection of the gross specimen. Also note thickening of preexisting bone trabeculae caused by appositional deposition of matrix by the tumour.

DNA copy numbers

Comparative genomic hybridization analysis reveals that chromosomal regions 3q26, 4q12-13, 5p13-14, 7q31-32, 8q21-23, 12q12-13, 12q14-15, and 17p11-12 are most frequently gained {1404,2033,2091}. Gain of 8q23 is seen in 50% of tumours {2033} and seems to be a sign of poor prognosis {2089}. Increased copy number of the MYC gene localized to 8q24 was detected by fluorescence in situ hybridization (FISH) in 44% of cases {2033}. The 17p amplicon is intriguing as it is rarely seen in other tumour types. The most frequent losses are seen at 2q, 6q, 8p, and 10p {1146, 2091}.

Loss of heterozygosity (LOH)

Chromosome arms 3q, 13q, 17p, and 18q are most frequently involved in LOH {1179}. As the incidence of LOH is high at 3q26.6-26.3, this area has been suggested to harbour a putative suppressor gene {1179}.

Molecular genetics

Target genes of recurrent amplifications
Amplifications at 1q21-23 and at 17p are frequent findings in conventional osteo-sarcoma {1146}. Several genes have been reported to be involved in the 1q21-23 amplicon {708,1435}. Similarly, a variety of genes in the 12q13-15 region are co-amplified {172,711, 1098,1490,1607,1796,1975,2095, 2329}. MDM2 {1205, 1607} and PRIM1 {2329} amplifications have been detected in 14-27% and 41% of osteosarcoma cases, respectively. In aggressive osteosarcomas CDK4 is most consistently amplified, alone or together with MDM2 {171,710,1307}. The amplification and overexpression patterns of CDK4, SAS, and MDM2 appear to differ from those in parosteal osteosarcoma {2305}. Recently, it was shown by FISH analysis that sequences, including CCND2, ETV6, and KRAS2, at 12p and MDM2 at 12q were differently amplified in low grade osteosarcomas (parosteal osteosarcoma) and high grade osteosarcomas {796}. Amplifications at 12p were seen in 1/5 low grade osteosarcomas in contrast to 9/19 high grade osteosarcomas.

Gene expression

Overexpression of MET {652,1804} and FOS {2302} has been reported in more than 50% of osteosarcoma cases, whereas MYC is overexpressed in less than 15% of cases {130,1208}. MYC, FOS, and cathepsin L have been shown to be overexpressed in a high proportion of relapsed tumours and metastases {761, 1655}. Bone morphogenetic protein-6 and bone morphogenetic

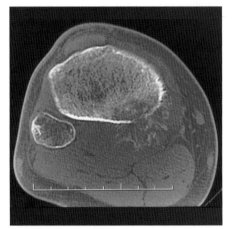

Fig. 11.20 Chondroblastic osteosarcoma. CT shows a mixed lytic / blastic lesion with evidence of ring-like (i.e., chondroid) calcifications.

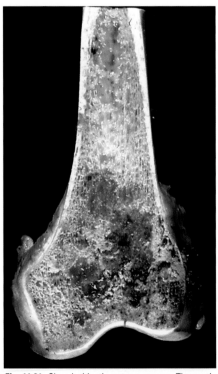

Fig. 11.21 Chondroblastic osteosarcoma. The cartilage component is sufficiently large and well organized to be clearly seen grossly. Note central blue grey cartilage. Peripheral areas with grey-tan tumour infiltrating cancellous bone.

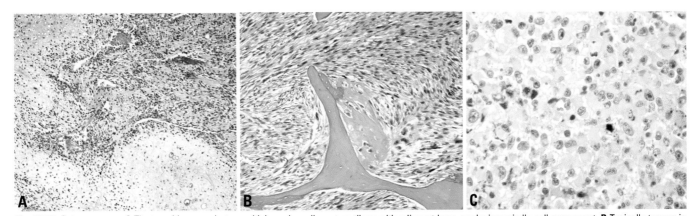

Fig. 11.22 Osteosarcoma. **A** The transition zone between high grade malignant cartilage with adjacent bone-producing spindle cell component. **B** Typically tumour is composed of fusiform spindle cells with minimal osseous matrix. Although anaplastic, cells may have minimal pleomorphism, be organized in herringbone arrangement and mimic fibrosarcoma. **C** Epithelioid osteosarcoma. A densely packed population of neoplastic cells with large eccentric nuclei and abundant eosinophilic cytoplasm imparts an over-all epithelioid or plasmacytoid appearance to the tumour.

°protein receptor 2 are expressed in more than 50% of osteosarcomas {858} and the *MAGE* genes in several cases {2050}.

Gene expression profiling

cDNA array analysis of osteosarcoma cell lines and primary tumours showed that *HSP90B* (heat shock protein 90b) and *PABPL1* (binding protein-like 1) were highly overexpressed, whereas *FN1* (fibronectin 1) and *THBS1* (trombospondin 1) were underexpressed {2290}.

Genetic susceptibilty

Hereditary retinoblastoma (RB) patients have a high risk of osteosarcoma development {550}. Such tumours are likely to show LOH at 13q and alterations of the *RB1* tumour suppressor gene. According to several studies, the frequency of *RB1* alterations in sporadic osteosarcoma has been found to vary between 30-40% {75, 1778,2116,2208,2304}. The prognosis for patients with *RB1* alterations seems to be poorer than for patients without *RB1* alterations {2208}.

Li-Fraumeni syndrome patients with a *TP53* germline mutation have an increased risk to develop a variety of tumours, including osteosarcoma. In sporadic osteosarcoma LOH at 17p and *TP53* mutations are seen in approximately 35% of the tumours {58, 313, 1349, 1459,1519,2117,2316}. The event-free survival rate has been reported to be lower in osteosarcoma patients with *TP53* alterations than in those without {2140}.

Prognostic factors

Untreated, conventional osteosarcoma is universally fatal. Aggressive local growth and rapid haematogenous systemic dissemination mark its course. Although metastases may affect many sites, pulmonary metastases are the most frequent site of clinically significant systemic disease. Bone is the second most frequent site of metastases, but this is largely a pre-terminal event.

The identification of prognostic factors has been an additive process in which factors have been investigated, identified and incorporated into an overall therapeutic strategy {1,207,274,426,453, 662,1327,1740,1835,1955,2098,2099}.

Traditionally, age, gender, location, tumour size, stage, and the results of various laboratory tests have been used in an effort to predict prognosis. However, response to pre-operative therapy is currently the most sensitive indicator of survival. At the same time, it is recognized that a single system does not apply to all cases. Unique biological aggressiveness, coupled with an inability to completely resect the tumour at certain sites (e.g., skull, spine) is one example. There are certain sites (e.g., jaw, pelvis) in which response to therapy does not appear to reflect prognosis despite the capacity for complete surgical tumour removal.

When treated by ablative surgery alone, survival is limited. With the development of effective multi-disciplinary therapy, significant changes have been introduced to the management of osteosarcoma.

The death of 80-90% of osteosarcoma patients with pulmonary metastases, despite the use of immediate ablative surgery and pre-surgical, radiographically normal lungs at the time of diagnosis implies that subclinical pulmonary micro-metastases are present in the vast majority of cases at presentation.

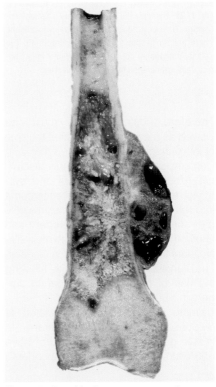

Fig. 11.23 Osteoblastic osteosarcoma, after pre-operative chemotherapy. Surgical specimen showing cystification and absence of luster, indicative of non-viable tumour (100% tumour necrosis).

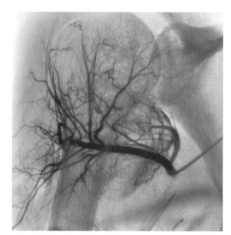

Fig. 11.24 Post-chemotherapy arteriogram. After two courses of therapy, there is almost complete disappearance of neovascularity, indicating a high probability of response to therapy.

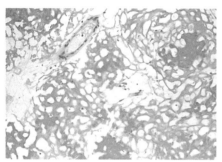

Fig. 11.25 Osteoblastic osteosarcoma after chemotherapy. Tumour-produced osseous matrix is present. There are no neoplastic cells ("cell drop-out"). The cellular component consists of occasional inflammatory cells, granulation tissue and capillaries.

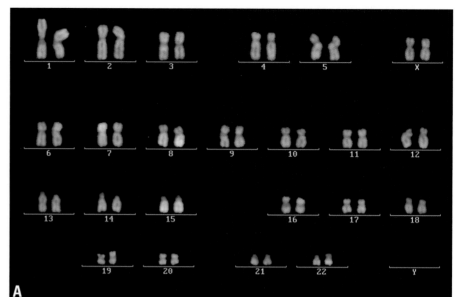

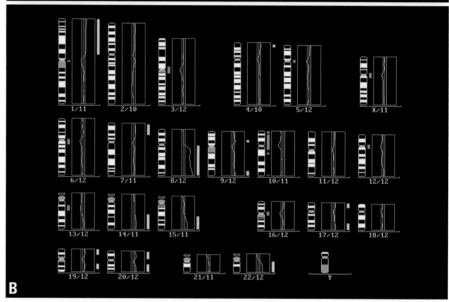

Fig. 11.26 Osteosarcoma. DNA copy number changes in high grade osteosarcoma detected by comparative genomic hybridization. **A** Hybridization of tumour DNA (green) and reference DNA (red) to DAPI (blue) counterstained metaphase chromosomes. Green areas, e.g., at 8q, indicate DNA copy number gain. **B** Green-to-red ratios for each chromosome area are measured using special software. The line in the middle indicates green-to-red ratio 1, and thresholds for losses (0.85) and gains (1.17) are indicated by red and green lines, respectively. Bars show chromosomal areas with copy number changes. Numerous chromosomal imbalances are detected, including amplification of 8q and 15q and loss of 10p and 13q.

Therefore, osteosarcoma must be viewed as a systemic disease at the time of initial diagnosis.

Contemporary therapy is multi-disciplinary, focusing on both local and systemic manifestations of osteosarcoma through the judicious use of multidisciplinary therapy incorporating surgery and chemotherapy. The use of such multi-disciplinary therapy has resulted in disease-free survival of 60-80%, while allowing the use of functional limb-sparing surgery in >80% of patients.

Ultimate survival is directly related to response to pre-operative therapy. In those patients whose tumours have >90% tumour necrosis (i.e., "responders")

long-term survival is generally 80-90%. In those cases, in which tumour necrosis is <90% (i.e., "non-responders") and there is no change in post-operative therapy, the survival is extremely poor; usually <15%. It has been demonstrated that, with

appropriate changes in post-operative therapy, significant numbers of non-responders can be salvaged and long-term survival in this group may be greatly improved; in some cases approaching that of responders {107,160}.

Telangiectatic osteosarcoma

T. Matsuno
K. Okada
S. Knuutila

Definition

A malignant bone-forming tumour characterized by large spaces filled with blood with or without septa. The roentgenogram typically shows a purely lytic destructive process without matrix mineralisation.

ICD-O code   9183/3

Synonyms

Malignant bone aneurysm, haemorrhagic osteosarcoma, aneurysmal bone cyst-like osteosarcoma.

Epidemiology

Telangiectatic osteosarcoma is a rare subtype, accounting for less than 4% of all cases of osteosarcoma. It most frequently occurs in the second decade of life and has a male predominance (1.5:1 male/female ratio) {2155}.

Sites of involvement

Most tumours occur in the metaphyseal region of long tubular bones. The distal femoral metaphysis is the single most common anatomic site, followed by the upper tibia and proximal humerus or proximal femur {2155}. Rare cases occurring in rib {1357}, skull {2261}, sacrum {1956}, and mandible {325} are reported. Recently, multicentric telangiectatic osteosarcoma has been reported {1658}.

Clinical features / Imaging

Clinical presentation is similar to conventional osteosarcoma. One characteristic clinical finding of this tumour is pathological fracture, being present in one-fourth of the cases {1432}. Massive bone destruction may explain the high rate of pathological fracture. In laboratory data, serum alkaline phosphatase level is elevated in one-third of the cases, being less frequent than in conventional osteosarcoma {106}.

Radiographically, the lesions show purely lytic, large bone destruction without distinct surrounding bony sclerosis. The tumours commonly show extension into soft tissues. Most of the lesions are located in the metaphysis, and usually extend into the epiphysis. The tumours often expand the cortex of bone and/or disrupt the cortex. Periosteal reactions including Codman's triangle and onion skin are frequent. The finding of significant sclerosis within the lesion militates against the diagnosis of telangiectatic osteosarcoma. On magnetic resonance images, a T1-weighted image shows heterogeneous low signal intensity, and a T2-weighted image shows high signal intensity with several cystic foci and fluid-fluid level with an extraskeletal extension of the tumour, similar to aneurysmal bone cyst.

Aetiology

Aetiology of telangiectatic osteosarcoma is unknown. Several cases associated with Paget disease of bone {532,1423} or retinoblastoma {280} have been reported in the literature.

Macroscopy

On gross examination, tumours show a dominant cystic architecture in the medullary space {1357}. The cystic portion of the tumour is filled incompletely with blood clot which is described as "a bag of blood". There is no fleshy or sclerotic tumour bone formation. Extensive irregular cortical erosion and/or complete disruption of cortical continuity with soft tissue mass are occasionally seen.

Histopathology

The tumour contains blood-filled or empty spaces separated by thin septa simulating aneurysmal bone cyst. A few of the tumours are more solid and have smaller cystic spaces. Sections taken at the edges of the lesions shows permeation of

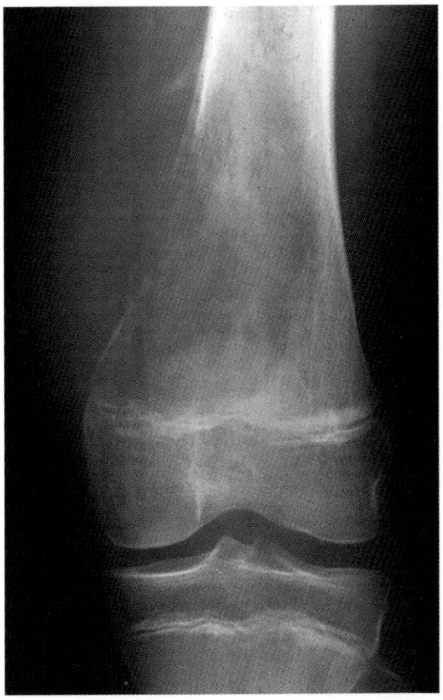

Fig. 11.27 Telangiectatic osteosarcoma. A purely lytic bone destruction is seen in the metaphysis of the distal femur. There is no surrounding bony sclerosis. Note the cortical bone destruction with periosteal reaction (Codman's triangle) and massive extension of the tumour into soft tissue.

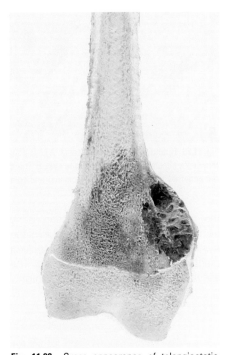

Fig. 11.28 Gross appearance of telangiectatic osteosarcoma with dominant cystic architecture, incompletely filled with blood clots ("a bag of blood"). There is no fleshy or sclerotic tumour bone formation. The tumour permeates into the surrounding medullary canal.

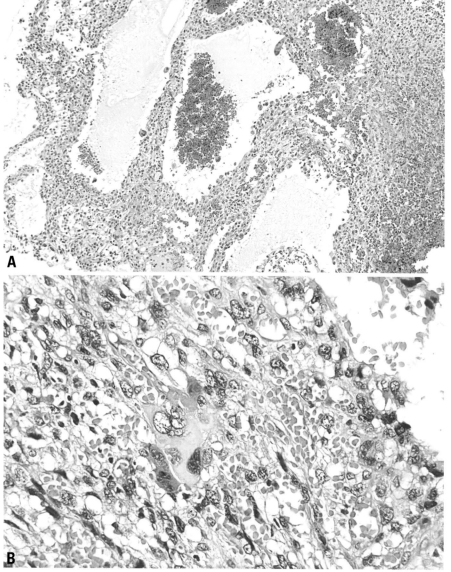

A

B

Fig. 11.29 Telangiectatic osteosarcoma. **A** Low-power microscopy reveals blood-filled or spaces separated by thin septa simulating aneurysmal bone cyst. **B** The cystic spaces are lined by benign-looking giant cells without endothelial lining. The septa are cellular and contain atypical mononuclear tumour cells.

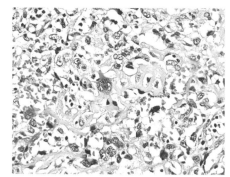

Fig. 11.30 Telangiectatic osteosarcoma. Highly malignant tumour cells produce minimal amounts of fine, lace-like osteoid.

haemorrhagic area. The amount of osteoid varies, but usually fine, and lace-like osteoid is observed in minimal amount. In fact, even if unmistakable osteoid is not seen on multiple sections, these tumours tend to make osteoid matrix when they metastasize. Cellular septe contain many benign looking multi-nucleated giant cells, and these features may lead to a mistaken diagnosis of benign or even malignant giant cell tumour. In small biopsy samples, the only finding may be that of a blood clot with a few malignant cells.

Genetics
Cytogenetic information exists for only four cases {263, 688, 965}. Three had highly complex chromosomal changes, and one had trisomy 3 as the sole change.
Mutations in the *TP53* and *RAS* genes, LOH at the *TP53*, *CDKN2A* and *RB1* loci, and amplification of the *MDM2* and *MYC* genes seem to be rare in telangiectatic osteosarcomas {1743}.

Prognostic factors
Prognosis in the modern era is similar to conventional osteosarcoma. {106,1357, 2155}. Telangiectatic osteosarcoma is exquisitely sensitive to chemotherapy (but this may not reflect an improved survival).

the tumour between pre-existing bony trabeculae. Higher-power view shows the cystic spaces lined by benign-looking giant cells without endothelial lining. The septa are cellular, containing highly malignant atypical mononuclear tumour cells. The tumour cells are hyperchromatic and pleomorphic with high mitotic activity including atypical mitoses. Rarely, noncohesive atypical cells are seen in

Small cell osteosarcoma

R. Kalil
J.A. Bridge

Definition

An osteosarcoma composed of small cells with variable degree of osteoid production.

ICD-O code   9185/3

Synonym

Osteosarcoma with small cells resembling Ewing sarcoma.

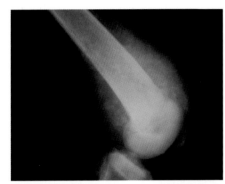

Fig. 11.31 Small cell osteosarcoma of distal femur in a 16 year-old patient. Aggressive roentgenographic image with lytic and blastic tumour tissue at the soft tissue compartment of the lesion and permeative pattern in the bone shaft.

Epidemiology

Small cell osteosarcoma comprises 1.5% of osteosarcomas {98,184,1529}. Patients range in age from 5 to 83, although most are in the second decade. There is a slight predilection for females, 1.1 to 1 {98,184,1340,1529}.

Sites of involvement

Over half of the tumours occurs in the metaphysis of long bones. Rarely multiple skeletal sites are involved {1529, 1953}.

Clinical features / Imaging

Most patients present with pain, swelling or both {1529}.
Symptoms are usually of short duration, but may be prolonged {98,184,1340, 1529}.
Roentgenograms show an aggressive process with destruction of the cortex.

There is always a lytic component, usually admixed with radiodense areas. Mineralized tissue is seen in most tumours, either intramedullary and/or in soft tissue tumour extension strongly suggesting a specific diagnosis of osteosarcoma {98,184,1340,1529}.
Although not distinctive, the diagnosis may be suggested when an osteoblastic tumour extends well down into the shaft of the bone with a permeative pattern {568}.

Macroscopy

The gross features of small cell osteosarcoma are indistinguishable from those of conventional osteosarcoma.

Histopathology

Small cell osteosarcoma is composed of small cells associated with osteoid production. Tumours are classified according to the predominant cell pattern: round cell type or short spindle cell type {98,1529}.

Nuclear diameter of round cells can range in size from very small to medium; the smaller ones comparable to those of Ewing sarcoma and the larger ones to large cell lymphoma {98}. The cells have scanty amounts of cytoplasm.
Nuclei are round to oval and the chromatin may be fine to coarse. Mitoses range from 3 to 5/HPF.
In the less frequent spindle cell type, nuclei are short, oval to spindle, have a granular chromatin, inconspicuous nucleoli and scanty amounts of cytoplasm.
Lace-like osteoid production is always present. Particular care must be taken to distinguish osteoid from fibrin deposits that may be seen among Ewing sarcoma cells.

Immunophenotype

There is no specific immunophenotype for small cell osteosarcoma. Tumour cells may be positive for CD99, vimentin, osteocalcin, osteonectin,

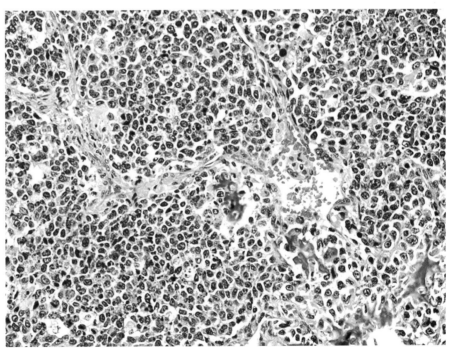

Fig. 11.32 Small cell osteosarcoma, small cell type. Osteoid production at lower right.

smooth muscle specific actin, Leu-7 and KP1 {508,513}.

Ultrastructure

Nuclei may be irregular or have smooth contours and, sometimes, contain large nucleoli. Cytoplasm is poorly differentiated and contains microfilaments, ribosomes, mitochondria and RER in variable amounts. Glycogen is present in 30% of cases. Small junctions are seen in closely apposed cells {518,2218}.

Matrix shows flocculent dense material in close apposition to tumour cell membranes, with subplasmalemmal densities in the adjacent cells, possibly a premineralisation stage of the matrix. These findings may also be seen in chondroid lesions, but never in Ewing sarcoma/ PNET group of tumours {1646}

Genetics

The 11:22 translocation of the Ewing family of tumours is not seen in this neoplasm.

Prognostic factors

Aside from the fact that small cell osteosarcoma itself has a slightly worse prognosis than conventional osteosarcoma, there are no particular histological or imaging findings related to prognosis {98,1529}.

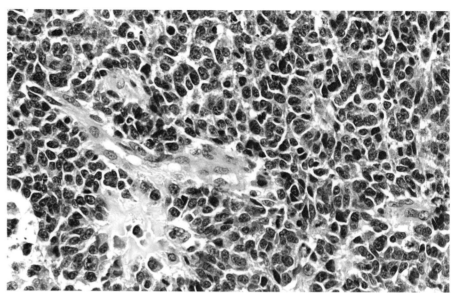
Fig. 11.33 Small cell osteosarcoma, epithelioid-like pattern. Osteoid production at lower left.

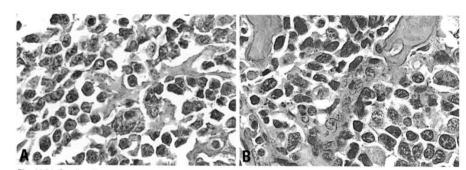
Fig. 11.34 Small cell osteosarcoma. **A** Small cell type. **B** Medium cell type.

Low grade central osteosarcoma

C.Y. Inwards
S. Knuutila

Definition
A low grade osteosarcoma that arises from the medullary cavity of bone.

ICD-O code   9187/3

Synonyms
Well differentiated intramedullary osteosarcoma, low grade intramedullary osteosarcoma, low grade intraosseous-type osteosarcoma.

Epidemiology
Low grade central osteosarcoma accounts for less than 1% of primary bone tumours and only 1-2% of all osteosarcomas {1468,2155,2158}. Males and females are equally affected. The peak incidence is in the second and third decades of life.

Sites of involvement
Approximately 80% of low grade central osteosarcomas are located in the long bones with a distinct predilection for the distal femur and proximal tibia {1186}. The femur is the most frequently involved bone (approximately 50%), followed by the tibia, which is the second most frequently involved bone. Flat bones are uncommonly affected {178,1186,2057, 2312}.

Clinical features / Imaging
Pain and / or swelling are the usual complaints. The duration of pain may be many months or even several years. The radiographic features of low grade central osteosarcoma are variable, however, they are worrisome enough to at least suggest the possibility of malignancy in most cases {345, 581,1186}. Nevertheless, there are examples where aggressive features are subtle or even impossible to detect. They tend to be large metaphyseal or diametaphyseal intramedullary tumours. It is not uncommon to see extension into the end of the bone when the epiphyseal plate is closed. Although the majority of tumours are poorly marginated, up to one-third may show intermediate or well defined margins suggesting an indolent or benign lesion. Trabeculation and sclerosis are also common findings that reflect the indolent nature of this tumour {345}. The radiographic density is variable, however, low grade central osteosarcomas typically contain areas of heavy mineralisation with regions of amorphous, cloud-like, or fluffy mineralisation {581,1186}. Cortical destruction is the most convincing radiographic feature in support of malignancy. The majority of low grade central osteosarcomas will show some degree of cortical disruption with or without soft tissue extension. Computed tomography and magnetic resonance imaging can be quite useful in delineating the extent of the tumour and identifying cortical abnormalities that are not evident on plain films.

Macroscopy
The cut surface of a low grade central osteosarcoma shows a grey-white tumour with a firm and gritty texture arising from within the medullary cavity. Cortical destruction with or without a soft tissue mass may also be seen.

Histopathology
Low grade central osteosarcoma is composed of a hypo- to moderately cellular fibroblastic stroma with variable amounts of osteoid production. The collagen-producing spindle cells are arranged in interlacing bundles that permeate surrounding pre-existing bony trabeculae and bone marrow similar to that of desmoplastic fibroma. While the tumour cells show some degree of cytological atypia, it is usually subtle. Nuclear enlargement and hyperchromasia are generally evident. Occasional mitotic figures are almost always identified.

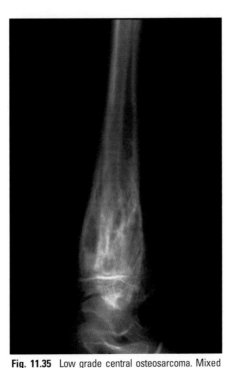

Fig. 11.35 Low grade central osteosarcoma. Mixed lytic and sclerotic lesion involving the distal third of the tibial diaphysis and metaphysis associated with expansion, suggesting a benign or low grade tumour.

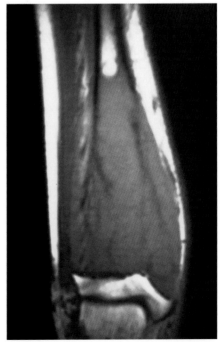

Fig. 11.36 Low grade central osteosarcoma. Coronal T2 weighted MRI illustrates extensive destruction of the distal third of the tibia and extraosseous soft tissue extension. In contrast, fibrous dysplasia typically would not have such aggressive radiographic features.

Variable patterns of bone production are found in low grade central osteosarcoma. Some tumours contain irregular anastomosing, branching, and curved bone trabeculae simulating the appearance of woven bone in fibrous dysplasia {715}. Others contain moderate to heavy amounts of bone present as long longitudinal seams of lamellar-like bone resembling parosteal osteosarcoma. Small scattered foci of atypical cartilage are occasionally seen. In addition, benign multinucleated giant cells have been reported in up to 36% of low grade central osteosarcomas. In 15-20% of cases progression to high grade spindle cell sarcoma occurs, most commonly at the time of tumour recurrence.

Genetics

The results of a CGH study indicate recurrent gains in minimal common regions at 12q13-14, 12p, and 6p21 {2088}. The low number of chromosomal imbalances in low grade central osteosarcoma is in sharp contrast with the complex aberrations seen in high grade osteosarcoma.
MDM2, *CDK4*, and *SAS* at the 12q13-15 amplicon have been reported to be amplified at frequencies of 35%, 65% and 15%, respectively {1747}.

Prognostic factors

Low grade central osteosarcoma behaves in a much more indolent fashion than conventional osteosarcoma. Nevertheless, it is associated with a high incidence of local recurrence after inadequate resections. Recurrences may exhibit a higher histological grade or

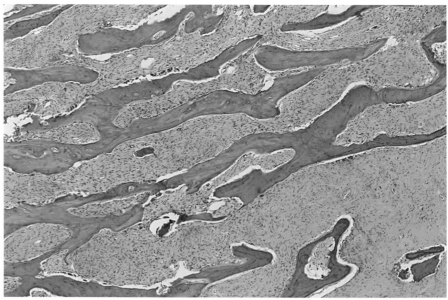

Fig. 11.37 Low grade central osteosarcoma. At low magnification, long, parallel seams of bone surrounded by a hypocellular spindle cell stroma are seen, resembling the pattern of parosteal osteosarcoma.

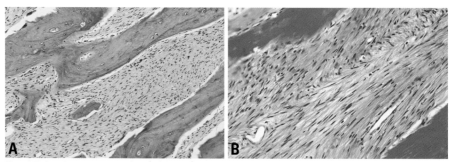

Fig. 11.38 Low grade central osteosarcoma. **A** Irregularly shaped spicules of bone surrounded by a spindle cell stroma with minimal atypia. Distinction fibrous dysplasia requires radiographic correlation. **B** At higher magnification, scattered cells with nuclear enlargement and hyperchromasia occur.

dedifferentiation with the potential for metastases {345,999,1186}. It is metastatic tumour from the higher grade recurrence that can lead to death in patients with low grade central osteosarcoma.

Secondary osteosarcomas

M. Forest
G. De Pinieux
S. Knuutila

Definition

Secondary osteosarcomas are bone forming sarcomas occurring in bones that are affected by preexisting abnormalities, the most common being Paget disease and radiation change, and rarely various other disorders.

ICD-O code   9180/3

Paget osteosarcoma

ICD-O code   9184/3

Synonym

Paget sarcoma.

Epidemiology

Incidence of sarcomatous changes in Paget disease is estimated to be 0.7-0.95%, and osteosarcomas represent 50-60% of Paget sarcomas {867,989, 1879,2263}. In most series, Paget osteosarcoma is more common in men (ratio 2:1), with an overall median age of 64 years: it accounts for more than 20% of osteosarcomas in patients older than 40 years of age.

This complication is usually observed in patients with widespread Paget disease (70%), but can occur in monostotic Paget disease as well.

Sites of involvement

Any bone affected by Paget disease has the potential to undergo sarcomatous change. Except for the high frequency in the humerus and the lower frequency in the vertebrae, osteosarcoma has the same distribution as uncomplicated Paget disease.

Approximately, two-thirds are seen in large limb bones (femur, humerus, tibia), one-third in the flat bones (pelvis, skull and scapula). 10-17% of all Paget osteosarcomas involve the skull.

Most tumours arise in the medulla; few are located near the periosteal surface of bone.

Multifocal osteosarcoma occurs in 17% of cases, usually involving the femur and the skull, superimposed on polyostotic Paget disease and may represent multiple primary tumours or metastatic spread.

Clinical features / Imaging

Clinical symptoms are a change in pain pattern, a swelling, and occasionally pathological fracture (12-20%, more commonly in the femur). Often, there is an elevation of alkaline phosphatase levels above those usually seen in Paget disease. On imaging, tumours with a lytic pattern are more frequent than a blastic or sclerotic appearance {2263}, with cortical disruption and a soft tissue mass. The affected bone shows radiographic features of Paget disease.

Macroscopy

The gross appearance is variable reflecting the patterns seen for conventional osteosarcoma. The non-neoplastic bone shows thickened bone trabeculae and cortical thickening.

Histopathology

Paget osteosarcomas are high grade sarcomas, mostly osteoblastic or fibroblastic osteosarcomas. A great number of osteoclast-like giant cells may be found {1879}. Telangiectatic and small cell osteosarcomas have been reported {2263}.

Genetics

Recent evidence suggests that predisposition to Paget disease may have a genetic component linked to a region of chromosome arm 18q {370,811,883}. In a study of 96 sporadic osteosarcomas frequent LOH was seen at chromosome arm 18q {1546}.

Prognostic factors

The prognosis is poor, especially for tumours located in the pelvic bones and the skull, with a five-year overall survival rate of 11% {2263}. Survival is shorter in cases of multifocal disease. Metastases are present in 25% of patients, at initial presentation (predominantly pulmonary or bone metastases).

There is a small fraction of long-term survivors after aggressive therapy (age less than 60 years, monostotic Paget disease, sarcomas arising in long bones) {867}.

Postradiation osteosarcoma

ICD-O code   9180/3

Synonyms

Postradiation sarcomas, radiation induced sarcoma.

Epidemiology

They constitute 3.4-5.5% of all osteosarcomas and 50-60% of radiation-induced sarcomas. It is estimated that the risk of developing osteosarcoma in irradiated bone is 0.03-0.8% {996,1334}.

Children treated with high-dose radiotherapy and chemotherapy are at the greatest risk. The prevalence of postradiation osteosarcomas is increasing as children survive treatment of their malignant disease {145,2190}.

Sites of involvement

Postradiation osteosarcoma can develop in any irradiated bone, but the most common locations are the pelvis and the shoulder region.

Clinical features / Imaging

The criteria for the diagnosis are well established: the affected bone may have been normal, contain a biopsy proven benign tumour or non-bone forming malignancy; history of prior radiation therapy and tumour developing in the path of the radiation beam; a symptom-free latent period (frequently long but may be as short as two years); a histologically proven osteosarcoma {996}.

The latent period is generally long (median of 11 years), and inversely related to the radiation dosage. Radiation doses are usually greater than 20 Gy; most sarcomas occur in association with doses of approximately 55 Gy.

Common symptoms are pain and swelling.

On imaging, the tumours are densely sclerotic or lytic lesions with a soft tissue mass. Radiation osteitis is present in about 50% of cases (trabecular coarsening and lytic areas in the cortex). Multicentric osteosarcomas have been reported as well as a few parosteal osteosarcomas {2115}.

Macroscopy
Similar to conventional osteosarcoma.

Histopathology
High grade osteosarcomas predominate. Histological changes of radiation osteitis may be present.

Genetics
Cytogenetic and DNA copy number changes are complex and similar to those in conventional osteosarcomas {1427}. Postradiation osteosarcomas frequently exhibit 3p loss cytogenetically {1427}. Sporadic and postradiation osteosarcomas differ in copy number changes by comparative genomic hybridisation {2094}. Whereas gains were more frequent than losses in sporadic tumours, the reverse was seen in radiation-associated sarcomas. Further-more, loss of 1p was rare (3%) in sporadic cases, but frequent (57%) in radiation-associated tumours. In one study, a high (58%) frequency of $TP53$ mutations was found {1532}.

Prognostic factors
The 5-year-cumulative survival rate is of 68.2% for patients with extremity lesions, 27.3% for patients with axial lesions {1005}.

The prognosis is worse for pelvic, vertebral and shoulder girdle locations.

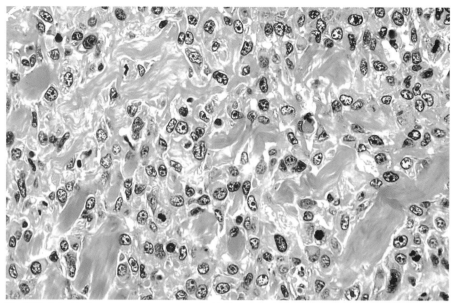

Fig. 11.39 Osteoblastic osteosarcoma associated with fibrous dysplasia of the femur.

Osteosarcoma in the course of various bone diseases

Osteosarcoma has been reported in association with a variety of conditions affecting bone. Many of the reports are of rare associations. The three associations deserving special attention are bone infarct, prosthetic joint and fibrous dysplasia. Infarct associated sarcomas most commonly show the histological pattern of malignant fibrous histiocytoma, however a minority are osteosarcomas. It has been suggested that the malignant transformation in large and multiple infarcts arises from the reparative process of osteonecrosis, but this view is disputed {503,2122}. Malignant tumours have been reported at the site of prosthetic replacements as well as at the site of prior internal fixation. The majority of such cases have shown a malignant fibrous histiocytoma morphology, but six cases of osteosarcoma in association with total hip replacements have been reported {271}. Osteosarcoma associated with fibrous dysplasia is most common in the setting of Albright syndrome {992,2074}. Many of the reported cases of osteosarcoma arising in fibrous dysplasia have also been complicated by radiation therapy {992,1822,2074}. There is nothing unique about the pathology or prognosis of secondary osteosarcoma arising in association with bone infarct, prosthesis or fibrous dysplasia.

Parosteal osteosarcoma

K.K. Unni
S. Knuutila

Definition
Parosteal osteosarcoma is a low grade osteosarcoma which arises on the surface of bone.

ICD-O code   9192/3

Synonyms
Juxtacortical osteosarcoma, juxtacortical low grade osteosarcoma.

Epidemiology
Although rare, parosteal osteosarcoma is the most common type of osteosarcoma of the surface of bone. It accounts for about 4% of all osteosarcomas. There is a slight female predominance and most patients are young adults, about 1/3 occurs in the 3rd decade of life {1599}.

Sites of involvement
About 70% involve the surface of the distal posterior femur. The proximal tibia and proximal humerus are also relatively commonly involved. Flat bones are uncommonly affected.

Clinical features / Imaging
Patients generally complain of a painless swelling; inability to flex the knee may be the initial symptom. Some patients complain of a painful swelling.
Roentgenograms show a heavily mineralised mass attached to the cortex with a broad base. The tumour has a tendency to wrap around the involved bone. Computerized tomograms and magnetic resonance images are useful in evaluating the extent of medullary involvement. The outermost portions of the tumour are usually less mineralised {185}. In some cases there may be an incomplete lucency between the tumour and the underlying bone.

Macroscopy
Parosteal osteosarcoma presents as a hard lobulated mass attached to the underlying cortex. Nodules of cartilage may be present. Occasionally, the cartilage will be incomplete cap-like, covering the surface and thus suggesting a diagnosis of osteochondroma. The periphery may be softer and seen to invade skeletal muscle. Invasion of the bone marrow may be seen in 25% of the cases. Soft, fleshy areas, if present, suggest dedifferentiation.

Histopathology
Parosteal osteosarcoma consists of well formed bony trabeculae seen in a hypocellular stroma. The bony trabeculae are arranged in a parallel manner and simulate normal bone {1025}. The trabeculae may or may not show osteoblastic rimming. The intertrabecular stroma is hypocellular. The spindle cells in the stroma show minimal atypia. In about 20% of the cases, the stroma is more cellular and the spindle cells show moderate atypia. About 50% of the tumours will show cartilaginous differentiation. This may be in the form of hypercellular nodules of cartilage

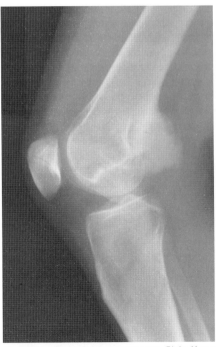

Fig. 11.40 Parosteal osteosarcoma. Plain X-ray shows a heavily mineralised mass attached to the posterior aspect of the distal femur not involving

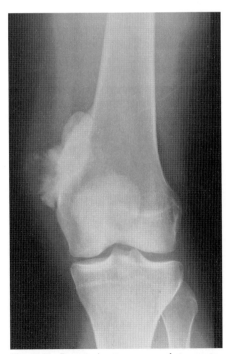

Fig. 11.41 Parosteal osteosarcoma Anteroposterior view of the knee showing a lobulated, heavily mineralised mass attached to the cortex.

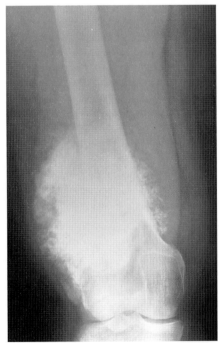

Fig. 11.42 Parosteal osteosarcoma. The formation of large, heavily mineralised masses surrounding the involved bone is common.

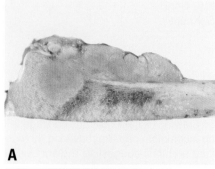

A

B

Fig. 11.43 Parosteal osteosarcoma. **A** Although much of the tumour is on the surface of the proximal tibia, there is clear-cut marrow involvement. **B** Gross specimen showing large amounts of chondroid differentiation. The marrow cavity, which is free of involvement, is seen at the bottom.

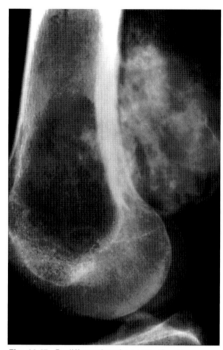

Fig. 11.45 Dedifferentiated parosteal osteosarcoma. The appearance of the lesion on the surface is that of a heavily mineralised mass, typical of parosteal osteosarcoma. There is a very destructive appearing lesion within the medullary cavity, which was the dedifferentiated component.

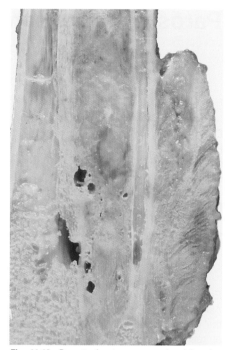

Fig. 11.46 Parosteal osteosarcoma involving the bones of the forearm. Much of the tumour has the appearance of classical parosteal osteosarcoma with fibrous areas. However, between the bones, there are soft areas representing dedifferentiation.

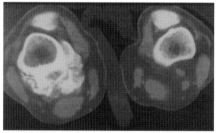

Fig. 11.44 Parosteal osteosarcoma. CT shows a mineralising mass. The marrow is free of involvement. This is the same case as shown in Fig. 11.42.

within the substance of the neoplasm or as a cap on the surface. When present, the cartilage cap is mildly hypercellular, and the cells show mild cytological atypia and lacks the 'columnar' arrangement seen in osteochondromas. There is, however, enchondral ossification as seen in osteochondroma. Unlike fatty and haematopoietic marrow, as seen in osteochondromas, there is spindle cell proliferation between the bony trabeculae. Large areas devoid of bone and rich in collagen similar to

desmoplastic fibroma may be present. About 15% of the tumours will show high grade spindle cell sarcoma (dedifferentiation). This may be at the time of the original diagnosis or, more often, at the time of recurrence {2289}. The areas of dedifferentiation may be osteosarcoma, fibrosarcoma or malignant fibrous histiocytoma.

Immunophenotype

There are no specific features helpful in diagnosis.

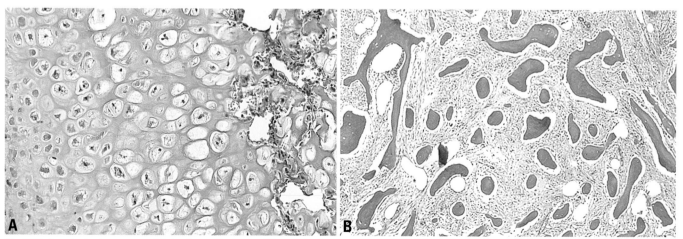

Fig. 11.47 Parosteal osteosarcoma. **A** Extensive cartilagineous differentiation is not uncommon. **B** Well-formed bony trabeculae in a hypocellular spindle cell stroma.

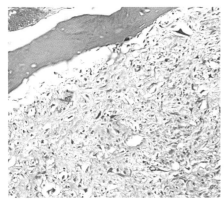

Fig. 11.48 Parosteal osteosarcoma. Area of dedifferentiation with pleomorphic appearing nuclei.

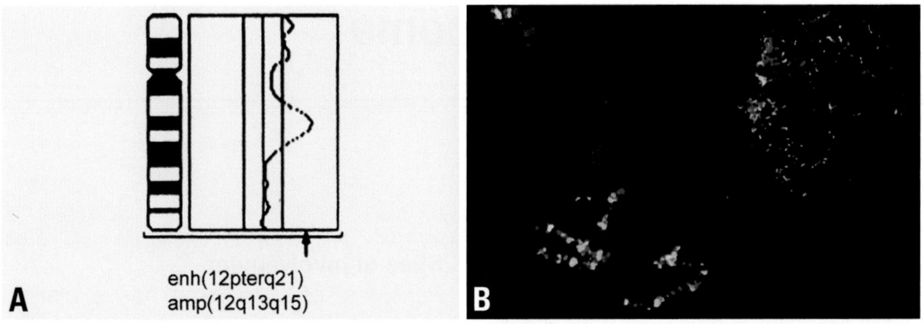

enh(12pterq21)
amp(12q13q15)

A

B

Fig. 11.49 Parosteal osteosarcoma. **A** CGH profile indicating gain at 12pterq21 with amplification 12q13q15. The arrow indicates the cutoff value of 1.5 for amplification (from J. Szymanska et al. {2071}). **B** MS-FISH from the same tumour shows a normal chromosome 12 (top left), ring, and large marker chromosome. FISH shows amplification of *KRAS2*, *CDK4*, and *MDM2*, respectively, whereas no copy number increase could be demonstrated on ETV6 (from D. Gisselsson et al. {796}).

Genetics

Chromosomal alterations in parosteal osteosarcomas are different from those in conventional osteosarcomas. Parosteal osteosarcomas are characterized by one or more supernumerary ring chromosomes, often as the sole alteration {1428, 1634,1961}. CGH studies indicate gain at 12q13-15 as the minimal common region of amplification in the rings {2071}.

The *SAS*, *CDK4*, and *MDM2* genes have been shown to be coamplified and overexpressed in a great proportion of cases {2305} and the incidence of the amplifications of these genes seems to be essentially lower in classical high grade osteosarcoma. Mutations in *RB1* {2208} or microsatellite instability {2087} have not been found to be present in parosteal osteosarcoma.

Prognostic factors

Prognosis is excellent with 91% overall survival at 5 years {1599}. Marrow invasion and moderate cytological atypia do not predict a worse prognosis. If incompletly excised the tumour may reccur and dedifferentiate. The presence of such dedifferentiated areas is associated with a prognosis similar to that of conventional osteosarcoma.

Periosteal osteosarcoma

A.G. Ayala
B. Czerniak

A.K. Raymond
S. Knuutila

Definition

Periosteal osteosarcoma, is an intermediate grade chondroblastic osteosarcoma arising on the surface of bone.

ICD-O code   9193/3

Synonyms

Juxtacortical chondrosarcoma, juxtacortical chondroblastic osteosarcoma.

Epidemiology

Periosteal osteosarcoma {644, 2013, 2155} accounts for less than 2% of all the osteosarcomas {2155,2156}.

Of the surface osteosarcomas, it is more common than high grade surface osteosarcoma, but about one-third as common as parosteal osteosarcoma {644,1600}. The peak incidence of periosteal osteosarcoma is in the second and third decades of life. There is a slight male predominance.

Sites of involvement

Periosteal osteosarcoma has a distinct predilection for the diaphysis or diaphyseal-metaphyseal area of the long bones, with the tibia and femur the most commonly involved bones, followed by the humerus {179,644,874,1792,2013, 2155,2156}. In the long bones, this tumour usually affects the anterior, lateral or medial portions of the shaft, but occasionally may surround the entire circumference of the bone. It can also involve the clavicle, pelvis, mandible, ribs and cranium {179,644,874,1792,2013,2155, 2156}. The case of a bilateral metachronous lesion has also been reported {979}.

Clinical features / Imaging

A painless mass or limb swelling is the most common initial complaint with pain or tenderness later developing in the affected area {179,644,2013,2156}. In most patients the complaints have lasted for less than 1 year and more than half of the patients have been symptomatic for about 6 months {644}.

This tumour, arising on the surface of a bone, displays nonhomogeneous, calcified spiculations that are disposed perpendicular to the the cortex and give an overall sunburst appearance. The lesion decreases in density from the cortical base to the surface, where the tumour has a relatively well demarcated advancing margin. Commonly, the cortex appears thickened as result of the production of a heavily ossified matrix. The bone spicules are variously calcified with fine and coarse calcification. A Codman's triangle is frequently present. Computed tomography and magnetic resonance imaging are very important in the evaluation of tumour size, integrity of the cortex, soft tissue extension and relationship to the neurovascular bundle.

Macroscopy

The tumour arises from the bone surface and may involve part of the bone or the entire circumference {644,2013, 2155,2156}. It has a conspicuous fusiform appearance when it involves the entire circumference of the shaft of a bone. A spiculated pattern arising perpendicular to the cortex is commonly seen grossly, with the longest spicules situated at the centre of the lesion; these

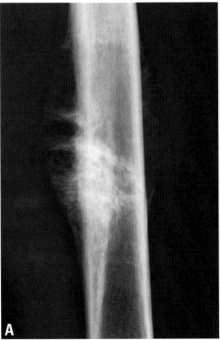
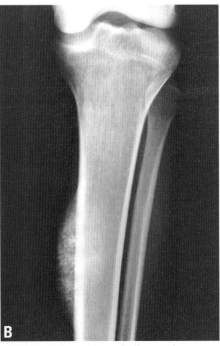

Fig. 11.50 Periosteal osteosarcoma. **A** Plain radiograph of femur shows a large, fusiform surface mass. Perpendicular to the cortex, there are multiple, parallel thin columns of calcified matrix. Focal lytic areas are also present. **B** The upper shaft of the tibia displays a well demarcated tumour arising from the cortical surface of the bone. Fluffy calcifications are present.

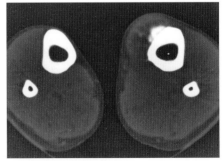

Fig. 11.51 Periosteal osteosarcoma. CT scans show a heavily ossified tibial mass arising from the cortex, covered by a larger, focally or minimally calcified soft tissue mass component.

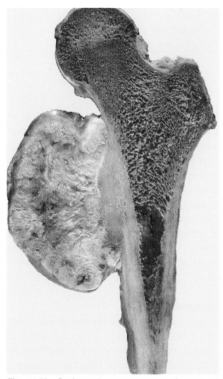

Fig. 11.52 Periosteal osteosarcoma of proximal femur. A broad based, mushroom-like, large surface tumour depicting a thickened ossified area blending in with the cortex. Covering this area there is a large soft tissue component depicting seemingly two layers of tissue. One is whitish-cartilaginous and the other is tan-yellow.

spicules gradually taper from the centre to the outer extremes of the lesion in all directions. A solid ossified mass is commonly seen adjacent to the cortex, while the periphery tends to be uncalcified or minimally calcified. Part of the tumour usually has the glistening, greyish appearance typical of cartilage. The advancing margin is generally well delineated by a capsule/ pseudocapsule that is the product a thickened periosteum. The bony mass merges imperceptibly with the cortex at its base, giving the appearance of a thickended cortex.

Histopathology

Histologically, periosteal osteosarcoma has the appearance of a moderately differentiated chondroblastic osteosarcoma {2155,2156}. The ossified mass is generally found arising from the cortex, to which it is intimately attached, and it is made up of relatively mature bone that has resulted from endochondral ossification. The cartilaginous component predominates, but elements of intermediate grade osteosarcoma are invariably present. The cartilaginous component may show varying degrees of cytological atypia.

The matrix may be myxoid. The bony spicule consists of elongated vascular cores surrounded by a calcified, osseous or chondro-osseous matrix, which in turn may be surrounded by non-calcified cartilaginous growth. The periphery of the tumour generally shows no calcification and is made up of fascicles of spindle cells. In these areas, there may be significant mitotic activity with abnormal figures. These areas may also contain lace-like osteoid.

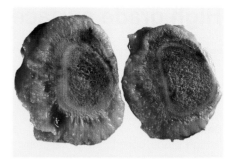

Fig. 11.53 Periosteal osteosarcoma of femur. These cross sections of the shaft of the femur depict a surface tumour involving the entire circumference of the bone. Calcified spicules impart a sunburst appearance. A glistening non-calcified tumour component covers the entire tumour. The medullary cavity is intact.

Genetics

Among four reported cases, one had +17 as the sole change {263}, and three had complex karyotypic changes {795, 965,2090}.

Prognostic factors

Although periosteal osteosarcoma is associated with a better prognosis than conventional osteosarcoma, it is still a malignant tumour with a tendency to recur and to metastasise {644,2013, 2155,2156}. Medullary involvement by the tumour may portend poorer prognosis. A recurrence rate of 70% has been reported for patients who underwent marginal excision {1341}. The rate of metastasis has been reported to be about 15% {644,1792,2155,2156}.

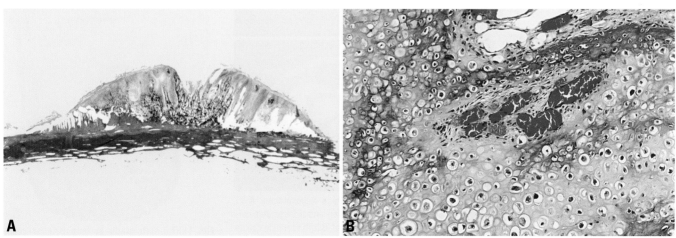

Fig. 11.54 Periosteal osteosarcoma. **A** A cross section of the tibial tumour which shows an ossified mass blending with and thickening the cortex and covered by an uncalcified component. **B** Typical appearance of chondroblastic grade 3 osteosarcoma. There are lobules of malignant-appearing cartilage with bone formation in the centre of the lobules.

High grade surface osteosarcoma

L. Wold
E. McCarthy
S. Knuutila

Definition
A high grade bone-forming malignancy which arises from the surface of the bone.

ICD-O code   9194/3

Synonyms
Juxtacortical osteosarcoma, surface osteosarcoma.

Epidemiology
High grade surface osteosarcoma comprises less than one percent of all osteosarcomas. The peak incidence is in the second decade, and the age distribution of patients at the time of diagnosis is similar to conventional osteosarcoma. There is a slight male predilection.

Sites of involvement
The femur is most commonly affected followed in frequency by the humerus and tibia.

Clinical features / Imaging
Patients with high grade surface osteosarcoma most commonly present with a mass and/or pain in the region of the tumour. The tumour radiographically presents as a surface, partially mineralised, mass extending into the soft tissues. The underlying cortex is commonly partially destroyed, and periosteal new bone is commonly present at the periphery of the tumour. Cross sectional imaging may show minimal medullary involvement, but the tumour is most commonly relatively well circumscribed at its soft tissue margin. The pattern of mineralisation present is variable depending upon the amount of chondroid and osseous matrix produced by the tumour.

Macroscopy
The tumour is situated on the surface of the affected bone and commonly erodes the underlying cortical bone. Tumours vary in consistency depending upon whether they are predominantly osteoblastic, chondroblastic, or fibroblastic. However, all tumours will have "soft" areas in them, a feature which helps separate this tumour from parosteal osteosarcoma. The surface of the tumour is commonly multilobulated, and the colour varies depending upon the amount of chondroid matrix, haemorrhage, and necrosis present.

Histopathology
These tumours show the same spectrum of features seen in conventional osteosarcoma. Regions of predominantly osteoblastic, chondroblastic, or fibroblastic differentiation may predominate. However, all tumours will show high grade cytological atypia and lace-like osteoid as seen in conventional osteosarcoma. Many tumours show regions rich in cytologically atypical spindle cells

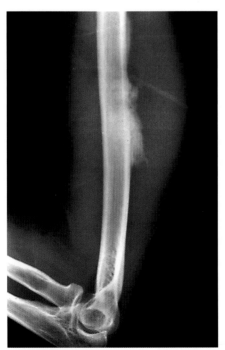

Fig. 11.55 High grade surface osteosarcoma in the middle portion of the humerus. The lesion is mineralised where it is attached to the bone but there is also a large unmineralised soft tissue mass.

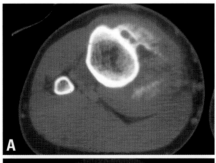
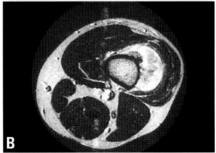

Fig. 11.56 High grade surface osteosarcoma. **A** CT showing focal mineralisation and a large unmineralised soft tissue component. **B** MRI scanning can be very sensitive in evaluating whether there is medullary involvement in surface tumours of bone. There is no medullary involvement in this case.

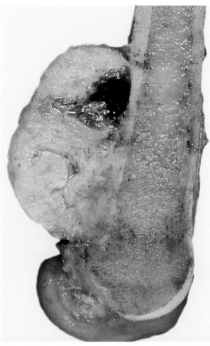

Fig. 11.57 High grade surface osteosarcoma involving the distal femur. The tumour is soft and fleshy.

with brisk mitotic activity evident in these regions. The pattern of osteoid production and the high grade cytological atypia evident in high grade surface osteosarcoma help to separate it from parosteal osteosarcoma. High grade surface osteosarcomas which show predominant chondroblastic differentiation may be confused with periosteal osteosarcoma. The degree of cytological atypia is greater in high grade surface osteosarcoma than in periosteal osteosarcoma, and the tumours also generally show larger regions of spindle cell morphology. Unlike same dedifferentiated parosteal osteosarcoma, low grade regions of tumour are not identified in high grade surface osteosarcoma.

Immunophenotype
Similar to conventional osteosarcoma.

Prognostic factors
As in conventional osteosarcoma the major prognostic feature is the response to chemotherapy.

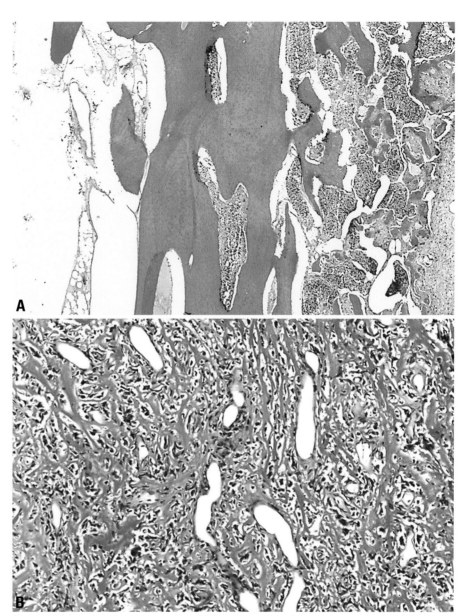

Fig. 11.58 High grade surface osteosarcoma. **A** The tumour produces large amounts of bone (right). The cortex (middle) and the medullary cavity (left) are uninvolved. **B** Wide vascular spaces bear resemblance to osteoblastoma, but the high grade cytologic atypia and the compact nature of the spindle cell proliferation help to distinguish high grade surface osteosarcoma from osteoblastoma.

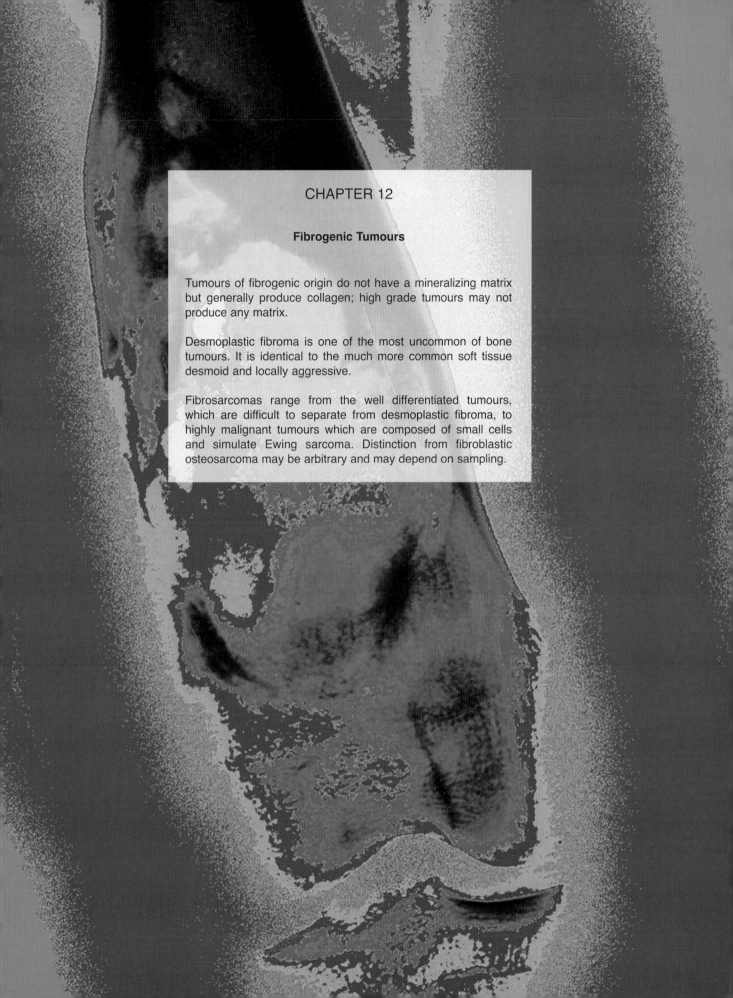

CHAPTER 12

Fibrogenic Tumours

Tumours of fibrogenic origin do not have a mineralizing matrix but generally produce collagen; high grade tumours may not produce any matrix.

Desmoplastic fibroma is one of the most uncommon of bone tumours. It is identical to the much more common soft tissue desmoid and locally aggressive.

Fibrosarcomas range from the well differentiated tumours, which are difficult to separate from desmoplastic fibroma, to highly malignant tumours which are composed of small cells and simulate Ewing sarcoma. Distinction from fibroblastic osteosarcoma may be arbitrary and may depend on sampling.

Desmoplastic fibroma of bone

V. Fornasier
K.P.H. Pritzker
J.A. Bridge

Definition

Desmoplastic fibroma is a rare, benign bone tumour composed of spindle cells with minimal cytological atypia and abundant collagen production.

ICD-O code

8823/0

Synonyms

Desmoid tumour of bone, intra-osseous counterpart of soft tissue fibromatosis.

Epidemiology

The incidence is approximately 0.1% of all primary bone tumours. It tends to occur in adolescent and young adults with near equal gender distribution.

Sites of involvement

Desmoplastic fibroma may involve any bone but is most frequent in the mandible.

Clinical features / Imaging

Patients present with a variety of symptoms. Some have pain, others present because of deformity or loss of function. Radiographically, desmoplastic fibroma is usually a well defined, radiolucent lesion that may expand the host bone. Intralesional trabeculation is frequent. Larger lesions may breach the periostium and extend into soft tissue. Such erosive, destructive pattern may mimic other, more aggressive lesions. Desmoplastic fibroma has low signal intensity in both T1 and T2 weighted MRI images. The extent of disease and margins are best assessed with CT and MRI.

Macroscopy

The tumour is firm and the cut surface is creamy-white with a variegated whorled pattern. The advancing surfaces of the lesion tend to be scalloped and apparently well defined. The tumour may extend into soft tissue.

Histopathology

The lesion is composed of spindle cells (fibroblasts/myofibroblasts) on a richly collagenous, variably hyalinized background. The degree of cellularity is variable but cellular atypia and pleomorphism are minimal or absent. Mitoses are rare.

Genetics

FISH analyses of desmoplastic fibroma suggest that trisomies 8 and 20 represent nonrandom aberrations in a subset of these lesions, analogous to similar findings in soft tissue desmoid tumours {267}.

Prognostic factors

The tumour behaves in a locally progressive/aggressive manner. Recurrence following curettage and resection are 72% and 17%, respectively {832}. Local relapse has been reported as late as eight years following primary surgery. There is a single reported case involving the spine that showed little detectable change over a follow up period of nine years without therapy {1482}.

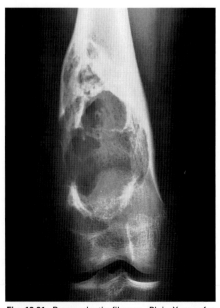

Fig. 12.01 Desmoplastic fibroma. Plain X-ray of a tumour involving the distal femur. The lesion is large, lobulated, and has a sclerotic rim.

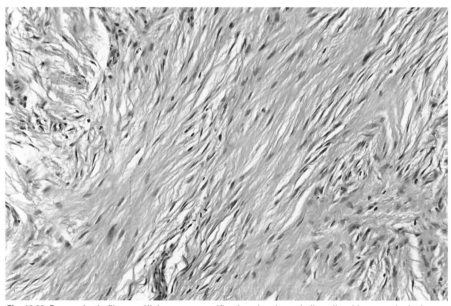

Fig. 12.02 Desmoplastic fibroma. High power magnification showing spindle cells without cytological atypia and large amounts of collagen.

Fibrosarcoma of bone

L.B. Kahn
V. Vigorita

Definition

A primary malignant spindle cell neoplasm of bone in which the tumour cells are typically organized in a fascicular or "herringbone" pattern.

ICD-O code   8810/3

Epidemiology

Precise epidemiological data pertaining to fibrosarcoma of bone is difficult to obtain due to inconsistent terminology usage for fibrosarcoma versus malignant fibrous histiocytoma.
Fibrosarcomas constitute up to 5% of all primary malignant bone tumours, with relatively uniform incidence over the second to sixth decades and equal gender distribution {991}. There have been occasional reports of cases occurring during infancy {167,425}.

Sites of involvement

Historical series indicate that fibrosarcomas most frequently involve the metaphyses of long bones. In one large series, the distal femur was involved in 48 of 102 of cases (47%) {2075}. Other frequent sites of involvement were the proximal femur (16%), distal humerus (14%) and proximal tibia (11%). A series of 130 cases also identified the distal femur as the most common site (21%) of involvement {991}.

Clinical features / Imaging

Pain and swelling are the usual symptoms. Up to one-third of patients have pathological fracture {1221}.
Radiographically, fibrosarcoma usually appears as a destructive geographic lesion, but may have an ill defined permeative, "moth eaten" appearance with cortical destruction and frequent soft tissue extension. A periosteal reaction is not infrequently present {2075}. The soft tissue extension may be better visualised by CT and MRI.

Aetiology

In most cases, the aetiology of fibrosarcoma of bone is not known. However, fibrosarcoma has been reported in association with a number of conditions including prior radiation therapy, Paget disease, giant cell tumour, osteochondroma, bone infarcts, chronic osteomyelitis, fibrous dysplasia, ameloblastic fibroma and hereditary bone dysplasia {85,644,886}.

Macroscopy

Well differentiated tumours produce large amounts of collagen, resulting in a firm consistency with a trabeculated, white cut surface and circumscribed margins. Poorly differentiated tumours have a softer, fleshy consistency with foci of necrosis; they vary in colour and are poorly marginated.

Histopathology

Histologically, fibrosarcoma of bone is composed of a uniformly cellular population of spindle shaped cells arranged in a fascicular or "herringbone" pattern with a variable amount of collagen production. Parts or all of the lesion may be more myxoid and such lesions have been labelled myxofibrosarcomas. Higher grade lesions tend to be more cellular with less collagen production, exhibit greater nuclear atypia and a higher mitotic count including abnormal mitoses than their better differentiated counterparts. Areas of necrosis may be seen.

Differential diagnosis

In cases with more severe cytological atypia, including tumour giant cells, fibrosarcoma may be difficult to distinguish from malignant fibrous histiocytoma. The presence of a storiform pattern and epithelioid type cells with "ground glass" cytoplasm would favour a diagnosis of malignant fibrous histiocytoma. In view of the identical clinical,

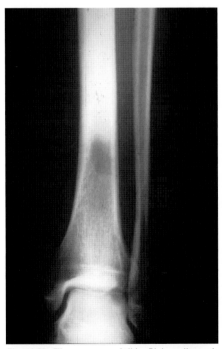

Fig. 12.03 Fibrosarcoma of tibia. Plain radiograph demonstrating ill defined purely osteolytic lesion involving distal third of tibia. The soft tissue extension of the tumour is not evident in this study.

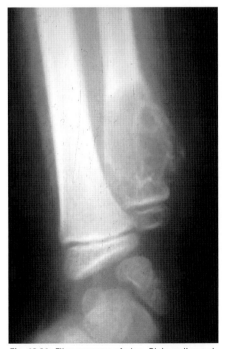

Fig. 12.04 Fibrosarcoma of ulna. Plain radiograph showing ill defined expansile osteolytic lesion of the metaphysis with cortical destruction on the medial aspect.

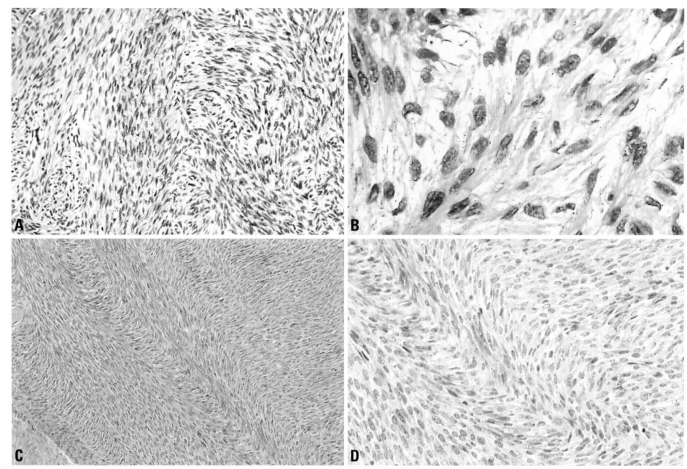

Fig. 12.05 Fibrosarcoma of tibia. **A** The fibrocytic cells are arranged in a haphazard fascicular rather than in the more typical "herring bone" pattern. **B** High power photomicrograph reveals a fairly uniform appearance of the neoplastic cells. The nuclei are ovoid, blunt-ended and have single small nucleoli and finely dispersed chromatin. Collagen fibres appear to emanate from the nuclear poles. **C** Fibrosarcoma illustrating the characteristic "herringbone" pattern. **D** High power appearance of the previous photomicrograph.

radiological and even prognostic features of these two lesions, some investigators have chosen to include them within the category of fibrosarcomas {2075}. Well differentiated fibrosarcoma is distinguished from desmoplastic fibroma by the presence of readily identifiable mitoses and high cellularity in the former and their extreme paucity or absence in the latter.

Prognostic factors

Two series have reported an overall 5-year survival approximating 34% {1647, 2075}. The most important prognostic factor is histological tumour grade. In one series, the 10 year survival was 83% in low grade and 34% in high grade fibrosarcoma {181}. Another series reported an overall 10-year survival rate of 28%, but there was a higher chance of survival (48%) in primary tumours originating from the cortical surface {991}. In the latter series, metastases occurred in 59/130 patients (45%), most frequently involving lung and other bones. In addition to poor histological differentiation, other ad- verse prognostic factors included age over 40 years and axial skeletal location {1647}.

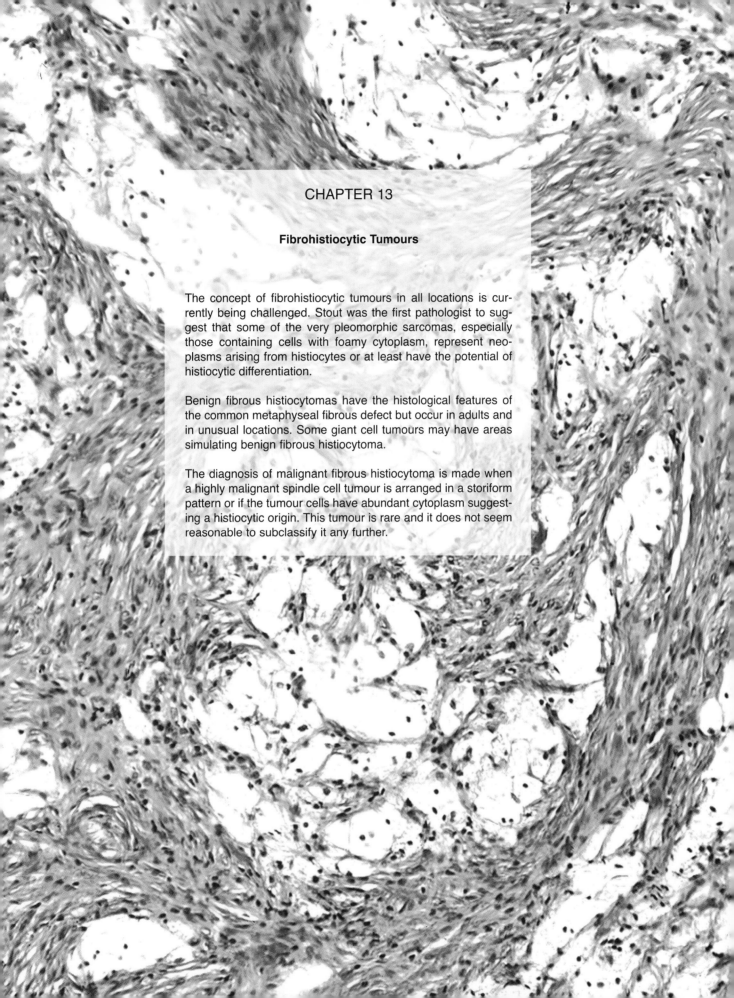

CHAPTER 13

Fibrohistiocytic Tumours

The concept of fibrohistiocytic tumours in all locations is currently being challenged. Stout was the first pathologist to suggest that some of the very pleomorphic sarcomas, especially those containing cells with foamy cytoplasm, represent neoplasms arising from histiocytes or at least have the potential of histiocytic differentiation.

Benign fibrous histiocytomas have the histological features of the common metaphyseal fibrous defect but occur in adults and in unusual locations. Some giant cell tumours may have areas simulating benign fibrous histiocytoma.

The diagnosis of malignant fibrous histiocytoma is made when a highly malignant spindle cell tumour is arranged in a storiform pattern or if the tumour cells have abundant cytoplasm suggesting a histiocytic origin. This tumour is rare and it does not seem reasonable to subclassify it any further.

Benign fibrous histiocytoma of bone

M. Kyriakos

Definition
A benign lesion of bone composed of spindle-shaped fibroblasts, arranged in a storiform pattern, with a variable admixture of small, multinucleated osteoclast-like giant cells. Foamy cells (xanthoma), chronic inflammatory cells, stromal haemorrhages and haemosiderin pigment are also commonly present.

ICD-O code   8830/0

Synonyms
Fibroxanthoma, fibrous xanthoma, xanthofibroma, xanthogranuloma.

Epidemiology
Benign fibrous histiocytoma is rare, with less than 100 reported cases. Patients have ranged in age from 6 to 74 years at diagnosis {110,180}, 60% being older than age 20 years, with a slight female prevalence.

Sites of involvement
Approximately 40% of benign fibrous hisiocytomas occur in the long bones, with femur and tibia most frequently involved. As many as 25% of cases involve the pelvic bones, in particular the ilium. However, this tumour may involve virtually any bone. In the long bones,

benign fibrous histiocytoma is centred in the epiphysis or diaphysis.

Clinical features / Imaging
Although some patients (~15%) are asymptomatic {180,583,1639}, in most (65%) the lesion causes pain which may be present for days {877} up to several years {364,1308,1468,1781}. Occasional patients present because of pathological fracture {365,506,939}.

Roentgenographically, benign fibrous histiocytoma (BFH) appears as a well defined, benign appearing, radiolucent medullary defect without matrix formation; internal trabeculation or pseudoseptations, may be evident {365}. Approximately two-thirds of the lesions have sclerotic margins, at times best seen with computed tomography {100, 180,723,877,959}. The lesion may thin and expand the cortex, however, a periosteal reaction is lacking in the absence of fracture {180,364,365,506, 723,765,959,1639,1781,2155}. Soft tissue extension is not present. Rarely, the lesion is less well defined, with indistinct borders, having a pattern suggestive of malignancy {939,2155}. At the end of a long bone it may be central or eccentric and be indistinguishable from a giant cell tumour (GCT) {1355,1875}. The diagno-

sis of benign fibrous histiocytoma should be considered in cases in which the clinical radiographic setting is also compatible with diagnoses of: metaphyseal fibrous cortical defect, non-ossifying fibroma or giant cell tumour of bone.

Macroscopy
Most lesions are 3.0 cm in diameter or smaller {100,110,364,583,1308,1484, 1639}, although cases up to 7.0 cm have been reported {723,2155}. The tumour tissue is usually firm, grey-white, and frequently contains irregular yellow to reddish brown foci.

Histopathology
The basic pattern of BFH consists of a stroma of spindle-shaped fibroblasts, arranged, at least focally, in a whorled, storiform pattern, among which a variable number of small, multinucleated, osteoclast-type giant cells are scattered. The spindle cell nuclei may be dark, thin and elongate, or round to oval and vesicular with a micronucleolus. In rare cases the stromal cells exhibit mild nuclear atypia justifying the term "atypical fibrous histiocytoma". There is no consensus as to how extensive or severe the degree of atypia should be to consider a low grade malignancy {1587,1840}. Foam (xanthoma) cells, with small, dark nuclei are frequently, but not always, found interspersed among the stromal cells either individually, or in small clusters or sheet-like masses. Scattered inflammatory cells, mainly lymphocytes, are present, occasionally situated in small, loose clusters. Mitotic figures may be evident but atypical forms are not present. Small stromal haemorrhages are common as are deposits of haemosiderin either as fine cytoplasmic granules within the stromal cells or small macrophages, or as large, extracellular clumps. Zones of ischaemic necrosis may occur secondary to fracture. The lesion is sharply demarcated from the adjacent uninvolved bone, scalloping it without permeation.

BFH must be distinguished from fibrohistiocytic degenerative or repair tissue that

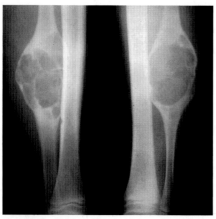

Fig. 13.01 Benign fibrous histiocytoma. A well defined, lytic lesion involves the mid- diaphysis of the fibula in a 10-year- old boy. The lesion expands and scallops the bone.

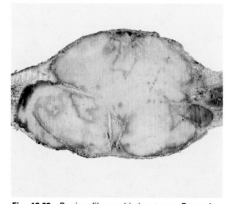

Fig. 13.02 Benign fibrous histiocytoma. Resection specimen of the same lesion (Fig. 13.01) shows a pale, cream-yellow cut surface with focal rust brown areas along its periphery. Marked cortical thinning and endosteal scalloping are evident.

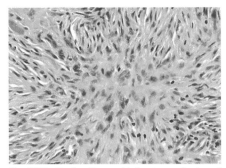

Fig. 13.03 Benign fibrous histiocytoma. Centre of storiform focus shows spindle cells, whose nuclei are elongated or oval with a fine chromatin pattern. Note intracytoplasmic haemosiderin.

occurs in other bone lesions, most notably and frequently in GCT of long bones {180,365,1468}. In an adult with a lytic, destructive lesion at the end of a long bone, careful search for residual foci of GCT must be made before making a diagnosis of BFH {180}.

BFH is histologically indistinguishable from non-ossifying fibroma (NOF), being separated from the latter only on clinical and radiological grounds {1875,2286}, i.e., its location in non-long bones, or lack of metaphyseal involvement if in a long bone; its usual occurrence in older patients; the presence of pain even in the absence of pathological fracture; and a radiological pattern that may lack the well defined, sclerotic, bubble-type margins typical of NOF.

Immunophenotype
There are no specific marker proteins.

Prognostic factors
The prognosis is excellent, surgical curettage / resection usually being curative.

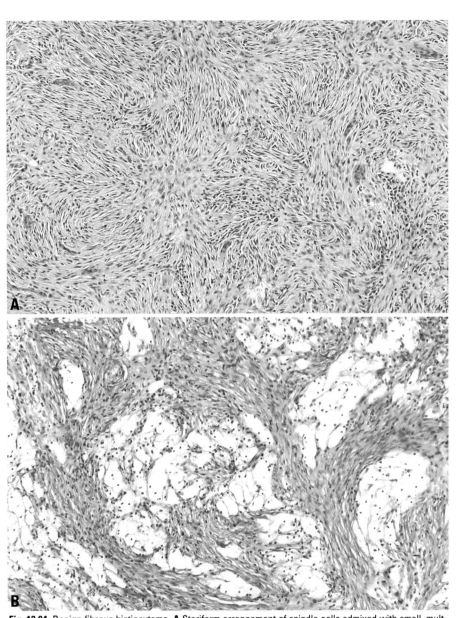

Fig. 13.04 Benign fibrous histiocytoma. **A** Storiform arrangement of spindle cells admixed with small, multinucleated osteoclast-like giant cells. Loose clusters of lymphoid cells are also present. **B** Clusters of foam cells with pale cytoplasm and small, dark nuclei are seen interspersed among whorled spindle cells. Such foam cells may be absent or so extensive as to dominate the lesion.

Malignant fibrous histiocytoma of bone

G.C. Steiner
G. Jundt
J.A. Martignetti

Definition
Malignant fibrous histiocytoma (MFH) defines a malignant neoplasm composed of fibroblasts and pleomorphic cells with a prominent storiform pattern.

ICD-O code   8830/3

Synonyms
MFH was initially described in the bone in 1972 by Feldman and Norman {647}, although similar tumours were earlier described in the soft tissue by Stout and co-workers in 1963 {1632} and 1964 {1589}. MFH has also been termed malignant histiocytoma, xanthosarcoma, malignant fibrous xanthoma and fibroxanthosarcoma.

Epidemiology
Males are more frequently affected than females. MFH of bone is a relatively rare tumour which represents less than 2% of all primary malignant bone lesions. The age of patients at the time of diagnosis is broad and usually varies from the 2nd to 8th decades, with a higher incidence in adults over 40 years of age. Approximately 10-15% of cases occur in patients less than 20 years of age. MFH can arise as a primary bone tumour or may develop secondary to pre-existing bone conditions such as Paget disease or bone infarct, or at the site of bone which was irradiated for the treatment of osseous or extraosseous tumours {503,997,1367}. Secondary MFH accounts for approximately 28% of all MFH {305,538,990, 1571,1648}.

Sites of involvement
Primary MFH predilects the long bones of the lower extremities, particularly the femur (30-45%), followed by tibia and humerus. The knee is a common location, with concurrent involvement of the distal femur and proximal tibia {193}. Among the trunk bones, the pelvis is most frequently involved. Almost all MFH are solitary lesions, but rare multifocal tumours have been reported {1367}.

Clinical features / Imaging
Clinically, most patients complain of pain and, less frequently, swelling that varies from 1 week to 3 years (average 7-9 months). Rarely, a pathological fracture may be the initial presenting symptom.
MFH in the long bones predilects the metaphyseal region with epiphyseal extension in some cases. Diaphyseal location is infrequent. The tumours are essentially osteolytic lesions, but sclerotic areas may be present. The margins are usually ill defined and a moth-eaten or permeative pattern of bone destruction can be observed. Some tumours have well defined borders. The cortex is commonly involved and destroyed by the tumour with often soft tissue extension. Periosteal reaction is not a frequent finding {1272,1522}.

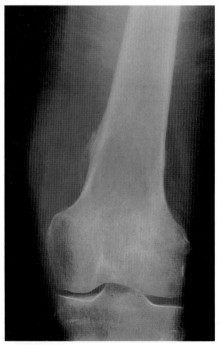

Fig. 13.05 Malignant fibrous histiocytoma of the distal femur, presenting as large, lytic lesion with ill defined margins and focal periosteal reaction.

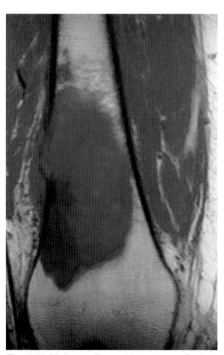

Fig. 13.06 Malignant fibrous histiocytoma. Sagittal T1-weighted MR image showing a large medullary lesion with focal soft tissue extension.

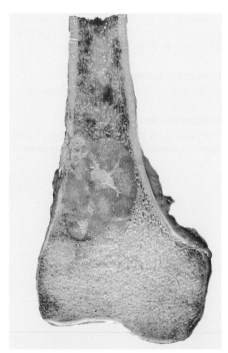

Fig. 13.07 Malignant fibrous histiocytoma. Greyish-white, circumscribed tumour with yellowish necrotic area, focally destroying the cortex (left).

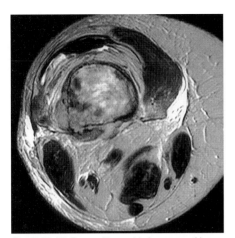

Fig. 13.08 Malignant fibrous histiocytoma of bone. Axial T2-weighted MR image demonstrating an inhomogeneous lesion with cortical destruction and soft tissue extension.

MFH occurring in metaphyseal location can be very aggressive {1522}. The radiographic features of primary MFH are nonspecific and in older patients can mimic lymphoma, myeloma or osteolytic metastases. In younger patients, osteosarcoma and Ewing sarcoma are included in the differential diagnosis. MRI usually helps to demonstrate the intra- and extraosseous extent of the tumour, but the imaging features are not specific to differentiate MFH from other tumours. However, the presence of an eccentric lytic and diaphyseal lesion with cortical destruction and soft tissue extension, or a metaphyseal lytic lesion that extends to the epiphysis but not to the subchondral bone, should raise suspicion of MFH {1272,1522}.

In secondary MFH arising in Paget disease and bone infarct, the radiographs indicate the presence of an underlying bone process in most cases.

Macroscopy

The gross appearance of this tumour is not characteristic. It varies in colour from tan to greyish-white, soft to firm in consistency. Areas of yellowish discolouration, necrosis and haemorrhage are frequently seen. The margins are irregular and often cortical destruction and soft tissue infiltration are present.

Histopathology

Microscopically, MFH consists mainly of a mixed population of spindle cells, histiocytoid and pleomorphic cells. Varying amounts of multinucleated giant cells of the osteoclast type are seen as well as foamy cells and chronic inflammatory cells. The nuclei of the tumour cells may be quite atypical, particularly in the malignant giant cells. Typical and atypical mitoses are present. There is a variability of cellular patterns within these tumours. A characteristic storiform pattern is commonly seen in the fibroblastic areas, in which bundles of spindle cells are arranged in a storiform or pinwheel pattern.

Different histological subtypes have been described in MFH of soft tissue and bone: storiform–pleomorphic, histiocytic, myxoid, giant cell, and inflammatory. The storiform-pleomorphic is the most common histological subtype in bone. The myxoid pattern is rare. Most MFH are high grade tumours, but a few low grade lesions have been reported {305,538, 990,1571,1648}.

Immunophenotype

Immunomarkers are of limited value in the diagnosis of MFH of bone. They are useful to rule out other malignant neoplasms that may resemble MFH such as leiomyosarcomas, metastatic carcinomas and melanomas {675}. Vimentin is strongly positive in tumour cells. Smooth muscle actin, indicative of myofibroblastic differentiation, may be focally positive. The presence of cytokeratin immunoreactivity in MFH is nonspecific. CD68 reactivity may be present in the tumour

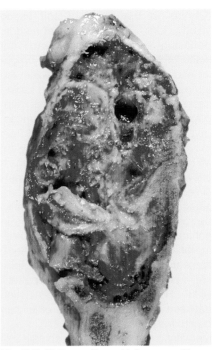

Fig. 13.09 Malignant fibrous histiocytoma of bone. Gross photograph of resected specimen shows yellowish brown, partly cystic tumour tissue.

cells but is not a specific marker for histiocytes and therefore of no diagnostic significance {69,2051}.

Differential diagnosis

MFH may have foci of osteoid or primitive bone formation at the periphery of the

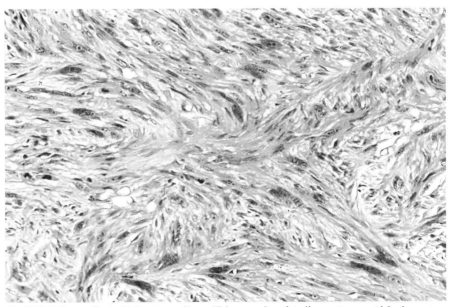

Fig. 13.10 Malignant fibrous histiocytoma of bone. High power view of storiform pattern containing large atypical tumour cells.

tumours in the areas of soft tissue involvement. This usually represents periosteal reactive bone and not osteosarcoma {990}. Also, foci of irregular and coarse collagen fibres within the tumour, which are present in some cases, can be misinterpreted as neoplastic osteoid. In these instances, detailed histological evaluation will help to rule out osteosarcoma, particularly the MFH-like variant of osteosarcoma, which shows unequivocal evidence of mineralised osteoid and bone {1528}. Fibrosarcoma often overlaps histologically, clinically and radiologically with MFH. In contrast to MFH, which contains pleomorphic cells and a storiform pattern, fibrosarcoma consists of bundles of spindle cells with a herringbone pattern {538}. However, histological distinction between one tumour and the other can be arbitrary.

Metastatic carcinoma with a spindle cell component and melanoma should be distinguished from MFH by the use of appropriate immunomarkers.

Genetics

In 5/7 sporadic MFHs, LOH was found for markers within the 9p21-22 region, and the minimally defined region of LOH could be narrowed down even further {1338}. Loss of the 9p21-22 region in bone MFH has previously also been noted using comparative genomic hybridization {1957}. The LOH results are in accord with mutation studies which suggest that CDKN2A is not the critical gene {2096}.

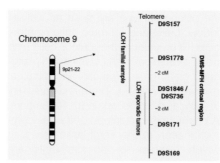

Fig. 13.11 Malignant fibrous histiocytoma of bone. Minimal region of deletion on chromosome arm 9p.

Genetic susceptibility

Diaphyseal medullary stenosis with malignant fibrous histiocytoma (DMS-MFH) is a rare, autosomal dominant bone dysplasia / cancer syndrome of unknown aetiology {85,886}. The skeletal phenotype is characterized by cortical growth abnormalities, including diffuse diaphyseal medullary stenosis with overlying endosteal cortical thickening, metaphyseal striations, and scattered infarctions and sclerotic areas throughout the long bones. Notably, malignant transformation has occurred in 13 of 40 patients in the five reported DMS-MFH families {85,886, 1337,1521,1583}. Malignant fibrous histiocytoma has been the consistent diagnosis in all the tumours studied.

Using a positional cloning strategy, the DMS-MFH gene was localized in three unrelated families to chromosome bands 9p21-22 with a maximal two-point LOD score of 5.49 {1337}.

Haplotype analysis narrowed the boundaries of the gene locus to an ~3 cM region. These results were independently corroborated in another DMS-MFH family {1521}.

Prognostic factors

MFH is a highly malignant neoplasm with frequent tendency to metastasis, particularly to the lungs (45-50%). The recommended treatment is wide surgical excision. In those patients with histologically high grade and resectable lesions, preoperative chemo therapy appears to be the standard of care. The chemotherapy regimen is similar to that used in osteosarcoma. The degree of tumour necrosis in the resected specimen after chemotherapy is apparently an important prognostic factor, as in the management of osteosarcoma {193,1648}. In patients with localized disease, the 5-year disease-free survival has been reported to be over 50% {246,1648}. Radiotherapy is used particularly in patients with inadequate surgical treatment.

Favourable prognostic factors are: younger age at manifestation (under 40 years); adequate surgical margins and histological low grade. Some authors report that a prominent chronic inflammatory infiltrate is associated with a better prognosis, as opposed to the presence of prominent desmoplasia with hyalinization {2325}. The histological subtype of the lesion does not affect the prognosis.

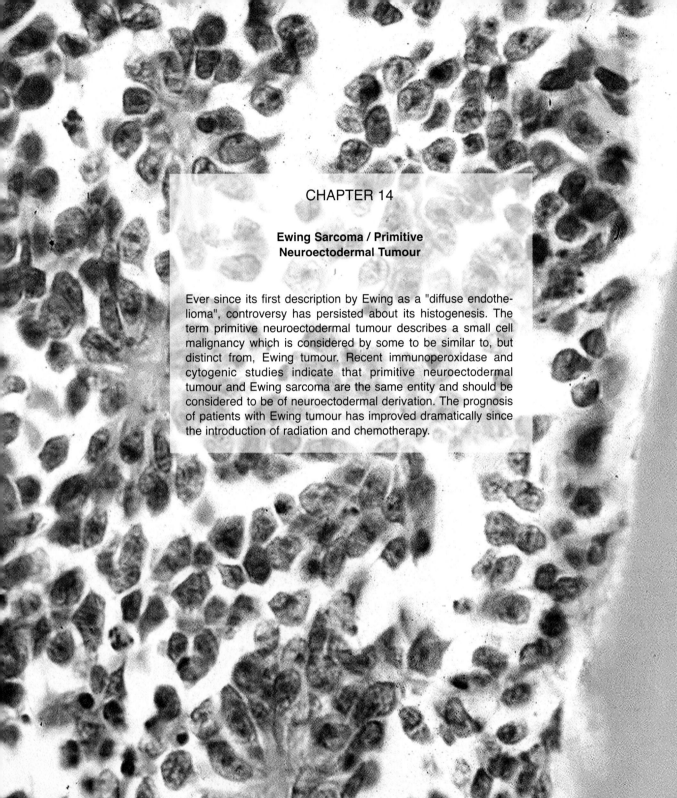

CHAPTER 14

Ewing Sarcoma / Primitive
Neuroectodermal Tumour

Ever since its first description by Ewing as a "diffuse endothe-
lioma", controversy has persisted about its histogenesis. The
term primitive neuroectodermal tumour describes a small cell
malignancy which is considered by some to be similar to, but
distinct from, Ewing tumour. Recent immunoperoxidase and
cytogenic studies indicate that primitive neuroectodermal
tumour and Ewing sarcoma are the same entity and should be
considered to be of neuroectodermal derivation. The prognosis
of patients with Ewing tumour has improved dramatically since
the introduction of radiation and chemotherapy.

Ewing sarcoma / Primitive neuroectodermal tumour (PNET)

S. Ushigome
R. Machinami
P.H. Sorensen

Definition

Ewing sarcoma and PNET are defined as round cell sarcomas that show varying degrees of neuroectodermal differentiation. The term Ewing sarcoma has been used for those tumours that lack evidence of neuroectodermal differentiation as assessed by light microscopy, immunohistochemistry, and electron microscopy, whereas, the term PNET has been employed for tumours that demontrate neuroectodermal features as evaluated by one or more of these modalities.

ICD-O codes

Ewing sarcoma   9260/3
PNET   9364/3
Askin tumour   9365/3

Synonyms

Ewing tumour, peripheral neuroepithelioma, peripheral neuroblastoma, Askin tumour.

Epidemiology

Ewing sarcoma / PNET is relatively uncommon accounting for 6-8% of primary malignant bone tumours and is less common than myeloma, osteosarcoma and chondrosarcoma. It is the second most common sarcoma in bone and soft tissue in children. Ewing sarcoma / PNET shows a predilection for males with the ratio of 1.4 to 1. Nearly 80% of patients are younger than 20 years, and the peak age incidence is during the second decade of life. Patients older than 30 are extremely uncommon. Ewing sarcoma / PNET rarely arises in Blacks.

Sites of involvement

Ewing sarcoma / PNET tends to arise in the diaphysis or metaphyseal-diaphyseal portion of long bones. The pelvis and ribs are also common locations. The skull, vertebra, scapula, and short tubular bones of hands and feet are rarely involved.

Clinical features / Imaging

Pain and a mass in the involved area are the most common clinical symptoms. Fever (remittent, about 38°C), anaemia, leukocytosis and increase in sedimentation rate are often seen. Pathological fracture is an uncommon complication. Radiographically, an ill defined osteolytic lesion involving the diaphysis of a long tubular bone or flat bone is the most common feature. Permeative or moth-eaten bone destruction often associated with "onion-skin" like multilayered periosteal reaction is characteristic. The cortex overlying the tumour is irregularly thinned or thickened. A large, ill-defined soft tissue mass is a frequent association in Ewing tumour. Expansile bone destruction with soap-bubble appearance might be seen.

MRI and CT study help demonstrate the extent of the tumour in the bone and soft tissue.

Macroscopy

The tumour in bone and soft tissue is tan–grey and often necrotic and haemorrhagic. Necrotic yellowish and semi-fluid tissue obtained from intramedullary or subperiosteal lesion at open biopsy might grossly be erroneously interpreted as pus by surgeons. Some soft tissue tumours may be associated with a large peripheral nerve.

Histopathology

The morphology of the tumour is variable. Most cases are composed of uniform small round cells with round nuclei containing fine chromatin, scanty clear or eosinophilic cytoplasm, and indistinct cytoplasmic membranes, whereas in others, the tumour cells are larger, have prominent nucleoli, and irregular contours {1540}. The cytoplasm of the tumour cells frequently contains PAS positive glycogen. In soft tissue tumours, the tumour cells rarely have a spindle cell morphology. In some cases Homer–Wright rosettes are present {2161}. Necrosis is common with viable

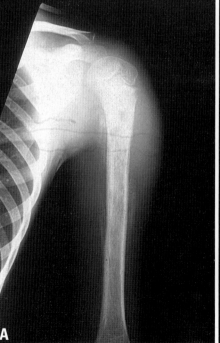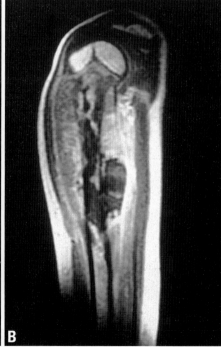

Fig. 14.01 Ewing sarcoma of the left humerus in a 6-year-old boy. **A** Periosteal new bone formation showing "onion-skin" appearance. **B** Axial T1-weighted MRI of the same lesion. Both intraosseous and extraosseous tumours are more clearly demonstrated than on plain X-ray.

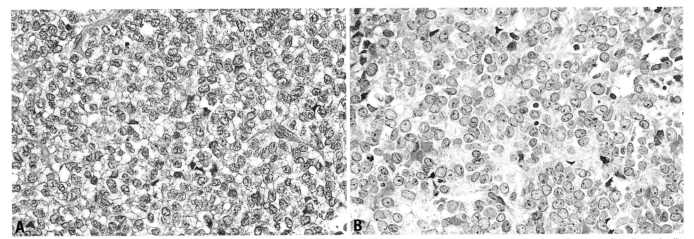

Fig. 14.02 Ewing sarcoma. **A** Uniform round cells with uniform round nuclei. **B** Histology of Ewing tumour / PNET predominantly composed of rosettes of small round cells and luminal fibrillary processes.

cells frequently perivascular in distribution.

Immunophenotype

CD99 is expressed in almost all cases in a characteristic membranous fashion, though it is not specific. Vimentin stains most tumour cells and neural markers such as neuron specific enolase (NSE), are frequently expressed. Ewing sarcoma / PNET has also been shown to stain with keratin in some cases.

Ultrastructure

Ewing sarcoma / PNET is composed of primitive round to oval tumour cells often with glycogen aggregates in the cytoplasm. Fine cytoplasmic processes are often observed. Primitive intercellular junctions are often seen. Neurosecretory granules (100-150 nm) and microtubules may be present.

Genetics

The Ewing family of tumours (EFT) is characterized by a recurrent t(11;22) (q24;q12) chromosomal translocation,

detectable in approximately 85% of the cases {96,2146,2257}. Secondary chromosomal aberrations, notably gains of chromosome arm 1q and chromosomes 8 and 12 occur in more than half of the cases. Molecular cloning of the t(11;22) breakpoints revealed an in-frame fusion between the 5' end of the *EWS* gene from chromosome band 22q12 with the 3' portion of the 11q24 *FLI1* gene, a member of the ETS family of transcription factors {497,1360}. It was subsequently found that another 10-15% of cases have a variant t(21;22)(q22;q12) translocation fusing *EWS* to a closely related ETS gene, *ERG* from chromosome band 21q22 {790,1995,2351}. In 1% or less of EFT cases, t(7;22), t(17;22), and t(2;22) translocations and inv(22) have been described that give rise to fusions between *EWS* and the *ETS* genes *ETV1*, *E1AF*, *FEV*, and *ZSG*, respectively {1038,1060,1693,2159}. Therefore, virtually all EFTs appear to express some form of *EWS/ETS* gene fusion {496}. Chimeric transcripts analysed to date all encode the N-terminal transcriptional

activation domain of EWS fused to the C-terminal DNA binding domain of the ETS partner (reviewed in {89}). EWS/FLI1 has potent oncogenic activity {1360}, and many studies have suggested that it and other EWS/ETS chimeric proteins function as aberrant transcription factors binding to ETS target genes {111,1242, 1361,1598}. In this regard, a number of up-regulated genes have been identified in EWS/FLI1 expressing cells {88, 248, 1359, 2110}. One target is suggested by the observation that EWS/ETS proteins down-regulate expression of the TGF-β type II receptor (TGFBR2), a putative tumour suppressor {865,1003}. TGF-β signalling induces apoptosis in many cell types, and, therefore, repression of TGFBR2 may provide EFT cells with a mechanism to avoid programmed cell death. Inactivation of the INK4a locus encoding the CDKN2A cell cycle inhibitor is the second most common genetic alteration in EFTs {1162}. The significance of this finding is underscored by the recent observation that loss of CDKN2A stabilises the EWS/FLI1 onco-

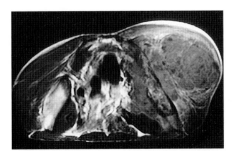

Fig. 14.03 Ewing sarcoma. MRI (T1 image) of pelvic tumour showing a huge soft tissue mass outside and inside the iliac wing.

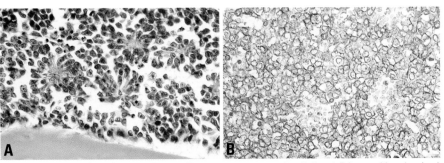

Fig. 14.04 Ewing sarcoma / PNET. **A** Rosette-like structures are occasionally found. **B** Immunohistochemi-cal expression of CD99 showing characteristic reactivity on the cell membranes.

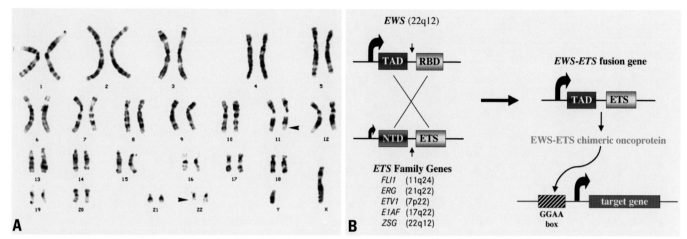

Fig. 14.05 Ewing sarcoma. **A** Karyotype showing the most common rearrangement, a translocation t(11;22)(q24;q12). Arrowheads indicate breakpoints. **B** Schematic diagram of *EWS-ETS* gene fusions in Ewing family of tumours.

protein {501}, and that *CDKN2A* mutations may be associated with poor outcome in EFTs {2228}.

Genetic diagnostic approaches include chromosome banding analysis, interphase fluorescence in situ hybridisation, RT-PCR assays, and Southern blotting. It is advisable to have available more than one diagnostic modality, to be able to confirm unexpected or discrepant results {126,549,1181,1204,1380,1694,1996}.

Detection of fusion transcripts in peripheral blood or bone marrow is a sensitive marker of minimal residual disease {462,

2252,2348}, although the clinical significance of such a finding remains to be determined {94,1380}

Prognostic factors

The prognosis in Ewing sarcoma / PNET has improved in the modern era of treatment and current survival rate is estimated to be 41%. Important prognostic features include the stage, anatomic location and the size of the tumour. Tumours, that are metastatic at the time of diagnosis, arise in the pelvis, and are large tend to do poorly. In addition to its diagnostic

utility, *EWS/ETS* fusion status also provides prognostic information. Further diversity of these rearrangements is conferred by different combinations of exons from *EWS* and its partner genes giving rise to variably sized chimeric proteins {2351}. Among loco-regional tumours with *EWS/FLI1* gene fusions, the most common so-called type 1 gene fusion (in which *EWS* exon 7 is fused to *FLI1* exon 6) has been reported to be associated with a better prognosis than cases with larger, less common, fusion types {460}.

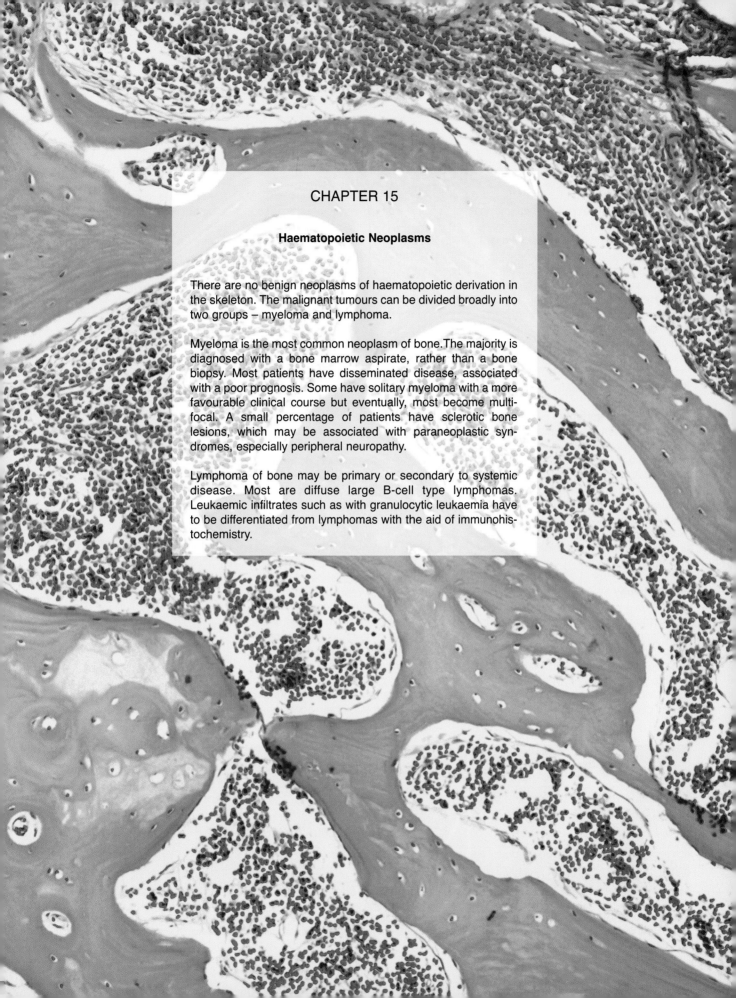

CHAPTER 15

Haematopoietic Neoplasms

There are no benign neoplasms of haematopoietic derivation in the skeleton. The malignant tumours can be divided broadly into two groups – myeloma and lymphoma.

Myeloma is the most common neoplasm of bone. The majority is diagnosed with a bone marrow aspirate, rather than a bone biopsy. Most patients have disseminated disease, associated with a poor prognosis. Some have solitary myeloma with a more favourable clinical course but eventually, most become multifocal. A small percentage of patients have sclerotic bone lesions, which may be associated with paraneoplastic syndromes, especially peripheral neuropathy.

Lymphoma of bone may be primary or secondary to systemic disease. Most are diffuse large B-cell type lymphomas. Leukaemic infiltrates such as with granulocytic leukaemia have to be differentiated from lymphomas with the aid of immunohistochemistry.

Plasma cell myeloma

F.J. Martinez-Tello
M. Calvo–Asensio
J.C. Lorenzo-Roldan

Definition

Plasma cell myeloma is a monoclonal neoplastic proliferation of plasma cells of bone-marrow derivation, usually multicentric, that eventually infiltrates various organs but rarely produces plasma cell leukaemia. It is characterized by osteolytic lesions, bone pain, hypercalcemia, a monoclonal gammopathy, and disorders due to depositon of abnormal immunoglobulin chains (amyloid) in various tissues, including kidney.

ICD-O code   9732/3

Synonyms and variants

Myeloma, multiple myeloma.
The following variants of plasma cell myeloma have been described {844}: non-secretory myeloma, indolent myeloma , smoldering myeloma, plasma–cell leukaemia (PCL), in addition to extramedullary plasmacytoma, and solitary plasmacytoma of bone. The exact distinction is based on clinical and radiographic features.

Epidemiology

Plasma cell myeloma is the most frequent tumour that occurs primarily in bone and the most common lymphoid neoplasm in Blacks and the second most common in Whites. It is rare in individuals younger than 40 years (less than 10%). Most patients are in the sixth and seven decades of life. The median age at diagnosis is 68 years in males and 70 in females. Both sexes are equally affected {512}.

Sites of involvement

The bones that contain haematologic marrow in adults are the most frequently involved: vertebrae, ribs, skull, pelvis, femur, clavicle and scapula {843,1850}.

Clinical features / Imaging

The extensive osteolytic skeletal lesions cause bone pain, pathological fractures, hypercalcemia and anaemia. The lumbar or thoracic spinal regions are most often affected by pain. Frequently a pathological fracture is the first symptom. Most fractures affect the spine. Neurologic symptoms due to spinal cord or nerve roots lesions, secondary to extraosseous extension of the tumour or pathological fracture, are frequently observed. Peripheral neuropathy is increasingly observed with the osteosclerotic variant of multiple myeloma but it is rare with classic plasma cell myeloma {2155}. Anaemia is a consequence of marrow destruction and renal damage with resultant loss of erythropoetin {122}. An M-component is found in the serum or urine in 99% of the patients. The monoclonal proteins are in 50% of the cases of the IgG class, 25-20% of the IgA class, and, rarely, of the IgM, IgD or IgE classes. Biclonal gammapathies are found in 1% and a monoclonal light chain (Bence-Jones protein) is found in the serum in 75% of the patients {1850}. Renal failure is the result of tubular lesions due to monoclonal light chain

Table 15.01
Diagnostic criteria for plasma cell myeloma.

Major criteria:
> Plasmacytoma on biopsy
> Marrow plasmacytosis (>30%)
> M component:
Serum IgG>3.5g/dl, IgA>2g/dl
Urine ->Ig/24 hr or kappa or lambda
(Bence Jones protein) without amyloidosis

Minor criteria:
> Marrow plasmacytosis (10-30%)
> M component present but less than listed above
> Lytic bone lesions
> Reduced normal levels of immunoglobulins (<50% normal: IgG <600mg/dl, IgA<100 mg/dl, IgM<50mg/dl)

The diagnosis of myeloma requires a minimum of one major and one minor criterion or three minor criteria, which must include the first two. These criteria must be present in a clinical setting of symptomatic and progressive disease.

From references {843,1850}.

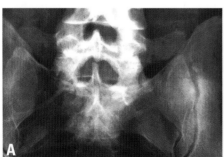
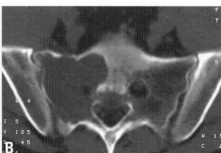
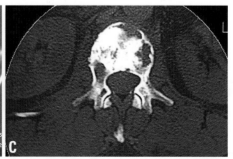

Fig. 15.01 Plasma cell myeloma. **A** Plain radiograph of the lumbo-sacral region of the spine shows a very light radiolucency of the right wing of the sacrum. **B** CT scan of the same patient, at the level of S2, shows loss of the cancellous bone of the right wing of the sacrum, of a large area of the vertebral body, and small scalloping of the endosteal surface of the cortical bone. **C** Patient with POEMS syndrome with multiple lesions in the skeleton. CT scan of L1 with extensive radiodense areas, and points of disruption in the anterior cortex.

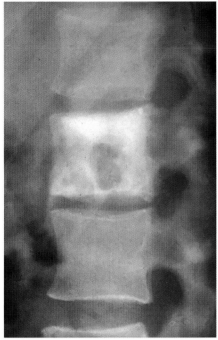

Fig. 15.02 Plasma cell myeloma. Patient with POEMS syndrome with multiple lesions in the skeleton. X-ray of the dorso-lumbar region of the spine showing marked radiodensity with a less radiodense central area. The discal space L1-L2 is typically diminished.

Erosions of the cortex are commonly observed but prominent periosteal new bone formation is not. Expansion of the affected bone may occur in bones with a small diameter, such as the ribs. The earliest and more severe changes are seen in the skull, vertebrae, ribs and pelvis. About 12-25% of patients have no detectable foci of bone destruction at presentation but may show generalised osteoporosis {2155}. Solitary myeloma lesions are also typically lytic and may also expand the bone. Infrequently the lesions in plasma cell myeloma may be sclerotic, which are typical for the very rare POEMS syndrome (polyneuropathy, organomegaly, endocrinopathy, monoclonal gammopathy, skin changes) {122, 871}. CT and MRI studies may discover a very subtle small lesion not visible on plain radiographs. The features of MRI are variable, because plasma cell myeloma does not involve the marrow in a homogeneous fashion and because the extent of fatty marrow replacement which varies with age. For differential diagnosis metastatic carcinoma, malignant lymphoma, and hyperparathyroidism have to be considered. The lesions of metastatic carcinoma and malignant lymphoma are usually positive on bone scan, whereas those of myeloma are usually not {538}.

Aetiology

The aetiology is largely unknown. Possible, but unproven, aetiologic factors include long standing chronic infections (chronic osteomyelitis, rheumatoid arthritis, etc.), exposure to low level radiation (radiologists, nuclear plant work-

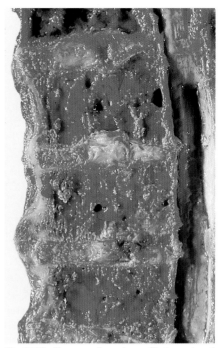

Fig. 15.03 Plasma cell myeloma. Photographs of gross autopsy specimens. The normal bone structure and bone marrow of the vertebral bodies are replaced by a gelatinous haemorrhagic tissue.

ers), and exposure to asbestos, pesticides, petroleum products, rubber, plastic and wood products {1851}. Some cases of POEMS syndrome have been associated with Kaposi sarcoma / human herpesvirus 8 infection {154,1467}.

Macroscopy

Biopsy or curettage samples show fragments of tan-grey soft tissue. At autopsy, soft pink or grey friable masses are the

proteinuria. The patients have often recurrent bacterial infections, partially because a decreased normal immunoglobulin production due to displacement by the neoplastic clone.

The myelomatous bone lesions are lytic, sharply demarcated lesions, being the consequence of replacement of bone trabeculae by tumour tissue, are not surrounded by a sclerotic zone and may reach 5 cm in its greatest diameter.

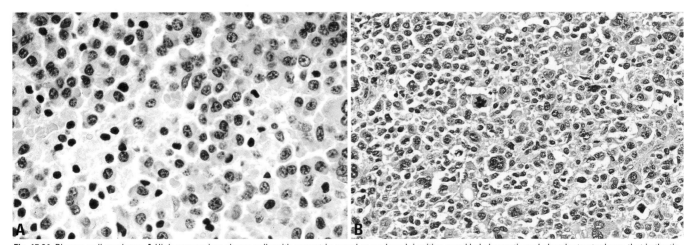

Fig. 15.04 Plasma cell myeloma. **A** High power view shows cells with eccentric round or oval nuclei, with a speckled chromatin and abundant cytoplasm, that in the tissue section stains pink. **B** Poorly differentiated plasma cell myeloma, showing cellular pleomorphism with frequent multinucleated cells and atypical mito-tic features, consistent with the term "anaplastic myeloma".

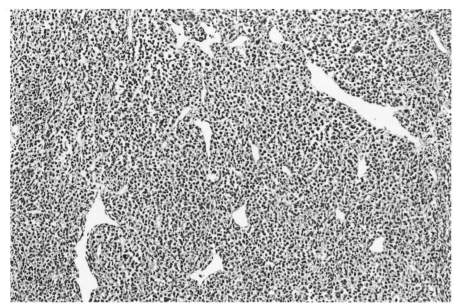

Fig. 15.05 Plasma cell myeloma. Low power appearance shows a rich vascular pattern. The tumour cells surround the vascular channels, simulating a haemangiopericytomatous pattern.

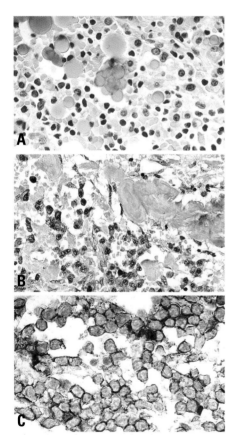

Fig. 15.06 Plasma cell myeloma. **A** A so called "Mott cell" is shown in the centre of the picture, with grape-like cytoplasmic inclusions. The cell is surrounded by numerous Russell bodies. **B** Plasma cell myeloma containing amyloid. Deposition of pale, waxy amorphous proteinaceous material in between neoplastic plasma cells (Congo red stain). **C** Immunoexpression of CD 138 in almost all neoplastic cells.

typical appearance. Diffuse involvement of bone marrow and discrete nodules are also common. Some plasma cell myelomas may simulate a lymphoma showing a fish-flesh appearance. It is quite common to see expansion of the affected bone and extraossous extension, collapse of one or several vertebral bodies and pathological fractures. Very infrequently the tumour masses have a grey, waxy appearance due to extensive amyloid deposition. Unusual cases have a combination of lytic and sclerotic changes.

Histopathology

Plasma cell myeloma is a neoplasm of round or oval cells of the plasma cell lineage showing a spectrum of variable features of cellular maturity that have prognostic significance. Well differentiated tumours show sheets of closely packed cells, that resemble normal plasma cells, with little intercellular matrix. In the histological sections these cells have abundant, dense eosinophilic cytoplasm and show distinct cell outlines. The nucleus is eccentric, with the chromatin clustered at the periphery, often showing a cartwheel appearance and a prominent nucleolus. Mitotic figures are rare in well differentiated plasma cell myeloma The cytological features are better observed in Giemsa stained preparations in which the cytoplasm is basophilic with a perinuclear

clear zone that correspond ultrastructurally to a well developed RER and a prominent Golgi centre, respectively. The tumour cells may accumulate immuno-globulins in the cytoplasm and show a morular appearance or "Mott cells". Extracellular globules of polymerized immunoglobulines, called Russell bodies, may be also observed. The cells of less differentiated tumours show nuclei with less clumping of the chromatin and enlarged nucleoli, and the cytoplasmic membrane becomes indistinct. The poorly differentiated plasma cell myeloma may show atypical cells, with occasional double nuclei, brisk mitotic activity and atypical mitotic figures making difficult to recognize the plasma cell nature of the cells.

Immunophenotype

Myeloma cells have the same features as normal plasma cells and express their own distinct antigen [plasma cell associated antigen (PCA, CD38)] {1270}. Plasma cell myeloma characteristically expreses monotypic cytoplasmic Ig and lacks surface Ig. In about 85% both heavy and light chains are produced, but in the remaining cases light chain only is expressed (Bence–Jones myeloma) {1178}. The monotypic expression of kappa or lambda immunoglobulin by the tumour cells establishes the diagnosis of malignancy {2169}. Myeloma cells frequently express the natural killer antigen CD56/58 which is not expressed in reactive plasma cells {405}. The majority of myelomas lack the pan-B antigens CD19 and CD20, while CD38 and the Ig-associated antigen CD79a are expressed in most cases {1270}, and CD138 {498} is a reliable marker for identifying and quantifying normal and tumoural plasma cells in paraffin sections. Myeloma cells may be positive for EMA {841}. Few cases may express CD10 {842} and occasionally plasma cell myeloma may show aberrant expression of myelomonocytic antigen {123}.

Prognostic factors

Multiple myeloma is generally an incurable disease (median survival 3 years; 10% survival at 10 years {560,1850}. A shorter survival time is associated with a higher stage {133,561}, renal insufficiency {133,561}, degree of marrow replacement by tumour cells {1154}, cellular immaturity and atypia {1851}, high Ki-67 proliferation antigen levels {842} and chromosome deletion of 13q14 and 17p13 {1682}. The lack or weak expression of CD56 delineates a special subset of plasma cell myeloma at diagnosis with a lower osteolytic potential and a trend to develop a PCL {138}. The prognosis is better in solitary lesions.

Table 15.02
Diagnostic criteria of solitary myeloma (plasmacytoma of bone).

Diagnostic criteria
> A single tumour in the bone marrow showing identical macroscopic, microscopic, immunophenotype and genetic features to those of plasma cell myeloma
> Solitary osteolytic lesion on radiological studies
> Absence of other lesions on complete skeletal radiographs
> No evidence of plasmacytosis in the bone marrow away of the solitary lesion

From references {137,719,834,1194,1260,1391}.

Malignant lymphoma

K.K. Unni
P.C.W. Hogendoorn

Definition
Malignant lymphoma is a neoplasm composed of malignant lymphoid cells, producing a tumefactive lesion within bone.

ICD-O code   9590/3

Synonyms
Reticulum cell sarcoma, primary non-Hodgkin lymphoma of bone, Hodgkin lymphoma.

Epidemiology
Malignant lymphoma involving bone is unusual, accounting for approximately 7% of all bone malignancies. Lymphomas involving bone account for about 5% of extranodal lymphoma. Radiographic studies {249} show that 16% of patients with lymphoma have evidence of bone involvement. Patients may be of any age group but there is a tendency to involve adults, especially older adults. There is a male predominance {943}.

Sites of involvement
Lymphoma affects portions of bone with persistent red marrow. The femur is the most commonly involved single site. The spine and the pelvic bones are other common sites. It is extremely unusual to see malignant lymphoma involving the small bones of the hands and feet. When malignant lymphoma presents in the spine or in the maxillary antrum, it is often difficult to know whether the process is primary in bone or in soft tissues.

Clinical features / Imaging
The majority of patients with lymphoma present with bone pain. Some patients present with a palpable mass. Neurological symptoms are common with involvement of the spine. Patients with primary lymphoma of bone rarely present with systemic or B symptoms, such as fever or night sweats. Occasionally, symptoms associated with hypercalcemia, such as constipation, lethargy and somnolence may be present {1512}. Lymphoma involving bone can be separated into four groups:
1) a single skeletal site, with or without regional lymph node involvement;
2) multiple bones are involved, but there is no visceral or lymph node involvement;
3) patients present with a bone tumour but work up shows involvement of other visceral sites or multiple lymph node at multiple sites;
4) the patient has a known lymphoma and a bone biopsy is done to rule out involvement of bone.
Groups 1 and 2 are considered primary lymphoma of bone.
The roentgenographic features are quite variable and somewhat non-specific. In the long bones, the diaphysis tends to be preferentially involved. The tumour tends to involve a large portion of the bone; it is not unusual to see destruction of up to half of the bone. Occasionally, the entire bone is destroyed. The process is poorly demarcated with a wide area of transition from normal bone. There may be variable sclerosis; rarely, the tumour is very sclerotic or entirely lytic. More commonly, however, it is a mixture of lysis and sclerosis. The cortex is frequently destroyed and there is a large soft tissue mass. In a flat bone, such as the pelvis, large areas of destruction with soft tissue extension on either side suggest a diagnosis of lymphoma. Periosteal new bone formation is unusual. A purely sclerotic lesion may be mistaken for Paget disease. If the cortex is not involved, the marrow destruction may not be obvious on plain roentgenograms. Radionuclide bone scan is almost always positive. Magnetic resonance images show signal abnormalities in the marrow,

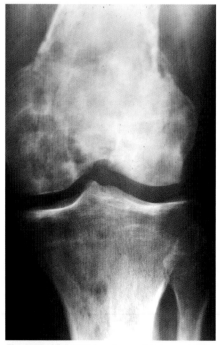

Fig. 15.07 Malignant lymphoma of femur and tibia. Note extensive lytic and sclerotic lesions.

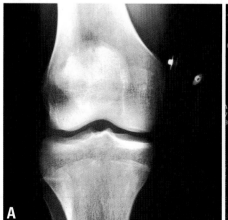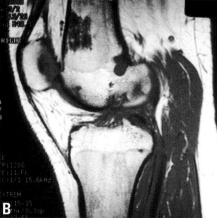

Fig. 15.08 Malignant lymphoma in a 15-year-old boy. **A** Plain roentgenogram does not reveal the lesion. **B** MRI of the same case shows multifocal involvement of bone with signal changes.

whereas the plain roentgenograms may be completely normal.

Macroscopy

It is unusual to see gross specimens of malignant lymphoma involving bone, because the treatment is usually with radiation and/or chemotherapy, following diagnoses made with needle biopsies. However, a portion of bone may be resected if the patient presents with a pathological fracture. Grossly, a large portion of bone is involved, with cortical destruction. The lesion has the soft fish-flesh appearance of lymphoma elsewhere in the body.

Histopathology

The majority of lymphomas involving the skeleton show a diffuse growth pattern. Although bone marrow involvement is not uncommon in follicular small cleaved cell lymphoma, it is unusual to have this type of lymphoma present as a destructive bone tumour. Similarly, chronic lymphocytic leukaemia rarely presents as a tumefactive process. Consequently, most skeletal lymphomas are diffuse large cell type. It has a very characteristic growth pattern similar to involvement elsewhere, and tends to leave behind normal structures, such as medullary bone and marrow fat cells and permeate between these structures. The bony trabeculae may appear normal or may appear thickened or irregular, even pagetoid. 92% of primary non-Hodgkin lymphoma of bone was found to be of the large B cell type and only 3% diffuse follicle centre cell, 3% anaplastic large cell and 2% immunocytoma {943}. The cytological features of the large B-cell type show quite a bit of variation including marked multilobation {1703}. The nuclei tend to be large and irregular with a cleaved appearance. There frequently is a mixture of small, medium and large cells, giving rise to a polymorphic appearance. Nucleoli may be prominent. The cytoplasm is not abundant but may be amphophilic. Fine reticulin fibres are present between individual tumour cells. Occasionally, this gives rise to thick, fibrous bands. Rarely a lymphoma will have so much fibrosis that the tumour cells may spindle, even showing a storiform pattern, leading to an erroneous diagnosis of a sarcoma. Another common finding is associated infiltrate of non-neoplastic small lymphocytes. One problem with the diagnosis of lymphoma in bone is that the cells tend to get crushed. One may not be able to identify individual tumour cells but see complete replacement of the marrow with DNA smears. This may be associated with a very fine fibrosis. If a bone biopsy shows such crush artefact, a diagnosis of malignant lymphoma should be suspected.

Hodgkin lymphoma may involve the skeleton as a manifestation of widespread disease and produce a tumour mass but primary manifestations are

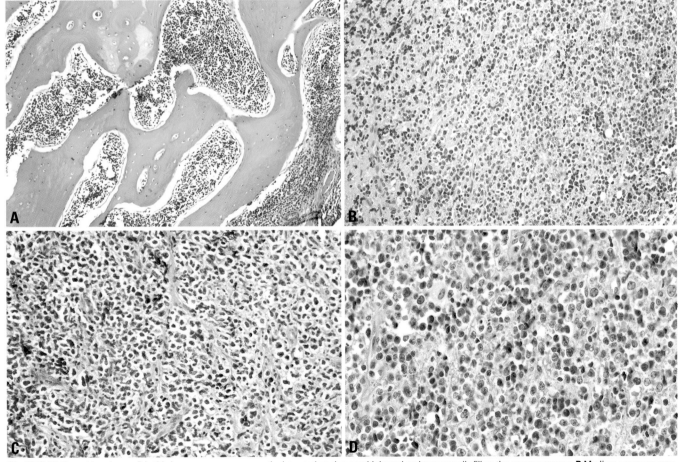

Fig. 15.09 Malignant lymphoma. **A** In this low power appearance, the bony trabeculae are thickened and tumour cells fill up the marrow spaces. **B** Medium power appearance of the neoplastic infiltrate. **C** In some cases lymphoma cells may cluster as shown in this photomicrograph. **D** Although nuclei are round and small there is more variation in size and shape of nuclei than is seen in Ewing sarcoma.

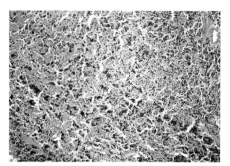

Fig. 15.10 Malignant lymphoma. Crush artefact is frequently present.

rare. Classical Reed-Sternberg cells with bi-lobed nuclei and prominent nucleoli are present but may be difficult to find. More commonly, one finds variants, such as large cells with large nuclei and prominent nucleoli. Variation in size and shape of the cells, especially the presence of plasma cells and eosinophils should alert one to the possibility of Hodgkin lymphoma. Areas of necrosis may be also prominent. Nodular sclerosing Hodgkin lymphoma and mixed cellularity are the usual types {1623}.

Leukaemic infiltrates may produce a tumour mass centred in bone. Patients with chronic or acute myelogenous leukaemia may present with destructive lesions of bone or granulocytic sarcoma {1390}. The clinical course may be indolent {2247}. Histological features of the infiltrating cells recapitulate the features of the systemic disease.

Immunophenotype

Immunoperoxidase stains have become indispensable in the recognition and subclassification of malignant lymphoma. Lymphomas involving bone are usually worked up in the same way as lymph node counterparts. Almost all primary lymphomas involving bone are B-cell neoplasms and hence stain with CD20 {943}. T-cell lymphomas and anaplastic large lymphomas are vanishingly rare. CD15 and CD30 stains recognize Reed-Sternberg cells of Hodgkin disease and myeloperoxidase reactions help support a diagnosis of granulocytic sarcoma.

Genetics

Specific studies on primary lymphomas of bone are lacking.

Prognostic factors

Although the prognosis of lymphoma has been reportedly associated with cell type {544} the most important prognostic indicator is the stage of the disease. Patients with the first two stages do remarkably well, whereas patients with stage 3 and stage 4 disease fare poorly {1626}. Recent data on primary non-Hodgkin lymphoma of bone show a 5-year overall survival of 61%, and 46% of patients progression free at 5 years, notwithstanding heterogeneous treatment in that series {943}. Patients at presentation older than 60 years have a worse overall survival and a worse progression-free period. Patients with the immunoblastic subtype have a worse survival than the centroblastic mono / polymorphic subtype or the centroblastic multilobated subtype. Tumour localization is not found to be a significant prognostic factor. According to the Ann Arbor classification there is no difference in survival between stage I and stage II tumours and just a trend towards worse prognosis in stage IV tumours {943}.

CHAPTER 16

Giant Cell Tumours

Almost any kind of lesion in bone can contain giant cells, some-times numerous. In order to qualify as a giant cell tumour, the neoplasm has to have a combination of round to oval mono-nuclear cells and more or less uniformly distributed giant cells. Moreover, the nuclei of the giant cells should be very similar to those of the mononuclear cells.

Giant cell tumours occur in skeletally mature individuals and there is a slight female predominance. The ends of long bones and the body of the vertebrae are typical sites. The tumour is locally aggressive, but distant metastases are uncommon. When metastases do occur, they rarely prove fatal and hence the term benign metastases is appropriate.

Malignant change in giant cell tumour is uncommon. A sarcoma may co-exist with a giant cell tumour (primary) or may arise at the site of a previously diagnosed giant cell tumour (secondary).

Giant cell tumour

R. Reid
S.S. Banerjee
R. Sciot

Definition
Giant cell tumour is a benign, locally aggressive neoplasm which is composed of sheets of neoplastic ovoid mononuclear cells interspersed with uniformly distributed large, osteoclast-like giant cells.

ICD-O code   9250/1

Synonym
Osteoclastoma.

Epidemiology
Giant cell tumour represents around 4-5% of all primary bone tumours, and approximately 20% of benign primary bone tumours. The peak incidence is between the ages of 20 and 45. Although 10-15% of cases occur in the second decade, giant cell tumour is seldom seen in skeletally immature individuals and very rarely in children below 10 years {299,538,1875,2155}. There is a slight female predominance in some large series. There is no striking racial variation, but there may be some geographic variation.

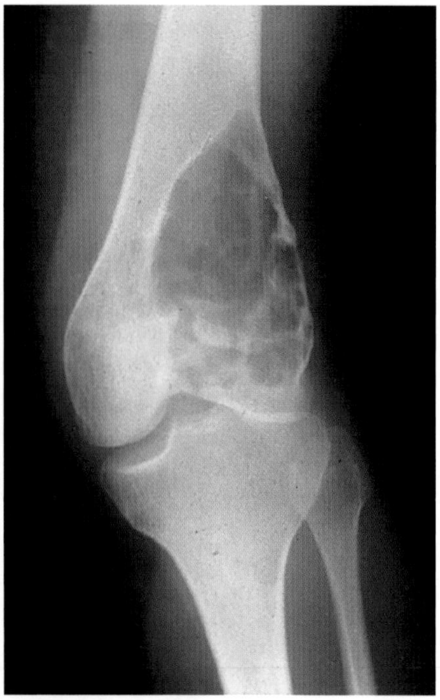

Sites of involvement
Giant cell tumours typically affect the ends of long bones, especially the distal femur, proximal tibia, distal radius and proximal humerus. Around 5% affect flat bones, especially those of the pelvis. The sacrum is the commonest site in the axial skeleton, while other vertebral bodies are less often involved. Fewer than 5% of cases affect the tubular bones of the hands and feet {200}. Multicentric giant cell tumors are very rare and tend to involve the small bones of the distal extremities.
Rarely, tumours with the morphology of giant cell tumour arise primarily within soft tissue {702}.

Clinical features / Imaging
Patients with giant cell tumour typically present with pain, swelling and often limitation of joint movement; pathological fracture is seen in 5-10% of patients. Plain X-rays of lesions in long bones usually show an expanding and eccentric area of lysis. The lesion normally involves the epiphysis and adjacent metaphysis; frequently, there is extension up to the subchondral plate, sometimes with joint involvement. Rarely, the tumour is confined to the metaphysis, usually in adolescents where the tumour lies in relation to an open growth plate, but occasionally also in older adults. Diaphyseal lesions are exceptional.
The margins of the lesion vary; this is the basis of a radiological grading/staging system {299}. Type 1, 'quiescent', lesions have a well-defined margin with surrounding sclerosis and show little, if any, cortical involvement. Type 2, 'active' tumours have well-defined margins, but lack sclerosis; the cortex is thinned and expanded. Type 3, 'aggressive' tumours have ill-defined margins often with cortical destruction and soft tissue extension. This grading system does not correlate well with histological appearances. On occasion, a giant cell tumour has a trabeculated 'soap-bubble' appearance. In the tubular bones of the hands and feet, the x-ray appearances are similar to those seen in long bones. Tumours of sacrum and pelvic bones are also lytic, commonly involve adjacent soft tissues and may affect sacro-iliac and hip joints.
There is seldom much reactive periosteal new bone formation. Only occasionally is radiologically evident matrix produced within the tumour, usually in long standing lesions.
CT scanning gives a more accurate assessment of cortical thinning and penetration than plain radiographs. MR imaging is most useful in assessing the extent of intra-osseous spread and defining soft tissue and joint involvement. Giant cell tumour typically shows low to intermediate signal intensity on T1 weighted images and intermediate to high intensity on T2 images. Large amounts of haemosiderin are often present giving areas of low signal in both modalities.

Macroscopy
The appearance of an intact specimen mirrors the radiological appearances in

Fig. 16.01 Giant cell tumour. Large, expansile area of lysis with a sclerotic border, cortical thinning, and extension to the subchondral plate.

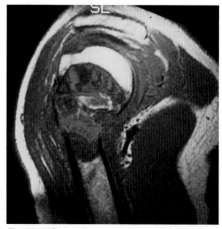

Fig. 16.02 Giant cell tumour of the proximal humerus. MRI shows a well demarcated lesion with focal destruction of cortex and extension into the epiphysis.

its eccentric location and fairly well defined area of bone destruction. This is often bounded by a thin and often incomplete shell of reactive bone. Although the tumour frequently erodes the subchondral bone to reach the deep surface of the articular cartilage, it seldom penetrates it. The tissue is usually soft and reddish brown, but there may be yellowish areas corresponding to xanthomatous change, and firmer whiter areas where there is fibrosis. Blood-filled cystic spaces are sometimes seen and, when extensive, this may cause confusion with an aneurysmal bone cyst.

Histopathology

The characteristic histopathological appearance is of round to oval polygonal or elongated mononuclear cells evenly mixed with numerous osteoclast-like giant cells which may be very large and contain 50 to 100 nuclei. The nuclei of the stromal cells are very similar to those of the osteoclasts, having an open chromatin pattern and one or two small nucleoli. The cytoplasm is ill-defined, and there is little intercellular collagen. Mitotic figures are invariably present; they vary from 2 to 20 per ten high power fields. Atypical mitoses are not, however, seen and their presence should point to a diagnosis of a giant cell rich sarcoma. Occasional binucleate and trinucleate cells are seen.

It is now generally accepted that the characteristic large osteoclastic giant cells are not neoplastic. The mononuclear cells, which represent the neoplastic component, are thought to arise from primitive mesenchymal stromal

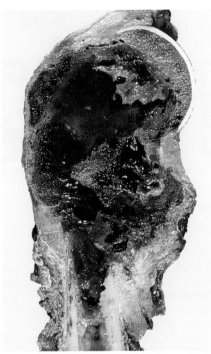

Fig. 16.03 Giant cell tumour. Large haemorrhagic tumour of the proximal humerus with extensive cortical destruction and soft tissue extension.

cells. They express RANKL, which stimulates formation and maturation of osteoclasts from osteoclast precursors {1814,2342}; these cells of monocyte lineage represent a second, minor, component of the mononuclear cells.

There are variations from these standard appearances. In some cases, the mononuclear cells are more spindle shaped, and they may be arranged in a storiform growth pattern. Commonly, small numbers of foam cells are present, and in rare cases this is the predominant pattern thus simulating a fibrous histiocytoma. There may be areas of fibrosis, while secondary aneurysmal bone cyst change occurs in 10% or so. Small foci of bone formation within the tumour are found, especially after pathological fracture or biopsy. When the tumour extends into soft tissue or is present in lung, the histological features are identical to the primary lesion, and there is often a peripheral shell of reactive bone. A striking feature, in one third of cases, is the presence of intravascular plugs, particularly at the periphery of the tumour; this does not appear to be of prognostic significance. Areas of necrosis are common, especially in large lesions. These may be accompanied by focal nuclear atypia which may suggest malignancy.

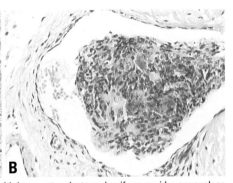

Fig. 16.04 Giant cell tumour. **A** Typical appearance with large osteoclasts and uniform ovoid mononuclear cells. **B** The vascular lumen contains a mixture of spindle and giant cells.

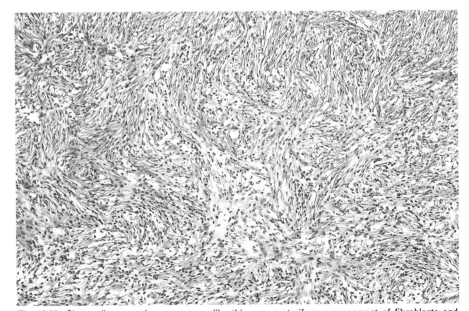

Fig. 16.05 Giant cell tumour. In some cases like this one, a storiform arrangement of fibroblasts and macrophages resembles a benign fibrous histiocytoma.

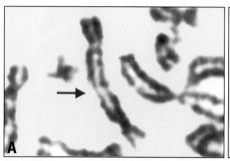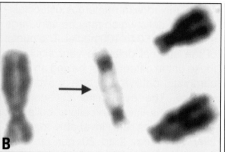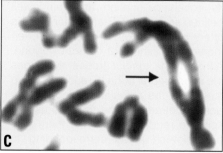

Fig. 16.06 Giant cell tumour. G-banded partial metaphase spreads (**A,B,C**). Telomeric associations are indicated by arrows.

Immunophenotype

The giant cells have the typical immunophenotype of normal osteoclasts, expressing markers of histiocytic lineage.

Genetics

Telomeric association is the most frequent chromosomal aberration. A reduction in telomere length (average loss of 500 base pairs) has been demonstrated in giant cell tumour cells when compared to leukocytes from the same patients {1898}. The telomeres most commonly affected are 11p, 13p, 14p, 15p, 19q, 20q and 21p {262,1644, 1909,2090,2343}. Giant cell tumours with a fibrohistiocytic reaction do not differ karyotypically from the others {1909}. This observation supports the hypothesis that these lesions are true giant cell tumours rather than a different en-tity like a fibroxanthoma. It is of interest that four cases of giant cell tumour also showed rearrangements in 16q22 or 17p13 {262,1488,1909}. These findings might indicate the possible presence of an associated aneurysmal bone cyst. It has been suggested that there is an association between the the presence or absence of chromosomal aberrations and clinical behaviour of giant cell tumours {262}.

Prognostic factors

Giant cell tumour is capable of locally aggressive behaviour and occasionally of distant metastasis. Histology does not predict the extent of local aggression. Following treatment by curettage, supplemented with bone grafting, cementation, cryotherapy, or instillation of phenol, local recurrence occurs in approximately 25% of patients. Recurrence is usually seen within 2 years. Block excision for lesions in small bones results in fewer local recurrences. Pulmonary metastases are seen in 2% of patients with giant cell tumours, on average 3-4 years after primary diagnosis {1947}. These may be solitary or multiple. Some of these metastases are very slow growing (benign pulmonary implants) and some regress spontaneously. A small proportion are progressive and may lead to the death of the patient.

Local recurrence, surgical manipulation and location in distal radius may increase the risk of metastasis {1350}. Histological grading does not appear to be of value in predicting which giant cell tumour will metastasise, providing that giant cell rich sarcomas have been excluded. True malignant transformation is rare {1346}, and often follows radiotherapy.

Malignancy in giant cell tumour

P.G. Bullough
M. Bansal

Definition
Malignancy in GCT is a high grade sarcoma arising in a giant cell tumour (primary) or at the site of previously documented giant cell tumour (secondary).

ICD-O code   9250/3

Synonyms
Malignant giant cell tumour, dedifferentiated giant cell tumour.

Epidemiology
Malignancy arising in a giant cell tumour can occur after treatment usually including radiation or de novo. Most sarcomas arise following radiation therapy. Primary malignant giant cell tumour is the least common type. Overall, malignant transformation can be expected in less than 1% of giant cell tumours. There is a slight female predominance and patients are generally about a decade older than patients with giant cell tumour.

Clinical features / Imaging
The recurrence of pain and swelling many years following treatment of a giant cell tumour should suggest the possibility of malignant transformation. The symptomatology of primary malignant giant cell tumour is non specific. In secondary malignant giant cell tumour plain roentgenograms show a destructive process with poor margination situated at the site of a previously diagnosed giant cell tumour, usually at the end of a long bone. Mineralization may be present. In primary malignancy in giant cell tumour, the tumour presents as a lytic process extending to the end of a long bone. Rarely the roentgenograms show typical features of giant cell tumour and a sclerotic destructive tumour juxtaposed to it.

Sites of involvement
Bones involved with giant cell tumour are also affected by malignancy in giant cell tumour. The distal femur and the proximal tibia are the most common sites. There have been no cases reported in the small bones of the hands and feet or the skull.

Macroscopy
The gross appearance of a secondary malignant giant cell tumour is that of any high grade sarcoma: a large fleshy white tumour with soft tissue extension. Primary malignant giant cell tumours occur at the ends of bones and have dark red or tan colour.

Histopathology
In secondary giant cell tumour the neoplasm is a high grade spindle cell sarcoma which may or may not produce osteoid. No residual giant cell tumour is usually present. In primary malignant giant cell tumour areas of conventional giant cell tumour with proliferations of round to oval mononuclear cells and multinucleated giant cells are present. There is an abrupt transition to a spindle cell tumour with marked cytological atypia. Multinucleated giant cell may or may not be present.

Prognostic factors
The prognosis in secondary malignant giant cell tumours is similar to that of a high grade spindle cell sarcoma. The prognosis in primary malignant giant cell tumours has been reported to be better {1536}. In this series of eight patients only one died of disease.

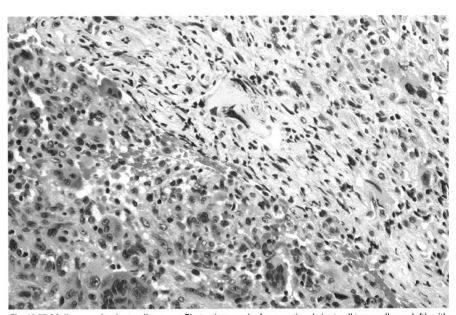

Fig. 16.07 Malignancy in giant cell tumour. Photomicrograph of conventional giant cell tumour (lower left) with mononuclear cells uniformly interspersed with multinucleated giant cells and an adjacent area of malignant anaplastic tumour cells (upper right).

CHAPTER 17

Notochordal Tumours

Notochordal tumours arise from remnants of the notochord and hence occur exclusively along the midline. Tumours which occur elsewhere may resemble chordomas.

The majority of the tumours occur in the sacrum or in the clivus. Involvement of the remainder of the spine is unusual. One of the characteristic histological features of chordoma is a lobulated growth pattern.

Chondroid chordomas occur exclusively in the base of the skull and show features of both low grade chondrosarcoma and chordoma. Some studies have indicated a better prognosis for this subtype.

Chordoma

J.M. Mirra
S.D. Nelson

C. Della Rocca
F. Mertens

Definition
Chordoma is a low to intermediate grade malignant tumour that recapitulates notochord.

ICD-O codes
Chordoma NOS   9370/3
Chondroid chordoma   9371/3
"Dedifferentiated" chordoma   9372/3

Epidemiology
Chordomas account for 1-4% of all primary malignant bone tumours. Chordoma most commonly presents after age 30, with the most common decade being the sixth (30% of patients). It is very rare under age 20 (1%). Male:female ratio is 1.8:1.

Sites of involvement
Axial spine (sacral 60%; spheno-occipital/nasal 25%; cervical 10%; & thoracolumbar 5%).

Clinical features / Imaging
The clinical features are related to the location and spread of the neoplasm. Being a slow-growing mass chordoma usually produces non specific symptoms for months to years before the diagnosis is made.

In the sacrococcygeal presentation pain is the most frequent symptom. It is usually referred to the lower back or tip of the spinal column. Constipation due to obstruction may develop. Almost all these neoplasms spread in the presacral area allowing physical detection by rectal examination. Nerve dysfunctions, such as anesthesia and paresthesia, are unusual and late manifestations. Those located in the spheno-occipital region are often associated with a chronic headache and symptoms due to compression of a cranial nerve. Ocular nerve involvement is the most frequent; compression and destruction of the pituitary gland may lead to endocrine disturbances; if spread is lateral a cerebellopontine angle tumour symptomatology can be evident. In case of spread inferiorly nasal obstruction, bleeding and even a nasal mass may appear.

Chordomas arising in the cervical, thoracic and lumbar spine usually produce symptoms related to nerve roots or spinal cord compression and / or a palpable mass can be present. Characteristically cervical chordoma may clinically manifest as a parapharyngeal mass. Clinically, most patients experience progressive pain, swelling and/or neurological deficits that may ultimately be incapacitating.

Radiologically, chordomas are typically solitary, central, lytic, destructive lesions of the axial skeleton {2058} They are almost always associated with a soft tissue mass and shards of bony detritus. Intratumoural calcification may be present particularly in sacral tumours. In the sacral area they tend to displace the bowel and/or bladder {1302}. MRI studies best visualise soft tissue extension and its relationship to anatomic structures. On MRI, T-1 weighted images are hypo- or isointense {418}, while T-2 weighted images are of high signal intensity {418,1551}.

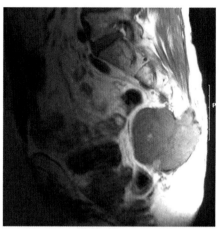

Fig. 17.01 Chordoma. T2 MRI showing a dark, lobulated, destructive mass in the sacrococcygeal region.

Macroscopy
Chordoma is a lobulated, glistening, greyish tan to bluish white, muco-gelatinous to friable, dark-red haemorrhagic tumour, generally from 5 to 15 cm. In most cases it is associated with extension beyond the contours of the bone into the surrounding soft tissues {418, 1468}.

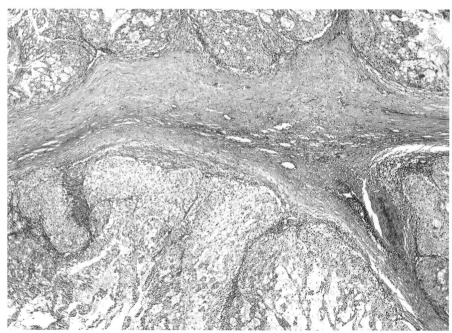

Fig. 17.02 Chordoma. Bands of fibrosis and lobularity typify this neoplasm on low power.

Histopathology

Chordomas are lobulated tumors, with individual lobules being separated by fibrous bands. The tumour cells are arranged in sheets, cords or float singly within an abundant myxoid stroma. They typically have an abundant pale vacuolated cytoplasm (the classic "physaliphorous cells"). They show mild to moderate nuclear atypia. There may be considerable variability in the appearance of the tumour from area to area. Mitoses are infrequent {1468}. In the chondroid variants, there are areas that may mimic hyaline or myxoid cartilage {925}. Chordoma associated with a high grade sarcoma is called a "dedifferentiated" chordoma {1398} or sarcomatoid chordoma {1506}. They account for less than 5% of all chordomas.

Immunophenotype

Chordomas are reactive with antibodies against S100 protein, pan-keratin, low molecular cytokeratins and Epithelial Membrane Antigen (EMA).

Genetics

Clonal chromosome aberrations have been detected in 16 cases {1477, 2082}. Nine of them had a hypodiploid stemline, with a chromosome number ranging from 33 to 44. Frequent numerical changes include loss of chromosomes 3, 4, 10, and 13, and the most commonly (half of the cases) deleted segments are 1p31-pter, 3p21-pter, 3q21-qter, 9p24-pter, and 17q11-qter. These results are in agreement with data obtained by comparative genomic hybridisation (CGH) {1880}. By CGH, also gains of chromosome arms 5q and 7q and chromosome 20 are frequently seen. The possibility of a tumour suppressor locus of significance for chordoma development at distal 1p is further strengthened by the finding of loss of heterozygosity at band 1p36 in sporadic as well as familial chordomas {1465}.

Prognostic factors

Prognosis has improved considerably with modern surgical techniques of resection especially with tumours of the sacrum {1051,2027} and even of mobile spine {210}. The chondroid variant has been reported to be associated with a better prognosis {925} although this

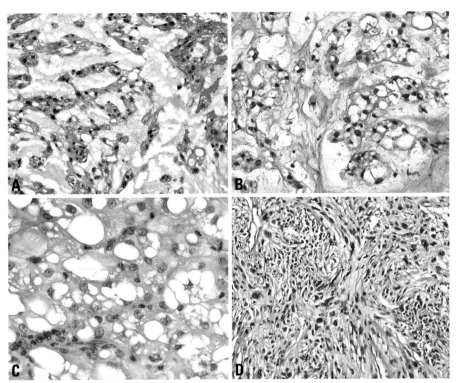

Fig. 17.03 Chordoma. A,B Chords of tumour cells in a myxoid background. Note occasional cells displaying a bubbly cytoplasm. C Some of the classic physaliphorous cells contain multiple intracytoplasmic bubbles that may cause nuclear indentations similar to those seen in lipoblasts. D Sarcomatoid, or "dedifferentiated" chondroma displaying prominent storiform architecture. Note the large, pleomorphic nuclei and the rather solid arrangement of cells without a prominent myxoid background.

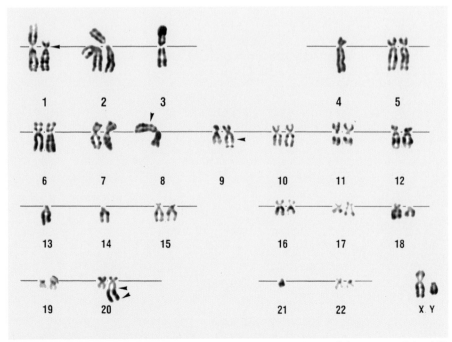

Fig. 17.04 Chordoma with complex karyotype, including the characteristic loss of chromosomes 3, 4 and 13. Arrowheads indicate breakpoints in structural rearrangements.

experience is not universal. Metastases to lung, bone, soft tissue, lymph node and skin occur, and are more frequent in patients with advanced disease.

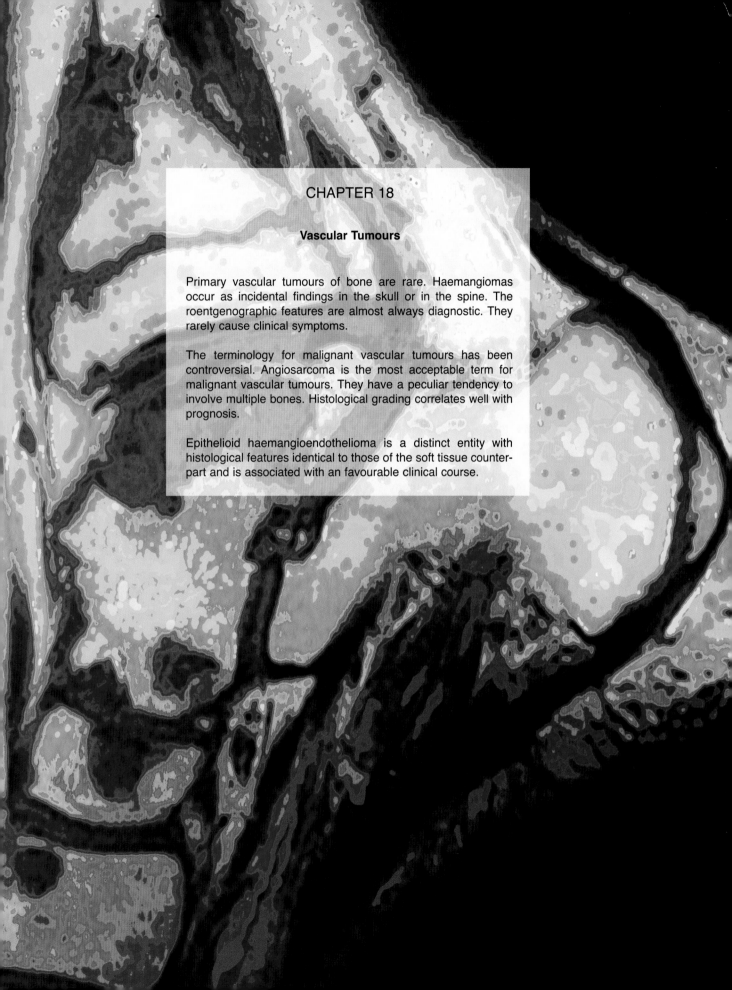

CHAPTER 18

Vascular Tumours

Primary vascular tumours of bone are rare. Haemangiomas occur as incidental findings in the skull or in the spine. The roentgenographic features are almost always diagnostic. They rarely cause clinical symptoms.

The terminology for malignant vascular tumours has been controversial. Angiosarcoma is the most acceptable term for malignant vascular tumours. They have a peculiar tendency to involve multiple bones. Histological grading correlates well with prognosis.

Epithelioid haemangioendothelioma is a distinct entity with histological features identical to those of the soft tissue counter-part and is associated with an favourable clinical course.

Haemangioma and related lesions

C.P. Adler
L. Wold

Definition
A benign vasoformative neoplasm or developmental condition of endothelial origin.

ICD-O code   9120/0

Synonyms
Capillary haemangioma, cavernous haemangioma, venous haemangioma, angioma, histocytoid haemangioma, angiomatosis.

Epidemiology
Haemangiomas are relatively common lesions; autopsy studies have identified them in the vertebrae of approximately 10% of the adult population {18}. However, clinically significant symptomatic tumours are very uncommon and account for less than 1% of primary bone tumours {539}. Haemangiomas occur at any age, but most are diagnosed during middle and late middle age with the peak incidence in the 5th decade of life {1875}. The male to female ratio is about 2:3 {18,539,1875,2153,2249}.

Sites of involvement
Vertebral bodies are the most common site, followed by the craniofacial skeleton, and then the long bones where they tend to involve the metaphyses {18,539,2249}.

Clinical features / Imaging
The majority of haemangiomas, especially those arising in the spine, are inci-dental radiographic findings. However, large vertebral tumours may cause cord compression, pain and neurological symptoms. Symptomatic tumours occuring elsewhere are painful and may cause a pathologic fracture. Haemangiomas present as a well demarcated lucent mass that frequently contains coarse trabeculations or striations. In flat bones like the calvarium, the tumour is expansile and lytic and produces a sunburst pattern of reactive bone formation. Clinically, indolent lesions frequently contain fat and sclerotic trabeculae on CT and MRI. Symptomatic tumours usually show loss of fat and reveal a low signal on T1-weighted images and a high signal on T2 {539,644,1280,1354,1875, 2287}.

Macroscopy
Haemangioma manifests as a soft well demarcated dark red mass. It may also have a honey-comb appearance with intralesional sclerotic bone trabeculae and scattered blood-filled cavities.

Histopathology
Haemangiomas have variable histological features. Capillary and cavernous haemangiomas are composed of thin-walled blood-filled vessels lined by a single layer of flat, cytologically banal endothelial cells. The vessels permeate the marrow and surround preexisting trabeculae. When capillary or cavernous haemangiomas involve a large localized

Table 18.01
Variants of haemangiomas.

Haemangioma:
    cavernous,
    capillary,
    epithelioid,
    histiocytoid,
    sclerosing
Papillary vegetant endothelial proliferation
    (Masson type)
Angiolymphoid hyperplasia with eosinophilia
    (Kimura disease)

Angiomatosis:
    non-aggressive: regional,
    disseminated: cystic angiomatosis
    aggressive: massive osteolysis
            (Gorham-Stout syndrome)

Osseous glomus tumour (glomangioma) Lymphangioma Lymphangiomatosis

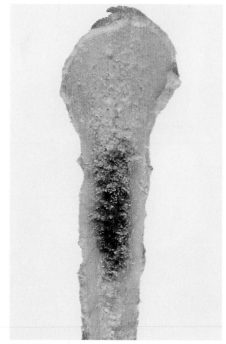

Fig. 18.02 Haemangioma of bone. Gross specimen of a tumour of the proximal fibula with a focus of brown-red appearance without marginal sclerosis.

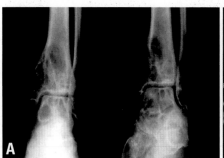 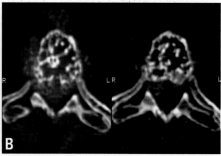

Fig. 18.01 Haemangioma of bone. **A** Plain radiographs show a lesion with multiple cystic defects within the distal tibia. **B** CT cross-sectional appearance of a vertebral haemangioma where the coarse trabeculae result in a "polka-dot" pattern.

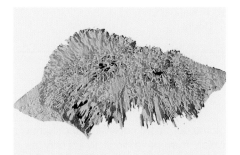

Fig. 18.03 Haemangioma of bone. The radiated spicules are demonstrated on this macerated specimen.

region or are widespread throughout the skeleton, it is known as angiomatosis. Gorham disease may be associated with a histological picture that resembles haemangioma. Epithelioid haemangioma is composed of large polyhedral neoplastic endothelial cells that have vesicular nuclei and abundant eosinophilic cytoplasm. Some tumour cells have round clear cytoplasmic vacuoles that may contain intact or fragments of red blood cells. Vacuoles in neighbouring cells often fuse forming vascular lumena. The epithelioid cells may line well formed vascular spaces or grow in solid cords or sheets. The stroma consists of loose connective tissue and may contain a mixed inflammatory infiltrate including eosinophils.

The vessels in lymphangioma are dilated, sinusoidal, filled with lymph fluid and lined by a single layer of flat, banal endothelial cells. The surrounding stroma may contain lymphocytes.

Immunophenotype
The endothelial cells uniformly express vimentin and many cells stain with antibodies to F. VIII, CD31, and CD34. Epithelial haemangiomas may also express keratins and EMA. FLI1 has also been observed in haemangiomas.

Ultrastructure
The endothelial cells contains Weibel-Palade bodies. Cytoplasmic filaments are abundant in epithelioid endothelial cells.

Prognostic factors
Haemangiomas have an excellent prognosis and have a low rate of local recurrence. Progression to an angiosarcoma is an extraordinarily rare event {528,611, 641,649,1628}.

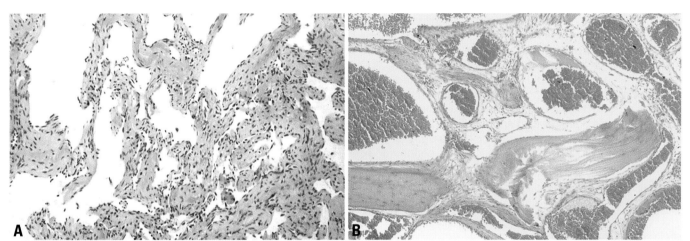

Fig. 18.04 Haemangioma of bone. **A** This bony haemangioma shows the morphology commonly associated with cavernous lesions which have been curetted. The spaces often become collapsed, and blood is no longer present because of the processing. **B** Histological pattern of a cavernous haemangioma showing broad thin-walled blood vessels, lined by a single layer of flat endothelial cells and filled with blood, within the medullary cavity between the bone trabeculas.

Angiosarcoma

A. Roessner
T. Boehling

Definition
Angiosarcomas of bone are composed of tumour cells which show endothelial differentiation.

ICD-O code   9120/3

Synonyms
Haemangiosarcoma, haemangioendothelioma, haemangioendothelial sarcoma, epithelioid angiosarcoma.

Epidemiology
Malignant vascular tumours of bone are very rare and account for less than 1% of malignant bone tumours. Age distribution shows a wide range with nearly equal distribution from the second to the eighth decade. Epithelioid haemangioendothelioma tends to occur during the second and third decades of life. Males and females are affected approximately equally.

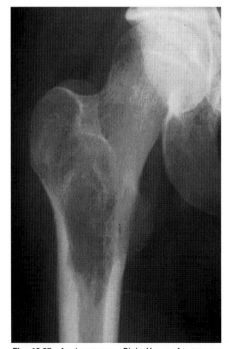

Fig. 18.05 Angiosarcoma. Plain X-ray of a tumour involving the proximal femur, featuring a purely lucent destructive process in the intertrochanteric region. The radiological appearance is nonspecific.

Sites of involvement
Malignant vascular tumours of bone show a wide skeletal distribution. They tend to affect the long tubular bones of the extremity and the axial skeleton, mainly the spine. These tumours reveal the tendency to develop multicentric lesions in bone. About a third of these lesions are multifocal.

Clinical features / Imaging
Malignant vascular tumours most commonly present as painful lesions which may be associated with a mass. Angiosarcoma usually develops purely lytic bone lesions. They are poorly marginated but can occassionally have a sclerotic rim. A soft tissue mass is often associated with less well differentiated tumours. The radiological appearence of epithelioid hemangioendothelioma is also non-specific. They also present as purely lytic lesions with varying degrees of peripheral sclerosis. Although the radiographic feature of malignant vascular tumours of bone are nonspecific, clustering of multifocal lesions in a single anatomic location suggests the diagnosis of a vascular neoplasm.

Aetiology
Angiosarcomas may arise at sites of prior radiation {338,452,1716}. The aetiology of the majority of malignant vascular tumours is unknown.

Macroscopy
Angiosarcomas are bloody and generally firm in their consistency. Necrosis is generally not observed. Epithelioid haemangioendotheliomas tend to be firm and tan-white. Both tumours can erode the cortex and extend into the soft tissue.

Histopathology
Tumour cells forming vascular spaces constitute the general histological feature of angiosarcoma of bone. Angiosarcoma of bone shows a wide range of histology, ranging from well differentiated cases mimicking haemangioma to poorly differentiated tumours which may be difficult to identify as a vascular tumour. Histo-logically, reactive bone formation can sometimes be observed in angiosarcoma of bone. This is more pronounced in the periphery, but can also be found in the more central portions of the lesion.

Poorly differentiated angiosarcomas are composed of more atypical endothelial cells. They exhibit very prominent nu clear atypia and a considerably increased number of mitoses with atypical mitotic figures. Formation of intraluminal buds can often be observed. Areas with necroses may be present. Some tumours may show epithelioid cytological features and mimic the appearance of metastatic carcinoma. Others show spindle cell cytological features and mimic other primary bone sarcomas.

Epithelioid haemangioendothelioma is composed of anastomosing cords, solid nests, and strands of endothelial cells that may sometimes form narrow vascular channels. The small capillary-sized tumour vessels can mimic small reactive vessels of granulation tissue. The epithelioid cells tend to have eosinophilic cytoplasm which may show vacuolization and sometimes signet ring-like appearance. Of remarkable significance is the

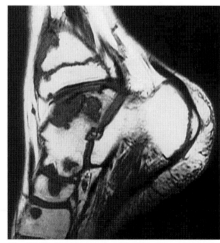

Fig. 18.06 Angiosarcoma. T2 MRI of a multicentric tumour involving multiple bones of the foot.

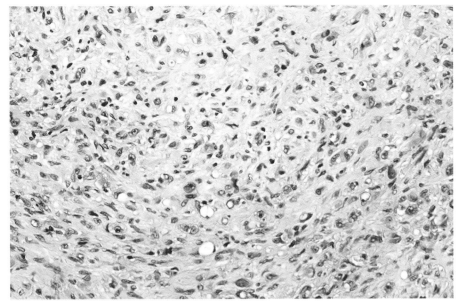

Fig. 18.07 Epithelioid haemangioendothelioma. The tumour cells are arranged in a cording fashion in a myxoid stroma. Note the occasional cytoplasmic vacuoles.

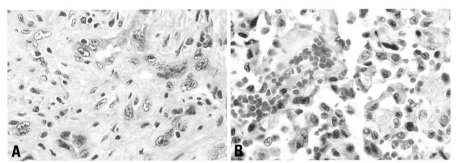

Fig. 18.08 A Epithelioid angiosarcoma. The tumour cells form anastomosing channels, have large nuclei and prominent nucleoli. **B** High grade angiosarcoma showing atypical cells with poorly formed papillae present within spaces.

myxoid and hyalinized appearance of the connective tissues stroma. The nuclei of the neoplastic cell show varying degrees of pleomorphism and anaplasia.

Immunophenotype
The endothelial cells uniformly express vimentin and many cells stain with antibodies to Factor VIII, CD31, CD34, and Ulex Europaeus. Epithelioid malignancies may also express cytokeratins and EMA {1134,2249}.

Ultrastructure
The endothelial cells contain Weibel-Palade bodies, but are generally difficult to find in poorly differentiated tumours. Cytoplasmic filaments are abundant in epithelioid neoplasms.

Genetics
Two epithelioid haemangioendotheliomas have shown an identical chromosomal translocation involving chromosomes 1 and 3 {1403}.

Prognostic factors
The histological degree of differentiation is the most significant factor in the prognosis of patients with malignant vascular tumours of bone {300,2288}. Some studies have also suggested that multifocal tumours show a survival advantage. This survival advantage may in part be related to the multifocal tumours showing better differentiation {1134,2142}.

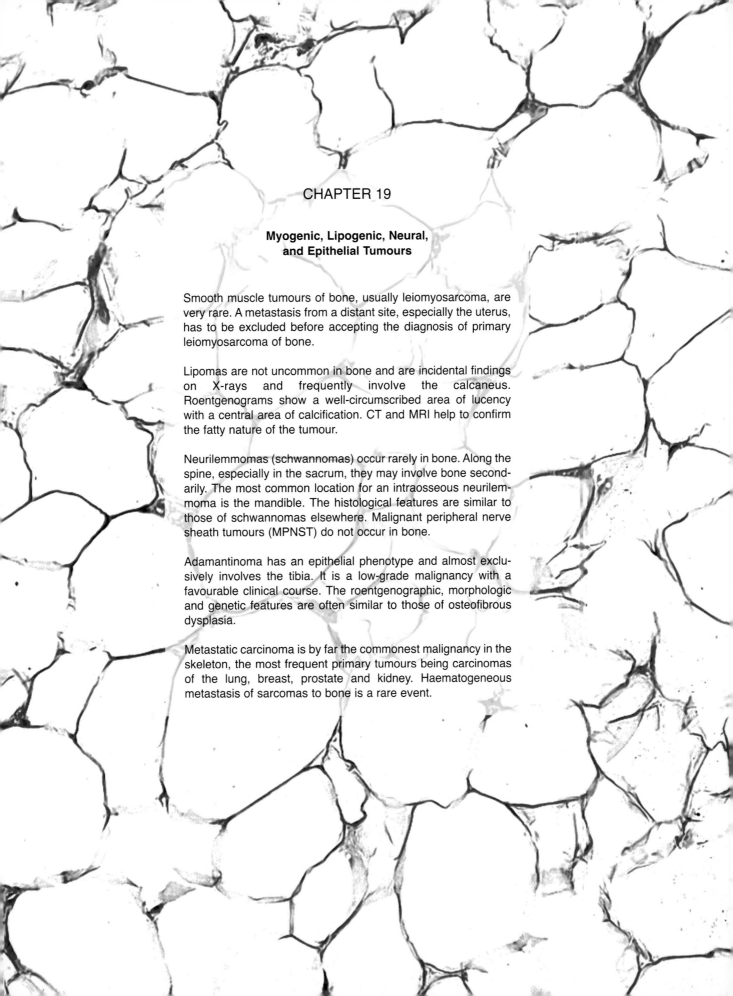

CHAPTER 19

Myogenic, Lipogenic, Neural, and Epithelial Tumours

Smooth muscle tumours of bone, usually leiomyosarcoma, are very rare. A metastasis from a distant site, especially the uterus, has to be excluded before accepting the diagnosis of primary leiomyosarcoma of bone.

Lipomas are not uncommon in bone and are incidental findings on X-rays and frequently involve the calcaneus. Roentgenograms show a well-circumscribed area of lucency with a central area of calcification. CT and MRI help to confirm the fatty nature of the tumour.

Neurilemmomas (schwannomas) occur rarely in bone. Along the spine, especially in the sacrum, they may involve bone secondarily. The most common location for an intraosseous neurilemmoma is the mandible. The histological features are similar to those of schwannomas elsewhere. Malignant peripheral nerve sheath tumours (MPNST) do not occur in bone.

Adamantinoma has an epithelial phenotype and almost exclusively involves the tibia. It is a low-grade malignancy with a favourable clinical course. The roentgenographic, morphologic and genetic features are often similar to those of osteofibrous dysplasia.

Metastatic carcinoma is by far the commonest malignancy in the skeleton, the most frequent primary tumours being carcinomas of the lung, breast, prostate and kidney. Haematogeneous metastasis of sarcomas to bone is a rare event.

Leiomyoma of bone

E. McCarthy

Definition
A benign spindle cell tumour of bone with smooth muscle differentiation.

Epidemiology
Leiomyomas of bone are very rare. Most patients are adults over age 30, although a child age 3 years has been reported. Males and females are equally affected {2166}.

Sites of involvement
The facial bones are most commonly affected by primary leiomyoma. The most common site is the mandible. In the extragnathic skeleton, the tibia is the most common site {2166}.

Clinical features
Patients present with pain. Radiologically, lesions are radiolytic, often multilocular. A sclerotic rim may be present. Occasionally there may be cortical expansion.

Macroscopy
Primary leiomyomas of bone are firm gray tan tumours. Most lesions are 3 cm or smaller in maximum dimension.

Histopathology
Histologically, leiomyomas of bone are identical to leiomyomas in other loca-tions. Uniform spindle cells are present in interlacing bundles. Mitotic figures are extremely rare. The cells are positive with immunohistochemical stains for smooth muscle actin and desmin. Occasionally, thick-walled blood vessels are present in a pattern identical to angioleiomyoma {2166}.

Prognostic factors
Local excision results in a complete cure.

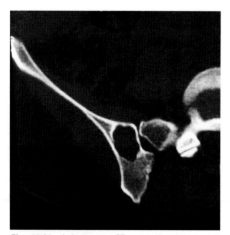

Fig. 19.01 Leiomyoma. CT scan showing a well defined lytic lesion with a sclerotic rim in the ilium.

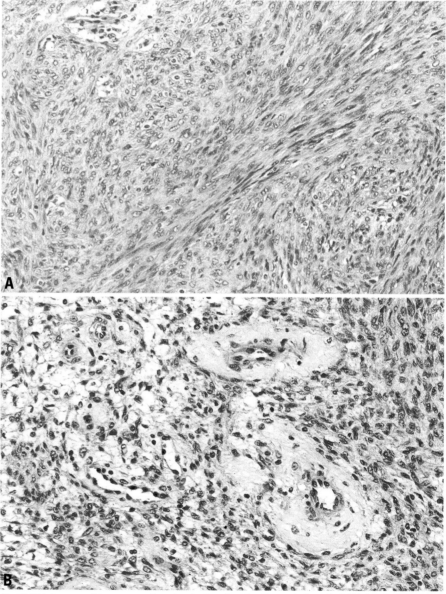

Fig. 19.02 Leiomyoma. **A** Low power view showing bundles of uniform spindle cells. **B** Thick walled vessels admixed with spindle cells in a pattern of angiomyoleiomyoma.

Leiomyosarcoma of bone

E. McCarthy

Definition
A very rare malignant spindle cell sarcoma of bone which shows smooth muscle differentiation with immunohistochemical or electron microscopic studies.

Epidemiology
Although the reported age range is from 9 to 87 years, the mean age is 44 years {165,1049,1932}. There is a slight male predominance.

Sites of involvement
Most lesions occur in the lower extremity around the knee, either in the distal femoral metaphysis or proximal tibial metaphysis. The craniofacial skeleton is the next most common area to be involved {68}.

Clinical features
Pain, present from 2 weeks to 1 year prior to diagnosis, is the most common symptom. Approximately 15% of patients present with pathological fracture.
Radiographically, it is an aggressive radiolytic lesion, with poorly defined margins, a permeative growth pattern, and cortical destruction. MRI shows a hypointense lesion on T1 and an iso-or hypointense lesion on T2 weighted studies {2056}.

Macroscopy
Lesions are grey to tan, firm or creamy masses, often with areas of necrosis or cystic degeneration. Despite a broad range in size, lesions average 6 cm in greatest dimension {68}. Cortical penetration is common.

Histopathology
Histologically, lesions are identical to leiomyosarcomas in other locations. Plump and pleomorphic spindle cells are arranged in bundles or fascicles. Mitotic figures are common. Often areas of necrosis are present. Smooth muscle differentiation is demonstrable by positive immunohistochemical staining for smooth muscle actin and desmin. Electron microscopic studies demonstrate fine filamentous actin fibrils in the cytoplasm.

Prognostic factors
Approximately 50% of patients develop metastases to the lungs within 5 years {68}. Ultimately, 50% of patients die from leiomyosarcoma of bone {1099}.

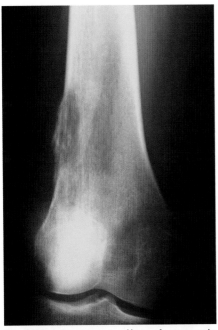

Fig. 19.03 Leiomyosarcoma. X-ray of a tumour in distal femur showing an aggressive, permeative lytic lesion with cortical destruction.

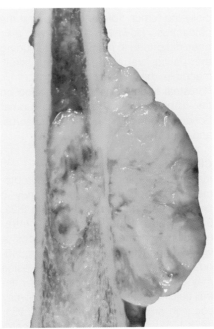

Fig. 19.04 Leiomyosarcoma. Macroscopy of the femoral lesion. Note both an intraosseous and an extraosseous component of the white fleshy tumour.

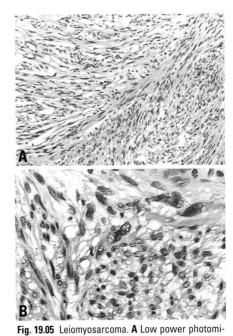

Fig. 19.05 Leiomyosarcoma. **A** Low power photomicrograph showing bundles of spindle cells.
B On high power magnification, note the cellular pleomorphism of the tumour cells.

Lipoma of bone

A.E. Rosenberg
J.A. Bridge

Definition

Lipoma of bone is a benign neoplasm of adipocytes that arises within the medullary cavity, cortex, or on the surface of bone.

Synonyms

Intramedullary lipoma, intracortical lipoma, ossifying lipoma, parosteal lipoma.

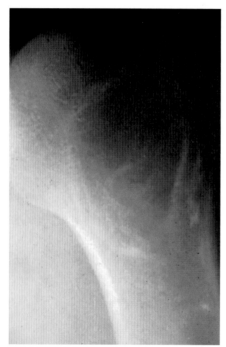

Fig. 19.06 Lipoma. Radiograph of intramedullary lipoma of humerus demonstrating an oval lytic lesion with a sclerotic rim.

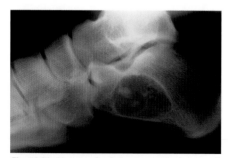

Fig. 19.07 Lipoma of calcaneous producing a well defined lytic lesion with central mineralization. Axial CT confirms the fatty nature of the lesion.

Epidemiology

Lipoma of bone is rare and accounts for less than 0.1% of primary bone tumours; their incidence is not known.

Intramedullary lipoma has a wide age range (2nd-8th decades) but most patients are approximately 40 years old at the time of diagnosis {1458}. Males are affected more frequently than females at a ratio of approximately 1.6:1 {1458}.

Parosteal lipoma usually develops during adulthood and most patients are in their 5th-6th decade of life at the time of diagnosis {1462}. There is a slight male predominance (9:7) {1462}.

Sites of Involvement

The vast majority of intraosseous lipomas arise within the medullary cavity and rarely develop in the cortex {2317}. They most commonly affect the metaphyseal regions of the long tubular bones, especially the femur, tibia and fibula and the calcaneus. However, they have also been described in many bones including the pelvis, vertebrae, sacrum, skull, mandible, maxilla, and ribs.

Parosteal lipomas generally develop on the diaphyseal surface of long tubular bones, especially the femur, humerus, and tibia {1462}.

Clinical features / Imaging

Intramedullary lipoma may be asymptomatic or produce achy pain. Rarely, it presents as a pathological fracture {822, 951, 1458}. Radiographically, intramedullary lipoma usually produces a well defined lytic mass that is surrounded by a thin rim of sclerosis. The lesion may also contain trabeculations or central calcifications. Bony expansion may occur in small caliber bones {822,951, 1458,1732}. CT shows that the fatty component has a low attenuation value similar to that of subcutaneus fat and on MRI the fat has high signal intensity on both T1 and T2 weighted images {1732}.

Parosteal lipoma is frequently asymptomatic and may present as a visible or palpable mass. Radiographs may reveal a radiolucent mass adjacent to the corti-cal surface that may show thickening or a periosteal reaction. Similar to intraosseous lipoma, the CT and MRI findings have the same features as subcutaneous fat except if there is calcification, cartilage or ossification within the lesion {1079,1752}.

Macroscopy

Intramedullary lipoma is usually 3-5 cm in size, is well defined, soft, and yellow. The surrounding bone is often sclerotic. Parosteal lipoma is usually 4-10 cm in greatest dimension, is well defined, soft and yellow. Some cases contain gritty spicules of bone or firm nodules of cartilage in the base or scattered throughout the mass.

Histopathology

Intramedullary lipoma is well defined and consists of lobules of mature-appearing adipocytes that may replace the marrow and encase preexisting bony trabeculae. The adipocytes have a single large clear cytoplasmic vacuole that displaces the crescent shaped nucleus to the periphery. Some tumours may demonstrate fat necrosis with foamy macrophages and fibrosis. In ossifying lipomas delicate trabeculae of woven and lamellar bone may be present throughout the tumour {121, 346}.

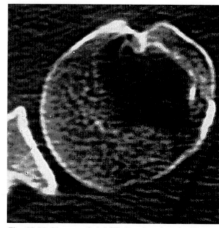

Fig. 19.08 Lipoma. Axial CT showing that the lipoma has the tissue density of fat.

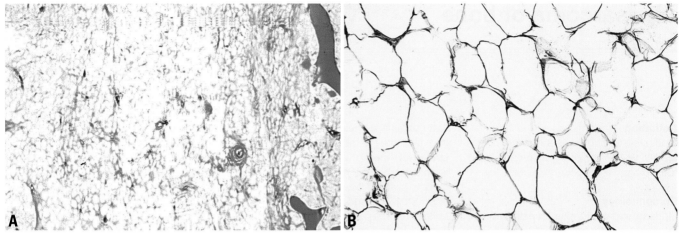

Fig. 19.09 A Well defined intramedullary lipoma composed of sheets of white adipocytes. **B** Parosteal lipoma composed of lobules of white fat cells.

Parosteal lipoma is also well defined and consists of lobules of mature appearing white adipocytes. The adipocytes have a single large clear cytoplasmic vacuole that displaces the crescent shaped nucleus to the periphery. Some cases may have bone with or without a hyaline cartilage in the base of the lesion or scattered throughout the mass in small islands {1462}.

Immunophenotype
The neoplastic fat expresses vimentin and S100 protein.

Genetics
The translocation t(3;12)(q28;q14) and its associated fusion transcript *HMGIC/LPP* characteristic of subcutaneous lipoma has been detected in a case of parosteal lipoma {255,1698}.

Prognostic factors
Lipoma of bone has an excellent prognosis and rarely recurs.

Liposarcoma of bone

A.E. Rosenberg

Definition
Liposarcoma of bone is a malignant neoplasm whose phenotype recapitulates fat.

Epidemiology
Liposarcoma of bone is an extraordinarily rare neoplasm. Most cases are described in the form of single case reports in older literature and the validity of the diagnosis in some cases has been questioned {457}. Liposarcoma of bone occurs in all age groups although the majority of patients are adults {15,457, 1090,2121}. Men are affected slightly more frequently than women.

Sites of involvement
Liposarcoma of bone usually develops in the long tubular bones especially the tibia and femur and has been reported to arise in the diaphysis, metaphysis, and epiphysis {15,457,1090,2121}.

Clinical features / Imaging
Liposarcoma of bone presents as a painful mass. Radiographically, the tumour manifests as a well defined or poorly defined mass {15,457,1090, 2121}.

Macroscopy
Most liposarcomas are large, lobulated, soft to firm and are yellow to tan-white in colour. Myxoid tumours may be glistening, slimy and mucinous.

Histopathology
The histological variants of liposarcoma reported in bone include well differentiated lipoma-like, myxoid and pleomorphic types {15,457,1090,2121}. Well differentiated lipoma-like liposarcoma consists of sheets of mature appearing adipocytes with scattered tumour cells having enlarged hyperchromatic nuclei. Some of these atypical cells are lipoblasts and are distinguished by cytoplasmic vacuoles that are round, clear, and scallop the nucleus. Myxoid liposarcoma consists of mildly atypical stellate and spindle cells enmeshed in a myxoid stroma that contains a finely arborizing vascular tree that has a plexiform pattern. Also scattered throughout the tumour are lipoblasts. Sheets of large pleomorphic cells in which the cytoplasm is either eosinophilic or filled with round clear vacuoles characterize pleomorphic liposarcoma. Mitoses are usually numerous.

Immunophenotype
There are no data regarding the immunophenotype of liposarcoma of bone.

Ultrastructure
The cytoplasm of the neoplastic cells contains membrane bound lipid droplets of varying size. Dilated rough endoplasmic reticulum and scattered mitochondria are also present {1650}.

Prognostic factors
Prognostic information regarding liposarcoma of bone is scant. Generally, the behaviour of the tumour should correlate with its histological grade.

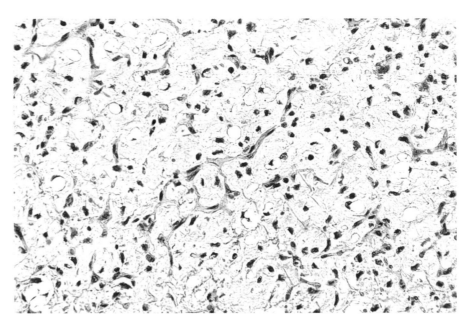

Fig. 19.10 Myxoid liposarcoma consisting of scattered spindle and stellate cells and occasional lipoblasts enmeshed in a frothy myxoid stroma that contains branching small caliber capillaries.

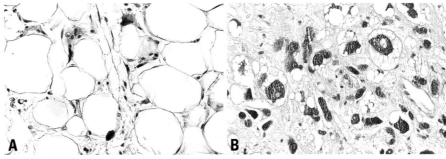

Fig. 19.11 A Well differentiated liposarcoma, lipoma-like type, containing mature appearing white fat cells and scattered adipocytes that have enlarged hyperchromatic nuclei. **B** Sheets of pleomorphic cells including lipoblasts characterize pleomorphic liposarcoma.

Schwannoma

K.K. Unni

Definition
Schwannoma is a benign neoplasm of Schwann cell origin arising within bone.

ICD-O code   9560/0

Synonyms
Neurilemmoma, neurinoma.

Epidemiology
Neurogenic tumours of bone are extremely uncommon. Although roentgenographic abnormalities may be found involving the skeleton in patients with

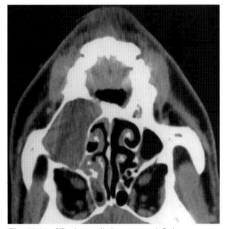

Fig. 19.12 CT of a well-demarcated Schwannoma of the maxilla.

neurofibromatosis, there are no well recognized examples of neurofibroma in bone. All benign neurogenic tumours in the skeleton are Schwannomas. They compose less than 1% of all benign tumours in the Mayo Clinic files (unpublished statistics, Unni, K. K.).

Sites of involvement
The mandible and the sacrum are the most common sites of involvement with neurilemmoma. In the mandible, the lesion almost always involves the mental foramen. When neurilemmoma involves the spine or the sacrum, it is frequently difficult to know whether the tumour is truly of bony origin.

Clinical features / Imaging
Most neurilemmomas are asymptomatic, incidental findings on roentgenograms. Occasionally, they produce pain and/or swelling.

Macroscopy
Schwannomas of bone are extremely well circumscribed and may show a fibrous capsule. They are tan to white and glistening. Foci of yellow discolouration may be seen.

Histopathology
Schwannoma is composed of spindle cells with wavy appearing nuclei. The nuclei frequently are arranged in a palisading fashion. Areas of hypocellularity may alternate with areas of hypercellularity. Focally, the nuclei may be enlarged and pleomorphic appearing. Mitotic activity is rare. Schwannomas are always diffusely and strongly positive with S100 protein.

Prognostic factors
Schwannomas are benign lesions and complete, but conservative surgical removal leads to cure. There are no examples of malignant transformation of neurilemmomas in bone.

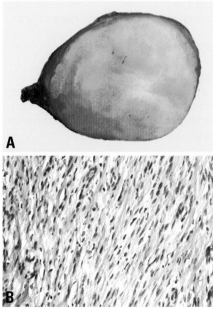

Fig. 19.13 A Encapsulated mandibular Schwannoma with tan and white areas. **B** Note the discrete tendency of spindle cell nuclei to palisade. The nuclei do not show cytological atypia.

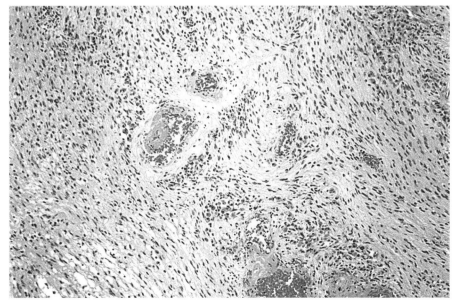

Fig. 19.14 Schwannoma. Note the hyalinization of vascular walls.

Adamantinoma

P.C.W. Hogendoorn
H. Hashimoto

Definition
A low grade, malignant biphasic tumour characterized by a variety of morphological patterns, most commonly epithelial cells, surrounded by a relatively bland spindle-cell osteo-fibrous component.

ICD-O code   9261/3

Synonyms
Adamantinoma of long bones, extragnathic adamantinoma, differentiated adamantinoma, juvenile intracortical adamantinoma.

Epidemiology
Adamantinoma comprises about 0.4% of all primary bone tumours {987,1503, 1518}. Patients present with this tumour from 3 up to 86 years, with a median age of 25-35 years. The youngest age group predominantly includes patients with osteofibrous dysplasia-like adamantino- ma, but very young patients with classic adamantinoma (age 3) and older ones with the osteofibrous dysplasia-like subtype (age 38) have been reported {918, 1502,2069}. There is a slight predominance in males.

Sites of involvement
The tibia, in particular the anterior (meta-) diaphysis, is involved in 85-90% of cases. In up to 10% this is combined with one or more lesions in the ipsilateral fibula as well. Rare other sites have been reported, especially the ulna.

Clinical features / Imaging
The main complaint is swelling with or without pain. Adamantinoma often displays a protracted clinical behaviour. Clinical symptoms like swelling or radiographic abnormality may last for more than 30 years prior to diagnosis, whereas local recurrences or metastases may develop years after primary, intralesional or marginal surgical treatment. On X-ray, typically a well circumscribed, cortical, (multi-)lobulated osteolytic lesion with intralesional opacities, septation and peripheral sclerosis is seen {217,987}. Multifocality within the same bone is regularly observed. The lesion commonly seems to remain intracortical and extends longitudinally, but may also destroy the cortex and invade the medullary cavity or surrounding periosteum and soft tissue. This is usually accompanied by lamellar or solid periosteal reaction. Aggressive tumours occasionally present as single large lytic lesions. MRI is useful to document multicentricity, the extension of the lesion, and eventual soft tissue involvement.

Macroscopy
Classic adamantinoma usually presents as a cortical, well-demarcated, yellowish-grey, lobulated tumour of firm to bony consistency with peripheral sclerosis. It may be a single lesion, but its multifocal appearance with apparently normal cortical bone lying in between is occasionally striking. Small lesions remain intracortical, and are usually white and gritty. Larger tumours show intramedullary extension and cortical breakthrough with soft tissue invasion in a minority of cases. Macroscopically detectable cystic spaces are common, filled with straw-coloured or blood-like fluid.

Histopathology
Classic adamantinomas are characterized by an epithelial and an osteofibrous component, that may be intermingled with each other in various proportions and differentiation patterns. The four main differentiation patterns of classic adamantinoma are basaloid, tubular, spindle cell, and squamous {2235}. The first two patterns are encountered most commonly, but all patterns may be present in one lesion. The spindle cell component is more often observed in recurrences, lining cystic spaces, and in metastases. The osteofibrous compo-

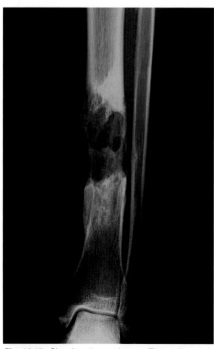

Fig. 19.15 Classic adamantinoma. The radiograph of the distal tibia shows an expansive, lobulated, lytic lesion with a defect of the outer surface of the cortex.

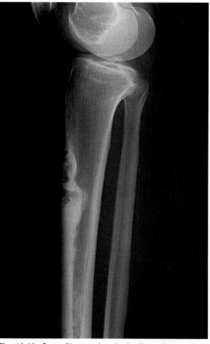

Fig. 19.16 Osteofibrous dysplasia-like adamantinoma. The lateral radiograph of the proximal aspect of the tibia shows a multilocular, lytic lesion with surrounding osteosclerosis of the anterior cortex.

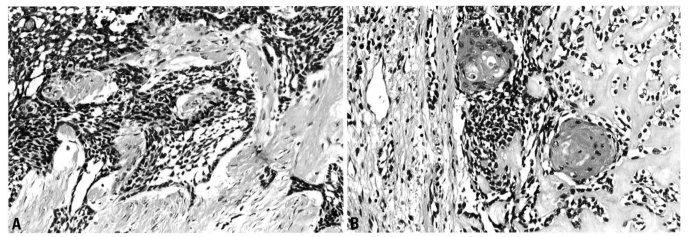

Fig. 19.17 Adamantinoma. **A** Basaloid pattern. Easily distuingishable epithelial fields without clear pallisading. **B** Squamoid pattern.

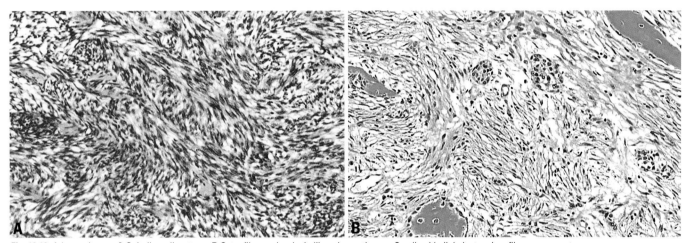

Fig. 19.18 Adamantinoma. **A** Spindle cell pattern. **B** Osteofibrous dysplasia like adamantinoma. Small epithelial clusters in a fibro-osseous stroma.

nent is composed of storiform oriented spindle cells. Woven bone trabeculae are usually present in or next to the centre of the lesion, prominently rimmed by osteoblasts, and with varying amounts of transformation to lamellar bone at the periphery of the tumour. Foam cells or myxoid change may be present, and mast cells or multinucleated giant cells are occasionally detected. Mitotic activity is usually low. A fifth histological pattern, the so-called osteofibrous dysplasia-like variant, is characterized by predominance of osteofibrous tissue, in which small groups of epithelial cells are only encountered by careful search or immunohistochemistry. The majority of classic and osteofibrous dysplasia-like adamantinomas display a "zonal" architecture. In classic adamantinoma, the centre is usually dominated by the epithelial component, and only few, small immature bone trabeculae are present in the fibrous tissue. Towards the periphery, the epithelial islands decrease to inconspicuous elements and the osteofibrous component gradually takes over with increasing amounts of woven bone trabeculae, transforming to lamellar bone. In osteofibrous dysplasia-like adamantinoma, the centre is occupied by fibrous tissue with scanty and thin immature woven bone trabeculae with epithelial elements. Small clusters of epithelial cells are the only feature which differentiate osteofibrous dysplasia-like adamantinoma from osteofibrous dysplasia.

Immunophenotype
The fibrous tissue is vimentin-positive. The epithelial cells show co-expression for keratin, EMA and vimentin. Chain-specific keratin expression {917,1050} revealed a predominantly basal epithelial cell differentiation, regardless of subtype, with widespread presence of basal epithelial cell keratins 5, 14, and 19. Also keratins 1, 13 and 17 are variably present. Keratins 8 and 18 are virtually absent. In classic adamantinomas, the epithelial component is surrounded by a continuous basement membrane, whereas less distinct epithelial islands show multiple interruptions or no surrounding basement membrane at all {919}. EGF/EGFR expression is restricted to the epithelial component. FGF2/FGFR1 is present in both components {242}.

Ultrastructure
Electron microscopic studies have confirmed the epithelial nature of adamantinoma, showing intracytoplasmic hemidesmosomes, tonofilaments, and microfilaments. Irrespective of histological subtype, the epithelial cells are bound by desmosomes and basement membranes have been found to surround the epithelial nests.

Genetics

Adamantinomas, classic as well as osteofibrous dysplasia-like, show recurrent numerical chromosomal abnormalities, mainly gain of chromosomes 7, 8, 12, and 19 {920,1058,1318,2004}. DNA flow cytometric and image cytometric studies showed that in aneuploid tumours, the aneuploid population was always restricted to the epithelial component {916}. *TP53* gene aberrations – as detected immunohistochemically or by loss of heterozygosity analysis - are restricted to the epithelial component of adamantinoma. There have been some cases reported with histological features of adamantinoma as well as Ewing sarcoma, sometimes called 'atypical' or 'Ewing-like' adamantinoma {741,1013, 1273,1400,1891,2178}.

Cytogenetic ana-lysis combined with FISH and RT-PCR of two cases formerly described as atypical or Ewing-like adamantinoma revealed an (11;22) translocation, typical for Ewing sarcoma {257}. Because of these findings these tumours were labelled "adamantinoma-like Ewing sarcoma". The t(11;22) translocation is not present in adamantinoma {908,1318}.

Prognostic factors

Risk factors for recurrence are intralesional or marginal surgery and extracompartmental growth {918,1050,1084, 1739}. Recurrence percentages after non-radical surgery may rise up to 90% {918,1050,1084}. Recurrence is associated with an increase in epithelium-to-stroma ratio and more aggressive

behaviour {918,1084,1503}. Besides, male sex {1050,1084}, females at young age {1503}, pain at presentation {1084}, short duration of symptoms {918,1084}, young age (<20 years) {918}, and lack of squamous differentiation of the tumour {918, 1084} have been associated with increased rates of recurrence or metastasis. Adamantinomas metastasise in 12-29% of patients with comparable mortality rates {918,1084,1503,1739}. Metastatic tumours are all classic adamantinomas, although rarely osteofibrous dysplasia-like adamantinomas may metastasise after recurrence and subsequent progression to classic adamantinoma {918}. The tumour spreads to regional lymph nodes and the lungs, and infrequently to skeleton, liver, and brain.

Metastases involving bone

N.A. Jambhekar
A. Borges

Definition

A tumour (usually malignant) involving bone, which has originated from another (distant) site.

Synonyms

Metastatic carcinoma, skeletal deposits, osseus metastasis, secondaries in bone, bony implants.

Epidemiology

The skeletal system is the third most common site to be involved by metastatic tumour after the lungs and liver {174}. Metastatic carcinomas are the most common malignant tumour affecting the skeleton {2154}. Over two-thirds of patients with bone metastasis are between 40-60 years of age {504}. Most metastases originate from common cancers namely breast, lung, prostate, kidney and thyroid gland which account for 93% of all deposits {504}. A complete radiographic and clinical search will

identify the primary site in up to 85% of cases {1812}.
Although metastases are rare in children, when they occur, they most often include neuroblastoma, rhabdomyosarcoma and clear cell sarcoma of kidney.

Sites of Involvement

Metastatic carcinomas involve bones with persistent red marrow such as vertebra, proximal femur ribs, sternum, pelvis, skull and shoulder girdle. Out of 114 histologically evaluated lesions 44.3% involved axial skeleton, 28.8% the appendicular skeleton and 26.9% involved multiple bones {504}. The lumbar spine {757,1872} and proximal femur {757} are favoured sites. Bones of the hands and feet are rarely involved {923, 1252,1433,1507,1925}.

Clinical features

Pain, swelling, fracture and neurological symptoms (spine) are common {278}.

Skull base metastasis may cause Collet-Sicard syndrome {1865}; hypercalcaemia may accompany osteolysis {1520}.
Plain radiographs reveal lytic, blastic or

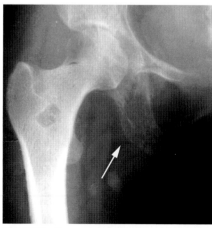

Fig. 19.19 Permeative destruction of bone by a metastasis (primary tumour unknown).

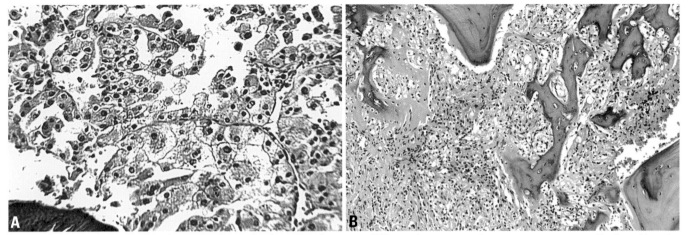

Fig. 19.20 A Metastatic renal cell carcinoma showing an alveolar and nesting pattern. **B** Metastatic prostate carcinoma; note monotonous small cells and irregular osteoid deposition.

mixed patterns {756}. Lung and breast deposits cause irregular lytic destruction, but are occasionally osteoblastic {1460, 1514}. Thyroid and kidney deposits are purely lytic; prostatic deposits are osteoblastic. Solitary metastasis {2120}, or an irregular periosteal reaction {1238, 1581} may simulate a primary bone sarcoma.

Plain radiographs are unreliable to detect vertebral deposits {707,1872} and despite gross evidence of spinal deposits in 36% of 832 autopsied patients dying of cancer, 26% had negative plain X-rays {1872}.

Bone scintigraphy is a sensitive method for the detection of skeletal metastases, because it covers the whole skeleton,

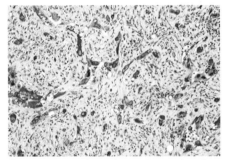

Fig. 19.21 Metastatic carcinoma. Scattered cytokeratin-positive tumour cells confirm the epithelial character of the lesion.

making it valuable for identifying the extent of the disease. CT scan is useful for guiding needle biopsies. MRI has also been used in some cases to detect and delineate metastases.

Aetiology

The location of the primary tumour and the local pattern of blood flow determine involvement of skeletal sites. The vertebral venous plexus (Batson's plexus) is a high volume, low pressure, valveless venous system independent of the pulmonary, portal and caval systems; it communicates directly with veins of the pelvis, proximal half of lower extremity, proximal half of upper extremity and head and neck {140}. Any increase in intrabdominal or intrathoracic pressure during exhalation or straining causes a backflow into the vertebral plexus bypassing the heart and lungs. This explains the preferential involvement of the vertebral and the proximal appendicular bones, and the occassional occurrence of extensive skeletal deposits despite lack of visceral involvement {1470}.

Macroscopy

The macroscopic appearance of skeletal metastasis varies depending upon the amount of bone produced in response to the tumour. Thus, osteoblas-

tic metastases from the breast are greyish white firm, whereas renal cell carcinoma produces soft haemorrhagic deposits.

Morphology

Metastatic tumours attempt to recapitulate the original tumour. Squamous carcinomas from most sites look alike, however, many adenocarcinomas such as renal cell, prostate and thyroid retain morphological similarities to the primary tumour. An accompanying fibroblastic, vascular, osteoblastic and osteoclastic response may be present. Sarcomatoid (spindle cell) carcinomas originating in the kidney or the lung may simulate a primary bone sarcoma.

Immunophenotype

Immunohistochemistry is useful when the diagnosis of metastatic carcinoma is straightforward but not distinctive enough to identify the primary site, or, when the differential is broad and includes sarcoma, carcinoma and melanoma {514}.

Prognostic factors

Bone metastasis usually heralds incurability and treatment is palliative. The outcome depends upon the primary site and the extent of disease.

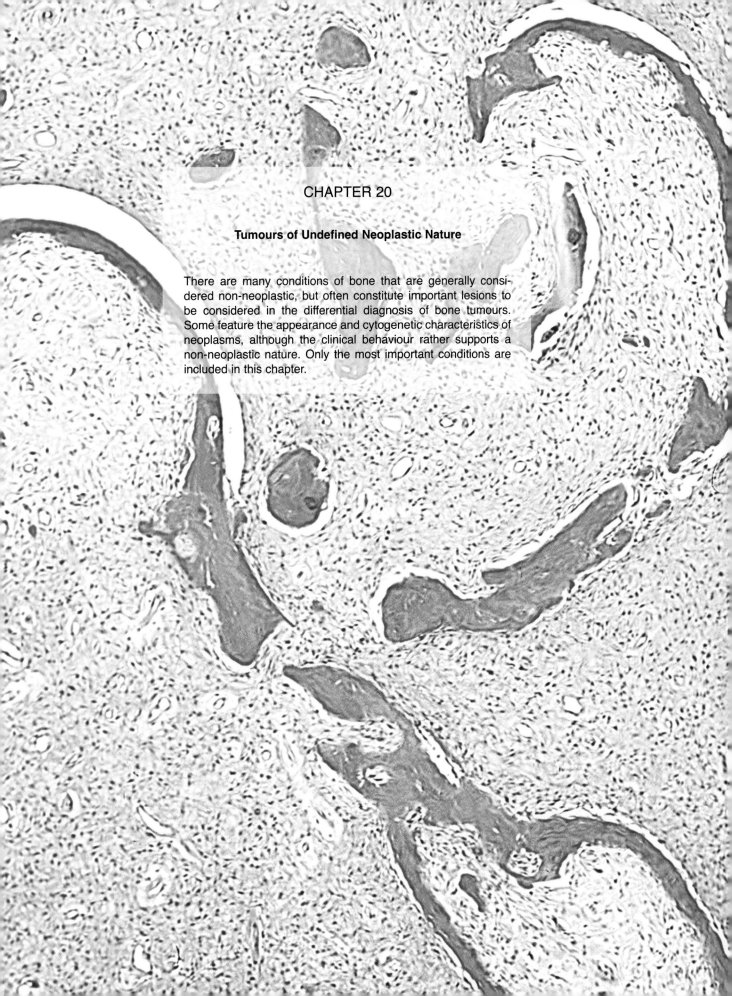

CHAPTER 20

Tumours of Undefined Neoplastic Nature

There are many conditions of bone that are generally considered non-neoplastic, but often constitute important lesions to
be considered in the differential diagnosis of bone tumours.
Some feature the appearance and cytogenetic characteristics of
neoplasms, although the clinical behaviour rather supports a
non-neoplastic nature. Only the most important conditions are
included in this chapter.

Aneurysmal bone cyst

A.E. Rosenberg
G.P. Nielsen
J.A. Fletcher

Definition
Aneurysmal bone cyst (ABC) is a benign cystic lesion of bone composed of blood filled spaces separated by connective tissue septa containing fibroblasts, osteoclast-type giant cells and reactive woven bone. ABC may arise de novo (primary ABC), or secondarily complicate other benign and malignant bone tumours (secondary ABC) that have undergone haemorrhagic cystic change.

Synonyms
Multilocular haematic cyst, giant cell reparative granuloma.

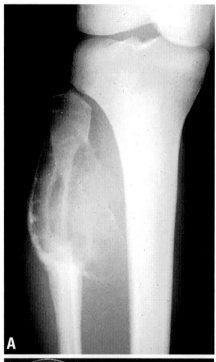

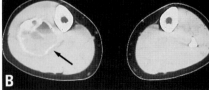

Fig. 20.01 Aneurysmal bone cyst. **A** Plain X-ray of an eccentric lytic mass of the proximal fibula. Note the peripheral shell of reactive bone. **B** CT of the same lesion (arrow).

Epidemiology
ABC affects all age groups, but is most common during the first two decades of life (median age approximately 13 years) and has no sex predilection {1345, 2200}. The estimated annual incidence is 0.15 per million individuals {1239}.

Sites of involvement
ABC can affect any bone but usually arises in the metaphysis of long bones especially the femur, tibia and humerus, and the posterior elements of vertebral bodies. Rare tumours whose morphology is identical to primary ABC of bone have also been described in the soft tissues {53}.

Clinical features / Imaging
The most common signs and symptoms are pain and swelling, which are rarely secondary to fracture. In the vertebrae it can compress nerves or the spinal cord and cause neurological symptoms. Radiographically, ABC presents as a lytic, eccentric, expansile mass with well defined margins. Most tumours contain a thin shell of subperiosteal reactive bone. Computed tomography and magnetic resonance imaging studies show internal septa and characteristic fluid-fluid levels created by the different densities of the cyst fluid caused by the settling of red blood cells {1173,2200}. In secondary ABC, CT and MRI may show evidence of an underlying primary lesion.

Macroscopy
ABC is a well defined and multiloculated mass of blood filled cystic spaces separated by tan white gritty septa. More solid areas can be seen which may represent either a solid portion of the ABC or a component of a primary tumour that has undergone secondary ABC-like changes.

Histopathology
ABC may arise de novo (primary ABC), or secondarily complicate other benign and malignant bone tumours (secondary ABC) that have undergone haemorrhagic cystic change {1281,1557,1699,1849, 1926}.

Primary ABC is well circumscribed and composed of blood filled cystic spaces separated by fibrous septa. The fibrous septa are composed of a moderately dense cellular proliferation of bland fibroblasts, with scattered multinucleated osteoclast-type giant cells and reactive woven bone rimmed by osteoblasts. The woven bone frequently follows the contours of the fibrous septa. In approximately 1/3 of cases the bone is basophilic and has been termed "blue bone", however, its presence is not diagnostic as it can be seen in other entities. Mitoses are commonly present and can be numerous, however, atypical forms are absent. Necrosis is rare unless there has been a pathological fracture. The solid variant of ABC has the same components as the septa and is very similar, if not identical, to giant cell reparative granuloma. Primary ABC accounts for approximately 70% of all cases {177,1859}.

The majority of secondary ABC develop in association with benign neoplasms, most commonly giant cell tumour of bone, osteoblastoma, chondroblastoma and fibrous dysplasia {1173,1345,2200}. However, ABC-like changes may also omplicate sarcomas, especially osteosarcoma.

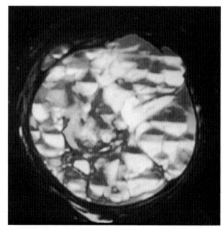

Fig. 20.02 Aneurysmal bone cyst. MRI of large destructive lesion of distal femur. Note numerous fluid-fluid levels.

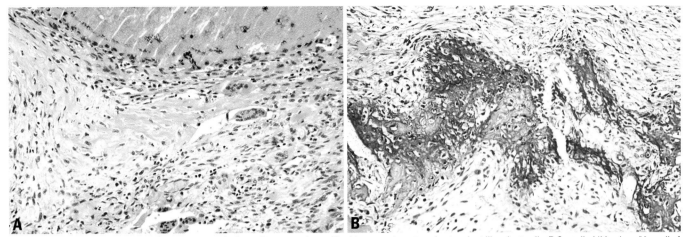

Fig. 20.03 Aneurysmal bone cyst. **A** Septa composed of reactive woven bone, fibroblasts, and scattered osteoclast-like giant cells. **B** So-called 'blue bone" in wall of the lesion.

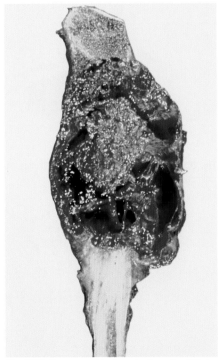

Fig. 20.04 Aneurysmal bone cyst of proximal fibula. The well-defined haemorrhagic multicystic mass has a prominent solid component in the centre.

Genetics

The most notable genetic feature is the characteristic rearrangement of the chromosome 17 short arm {1645}. The chromosome 17 rearrangements are often in the form of balanced translocations, in which material is exchanged with the long arm of chromosome 16. However, there are many variations on this theme, and at least five different chromosomes can serve as translocation partners with chromosome 17 {435,938,1645,1909,2281,2311}. The cytogenetic analyses invariably reveal normal metaphases along with those bearing the translocations. Therefore, the translocations can be assumed to result from acquired aberrations, arising in cytogenetically normal precursor cells. The cytogenetic findings provide compelling evidence that many aneursymal bone cysts are clonal proliferations, with activation of a 17p oncogene playing a key role in their tumourigenesis. The mechanisms of oncogene activation appear to be heterogeneous, as shown by the different types of 17p rearrange-ment, and as evidenced by the absence of 17p rearrangement in some cyto-genetically abnormal aneursymal bone cysts {135,435,938,1645,1909,2281, 2311}. It is also striking that these varied, but related, cytogenetic abnor-malities have been reported across the entire clinicopathological spectrum of aneursymal bone cysts. Chromosome 16 rearrangement was identified in a solid variant aneursymal bone cyst, whereas chromosome 17 rearrangement was found in an extra-osseous case {435}. Hence, it appears that there are generalisable transforming mecha-nisms, that are utilised irrespective of histological subtype or site of origin.

Prognostic factors

ABC is a benign potentially locally recurrent lesion. The recurrence rate fol-lowing curettage is variable (20-70%). Spon- taneous regression following incomplete removal is very unusual. Rare cases of apparent malignant trans-formation of ABC have been reported {1197}.

Simple bone cyst

R.K. Kalil
E.S. Araujo

Definition
An intramedullary, usually unilocular, bone cyst (cavity) filled with serous or sero-sanguineous fluid.

Synonyms
Solitary bone cyst; unicameral bone cyst; juvenile bone cyst; essential bone cyst.

Epidemiology
Males predominate in a ratio of 3:1. About 85% of patients are in the first two decades of life.

Sites of involvement
There is a predilection for long bones, proximal humerus, proximal femur and proximal tibia accounting for up to 90% of cases. Pelvis and calcaneus are also common locations in older patients.

Clinical features / Imaging
Simple bone cyst can produce pain and swelling but, more frequently, patients present with a pathological fracture.

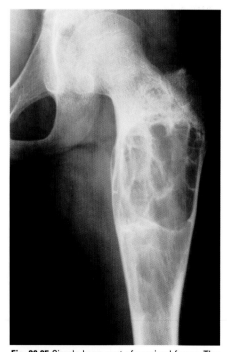

Fig. 20.05 Simple bone cyst of proximal femur. The lesion does not expand the bone.

Roentgenograms show a metaphysio-diaphyseal lucency, extending up to epiphyseal plate, with little or no expansion of bone; marginal sclerosis is absent or very thin. The cortex is usually eroded and thin, but is intact unless pathological fracture has occurred. There can be partial or complete septations of the cavity. MRI usually confirms its fluid content, that can be bloody in fractured lesions {1328}.

Aetiology
Growth defect at the epiphyseal plate has been postulated, or that a venous blood flow obstruction causes the simple cyst {342}.

Macroscopy
The cystic cavity is usually filled with serous or sero-sanguineous fluid. The inner surface of the cyst shows ridges separating depressed zones covered by a layer of thin membrane. Partial septae may be seen.
The occasionally curetted specimen consists of fragments of a usually thin, whitish membrane that may be attached at one surface to bone spicules.

Histopathology
The inner lining and septae of the cyst consist of connective tissue that can, occasionally, contain foci of reactive new bone formation, haemosiderin pigment and scattered giant cells. Fibrinous deposits are often seen. Some of these are mineralized, resembling cementum. Occasionally, histological features of fracture callus may be prominent. Rare "solidified" cases of simple bone cyst have been described in older subjects.

Genetics
A highly complex clonal structural rearrangement involving chromosomes 4, 6, 8, 16, 21 and both chromosomes 12 has been described in a surgically resected solitary bone cyst in an 11-year-old boy {2195}.

Prognostic factors
Recurrence is reported at 10-20% of cases, especially in children. Growth arrest of the affected bone and avascular necrosis of the head of the femur after pathological fracture can occur {2022}. Spontaneous healing after fracture has been described {52}.

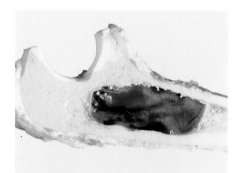

Fig. 20.06 Simple bone cyst of proximal ulna. A unilocular cyst contains fibrin clot.

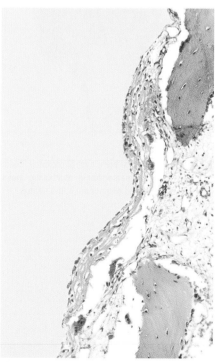

Fig. 20.07 Simple bone cyst. The lining is usually inconspicuous and contains scattered spindle cells and giant cells.

Fibrous dysplasia

G. Siegal
P. Dal Cin
E.S. Araujo

Definition
Fibrous dysplasia (FD) is a benign medullary fibro-osseous lesion which may involve one or more bones.

Synonyms
Fibrocartilagenous dysplasia, generalized fibrocystic disease of bone.

Epidemiology
Fibrous dysplasia occurs in children and adults world-wide and affects all racial groups with an equal sex distribution. The monostotic form is six times more common than polyostotic fibrous dysplasia.

Sites of involvement
The gnathic (jaw) bones are the most common site of involvement in surgical series (because they are often symptomatic) {1596}. In women, long bones are more often involved, whereas ribs and the skull are favoured sites in men {2154}. In the monostotic form, about 35% of cases involve the head, a second 1/3 occur in the femur and tibia, and an additional 20% in the ribs. In the polyostotic form, the femur, pelvis, and tibia are involved in the majority of cases {890}.

Clinical features / Imaging
Fibrous dysplasia may present in a monostotic or polyostotic form, and in the latter case, can be confined to one extremity or one side of the body or be diffuse. The polyostotic form often manifests earlier in life than the monostotic form {890}. The lesion is often asymptomatic but pain and fractures may be part of the clinical spectrum {333}. Fibrous dysplasia may also be associated with oncogenic osteomalacia {1660}.
The polyostotic form of fibrous dysplasia is intimately associated with McCune-Albright syndrome, in which there are endocrine abnormalities and skin pigmentation. There is also a relationship between fibrous dysplasia and intramuscular myxomas (Mazabraud syndrome) {630}.
Rontgenographic studies often show a non-aggressive geographic lesion with a ground glass matrix. There is generally no soft-tissue extension, and a periosteal reaction is not seen unless there is a complicating fracture. CT scans and MRI further delineate these features and better define the extent {422,1035,2118}.

Aetiology
Activating mutations of the G proteins have been identified in both the monostotic and polyostotic forms and may be aetiologically important.

Macroscopy
The bone is often expanded and the lesional tissue has a tan grey colour with a firm-to-gritty consistency. There may be cysts, which may contain some yellow-tinged fluid {1948}. When cartilage is present, it often stands out as sharply circumscribed of blue-tinged translucent material {2154}.

Histopathology
The lesion is generally well circumscribed and composed of fibrous and osseous components; which are present in varying proportions from lesion to lesion and also within the same lesion. The fibrous component is composed of cytologically bland spindle cells with a low mitotic rate. The osseous component is comprised of irregular curvilinear trabeculae of woven (or rarely lamellar) bone. Occasionally, the osseous component may take the form of rounded psammomatous or cementum-like bone. Secondary changes such as foam cells,

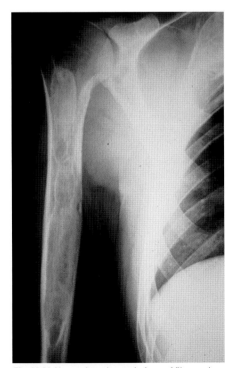

Fig. 20.08 X-ray of a polyostotic form of fibrous dysplasia. There is a well defined lucency with sclerotic margins.

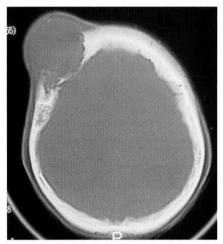

Fig. 20.09 CT of skull with fibrous dysplasia. In flat bones the process is often expansile.

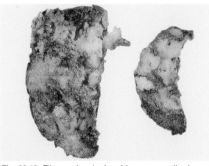

Fig. 20.10 Fibrous dysplasia with gross cartilaginous components.

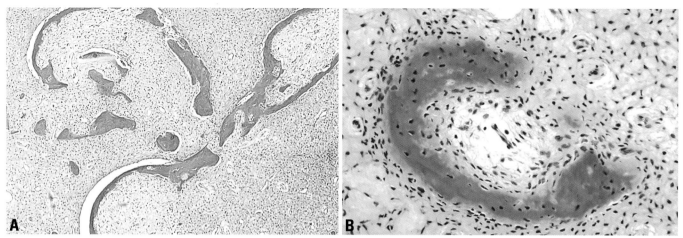

Fig. 20.11 Fibrous dysplasia. **A** Characteristic C shaped bony spicules with hypocellular spindle cell stroma. **B** High power appearance showing the typical appearance of bone which seems to be dissected by spindle cell proliferation. Note that there is no osteoblastic rimming.

multinucleate giant cells, a secondary aneurysmal bone cyst or myxoid change may occur.

Genetics
Activating mutations in the *GNAS1* gene, encoding the alfa subunit of stimulatory G protein, has been demonstrated in monostotic as well as polyostotic fibrous dysplasia {382} (see also chapter on McCune-Albright syndrome).

Clonal chromosome aberrations have been reported in eight of eleven investigated cases, suggesting that this entity is neoplastic in nature {439}. The only recurrent changes described so far are structural rearrangements involving 12p13 and trisomy 2 (three cases each).

Prognostic factors
The prognosis of patients with FD is good. Malignant transformation occurs, but rarely.

Osteofibrous dysplasia

V.J. Vigorita
B. Ghelman
P.C.W. Hogendoorn

Definition
Osteofibrous dysplasia (OFD) is a self-limited benign fibro-osseous lesion of bone characteristically involving cortical bone of the anterior mid-shaft of the tibia during infancy and childhood.

Synonyms
Kempson-Campanacci lesion, cortical fibrous dysplasia.

Epidemiology
The lesion is more commonly seen in boys during the first two decades of life with a precipitous drop-off thereafter, OFD has been reported in neonates, but is extremely rare after skeletal maturation.

Sites of involvement
The proximal or middle-third of the tibia is the most frequent site of involvement {301}. Lesions can be bilateral with ipsilateral or contralateral involvement of the fibula. Other sites include the ulna and radius {1055}. Multifocal or large confluent lesions oriented longitudinally along the cortical axis are not unusual.

Clinical features / Imaging
The lesion is rare after the age of 15. The most common presenting symptoms are swelling or a painless deforming bowing of the involved segment of the limb. OFD is typically epicentered in the cortical bone but may involve the medullary cavity by extension. Although slow growth is characteristic of OFD, some lesions are aggressive and may involve the entire bone with significant bowing deformity. Often well demarcated, it is associated with a thinning, expanding or even missing cortex. The expanding cortex is often sclerotically rimmed near the medullary bone. Separate or confluent oval-shaped, scalloped, saw-toothed or bubbly multiloculated lytic lesions are often noted. Perilesional sclerosis may be considerable. The radiodensity of the interior of the lytic foci are typically more radiodense than soft tissue. Periosteal reactions and soft tissue extensions are unusual. Bone scans are typically hot. CT scans classically delineate a cortical epicentre to the lesion not breaking through into the soft tissue and demarcated from medullary bone by sclerosis. MRI findings show high intensity lesions on T2 weighted images and mixed signals on T1 and fat suppressed images.

Aetiology
The occurrence of so-called OFD-like adamantinoma, to be distinguished from classic epithelium-rich adamantinoma but differentiated from OFD with difficulty, raises the possibility of an association between OFD and adamantinoma {112, 918,1188}. Some cases of OFD may arise de novo and are not related to adamantinoma.

Macroscopy
OFD is solid with a whitish, yellowish or reddish colour and soft or gritty texture blending into the surrounding host bone. The periosteum often appears intact but the cortex is thin or absent. The medullary extension is usually demarcated by a sclerotic rim.

Histopathology
The histopathologic findings in OFD are irregular fragments of woven bone often rimmed by lamellar layers of bone laid down by well defined osteoblasts. Osteoclasts may be present. The fibrous component consists of bland spindle cells with collagen production and a matrix that varies from a myxoid component to one that is moderately fibrous. Mitoses are extremely rare. A zonal architecture has been delineated with thin spicules and woven bone or even fibrous tissue predominating in the centre of the lesion with more abundant anastomosing and lamellar bone peripherally, the latter often blending

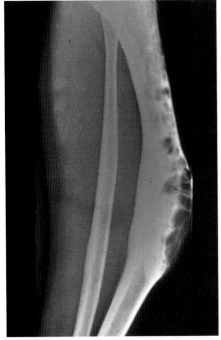

Fig. 20.12 Osteofibrous dysplasia. Expansile lucent, longitudinally-oriented tibial lesion surrounded by sclerosis and thinning of the anterior cortex of the diaphysis of the tibia. Note the anterior bowing of the tibia.

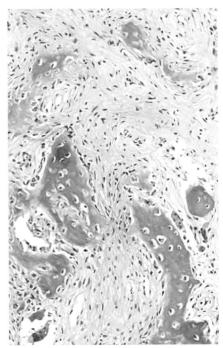

Fig. 20.13 Osteofibrous dysplasia. Low power magnification of the lesion featuring hypocellular spindle cell proliferation and spicules of bone. The bony spicules display prominent osteoblastic rimming.

Table 20.01
Chromosomal abnormalities in osteofibrous dysplasia.

No./Author	Age/sex	Tumour (type)	Karyotype abnormality
1 Bridge {256}	11,M	OFD (R)	47,XY,+12 (FISH: also +8,+20)
2 Bridge {256}	19,M	OFD (R)	49,XY,+7,+8,+22
3 Bridge {257}	18,F	OFD (P/R)	52,XX,+5,+7,+7,+8,+21,+21
P, primary tumour; R, recurrence, FISH: fluorescence in situ hybridization. Cases 1/2:keratin-negative OFDs.			

into the surrounding host bone {298}. Secondary changes of hyalinization, haemorrhage, xanthomatous change, cyst formation and foci of giant cells are rare. Cartilage or clusters of epithelial cells are absent.

Immunophenotype
Osteofibrous dysplasia is positive for vimentin and occasionally so for S100 and Leu7. Isolated cytokeratin positive mast cells have been mentioned.

A tumour should be defined as OFD-like adamantinoma when keratin-positive epithelial cells are found {918,1534}.

Genetics
Numerical chromosomal abberations, especially trisomy 7 and 8 have been demonstrated {256, 267}, as well as FOS and JUN proto-oncogene products.

Mutations of the alpha-subunit of signal transducing G-proteins with an increase in cyclic AMP formation are specifically absent {1845}.

Prognostic factors
The natural history of osteofibrous dysplasia is that of gradual growth during the first decade of life with stabilization at about 15 years of age followed by healing or spontaneous resolution. The progression of OFD-like adamantinoma (or 'OFD with keratin positive cells') to classic adamantinoma has been shown in a few patients {562,918, 1041,2016}. In many others, there is at least strong suggestion of a progression {381,2157, 2235}.

OFD-like adam- antinoma seldom progresses to classic adamantinoma.

Langerhans cell histiocytosis

B.R. De Young
K.K. Unni

Definition
Langerhans cell histiocytosis is a neoplastic proliferation of Langerhans cells.

ICD-O codes
Langerhans cell histiocytosis,
NOS   9751/1
Langerhans cell histiocytosis,
unifocal   9752/1
Langerhans cell histiocytosis,
multifocal   9753/1
Langerhans cell histiocytosis,
disseminated   9754/3

Synonyms
Eosinophilic granuloma, Langerhans cell granulomatosis, histiocytosis X. Clinical variants have been referred to as Hand-Schuller-Christian disease and Letterer-Siwe disease.

Incidence
Langerhans cell histiocytosis (LCH) is a relatively rare disorder, accounting for less than 1% of all osseous lesions. LCH involving bone has been reported in a wide age distribution ranging from the first months to the 8th decade of life with 80-85% of cases seen in patients under the age of 30, and 60% under the age of 10. Males are affected twice as often as females {1026,1253,1259,2253}.

Sites of involvement
Although any bone may be involved, there is a predilection for LCH to involve the bones of the skull, notably the calvarium. Other frequently involved sites include the femur, the bones of the pelvis, and the mandible {1259,2253}. In adults, the rib is the most frequent site of involvement {2253}. Monostotic disease is much more common than polyostotic.

Clinical features / Imaging
Pain and swelling of the affected area occur most commonly. Other findings are related to the bone involved. In cases of temporal bone involvement, the presenting features can show significant clinical overlap with otitis media or mastoiditis. With mandibular involvement, loosening or loss of teeth can be encountered. Vertebral body disease may result in compression fracture and possible neurological impairment. In adults, the lesion can present as an incidental finding on imaging studies.

Early lesions may appear very aggressive radiographically. Roentgenograms generally show a purely lytic, well demarcated lesion, usually associated with thick periosteal new bone formation. Skull lesions are sometimes described as representing a "hole in a hole" due to uneven involvement of the two osseous tables. In the vertebrae, the body is involved producing collapse giving rise to vertebra-plana.

Macroscopy
The involved tissue is soft and is red in colour.

Histopathology
The diagnosis depends on the recognition of Langerhans cells, which are intermediate size with indistinct cytoplasmic

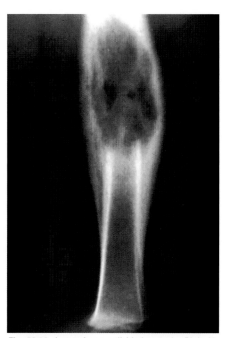

Fig. 20.14 Langerhans cell histiocytosis. Plain X-ray showing lucency in the shaft of the femur associated with thick periosteal new bone formation.

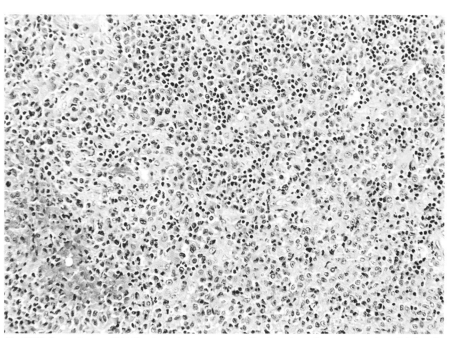

Fig. 20.15 Langerhans cell histiocytosis. Low power magnification shows loose aggregates of histiocytic appearing cells in a mixed inflammatory background with prominent eosinophilia and evidence of recent haemorrhage.

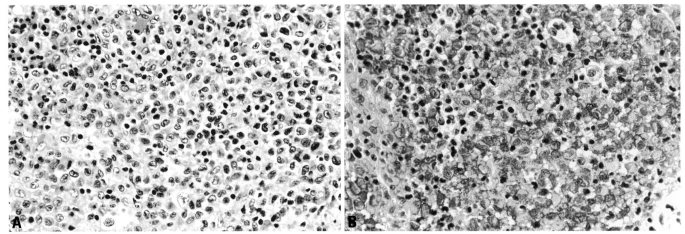

Fig. 20.16 Langerhans cell histiocytosis. **A** High power photomicrograph depicting Langerhans cells with ovoid to reniform nuclei with irregular notches and grooves. **B** Langerhans cells show distinct membrane based immunoreactivity for CD1a.

borders, eosinophilic to clear cytoplasm with oval nuclei which frequently are indented, irregular in outline, and typically possess nuclear grooves. Chromatin is either diffusely dispersed or condensed along the nuclear membrane. In osseous LCH, the Langerhans cells are found in nests or clusters. Diffuse sheet-like architecture is rare, and, if present, should raise the suspicion of haematolymphoid malignancy. The Langerhans cells are frequently admixed with inflammatory cells including large numbers of eosinophils, as well as lymphocytes, neutrophils and plasma cells. Necrosis is common and does not portend an aggressive clinical course. Multinucleat-ed osteoclast-like giant cells and occasionally lipid laden histiocytes may be present. The cells of LCH can exhibit a relatively brisk mitotic rate, with up to 5-6 mitoses per 10 high power fields.

Immunohistochemistry
Langerhans cells have a characteristic immunophenotype which includes expression of membrane based CD1a {584} and S100 protein in both a nuclear and cytoplasmic pattern {1530}. These cells typically fail to express CD45.

Ultrastructure
Langerhans cells contain unique intracy-toplasmic "tennis racket" shaped inclu-sions known as Birbeck granules which are thought to arise from the cell membrane.

Genetics
Studies of X-chromosome inactivation demonstrated that LCH is clonal {2275}.

Prognostic factors
The prognosis for patients with either monostotic or limited polyostotic disease is good. Death can result from LCH, but this is a rare event and is associated only with the disseminated forms of the disease and usually occurs in younger individuals less than three years at diagnosis and with visceral involvement.

Erdheim-Chester disease

T.N. Vinh
D.E. Sweet

Definition

Erdheim-Chester disease (ECD) is a rare histiocytosis characterized by infiltration of skeleton and viscera by lipid laden histiocytes leading to fibrosis and osteosclerosis.

Synonyms

Lipogranulomatosis, lipoidgranulomatosis, lipid (cholesterol) granulomatosis, polyostotic sclerosing histiocytosis.

Epidemiology

The disease demonstrates a slight male predominance with a peak incidence in the 5th through the 7th decades (age range is 7 to 84 years; mean age 53) {2203}.

Sites of involvement

ECD predominantly affects the major long bones of the extremities; but flat bones can also be involved {306,664, 1138}. Extraskeletal manifestations occur in more than 50% of cases, e.g. kidney/retroperitoneum, heart/pericardium, and lung.

Clinical features / Imaging

General symptoms consist of mild bone pain, occasionally associated with soft tissue swelling, fever, weight loss, and weakness. Other manifestations include exophthalmos, diabetes insipidus, kidney failure, cardiac, pulmonary, or neurological symptoms, eyelid xanthomas, and hepatosplenomegaly {627,1091, 1218,2045,2203}. Despite the impressive lipid laden histiocytic infiltration, the serum lipid profile is relatively normal.

The radiographic picture of ECD is unique and includes bilateral, symmetric, patchy or diffuse sclerosis of the medullary cavity of major long bones, with relative epiphyseal sparing {1785}. One third of cases have a mixed osteolytic and sclerotic pattern {276,1463, 2045}. The sclerotic lesions show increased uptake on bone scan. CT scan serves to detect orbital, dural, and retroperitoneal lesions. On MRI the lesion is of low signal intensity on T1-weighted sequences, enhances intensely after gadolinium injection {2299}, and gives mixed signal intensity on T2-weighted sequences {118,2045}.

Macroscopy

On gross examination, the lesions appear as sulphur-yellow and variably firm.

Histopathology

The histology consists of a diffuse infiltration of marrow by foamy histiocytes associated with dense fibrosis, lymphocytes, plasma cells and Touton giant cells. There is massive reactive sclerosis of cortical and cancellous bone with irregular cement lines.

Immunophenotype

Immunohistochemistry confirms the monocyte/macrophage lineage of the lipid laden foamy histiocytes and giant cells by their expression for lysozyme, Mac387, CD68 (Kp-1), CD4 {2168}, alpha-1-antichymotrypsin, alpha-1-antitrypsin and S100 protein (variable) {1615}. They are negative for CD1a.

Ultrastructure

Electron microscopy shows a predominance of histiocytes with indented nuclei, abundant intracytoplasmic lipid vacuoles and sparse mitochondria, lysosomes, and endoplasmic reticulum. Birbeck granules are absent {664}.

Prognostic factors

The majority of patients eventually die within 3 years of renal, cardiovascular, pulmonary, or CNS complications {2203}.

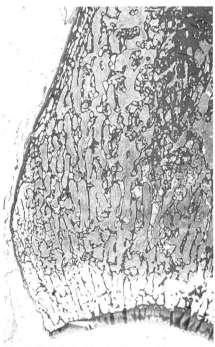

Fig. 20.18 Erdheim-Chester disease. Macrosection of tibia showing medullary sclerosis, which abruptly ends at the physis.

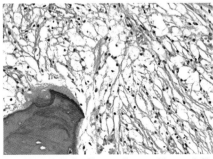

Fig. 20.19 Erdheim-Chester disease. Marrow infiltration by numerous foamy histiocytes associated with dense fibrosis.

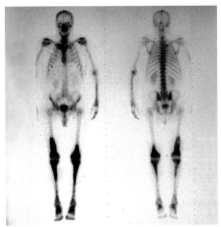

Fig. 20.17 Erdheim-Chester disease. Bone scan highlights the increased uptake throughout the entire length of the bones involved.

Chest wall hamartoma

E.F. McCarthy
H. Dorfman

Definition

Chest wall hamartoma is a non-neoplastic proliferation of mesenchymal tissue, predominantly cartilage, admixed with aneurysmal bone cyst elements. The lesion develops during fetal life and presents at or shortly after birth with an extrapleural mass arising from the rib cage.

Synonyms

Vascular hamartoma of infancy, mesenchymal hamartoma of the chest wall, mesenchymoma.

Epidemiology

The lesion is rare. To date only 59 cases have been documented. In approximately 40% of cases, the mass is apparent at birth. However, most cases present between ages one month to one year {97}. Less frequently, lesions may present in children up to age eight. One adult aged 26 was diagnosed with a chest wall hamartoma {531}. The lesion has also been diagnosed in utero with CT scans or ultrasound {1351,1807}.

Sites of involvement

The lesion is an intrathoracic and extraplural mass and arises from one or more ribs. Almost always, the posterior or lateral portions of the rib are affected.

Rarely, the lesion may be multifocal or bilateral in the chest cavity {2132}.

Clinical features

Chest wall hamartoma presents as a mass or fullness of the rib cage. Most often, the bulk of the mass is intrathoracic. As a result, infants frequently develop respiratory distress.

Radiographically, chest wall hamartoma is a partially mineralized mass arising from the inside of the rib cage and extending into the chest cavity. The involved rib is partially destroyed, and adjacent ribs are deformed. CT images show an expansile mass and partial rib destruction. Magnetic resonance images shows alternating areas of high and low signal on T1 and T2 sequences, reflecting both solid and cystic components {1886}.

Macroscopy

Lesions range from 3 to 7 cm in maximum dimension. Cut surface reveals grey to white solid areas adjacent to cystic cavities filled with blood.

Histopathology

Solid areas consist primarily of mature hyaline cartilage, although areas resembling chondroblastoma may be present. The cartilage often shows enchondral ossification. Areas with fibroblast-like cells are also present. Cystic areas show features typical of aneurysmal bone cyst: blood-filled lakes are bounded by fibrous septae which contain reactive bone and osteoclast-like giant cells.

Prognostic factors

Complete surgical removal of the affected ribs results in cure. Scoliosis is an occasional complication of surgery. Rarely untreated patients may die of respiratory insufficiency {1379}. However, most unoperated lesions remain stable. Spontaneous regression has also been reported {721}.

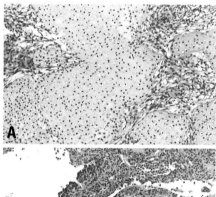

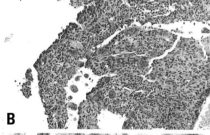

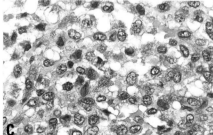

Fig. 20.22 Chest wall hamartoma (A) showing the typical chondroid matrix. B Histology similar to that of a conventional aneurysmal bone cyst with blood-filled lakes separated by septae composed of stromal cells and multinucleated giant cells. C Immature chondroblastoma-like cells.

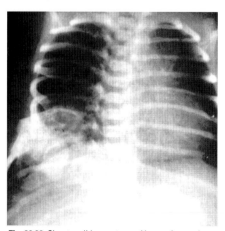

Fig. 20.20 Chest wall hamartoma. X-ray of a newborn showing a lesion in the right lower rib cage, involving several ribs and projecting into the chest cavity.

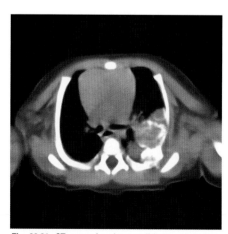

Fig. 20.21 CT scan of a chest wall hamartoma in a three-day-old infant involving the inner aspect of a rib. The lesion has a radiodense component.

CHAPTER 21

Congenital and Inherited Syndromes Associated with Bone and Soft Tissue Tumours

During the past decade, rapid progress has been made in our understanding of how inherited genetic aberrations may influence cancer risk. A large number of neoplasia-associated syndromes following Mendelian inheritance has been defined both clinically and at the DNA level, providing a solid basis for genetic counselling of patients and their families. The identification of specific genes involved in inherited cancer predisposition provides, in addition, important insights into genetic pathways involved in the development of sporadic neoplasia.

Although inherited susceptibility accounts for only a minority of all bone and soft tissue tumours, several syndromes and disorders have been identified, and for many of them the underlying genetic cause has been identified. In the attached Table, well characterized familial disorders associated with bone and soft tissue tumours are listed, including congenital malformation syndromes in which no clear pattern of inheritance has as yet been noted.

On the following pages, a more detailed description of the clinical, histopathological, and genetic data is provided for those syndromes that are well characterized at the DNA level, or for which the associated neoplasms display features that are distinct from those of their sporadic counterparts. Cowden disease, Li-Fraumeni syndrome and neurofibromatosis type 1 and 2 have been dealt with in the WHO Classification of Tumours of the Nervous System.

Table 21.01
Congenital syndromes associated with bone and soft tissue tumours.

OMIM[a]	Disorder[b]	Inheritance	Locus[c]	Gene	Bone and soft tissue tumours
103580	Albright hereditary osteodystrophy	AD	20q13	GNAS1	Soft tissue calcification and osteomas
153480	Bannayan-Riley-Ruvalcaba syndrome	AD	10q23	PTEN	Lipomas, haemangiomas
130650	Beckwith-Wiedemann syndrome	Sporadic/AD	11p15	Complex, incl. CDKN1C and IGF2	Embryonal rhabdomyosarcomas, myxomas, fibromas, hamartomas
210900	Bloom syndrome	AR	15q26	BLM	Osteosarcomas
160980, 605244	Carney complex	AD	17q23-24 2p16	PRKAR1AK -	Cardiac and other myxomas, melanocytic schwannomas
112250	Diaphyseal medullary stenosis with malignant fibrous histiocytoma	AD	9p21-22	-	Malignant fibrous histiocytomas of bone
151623	Li-Fraumeni syndrome	AD	17p13 22q11	TP53 CHEK2	Osteosarcomas, rhabdomyosarcomas and other soft tissue sarcomas
151800	Lipomatosis, symmetrical	Sporadic	-	-	Lipomas, lipomatosis of the head and neck
166000	Maffucci syndrome	Sporadic	-	-	Enchondromas, chondrosarcomas, spindle cell haemangiomas, haemangiomas, angiosarcomas
-	Mazabraud syndrome	Sporadic	20q13	GNAS1	Polyostotic fibrous dysplasia, osteosarcomas, intramuscular myxomas
174800	McCune-Albright syndrome	Sporadic	20q13	GNAS1	Polyostotic fibrous dysplasia, osteosarcomas
133700, 133701	Multiple osteochondromas, non-syndromic	AD	8q24, 11p11-12	EXT1 EXT2	Osteochondromas, chondrosarcomas
228550	Myofibromatosis	AR	-	-	Myofibromas
162200	Neurofibromatosis type 1	AD	17q11	NF1	Neurofibromas, malignant peripheral nerve sheath tumours
101000	Neurofibromatosis type 2	AD	22q12	NF2	Schwannomas
166000	Ollier disease (enchondromatosis)	Sporadic	3p21-22	PTHR1	Enchondromas, chondrosarcomas

OMIM[a]	Disorder[b]	Inheritance	Locus[c]	Gene	Bone and soft tissue tumours
167250; 602080	Paget disease of bone, familial	AD	18q21 5q31 5q35	*TNFRSF11A* - -	Osteosarcomas
176920	Proteus syndrome	Sporadic	-	-	Lipomas
180200	Retinoblastoma	AD	13q14	*RB1*	Osteosarcomas, soft tissue sarcomas
601607	Rhabdoid predisposition syndrome	AD	22q11	*SMARCB1*	Malignant rhabdoid tumours
268400	Rothmund-Thomson syndrome	AR	8q24	*RECQL4*	Osteosarcomas
180849	Rubinstein-Taybi syndrome	AD	16p13	*CREBBP*	Myogenic sarcomas
138000	Venous malformations with glomus cells	AD	1p21-22	-	Glomus tumors
277700	Werner syndrome	AR	8p11-12	*WRN*	Various bone and soft tissue sarcomas

a OMIM = entry number in McKusick's Online Mendelian Inheritance in Man {1376}.
b Syndromes associated with tumours affecting only the skin or parenchymatous organs are not included.
cAD = autosomal dominant; AR = autosomal recessive.

Familial adenomatous polyposis

M. Nilbert
C.M. Coffin

Definition
Familial adenomatous polyposis (FAP) is characterized by the development of multiple colorectal polyps, which are premalignant lesions with a strong tendency to progress into carcinomas. Gardner syndrome, characterized by colorectal polyps as well as extracolonic manifestations such as dental abnormalities, osteomas, epidermoid cysts and desmoid tumours, was initially considered a separate entity, but has now been recognized as a variant of FAP. FAP is caused by mutations in the adenomatosis polyposis coli (*APC*) gene on chromosome 5.

OMIM number   175100

Synonyms
Bussey-Gardner polyposis, adenomatous polyposis coli, familial polyposis coli, familial multiple polyposis, etc.

Incidence
Estimates of the incidence of FAP vary between 1/7,000 and 1/30,000 {1033}. Whereas dental abnormalities and osteomas occur in more than half of the patients, desmoid tumours and epidermoid cysts develop in a minority of the patients. Overall, FAP accounts for less than 1% of all colorectal cancers.

Diagnostic criteria
The diagnosis of FAP requires 1) at least 100 colorectal adenomas or 2) a

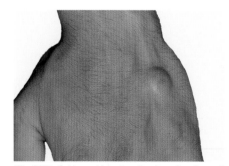

Fig. 21.01 Epidermoid cyst on the dorsal surface of the hand of a patient with familial adenomatous polyposis.

germline, disease-causing mutation of the *APC* gene or 3) a family history of FAP and at least one of the following: epidermoid cysts, osteomas or desmoid tumour. Other types of extracolonic manifestations are associated with FAP, including adenomatous polyps of the upper gastrointestinal tract, congenital hypertrophy of the retinal pigment epithelium (CHRPE), an increased risk of hepatoblastoma and tumours of the endocrine system, most commonly papillary carcinoma of the thyroid. Furthermore, an association with brain tumours, especially medulloblastomas, occurs in the Turcot syndrome, which in two-thirds of the cases is caused by *APC* mutations. In familial infiltrative fibromatosis (OMIM No. 135250), which is also caused by germline mutations of *APC*, there is an inherited predisposition to desmoid tumours, but only few or no colonic polyps.

Clinical features
Colorectal adenomas usually develop into endoscopically detectable lesions at 10-20 years of age and increase in number and size over time. Untreated FAP patients develop colorectal cancer at a median age of about 40 years. FAP patients should be screened with endoscopy with 1-2 year intervals from 10-15 years of age up to 40 years of age and prophylactic colectomy is performed when adenomas are detected. Extraintestinal manifestations, in particular epidermoid cysts, dental abnormalities, osteomas and CHRPE often preceed the development of adenomas and may serve as clinical markers of FAP.

Bone and soft tissue tumours
The description of Gardner syndrome in the 1950's highlighted the association of familial polyposis coli with a spectrum of extracolonic manifestations, including lesions of soft tissue and bone {766-769}. The most commonly encountered bone and soft tissue lesions are osteomas, cortical thickening of bone, epi-

dermoid cysts, and desmoid-type fibromatoses {766,768,1544,1606,1705}. In addition to these lesions, a variety of other soft tissue masses have been clinically described, with varying extents of pathological analysis. These include ill defined connective tissue masses, "lipomas" {1705}, "fibrous dysplastic lesions" {1544}, "familial infiltrative fibromatosis" {1913}, fibromatous mesenteric plaques {363}, juvenile nasopharyngeal angiofibroma {784}, Gardner fibroma {2227}, and rhabdomyosarcoma {84}.

The association of desmoids, including those with childhood onset, with adenomatous polyposis of the coli is now well recognized {175,312,361,362,566,768, 769,1032,1068,1913}. The incidence of desmoid tumours in patients with polyposis has been estimated to be around 10%. Pathological features of desmoid-type fibromatosis are described elsewhere in this book (see page 83). Particular *APC* mutation types are associated with a higher frequency of desmoid tumours {175, 312, 859, 931, 957, 1015,1047,1137,1286,1685,1799,1993}. The Gardner fibroma {2227}, described elsewhere in this book (see page 76), is similar to the fibromatous mesenteric plaques reported in patients with adenomatous polyposis coli {363}. These lesions are associated with development of desmoid-type fibromatosis in the same site, either following surgery or de novo {361,2227}. Recognition of the Gardner fibroma in childhood can serve as the sentinel event for diagnosis of adenomatous polyposis of the colon {2227}. Juvenile nasopharyngealangiofibroma has also been reported in association with adenomatous polyposis of the colon {8,10,784}. However, some have questioned whether this association is coincidental or whether it is actually related to another alteration of the *APC* gene {850}. Rhabdomyosar-coma has been reported in rare instances in individuals or families with adenomatous polyposis of the colon {84,1299}, but it is unclear whether this is a sporadic occurrence or another syndromic

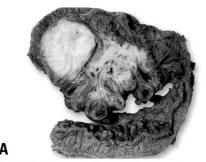
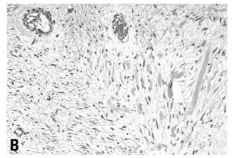

Fig. 21.02 Mesenteric fibromatosis (desmoid tumour) in a patient with FAP. **A** The lesion entraps loops of small intestine. **B** Histopathology is dominated by collagen bands and small vessels.

manifestation.

Bone lesions associated with adenomatous polyposis of the colon are entirely benign and are viewed as dysplasias. Multiple osteomas formed by membranous ossification, especially of calvarial and mandibular surfaces, characterize the "ivory exostosis" of Gardner syndrome {285, 331, 1075, 1690}. Histologically, the Gardner osteoma is a nodular excrescence of mature lamellar bone involving the cortical surface, especially the outer table of the skull, the mandibular cortex, or rarely other sites. Like desmoid fibromatosis, particular *APC* gene mutations are associated with more severe osseous manifestations {451, 1180, 2080}. Diffuse craniofacial sclerotic bone changes and dental malformations are also encountered. The bony lesions of adenomatous polyposis of the colon do not evolve into other benign neoplasms, such as osteoblastomas, or into malignant lesions.

Genetics

Germline mutations of the *APC* gene is the only identified cause of FAP. FAP is autosomally dominantly inherited with an almost complete penetrance. However, at least one-fifth of the patients lack a family history and are thus assumed to carry de novo mutations of the *APC* gene {204}.

Gene structure
The *APC* gene was in 1986 localized to 5q21-22 through observation of a patient with polyposis and a constitutional interstitial deletion of 5q followed by an establishment of linkage to this locus in several FAP kindreds {940, 1241}. The *APC* gene was isolated in 1991 and was found to be mutated in the germline of patients with FAP {840, 1123}. The gene spans 120 kb, is composed of 15 coding exons and contains an open reading frame of 8,538 bp. Several alternatively spliced forms of *APC* with different 5´regions have been identified.

Gene expression
The 2,843 amino-acid APC protein is ubiquitously expressed in most normal tissues with the highest expression found in the central nervous system. APC is a multifunctional protein with several functional domains through which APC exerts its main function as a negative regulator of the Wnt signalling pathway {312,693,921,1819}. Normal Wnt signalling inhibits the function of glycogen synthase 3ß (GSK3B), dephosphorylates axin / conductin and thereby targets ß-catenin for degradation. ß-catenin is involved in the cytoskeletal organisation with microtubule binding and in cell adhesion through interaction with E-cadherin. *APC* mutations, presumably trough loss of binding sites and degradation sites for ß-catenin lead to intracellular accumulation of ß-catenin, which is transferred to the nucleus and through interaction with transcription factors of the TCF/LEF family regulates expression of downstream target genes such as *MYC* and *CCND1* {2011, 2104}. The C-terminal mediates binding to microtubule-associated proteins of the EB1/RP1 family. Truncated APC thereby promotes chromosomal instability through disrupted interaction between the kinetochores and the spindle microtubules {693}.

Mutations
Analyses of the *APC* gene in patients with FAP reveal mutations in about 80% of the kindreds examined, and the remaining patient are likely to carry *APC* gene mutations leading to large deletions or impaired protein expression. Over 95% of the mutations identified result in protein truncation, which largely result from nonsense point mutations or deletions causing frameshifts. Genotype-phenotype correlations exist;

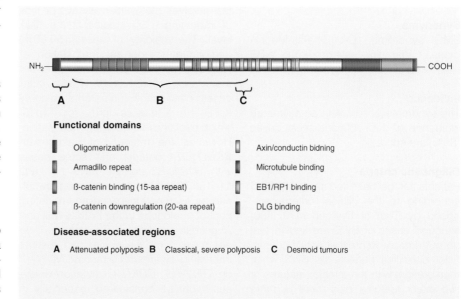

Fig. 21.03 Functional and disease-related domains of the *APC* gene. ß-catenin binding is achieved through the 15-amino acid and 20-amino acid repeat-containing regions and the C-terminal of APC which interacts with microtubule-associated proteins of the EB/RP family and with DLG, a human homologue of the Drosophila discs large tumour suppressor protein. Mutations between codons 1403 and 1578 have been associated with the extracolonic manifestations, e.g. desmoid tumours.

truncating mutations in the 5′ end of the gene have been associated with attenuated FAP, mutations in the central region of gene, including the mutational hotspot at codon 1309, are associated with multiple polyps at young age, and mutations between codons 1444 and 1578 are associated with an increased incidence of desmoid tumours {451, 1124, 2011}. However, patients with identical mutations can develop dissimilar clinical features and the genotype clinically serves as a risk determinant rather than as an absolute predictor of the extent of the disease.

Beckwith-Wiedemann syndrome

M. Mannens

Definition
The Beckwith-Wiedemann syndrome (BWS) is a complex overgrowth disorder caused by a number of genes that are subject to genomic imprinting. A high incidence of solid childhood tumours, including rhabdomyosarcoma, is seen in patients that present with BWS.

OMIM number   130650

Synonyms
EMG syndrome (Exomphalos-Macro-glossa-Gigantism syndrome), WBS (Wiedemann-Beckwith syndrome).

Incidence
The syndrome occurs with an estimated incidence of 1:13,700 and most cases (85%) are sporadic.

Diagnostic criteria
Patients can be classified as having BWS according to the clinical criteria proposed by Elliot or DeBaun {479, 580} although cases of BWS are known that do not comply with either set of criteria. Elliot classifies patients as BWS when they present with three major features or two major features plus three or more minor features (major features: anterior abdominal wall defects, macroglossia and pre- and/or postnatal growth > 90th centile; Minor features: ear creases or pits, naevus flammeus, hypoglycaemia,

nephromegaly and hemihypertrophy). DeBaun is less strict in his classification i.e. two or more of the five most common features (macroglossia, birth weight > 90th percentile, hypoglaecemia in the first month of life, ear creases/pits and abdominal wall defects).

BWS can be diagnosed in the laboratory by chromosome banding analysis (< 5%) or DNA-diagnostics. The current major test involves methylation assays or loss of imprinting (LOI) studies at the RNA level. The majority of cases (50-80%) demonstrates aberrant methylation of *KCNQ1OT1*, with or without aberrant methylation of *IGF2/H19*. These latter cases often show uniparental disomy (UPD), in a mosaic form, for 11p15, which explains this aberrant methylation. However, the majority of cases with *KCNQ1OT1* defects and some cases with *H19/IGF2* defects have no UPD 11p15. Therefore, an imprinting switch can be assumed involving an imprinting centre, analogous to the Prader-Willi and Angelman syndromes. The current data are most compatible with two distinct imprinting centres for either *KCNQ1OT1* or *IGF2/H19*. *CDKN1C* mutation analyses might be considered, especially in familial cases of BWS. The increased tumour risk for BWS patients seems to be associated with UPD in general and *H19* methylation defects in particular. *KCNQ1OT1* methylation defects only

seem to be a favourable prognostic factor since tumours are not, or only very rarely associated with this group of patients. Recurrence risks for a second pregnancy can be assessed with UPD studies. In case of a UPD in a mosaic form, there is no increased recurrence risk for BWS in a second pregnancy since the genetic defect occurred post-fertilisation.

Clinical features
The BWS is a disorder first described by Beckwith in 1963 at the 11th annual meeting of the Western Society for Pediatric Research. Later, Wiedemann and Beckwith described the syndrome in more detail {149, 2266}. BWS is characterized by a great variety of clinical features, among which are abdominal wall defects, macroglossia, pre- and postnatal gigantism, earlobe pits or creases, facial nevus flammeus, hypoglycemia, renal abnormalities and hemihypertrophy.

Tumours
BWS patients have a risk of 7.5% for the development of (mostly intra-abdominal) childhood tumours. Tumours most frequently found are Wilms' tumour, adrenocortical carcinoma, embryonal rhabdomyosarcoma, and hepatoblastoma. Also myxomas, fibromas, and chest wall hamartomas have been reported to occur at increased frequencies.

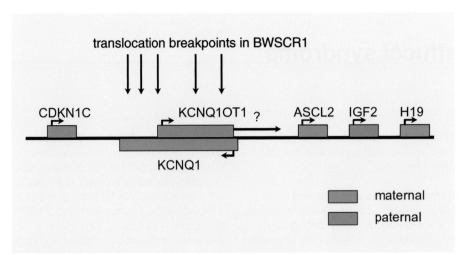

Fig. 21.04 Imprinted genes on 11p15 involved in BWS. The parental expression (imprinting) of these genes is indicated.

Genetics

BWS is caused by genetic changes in chromosome band 11q15, as shown by linkage studies, and the detection of chromosome abnormalities, LOI, and gene mutations. The syndrome is subject to genomic imprinting since maternal transmission seems to be predominant. In addition, chromosomal translocations are of maternal origin, duplications and UPD of paternal origin. All hitherto known causative genes are imprinted. The translocation breakpoints on chromosome 11 map to three distinct regions within 11p15.3-pter. Beckwith-Wiedemann syndrome chromosome region 1 (BWSCR1) near *INS/IGF2*, BWSCR2 5 Mb proximal to BWSCR1, and BWSCR3 2 Mb even more proximal {967}. This already points to genetic heterogeneity but also at the clinical level there seems to be heterogeneity. Chromosomal translocations in BWSCR1 and BWSCR3 are associated with the classical BWS phenotype and BWSCR2 with minor BWS features but pronounced hemihypertrophy. BWSCR 1 and BWSCR2 have been cloned and genes isolated from these regions were shown to be involved in the development of this disorder. All genes involved are subject to genomic imprinting {1326, 2023}.

BWSCR1

This region consists of a number of imprinted genes. All known translocation breakpoints disrupt *KCNQ1*, a gene coding for a potassium channel in-volved also in inherited cardiac arrhythmia syndromes. This imprinted gene, however, is most likely not directly involved in BWS. A gene transcribed in the antisense orientation of *KCNQ1* clearly is. This gene, *KCNQ1OT1*, shows aberrant methylation in 50-80% of BWS cases. It does not code for a protein and may function through its RNA. *CDKN1C* is an inhibitor of cyclin-dependent kinases. Heterozygous mutations have been identified in about 20% of BWS patients in two studies. Others, however, have not been able to confirm this mutation frequency. Although not a major cause of BWS, it is possible that in certain countries, e.g., in Asia, the mutation frequency is elevated. In addition, it has been reported that this gene is more frequently involved in familial cases of BWS. *CDKN1C* mouse models revealed some of the clinical BWS features such as omphalocele and renal adrenal cortex anomalies. In humans, *CDKN1C* also seems to be more frequently associated with abdominal wall defects. Another strong candidate for involvement in the aetiology of BWS is *IGF2*. Mouse models overexpressing Igf2 displayed a phenotype overlapping with the BWS phenotype. Loss of *IGF2* imprinting is often seen in BWS patients. Down-stream from *IGF2* lies *H19*, again a non-coding gene. The expression of *IGF2* and *H19* seems to be linked. *H19* is important for the maintenance of the imprinting status of *IGF2*. Mouse studies underline the link between *IGF2* and *H19* expression and overgrowth phenotypes were found. *H19* loss of imprinting is frequently seen in BWS cases although not always in combination with *IGF2* LOI. Finally, a gene called *ASCL2* is localized to the 11p15-imprinted region. Although no direct involvement in the BWS aetiology is known, this gene might account for the fact that most, if not all, BWS cases with UPD present in a mosaic form. The mouse homologue codes for a transcription factor, which is expressed during early mouse development and is essential for the development of the placenta. Therefore, also in humans, complete lack of expression might be lethal.

BWSCR2

Two patients define this second chromosomal region, one of whom developed a Wilms tumour {34}. Both translocations in 11p15.4 disrupt a paternally imprinted zinc-binding finger gene *ZNF215*. Parts of the 3' end of this gene are transcribed from the antisense strand of a second zinc-finger gene, *ZNF214*. Although putative mutations in these genes in other sporadic BWS cases were found, their involvement in BWS needs to be further elucidated by functional studies.

More detailed information on the structure and expression of genes involved in BWS could be found at: http://www.infobiogen.fr/services/chromcancer/Kprones/Beckwith WiedemannID10037.html {1325}.

Enchondromatosis:
Ollier disease and Maffucci syndrome

F. Mertens
K. Unni

Definition
Ollier disease is a developmental disorder characterized by the occurrence of multiple cartilaginous masses, particularly affecting the short and long tubular bones of the limbs. When cutaneous, soft tissue or visceral haemangiomas are also present, the disorder is referred to as Maffucci syndrome.

OMIM number   16600L {1376}

Synonyms
Ollier disease is also referred to as multiple enchondromas or dyschondroplasia.

Incidence
Rare, but exact incidence is unknown. Enchondromatosis has been described in many different ethnic groups, and there is no significant gender bias.

Diagnostic criteria
The diagnosis is based on the roentgenographic appearance and clinical features. No distinctive genetic or biochemical marker for either Ollier disease or Maffucci syndrome has as yet been identified.

Clinical features and tumours
Ollier disease usually manifests already in early childhood, commonly presenting as swelling of the fingers. Enchondromas in the metaphyseal regions of long bones may also result in deformity and limb asymmetry, as well as pathological fractures. Although careful examination will reveal that the vast majority of patients have bilateral enchondromatosis, there is a tendency for one side of the body to be more severely affected. The extent of a patient's orthopedic complications, which is highly variable and difficult to predict, is largely dependent on the number and skeletal distribution of enchondromas.

The enchondromas primarily affect the short and long tubular bones of the extremities, but flat bones, such as the pelvis and ribs, may be involved. The craniofacial bones and vertebrae, however, are usually spared. With few exceptions, the enchondromatous lesions stop growing at puberty. Continued or renewed growth in adults should raise the suspicion of malignancy. Whereas sarcomatous transformation of solitary enchondromas is rare, patients with Ollier have a markedly increased risk, ranging from 15 to 30%, of developing malignant bone tumours, in particular chondrosarcomas {1274,1901}. Some patients even develop multiple sarcomas {303}.

Most patients with Maffucci syndrome present at birth or in early childhood with cavernous haemangiomas, varying in size from a few millimetres to several centimetres, that are typically located in the dermis or subcutaneously on the distal parts of the limbs. However, haemangiomas may also be found in internal organs. In addition, spindle cell haemangioma, a vascular lesion with a high propensity for local recurrence but no potential for metastasis, is overrepresented among patients with Maffucci syndrome {639,1688}.

The skeletal features in Maffucci syndrome are indistinguishable from those in Ollier disease, but the risk of developing chondrosarcoma is possibly even higher among patients with Maffucci syndrome, with incidence figures reaching 20-30% in some series {1067,2055}. An increased incidence has also been suggested for other malignancies, including angiosarcomas, brain tumours, and tumours of the hepatobiliary system {538, 1901}, as well as certain benign tumours. In both forms of enchondromatosis, careful surgical and orthopedic intervention may avoid or minimise deformities. Furthermore, all patients should be instructed to pay close attention to signs or symptoms heralding malignant transformation.

The more widespread the disease, the greater is the likelihood for malignant transformation {538}. The prognosis for patients developing secondary chondrosarcoma is similar to that for patients with sporadic chondrosarcomas, and depends on tumour size and location, and histological malignancy grade {1230}.

Roentgenographic features
Roentgenographic features of Ollier disease and Maffucci syndrome are similar except for the presence of phleboliths in the soft tissue haemangiomas in the latter condition. The cartilage present has expansile masses at the metaphyseal region with calcification in the form of longitudinal striation.

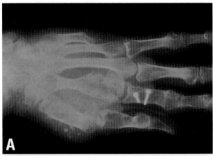
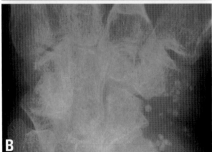

Fig. 21.05 Enchondromas and calcified thrombi in soft tissue haemangiomas in the left hand of a patient with Maffucci syndrome.

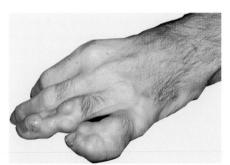

Fig. 21.06 Multiple enchondromas causing swelling and angular deformity in the left hand of a patient with Ollier disease.

Microscopic features

The cartilage in enchondromas is present as well circumscribed nodules in the medullary cavity and occasionally on the surface. The matrix does not show myxoid change. The lesion is hypercellular and the chondrocyte nuclei are enlarged and irregular.

Genetics

Most cases of enchondromatosis are sporadic, but families with multiple affected members have been reported, possibly suggesting autosomal dominant inheritance with reduced penetrance {1376}. Molecular genetic analysis of a high grade chondrosarcoma from a patient with Ollier disease revealed loss of heterozygosity for the chromosomal bands harbouring the *RB1* and *CDKN2A* tumour suppressor genes as well as TP53 overexpression, but none of these changes were found in tissue from an enchondroma {243}.

Recently, a study of patients with Ollier disease revealed mutations of the *PTHR1* gene, encoding a receptor for parathyroid hormone and parathyroid hormone-related protein (PTH/PTHrP), in two of six cases; in one as a germline mutation, and in one as a somatic mutation in enchondroma tissue {968}. The detected mutation, resulting in an R150C substitution in the extracellular domain of PTHR1, was shown to cause increased cAMP signalling, which is analogous to the situation in Jansen metaphyseal chondrodysplasia (OMIM 156400), an autosomal dominant disorder sharing some radiographic and histological features with Ollier disease. The hypothesis that a mutant PTH/PTHrP receptor could delay the differentiation of proliferating chondrocytes by constitutively activating Hedgehog signalling {1885} was further substantiated by studies of transgenic mice carrying the same R150C *PTHR1* mutation {968}. The R150C substitution could not be detected in a series of 50 sporadic chondrosarcomas {968}.

McCune-Albright syndrome

M.M. Cohen, Jr.
G.P. Siegal

Definition

McCune-Albright syndrome (MAS) is a sporadically occurring disorder consisting of polyostotic fibrous dysplasia, café-au-lait spots, and hyperfunctioning endocrinopathies. The syndrome is caused by mutations in the *GNAS1* gene.

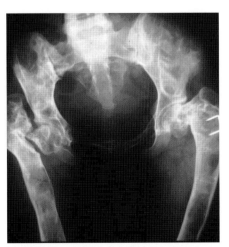

Fig. 21.07 Fibrous dysplasia in Albright syndrome.

OMIM number   174800L

Incidence

No accurate incidence has ever been determined for MAS. Fibrous dysplasia may occur without MAS and the overwhelming majority of these cases are monostotic. Polyostotic fibrous dysplasia occurs much less frequently and about 3% of the these cases represent MAS {382,383}.

Diagnostic criteria

Polyostotic fibrous dysplasia, café-au-lait spots, and hyperfunctioning endocrinopathies {31-33,1375}.

Clinical features

Cardinal features include café-au-lait spots, polyostotic fibrous dysplasia, multiple endocrinopathies including sexual precocity, pituitary adenoma, and hyperthyroidism. There is high expression of the *FOS* proto-oncogene in cells populating the bone marrow spaces. Many other abnormalities are found with low frequency: gastrointestinal polyps; hyperplasia of the thymus, spleen, and pancreatic islet cells; hepatobiliary disease; cardiac disease; failure to thrive; metabolic acidosis; abnormalities in serum electrolytes, glucose, or insulin

Table 21.02
GNAS1 mutations in solitary, sporadic neoplasms.

Neoplasm
Osteosarcoma
Pituitary adenoma
Thyroid adenoma
Thyroid carcinoma
Parathyroid adenoma
Leydig cell tumour
Ovarian cyst
Intramuscular myxoma*
Breast carcinoma

* Mazabraud syndrome, the combination of polyostotic fibrous dysplasia and intramuscular myxomas, is also caused by *GNAS1* mutations. From Cohen {382}

Table 21.03
Mutations in the *GNAS1* gene.

Disorder	Exon	Nucleotide Change	Amino Acid Substitution
McCune-Albright syndrome	8	C → T	Arg201Cys
	8	G → A	Arg201His
Polyostotic fibrous dysplasia	8	C → T	Arg201Cys
Monostotic fibrous dysplasia	8	C → T	Arg201Cys
	8	G → A	Arg201His
Panostotic fibrous dysplasia	8	C → A	Arg201Ser
Solitary pituitary adenoma	8	C → T	Arg201Cys
	8	G → A	Arg201His
	8	C → A	Arg201Ser
	9	A → G	Gln227Arg
	9	G → T	Gln227His

From Cohen and Howell {383}

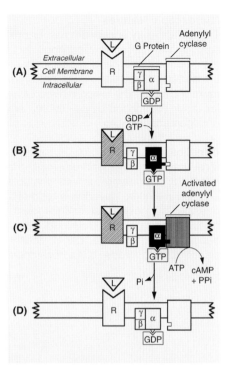

Fig. 21.08 (A) G protein composed of α, β, and γ subunits. This is the inactive form. B) Ligand (L) binding produces conformational change in receptor (R) and guanosine diphosphate (GDP) is replaced by guanosine triphosphate (GTP), resulting in dissociation of the α subunit. (C) Binding of α subunit to adenylyl cyclase activates 3',5'-cyclic adenosine monophosphate (cAMP) from adenosine triphosphate (ATP). (D) Hydrolysis of GTP to GDP by GTPase, causing dissociation of the α subunit from adenylyl cyclase and binding to the β and γ subunits, the inactive form. Ligand binding causes repetition of the cycle {383}.

levels; hyperphosphaturic hypophosphatemia; osteo-sarcoma (4%); developmental delay; microcephaly; and sudden or premature death {302,382,383, 392,1936}.

Bone and soft tissue tumours

As noted above, one of the primary pathological conditions which defines MAS is polyostotic fibrous dysplasia. Other benign lesions associated with this condition include mucoceles of the head and neck {547,745}, simple (unicameral) bone cysts {1001,1129} and aneurysmal bone cysts {76, 1288,1759}. Perhaps the best known concordance is with soft tissue, usually intramuscular, myxomas, known as the Mazabraud syndrome {2108}. Interestingly, activating mutation in the *GNAS1* gene have been detected in myxoma cells {1605}, but not in leukocytes or fibroblasts, from patients with Mazabraud syndrome.

Malignant bone tumours have also been associated with the fibrous dysplasia seen in MAS. Osteosarcoma, and possibly also conventional and dedifferentiated chondrosarcoma, appear to occur with increased frequency {212, 872, 932, 1282, 1630, 1725, 1823}. Although other sarcomas, including fibrosarcoma and malignant fibrous histiocytoma, have been linked to fibrous dysplasia {1822}, these have not been reported in patients with MAS.

Individuals with MAS are also susceptible to endocrine tumours, including adrenocortical and pituitary tumours {1133,1637}.

Genetics

McCune-Albright syndrome (MAS) is caused by mutations in the *GNAS1* gene located in chromosome band 20q13. *GNAS1* (guanine nucleotide-binding protein, α-stimulating activity polypeptide 1) encodes the G-protein α stimulatory subunit ($G_s\alpha$), a component of heterotrimeric G-protein complexes.

Gene function

G proteins (guanine nucleotide proteins) are a family of molecules composed of three subunits designated α, β, and γ. The function and specificity of each G protein is determined by the α subunit, which is unique for each type. The β and γ subunits tend to be more homogeneous. Like all G proteins, the inactive form of $G_s\alpha$ contains bound GDP (guanosine diphosphate). A GPCR (G protein-coupled receptor) facilitates the exchange of bound GTP (guanosine triphosphate) for GDP producing the active form {382,383}.

Adenylyl cyclase is activated following ligand-binding to G-protein-coupled receptor. Ligand-binding (B) produces a conformational change in the receptor and GDP is replaced by GTP, which results in dissociation of the a subunit.

Binding of the active form of the α subunit to adenylyl cyclase (C) activates this enzyme, resulting in the formation of cAMP from ATP. Hydrolysis of GTP to GDP is catalysed within seconds by the intrinsic GTPase (guanosine triphosphatase) activity of $G_s\alpha$ which causes dissociation of the a subunit from adenylyl cyclase and binding to the β, and γ subunits, resulting in the inactive form {382,383}.

Mutations

MAS, polyostotic fibrous dysplasia (PFD), monostotic fibrous dysplasia (MFD), and solitary pituitary adenoma (PA) have the same causal genesis – a ligand-independent, activating *GNAS1* mutation in the a subunit of stimulatory G protein ($G_s\alpha$). Mutations are located near the site which interacts with the γ-

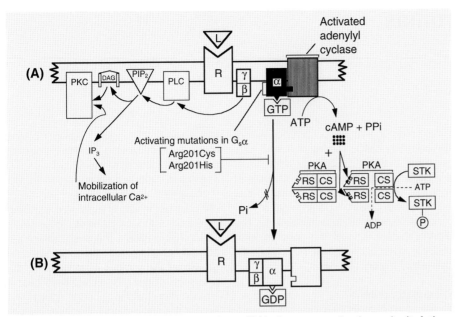

Fig. 21.09 (A) Activating mutations (Arg201Cys or Arg201His) in the gene encoding the α subunit of stimulatory G protein (G$_s$α), causing inappropriate stimulation of adenylyl cyclase interfering with hydrolysis of GTP by GTPase to GDP. The PKA pathway (protein kinase A or cAMP-dependent protein kinase pathway) is shown on the right. The PKC pathway (protein kinase C pathway) is shown on the left. Because the α subunit (G$_s$α) cannot dissociate from adenylyl cyclase, cAMP is overproduced which, in turn, overactivates the PKA pathway. PKA is composed of two regulatory subunits (RS) that have binding sites for cAMP, and two catalytic subunits (CS) that, when dissociated, phosphorylate serine/threonine kinases (STK). The dissociated βγ subunit overactivates the PKC pathway. PLC (phospholipase C) cleaves PIP2 (phosphatidylinositol bisphosphate) into two intracellular messengers: DAG (diacylglycerol) and IP3 (inositol trisphosphate). The latter triggers the release of sequestered calcium ions (Ca2+) which together with DAG activate PKC {383}.

phosphate of GTP, thus interfering with hydrolysis of GTP to GDP. Because G$_s$α cannot dissociate from adenylyl cyclase and bind to G$_{β}$γ, adenylyl cyclase remains active, producing increased cAMP activity which results in the pathology of MAS, PFD, MFD, and PA {382,383,1934,1936,1937,2230}. *GNAS* mutations have also been recorded in various solitary tumours {382}.

MAS, PFD, MFD, and PA occur sporadically. Mutations in the *GNAS1* gene occur postzygotically in a somatic cell. Clinical manifestations are variable in distribution and appearance. More generalized vs. more localized expression depends on (a) how small or how large the cell mass is during embryogenesis when the mutation occurs, and (b) where in the cell mass the mutation occurs {382, 383}.

GNAS1 mutations for MAS, PFD, MFD, and PA are of the gain-of-function type. It should be carefully noted that *GNAS1* mutations of the loss-of-function type are found in endocrine disorders characterized by hormone resistance, such as type 1a pseudohypothyroidism, glucocorticoid deficiency, and nephrogenic diabetes insipidus {1934}.

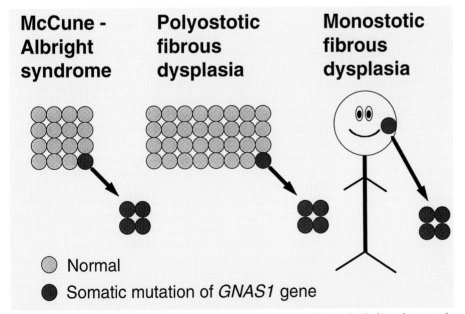

Fig. 21.10 How mutations cause McCune-Albright syndrome, polyostotic fibrous dysplasia, and monostotic fibrous dysplasia depend on when during embryonic development or during postnatal life the mutation occurs. Somatic mutation in a small cell mass is likely to result in McCune-Albright syndrome. Mutation in a larger cell mass may result in polyostotic fibrous dysplasia. A mutation in postnatal life – during infancy, childhood, or adult life – may result in monostotic fibrous dysplasia {383}.

Multiple osteochondromas

J.V.M.G. Bovée
P.C.W. Hogendoorn

Definition
Multiple osteochondromas (MO) is an autosomal dominant condition. It is genetically heterogeneous and is caused by mutations in one of the *EXT* genes.

OMIM numbers
According to the gene involved, the following OMIM numbers have been assigned:

EXT1	133700
EXT2	133701
EXT3	600209
TRPS2 / Langer Giedion syndrome	150230
Potocki-Shaffer syndrome	601224

Synonyms
EXT, diaphyseal aclasis, (multiple hereditary) osteochondromatosis, multiple cartilaginous exostoses, hereditary multiple exostoses.

Incidence
The solitary (sporadic) form of osteochondroma is approximately 6 times more common than the occurrence within the context of MO. The incidence of MO is approximately 1:50,000 persons within the general population {1887}. Males are more often affected (male: female ratio 1.5:1) {1236, 2265}, due in part to an incomplete penetrance in females {1236}. Approximately 62% of the patients with multiple osteochondromas have a positive family history {1236}.

Diagnostic criteria
A diagnosis of multiple exostoses can be made when radiologically at least two osteochondromas of the juxta-epiphyseal region of long bones are observed {1236}. MO is diagnosed in case of a positive family history and/or a proven germline mutation in one of the *EXT* genes.

Clinical features
Osteochondromas develop and increase in size in the first decade of life, ceasing to grow when the growth plates close at puberty. They are pedunculated or sessile (broad base) and can vary widely in size. The majority are asymptomatic and located in bones that develop from cartilage, especially the long bones of the extremities, predominantly around the knee. The number of osteochondromas may vary significantly within and between families. In addition, in the majority of MO patients bone remodelling defects are observed resulting in deformities of the forearm (shortening of the ulna with secondary bowing of radius) (39-60%) {1887, 1929}, inequality in limb length (10-50%) {1887, 1929}, varus or valgus angulation of the knee (8-33%) {1887, 1929}, deformity of the ankle (2-54%) {1887, 1929} and disproportionate short stature (37-44%) {1236, 2265}. It has long been thought that these abnormalities are the result of skeletal dysplasia, although recent evidence indicates that osteochondromas are neoplastic (see chapter 10), and it has been suggested that the growth retardation in MO may result from the local effects of enlarging osteochondromas {1717}. Moreover, the severity of angular deformity was found to be correlated with the number of sessile osteochondromas {309}.

The most important complication of MO is malignant transformation of an osteochondroma, which is estimated to occur in 0.5-3% of MO patients {815, 1236, 1695, 1887, 2265}. The suspicion of secondary chondrosarcoma is indicated by growth of the tumour after puberty, the presence of pain, or a thickness over 1 cm of the cartilaginous cap in adults. The size of the cartilaginous cap can be well established with T2-weighted MR imaging. There are no universally accepted guidelines for surveillance of individuals with MO so far.

Other complications of the osteochondromas include osseous and cosmetic deformities, fracture, bursa formation, arthritis (14%) {2265}) and impingement on adjacent tendons, nerves (23%) {2265}, vessels (11%) {2265} or spinal cord (<1%) {2187, 2265}.

Bone and soft tissue tumours
Hereditary osteochondromas and secondary peripheral chondrosarcomas developing within the cartilaginous cap of hereditary osteochondromas are histopathologically similar to their sporadic counterparts. Morphologically two types of osteochondroma can be recognized: broad based sessile cases with irregular cartilaginous linings and those with a well defined cartilaginous cap. Both may occur within and outside the context of MO. Malignant transformation of osteochondroma leads to a secondary peripheral chondrosarcoma in 94% of the cases {2276}. Very rare cases of other sarcomas developing in osteochondroma have been described, most often in solitary cases of osteochondroma {56, 1214, 1576, 1902, 1968, 2181} including osteosarcomas, and spindle cell sarcomas {1214, 1356}. These tumours develop in the stalk of the osteochondroma, in contrast to secondary peripheral chondrosarcomas, which develop in the cap of the pre-existing osteochondroma. A few cases of MO

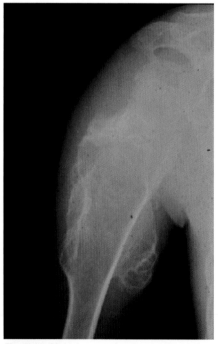

Fig. 21.11 Multiple osteochondromas in a patient with hereditary multiple osteochondromas.

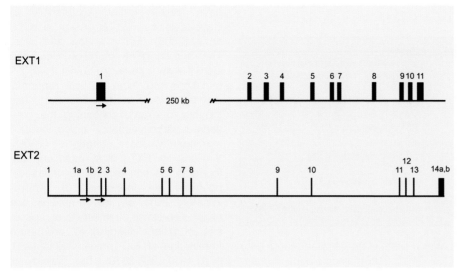

Fig. 21.12 Genomic structure of the *EXT1* and *EXT2* genes.

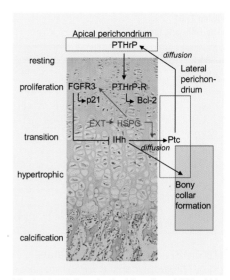

Fig. 21.13 706 Hypothesized function of EXT within the normal early embryonic growth plate.

patients have been reported to develop other sarcomas as well {239, 2139}. These osteosarcomas and spindle cell sarcomas (malignant fibrous histiocytomas and fibrosarcomas) display an indistinguishable phenotype from their non osteochondroma-related counterparts. Even more rare is the occurrence of "conventional" dedifferentiated peripheral chondrosarcoma, in which case the osteochondroma gives rise to peripheral low grade chondrosarcoma that in turn "dedifferentiates" into a high grade sarcoma that may appear as fibrosarcoma, malignant fibrous histiocytoma or osteosarcoma {183}. No soft tissue neoplasms are described within the context of MO.

Genetics
MO is a genetically heterogeneous disorder for which two genes, *EXT1* and *EXT2* located respectively at 8q24 and 11p11-p12, have been isolated {20, 395, 2031, 2310}. Additional linkage to chromosome arm 19p has been found, suggesting the existence of an *EXT3* gene {1229}. Loss of heterozygosity however is absent at this locus {236, 924, 1760} and the gene has never been identified. Three new genes, *EXTL1*, *EXTL2* and *EXTL3* have been identified based on their homology with the *EXT1* and *EXT2* genes {2180, 2283,2309}. However, no association with disease has been documented.
Both *EXT* genes are involved in a contiguous gene deletion syndrome. Patients carrying a deletion of 8q24

demonstrate the Langer-Giedion syndrome (LGS or trichorhinophalangeal syndrome type II (TRPS2; OMIM 150230), which is characterized by craniofacial dysmorphism and mental retardation in addition to multiple osteochondromas {975,1297,1298,1491}. LGS is due to loss of functional copies both of the *TRPS1* gene, encoding a zinc-finger protein {1491}, and the *EXT1* gene at 8q24 {975,1298}. Trichorhinophalangeal syndrome type I (TRPS1) (OMIM 190350) is similar to LGS although multiple osteochondromas are absent. Patients carrying a deletion of 11p11.2-p12 demonstrate Potocki-Shaffer syndrome (proximal 11p deletion syndrome {2307}, DEFECT11, 11p11.2 contiguous gene deletion syndrome). These patients demonstrate enlarged parietal foramina, multiple osteochondromas, and sometimes craniofacial dysostosis and mental retardation {134,1721}. The syndrome is caused by deletion of *EXT2* and probably of *ALX4*; haploinsufficiency of the latter was shown to potentially cause enlarged parietal foramina {134, 2303}.

Gene structure
The *EXT1* gene was identified by positional cloning {20}. The gene is composed of 11 exons, and spans approximately 350 kb of genomic DNA {1296}. The cDNA has a coding region of 2238 bp {20}. The promoter sequence is characteristic of a housekeeping gene {1296}. A mouse-homologue is found on mouse chromosome 15 with a very high

level of sequence homology {1266, 1279}. Additional homologues have been identified in Caenorhabditis elegans {369} and Drosophila melanogaster {156}.
The *EXT2* gene was also identified by positional cloning {2031,2310} and contains 16 exons, two of which (1a and 1b) are alternatively spliced {369}. The gene spans approximately 108 kb of genomic DNA {369}. The cDNA consists of approximately 3 kb, defining a single open reading frame of 2154 bp. The mRNA demonstrates alternative splicing {2031,2310}. A highly significant similarity with the *EXT1* gene product has been found, especially in the carboxy terminal region {2031,2310}. Homologues are found on mouse chromosome 2 {369, 2032} and in Caenorhabditis elegans {369}.

Gene expression
Both *EXT1* and *EXT2* mRNA is ubiquitously expressed {20, 2031, 2310}. A high level of expression of *Ext1* and *Ext2* mRNA has been found in developing limb buds of mouse embryos {1265, 2032} and expression was demonstrated to be confined to the proliferating and prehypertrophic chondrocytes of the growth plate {2030}. The gene products, exostosin-1 (*EXT1*) and exostosin-2 (*EXT2*), are endoplasmic reticulum localized type II transmembrane glycoproteins which form a Golgi-localized hetero-oligomeric complex that catalyzes heparan sulphate (HS) polymerisation

Table 21.04
The *EXT* gene family.

Gene	Chromosomal localization	Associated disease	Function: *glycosyltransferase activity involved in heparan sulphate (HS) biosynthesis:*
EXT1	8q24 {907}	MO	HS chain elongation {1267, 1372, 1954}
EXT2	11p11-p12 {977,961}	MO	HS chain elongation {1267, 1372, 1954}
EXTL1	1p36.1 {971}	Unknown	HS chain elongation {1108}
EXTL2	1p11-p12 {976}	Unknown	HS chain initiation {1127}
EXTL3	8p12-p22 {966}	Unknown	HS chain initiation and elongation {1108}

{1267,1372,1373,1954}. Heparan sulphate proteoglycans (HSPG) are large macromolecules composed of heparan sulphate glycosaminoglycan chains linked to a protein core. Four HSPG families have been identified: syndecan, glypican, perlecan and isoforms of CD44. HSPGs are required for high-affinity binding of fibroblast growth factor to its receptor {1275}. Furthermore, an *EXT1* homologue in Drosophila (tout-velu, Ttv) has been shown to be required for diffusion of an important segment polarity protein called Hedgehog (Hh) {156, 2107, 2126}, a homologue of mammalian Indian Hedgehog (IHh). It is therefore hypothesized that *EXT* mutations affect FGF and IHh signalling within the normal growth plate.

Mutations

The *EXT1* gene was reported to show linkage in 44%-66% of the MO families {1235, 1761}, whereas *EXT2* would be involved in 27% {1235}. Germline mutations of *EXT1* and *EXT2* in MO patients have been studied extensively in Caucasian as well as Asian populations {2306} (For overview see also: The human gene mutation database Cardiff www.hgmd.org {1176}). In *EXT1*, mutations are more or less randomly distributed over the first 6 exons, while the last 5 exons, containing the conserved carboxyterminal region, contain significantly less mutations {2306}. Similarly, in *EXT2* most mutations are found in the first exons. No mutational hotspots are found {2306}. Approximately 80% of the mutations are either non-sense, frameshift, or splice-site mutations leading to premature termination of EXT proteins {714,1656, 1761,1917,2308,2313}. The majority of missense mutations also lead to defective EXT protein function {340}.

Loss of the remaining wildtype allele has been demonstrated {238}, indicating that the *EXT* genes act as tumour suppressor genes. The limited number of genotype-fenotype correlational studies performed so far provide no uniform data {309,714}. The risk of malignant transformation would be higher in patients carrying *EXT1* mutations {714}.

Retinoblastoma syndrome

W.K. Cavenee
T. Hadjistilianou

O. Bögler
I.F. Newsham

Definition

Retinoblastoma (RB) is a malignant tumour originating from the embryonic neural retina. Familial retinoblastoma is typically bilateral, caused by a germline mutation in the *RB1* tumour suppressor gene and is often associated with the development of second site primary tumours, including osteosarcoma, fibrosarcoma, chondrosarcoma, Ewing sarcoma, pinealoblastoma, epithelial tumours, leukaemia, lymphoma, mela-noma and brain tumours.

OMIM number   180200 {1376}

Synonym

Retinoblastoma / osteogenic sarcoma syndrome.

Incidence

Retinoblastoma, the most common intraocular tumour of children, has a worldwide incidence between 1/3500 and 1/25000 with no significant differences between the sexes or races {28, 147,511,1856}.

Diagnostic criteria

Presentation is a white, pink-white, or yellow-white pupillary reflex termed "leukocoria" resulting from replacement of the vitreous by tumour, or by a large tumour growing in the macula {718}. Another common symptom, strabismus (exotropia or esotropia), can occur alone or associated with leukocoria. Less frequent presenting signs include a red, painful eye with secondary glaucoma, low-vision orbital cellulitis, unilateral mydriasis, and heterochromia {2346}. The tumour can be difficult to differentiate from a variety of simulating lesions such as persistent hyperplastic primary vitreous, retrolental fibroplasia, Coats disease, Toxocara canis infection, retinal dysplasia, or chronic retinal detachment {582,976}. These can be distinguished using CT, MRI, ultrasonography or fine-needle aspiration biopsy and a careful history of the family and affected child {582}.

Clinical features

Retinoblastoma can be unifocal or multifocal. In bilateral cases, one eye is usually in a more advanced stage, while the contralateral eye has one or more tumour foci. The average age at diagnosis is 12 months for bilateral and 18 months for unilateral cases, with 90 percent of the cases diagnosed before the age of 3 {29, 1157,1860,2123}. Retinoblastoma can be a part of the 13q-deletion syndrome in association with moderate growth and mental retardation, broad prominent nasal bridge, short nose, ear and dental abnormalities, and muscular hypotonia {38,717}.

Trilateral retinoblastoma describes the association between bilateral retinoblastoma and midline brain tumours, usually in the pineal region {554}. Pineal tumours resembling well differentiated retinoblastomas are also called ectopic retinoblastoma. CT scanning and MRI have reduced the misinterpretation of pineal tumours as intracranial spread of retinoblastoma {2346}. This is clinically important since ectopic intracranial retinoblastoma requires therapy to the whole neuraxis as well as high-dose equivalent radiotherapy to the primary tumour.

Pathology of retinoblastoma

Retinoblastoma occurs as a mass between the choroid and retina (exophytic) or bulge from the retina toward the vitreous (endophytic). Most advanced tumours show both patterns of growth. The tumour is histologically characterized by rosettes and fleurettes, which are believed to represent maturated or differentiated neoplastic cells. Rosettes are spherical structures (circular in section) of uniform cuboidal or short columnar cells arranged about a small round lumen (Flexner-Wintersteiner rosette) or without any lumen (Homer-Right rosette). The latter also appears in other neuro-ectodermal tumours such as medulloblastoma. Fleurettes are arranged with short, thin stromal axes surroun-

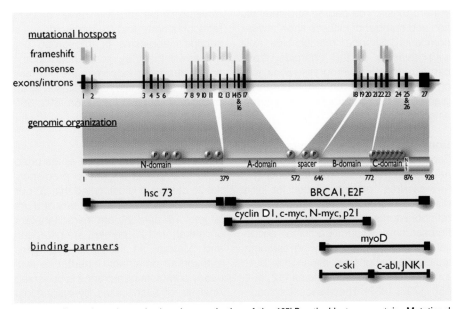

Fig. 21.14 Genomic and protein domain organization of the 105kD retinoblastoma protein. Mutational hotspots for frameshift and nonsense mutations are identified above individual exons. Examples of some of the known cellular binding proteins and their region of interaction are depicted below the protein domains. Sites of phosphorylation are also noted.

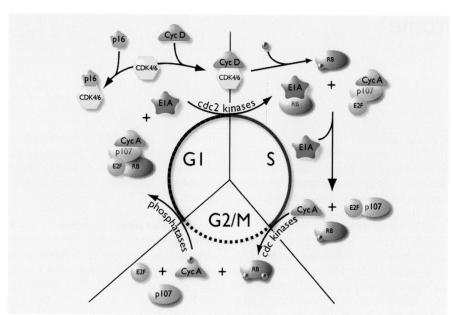

Fig. 21.15 Regulation of the cell cycle through oscillating phosphorylation of the p105 retinoblastoma protein.

ded by differentiated neoplastic cells with their apical part facing the externum. Tumours can be necrotic, with surviving cells around blood vessels, creating "pseudo-rosettes." Calcified foci and debris from nucleic acids can be found in necrotic areas giving rise to basophilic vessel walls {29, 1860, 2123}.

Growth patterns and other histological parameters are not useful for determining prognosis. The degree of differentiation and number of mitoses show a weak correlation. Stronger relationships exist with invasion of the choroids, optic nerves and sclera. Progressive invasion of the eye coats, even in the horizontal plane, is highly informative for determining prognosis {1157, 2123}.

Bone and soft tissue tumours

Second-site primary malignant tumours refer to nonmetastatic tumours arising in "disease-free" patients treated for initial disease. Tumours associated with retinoblastoma include osteosarcoma, fibrosarcoma, chondrosarcoma, epithelial malignant tumours, Ewing sarcoma, leukaemia, lymphoma, melanoma, brain tumours, and pinealoblastoma {12, 502, 550, 1793, 1837}. These second tumours are classified into five groups: (a)

tumours in the irradiated area, (b) tumours outside and remote from the irradiated area, (c) tumours in patients not receiving radiotherapy, (d) tumours unable to be determined as primary or metastases, and (e) tumours in members of retinoblastoma families who were free of retinal tumours. Two important observations have emerged from analysing these patients: (a) the great majority of children in whom second neoplasms develop have or will have bilateral retinoblastoma, and (b) the incidence of second neoplasms in this group was similar whether they received radiation or not. Osteogenic sarcomas are the most frequent second site neoplasms in all the published series {12, 336a, 502, 550, 1720a, 1723a, 1793, 1837}.

Genetics

Retinoblastoma has served as the prototypic example of a genetic predisposition to cancer. It is estimated that 60 percent of cases are nonhereditary and unilateral, 15 percent are hereditary and unilateral, and 25 percent are hereditary and bilateral. In the latter two types, autosomal dominant inheritance with nearly complete penetrance is observed. Analysis of such cases by epidemiological / cytogenetic {716, 941, 1145, 2006,

2017, 2044}, molecular genetic {317, 318} and molecular biological {558, 969} methods suggests as few as two required stochastic mutational events in the *RB1* locus for tumour formation. The first mutation can be inherited through the germ line or somatically acquired, whereas the second occurs somatically in either case. *RB1* locus inactivation is also found in non-hereditary retinoblastoma {552}, osteogenic and other sarcomas occurring as second primary tumours in retinoblastoma patients and some primary sarcomas in the absence of retinoblastoma involvement {724, 882}.

Gene structure and expression

The *RB1* locus in chromosome band 13q14.1 {317, 716, 2006, 2044} encompasses 200 kb of genomic DNA organized into 27 exons {228, 744, 1233}. The 105 kD RB1 protein is ubiquitously expressed in normal human and rodent tissues, including brain, kidney, ovary, spleen, liver, placenta, and retina. RB1 is differentially phosphorylated {1234}, with the unphosphorylated form predominantly found in the G1 stage of the cell cycle, and an initial phosphorylation occurring at the G1/S boundary {284, 482}. Viral proteins bind the p105RB protein {481, 564, 2262} using regions necessary for their transforming function. Over 100 intracellular pRB binding proteins have also been identified including E2F transcription factors, tumour suppressor BRCA1 and the RB-like proteins p107 and p130 {1508}. Complexing of the two latter factors also oscillates in a cell-cycle-dependent manner linking the tumour-suppressing function of RB1 with transcriptional regulation.

Mutations

Mutations that result in loss of RB1 function have been described for retinoblastoma patients and their tumours at the DNA, RNA, and protein levels. RB1 alterations have also been detected in a variety of clinically related second-site primary tumours including osteosarcoma, as well as other non-secondary tumours such as breast and small-cell lung carcinoma. Detection of *RB1* mutations provides for accurate prenatal risk assessment {319, 970, 2267, 2318}.

Rothmund-Thomson syndrome

N.M. Lindor

Definition

Rothmund-Thomson syndrome (RTS) is a constellation of various skin abnormalities, skeletal defects, juvenile cataracts, premature ageing, and a predisposition to osteosarcoma, skin cancer, and other tumours. At least a subset of cases are caused by inherited mutations in the *RECQL4* helicase gene.

OMIM number   268400

Synonym

Poikiloderma congenitale.

Incidence

RTS is a rare, autosomal recessive disorder. The exact incidence is unknown, but more than 250 cases have been reported in the world literature from a variety of ethnic backgrounds. A slight male preponderance (M:F = 2:1) has been reported {2212}.

Diagnostic criteria

Specific criteria for the diagnosis of RTS have not been established. The diagnosis is based upon clinical findings, the identification of *RECQL4* in a subset of

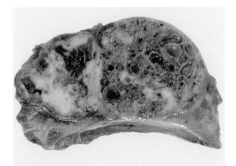

Fig. 21.16 Osteosarcoma of the rib in a patient with Rothmund-Thomson syndrome.

cases, and laboratory tests that can exclude some other, similar disorders.

Clinical features

The cardinal feature of RTS is a sun-sensitive erythematous rash that typically appears during the first 6 months. It usually starts in the face and then spreads to the buttocks and extremities. With time, the rash enters a chronic phase resulting in skin atrophy, telangiectasias, and marbleized mixed hyper- and hypopigmentation (poikiloderma) {1735, 2198, 2199, 2212}. Other features associated with RTS include short stature (~2/3 of the cases), premature greying and loss of hair (50-65%), sparse eyebrows/lashes (60-75%), juvenile cataracts (7-50%), photosensitivity (35%), radial ray anomalies (>20%) and other bony abnormalities, dystrophic nails and teeth, hypogonadism, and hypersensitivity to cytotoxic drugs and radiotherapy {1735, 2198, 2199, 2212}. RTS does not seem to be associated with intellectual or immunological impairment. There are no specific or consistently identifiable laboratory features in RTS. There have been several reports of acquired, clonal somatic mosaicism for chromosome abnormalities, especially trisomies, isochromosomes, and translocations frequently involving chromosome 8, often found in fibroblast cultures {1269}. There is no evidence of mismatch repair deficiency in the form of tumour microsatellite instability, as seen in tumours associated with the hereditary non-polyposis colon cancer syndrome, due to germline mutations in genes of the DNA mismatch repair complex). Furthermore, there is no increase in chromosomal sister-chromatid exchange rates (as seen

in Bloom syndrome), no excess of bleomycin-induced chromosome breakage (as seen in ataxia telangiectasia), and no chromosomal radial formation with mitomycin-C exposure (as seen in Fanconi anaemia). Ultraviolet sensitivity studies have yielded inconsistent results.

Bone and soft tissue tumours

Osteosarcomas, involving any bone and especially in non-common sites, have been reported to occur in up to one third of the patients, with a median age of diagnosis at 11.5 years {2212}. Also cutaneous malignancies, in particular squamous cell carcinomas, have been reported to be overrepresented in RTS {1735, 2212}.

Genetics

At least a subset of the cases of RTS are caused by mutations in the *RECQL4* (also known as *RECQ4*) helicase gene in chromosome band 8q24.3 {1128}. Only a small number of patients has as yet been investigated, with mutations being detected in approximately 40% of the cases {749}. The *RECQL4* gene has a predicted protein product of 1208 amino acids. It is highly expressed in the thymus and testis with low levels of intranuclear expression in multiple other tissues. *RECQL4* mutation analysis is available only in specialized centres. Mutations have included frameshift mutations, nonsense mutations, and deletions including part of the consensus helicase domain. This gene is homologous to the genes that cause Bloom syndrome and Werner syndrome, which might explain some of the clinical overlap {749}.

Werner syndrome

R.J. Monnat, Jr.

Definition

Werner syndrome (WS) is a rare, autosomal recessive genetic instability syndrome and is caused by mutations in the *WRN* gene. Affected patients develop a prematurely aged appearance in the second and third decades of life, and are at increased risk of developing both neoplastic and non-neoplastic diseases. Tumours include soft tissue sarcomas, thyroid carcinoma, malignant melanoma, meningioma, haematological neoplasms, and osteosarcoma. The most common causes of death are cancer and atherosclerotic cardiovascular disease.

OMIM number   277700

Synonym
Progeria of the adult.

Incidence

WS patients have been identified worldwide {819}. Estimates of the frequency or prevalence of WS, obtained by case counting and from consanguinity data, range from 1/22,000 to 1/10⁶ (reviewed in {1883}). The frequency of WS in different countries is strongly influenced by the presence of founder mutations and the frequency of consanguinity or inbreeding. The range of frequency estimates also undoubtedly reflects the variable and delayed development of the WS clinical phenotype {604, 819}, with consequent underdiagnosis.

Clinical features and diagnostic criteria

The most consistent clinical findings develop after age 10. These include bilateral cataracts, dermatological pathology resembling scleroderma, short stature and premature greying and loss of scalp hair {604,819}. There may be affected siblings as well as evidence of parental consanguinity (3rd cousin or closer). Additional, less consistent findings include diabetes mellitus, hypogonadism, osteoporosis, soft tissue calcification, premature atherosclerotic cardiovascular disease, high pitched, 'squeeky', or hoarse voice and flat feet.

A definite diagnosis can be established on clinical grounds when all of the consistent features and at least two additional findings are present. Additional diagnostic aids include evidence of elevated 24 hr urinary hyaluronic acid secretion; loss of WRN protein from fibroblasts or peripheral blood lymphocytes; and mutations in the *WRN* gene on chromosome arm 8p.

A clinical scoring system has been devised to identify more reliably definite, probable or possible WS patients. Additional information on this scoring system and the clinical diagnosis of WS can be found on the International Registry of Werner Syndrome Web site:
www.pathology.washington.edu/research/werner/registry/diagnostic.html

Table 21.05
Histopathological spectrum of neoplasia in Werner syndrome.
A wide spectrum of neoplasms has been identified in Werner syndrome (WS) patients, who are clearly at elevated risk of developing one or more of the neoplasms listed in the left column ('frequent'). These neoplasms represent 71% of all neoplasms reported in WS patients. WS patients may be at elevated risk of developing neoplasms listed in the right column, although the number of affected patients is too small in most cases to firmly establish this suspicion. A total of 257 neoplasms were represented in this analysis {820, 1494} (Y. Ishikawa, personal communication). The percentage of neoplasms from this analysis in each column or tumour type is indicated in parentheses.

Frequent (71%)	Less common (29%)
Soft tissue sarcomas (15.5% of cases) malignant fibrous histiocytoma leiomyosarcoma fibrosarcoma malignant schwannoma synovial sarcoma rhabdomyosarcoma	**Non-melanoma skin cancer (5.8%)** **Hepatobiliary carcinomas (5.3%)** hepatocellular cholangiocarcinoma gallbladder
Thyroid carcinomas (14%) follicular papillary anaplastic	**Genito-urinary (4.8%)** bladder carcinoma uterine/ovarian carcinoma renal cell carcinoma prostate carcinoma seminoma
Malignant melanoma (12.6%) acral lentigenous melanoma mucosal malignant melanoma	**Gastro-intestinal carcinoma (4.3%)** gastric oesophagus pancreas colon
Meningioma (11.1%) benign multiple / malignant	**Breast carcinoma (3.9%)** **Oro-pharyngeal carcinoma (2.4%)**
Haematological (11.1%) acute myelogenous leukaemias (M1-5) erythroleukaemia (M6) megakaryocytic leukaemia (M7) myelofibrosis/myelodysplasia aplastic anaemia	
Osteosarcoma (6.3%)	

Neoplastic disease spectrum

WS patients are at increased risk of developing both sarcomas and epithelial neoplasms {820, 1494}. The elevated risk of neoplasia is selective, and includes the following neoplasms in order of decreasing frequency: soft tissue sarcomas, thyroid carcinoma, meningioma, malignant melanoma, malignant or pre-neoplastic haematological disease and osteosarcoma. Many other neoplasms, including common adult epithelial malignancies, have been observed in WS patients. However, it is not clear whether the risk of developing these neoplasms is elevated above population controls. This histo-pathological spectrum of neoplasms overlaps with, though is distinct from, that observed in patients with two other RecQ helicase deficiency syndromes, Bloom syndrome and Rothmund-Thomson syndrome {1494}.

Several features of neoplasia in WS patients indicates that this human RecQ helicase deficiency syndrome is a heritable cancer predisposition: patients develop neoplasms at a comparatively early age; often have unusual sites of presentation (e.g., osteosarcoma of the patella) or less common histopathologic subtypes (e.g., follicular as opposed to papillary thyroid carcinoma); and can have multiple concurrent or sequential neoplasms, e.g., thyroid carcinoma and osteosarcoma. Estimates of the increased risk of neoplasia in WS patients range from 30-fold elevated overall lifetime risk across all tumour types to 1000-fold elevated risk for acral lentigenous melanoma.

Soft tissue sarcomas that have been identified in WS patients include malignant fibrous histiocytoma, malignant peripheral nerve sheath tumour, fibrosarcoma, rhabdomyosarcoma, lipo-sarcoma, and synovial sarcoma. Three histological subtypes of thyroid carcinoma have been reported in WS patients (follicular, papillary and anaplastic), with a predominance of the less common follicular variant. There has been no reported case of medullary thyroid carcinoma in a WS patient. The risk of malignant melanoma is confined almost exclusively to the relatively rare variants that arise on the palms and soles (acral lentigenous melanoma) or in mucosa of the nasal cavity or esophagus. Melanoma risk is most clearly elevated in Japanese WS patients {820}.

The spectrum of haematological disease in WS includes acute myelogenous leukaemia (M1-5), erythroleukaemia (M6) and megakaryocytic leukaemia (M7); atypical leukemia arising in the context of myelodysplasia; and the premalignant conditions myelodysplasia, myelofibrosis, and aplastic anaemia. The elevated risk of developing marrow-associated pre-malignant or malignant disease may be related to the progressive accumulation of genetic damage in bone marrow cell lineages {1509}.

Genetics

WS is an autosomal recessive disease: no cases are known to have been acquired or to have been caused by other agents. WS constitutes, together with Bloom syndrome and Rothmund-Thomson syndrome, a group of inherited human genetic instability / cancer predisposition syndromes that result from loss of function of a human RecQ helicase protein.

Gene structure and expression

The *WRN* gene consists of 35 exons in a 165 kb region of chromosome region 8p11-12 {2331}.

Two stable RNAs are encoded by the *WRN* gene, and the shorter, of 5.8 kb, is ubiquitously expressed at varying levels in many cell types, tissues and organs {2331}. The 162 kDa WRN protein is readily detectable in cell lines and tissue samples from normal individuals and heterozygous carriers of single mutant copies of the *WRN* gene by Western blot analysis {1510}. No systematic study of the level of expression of WRN protein as a function of cell type or of development has as yet been published. The WRN protein encodes both DNA helicase and exonuclease activities {1931}, and is likely to play an important physiologic role in homologous recombinational repair in human somatic cells {1728}.

Mutations

WS is an autosomal recessive disease, and thus patients have mutations in both *WRN* alleles. Virtually all of the *WRN* patient mutations thus far identified truncate the *WRN* open reading frame, lead to protein reduction or loss from patient cells and thus can be detected by Western blot analysis {821,1510}. Further mutation characterization can be performed by a combination of mutation-specific allele identification and / or DNA sequencing. Mutation analysis can be especially helpful in the diagnosis of WS in young patients, where the diagnosis is suspected but the clinical phenotype may be incompletely developed. A HUGO Locus-Specific *WRN* Mutational Database summarizes patient mutation data and mutation designations, polymorphism data, and related clinical data and cross-references these to the primary literature (www.pathology.washington.edu/research/werner/ws_wrn.html) {1511}. Additional information on *WRN* mutation analysis for the purpose of confirming a diagnosis of Werner syndrome can be obtained through the International Registry of Werner Syndrome Web site (www.pathology.washington.edu/research/werner/registry/diagnostic.html).

Contributors

Dr. Fadi ABDUL-KARIM
Institute of Pathology
University Hospitals of Cleveland
2085 Adelbert Road
Cleveland OH 44122
USA
Tel. +1 216 844 1807
Fax +1 216 844 1810
fwa@po.cwru.edu

Dr. Claus-Peter ADLER
Institute of Pathology
University of Freiburg i. Br.
Alberstrasse 19
Freiburg
GERMANY
Tel. +40 761 203 6741
Fax +40 761 203 6790
adlerc@ukl.uni-freiburg.de

Dr. Cristina R. ANTONESCU*
Dept. of Pathology
Memorial Sloan-Kettering Cancer Center
1275 York Avenue
New York, NY 10021
USA
Tel. +1 212-639-5721
Fax +1 212-717-3203
antonesc@mskcc.org

Dr. Alberto AYALA
Dept. of Pathology
UTMDACC-Pathology-Box 85
1515 Holcombe Boulevard
Houston, TX 77030
USA
Tel. +1 713 792 3151
Fax +1 713 792 4049
aayala@mdanderson.org

Dr. Patrizia BACCHINI
Istituto Rizzoli
University of Bologna
Via Di Barbiano 1/10
40136 Bologna
ITALY
Tel. +39 051 6366 593
Fax +39 051 6366 592
patrizia.bacchini@ior.it

Dr. S. S. BANERJEE
Dept. of Pathology
Christie Hospital
Wilmlslow Road, Withington
Manchester, M20 4BX
UNITED KINGDOM
Tel. +44-161-446-3000
Fax +44-161-446-3000
liz.ryan@christie-tr.nwest.nhs.uk

Dr. Manjula BANSAL
Dept. of Orthopaedic Pathology
The Hospital for Special Surgery
535 East 70th Street, Room 237
New York, NY 10021
USA
Tel. +1 212 606 1105
Fax +1 212 606 1910
bansalm@hss.edu

Dr. Frederic BARR
Dept. of Pathology & Laboratory Medicine
University of Pennsylvania
School of Medicine
Philadelphia, PA 19104-6082
USA
Tel. +1 215 898 0884
Fax +1 215 898 4227
barrfg@mail.med.upenn.edu

Dr. Alfred BEHAM
Institute of Pathology
University of Graz, Medical School
Auenbruggerplatz 25
A-8036 Graz
AUSTRIA
Tel. +43-316-3804410
Fax +43-316-373890
alfred.beham@kfunigraz.ac.at

Dr. Franco BERTONI*
Anatomia ed Istologia Patologica
Istituto Rizzoli
Via Di Barbiano 1/10
40126 Bologna
ITALY
Tel. +39 051 6366 593
Fax +39 051 6366 592
franco.bertoni@ior.it

Dr. Beata BODE-LESNIEWSKA
Institut für Klinische Pathologie
Universitätsspital Zürich
Schmelzbergstrasse 12
CH-8091 Zürich
SWITZERLAND
Tel. +41 1 255 40 51
Fax +41 1 255 25 51
beata.bode@pty.usz.ch

Dr. Oliver BÖGLER
Dept. of Neurosurgery and
Hermelin Brain Tumor Center
Henry Ford Hospital
2799 West Grand Boulevard
Detroit, MI 48202, USA
Tel. +1 313 916 7293
Fax +1 313 916 9855
oliver@bogler.net

Dr. Tom BÖHLING
Dept. of Pathology
Haartman Institute, University of Helsinki
Haartmansgatan 3, POB 21
SF-00014 Helsinki
FINLAND
Tel. +358 9 1912 6419
Fax +358 9 1912 6700
tom.bohling@helsinki.fi

Dr. Anita BORGES
Dept. of Pathology
Tata Memorial Hospital
Parel
Bombay 400 012
INDIA
Tel. +91-22-446-8134
Fax +91-22-414-6937
anitaboges@hotmail.com

Dr. Judith V.M.G. BOVÉE
Dept. of Pathology
Leiden University Medical Center
Albinusdreef 2, L1-Q, Postbox 9600
2300 RC Leiden
THE NETHERLANDS
Tel. +31 71 5266 507
Fax +31 71 5248 158
j.v.m.g.bovee@lumc.nl

Dr. Julia A. BRIDGE*
Dept. of Pathology/Microbiology
985440 Nebraska Medical Center
Omaha, NE 68198-5440
USA
Tel. +1 402 559 7212
Fax +1 402 559 6018
jbridge@unmc.edu

Dr. Peter BULLOUGH
Dept. of Orthopaedic Pathology
The Hospital for Special Surgery
535 E. 70th Street, Rm. 244B
New York, NY 10021
USA
Tel. +1 212 606 1341
Fax +1 212 606 1910
bulloughp@hss.edu

Dr. Eduardo CALONJE*
St. John's Institute of Dermatology
St. Thomas' Hospital
Lambeth Palace Road
SE1 7EH London
UNITED KINGDOM
Tel. +44-207-9289292 ext. 1383
Fax +44-207-9228347
jaime.calonje@kcl.ac.uk

Dr. Miguel CALVO-ASENSIO
Jefe De Patologia
Osteoarticular
San Pablo, 4
28230 Las Rozas, Madrid
SPAIN
Tel. +34 1 637 24 47
Fax +34 1 710 40 22
dr_mcalvo@yahoo.es

Dr. Webster K. CAVENEE
Ludwig Institute for Cancer Research
University of California, San Diego
9500 Gilman Drive
La Jolla, CA 92093-0660
USA
Tel. +1 858 534 7802
Fax +1 858 534 7750
wcavenee@ucsd.edu

Dr. John K.C. CHAN
Dept. of Pathology
Queen Elizabeth Hospital
Wylie Road
Kowloon, Hong Kong
HONG KONG
Tel. +852-2958-6830
Fax +852-2385-2455
jkcchan@ha.org.hk

Dr. Cheryl M. COFFIN*
Dept. of Pathology
University of Utah, School of Medicine
100 North Medical Drive
Salt Lake City, UT 84113
USA
Tel. +1 801-588-3165
Fax +1 801-588-3169
pcccoffi@ihc.com

Dr. M. Michael COHEN JR
Dept.s of Oral and Maxillofacial Sciences,
Pediatrics, Community Health and
Epidemiology, Dalhousie University
Halifax, Nova Scotia B3H 3J5
CANADA
Tel. +1 902 494 6412
Fax +1 902 494 6411
michael.cohen@dal.ca

Dr. Jean-Michel COINDRE*
Pathologie
Institut Bergonié
180, Rue de Saint-Genès
33076 BORDEAUX Cedex
FRANCE
Tel. +33 556 333333
Fax +33 556 330438
coindre@bergonie.org

Dr. Bogdan CZERNIAK
Dept.of Pathology
University of Texas
M.D. Anderson Cancer Center
1515 Holcombe Boulevard, Box 85
Houston, TX 77030-4095
USA
Tel. +1 713/794-1025

Dr. Paola DAL CIN*
Dept. of Pathology
Brigham and Women´s Hospital
75 Francis Street
Boston, MA 02115-6195
USA
Tel. +1 617 732 7981
Fax +1 617 975 0945
pdalcin@partners.org

Dr. Diederik R.H. DE BRUIJN
UMC St Radboud
Postbus 9101
417 Antropogenetica
6500 HB Nijmegen
THE NETHERLANDS
Tel. +31 24 361 41 07
Fax +31 24 354 04 88

---

* The asterisk indicates participation
in the Working Group Meeting on the
WHO Classification of Tumours of Soft
Tissue and Bone that was held in Lyon,
France, April 24-28, 2002.

Dr. Gonzague DE PINIEUX
Dept. of Pathology
Groupe Hospitalier Cochin
27, rue du Fg Saint-Jacques
75679 Paris, Cedex 14
FRANCE
Tel. +33 (1) 58 41 14 71 / 1481
Fax +33 (1) 58 41 14 80
gonzague.de-pinieux@cch.ap-hop-paris.fr

**Dr. Nicolas DE SAINT-AUBAIN
SOMERHAUSEN**
Service d'Anatomie Pathologique
Cytologie, Cytogénétique
Institut Jules Bordet, Rue Héger-Bordet 1
1000 Bruxelles, BELGIUM
Tel. +32 475 499 814
Fax +32 254 132 81
nicolas.desaintaubain@skynet.be

Dr. Barry R. DE YOUNG
Dept. of Pathology
University of Iowa Hospitals & Clinics
Room 5238 RCP, 200 Hawkins Drive
Iowa City, IA 52242
USA
Tel. +1 319 356 3264
Fax +1 319 384 8054
deyoungb@uihc.uiowa.edu

Dr. Angelo P. DEI TOS*
Dept. of Pathology
Regional Hospital of Treviso
Piazza Ospedale 1
31100 Treviso
ITALY
Tel. +39 0422 322707
Fax +39 0422 322663
apdeitos@ulss.tv.it

Dr. Carlo DELLA ROCCA
Dipartimento di Medicina
Sperimentale e Patologia
Viale Regina Elena 324
00161 Roma
ITALY
Tel. +39 06 499 70 731
Fax +39 06 446 36 52
carlo.dellarocca@uniroma1.it

Dr. Howard DORFMAN*
Dept. of Orthopaedic Surgery
Albert Einstein College of Medicine
111 East 210th Str.
Bronx, NY 10467
USA
Tel. +1 718 920 5622
Fax +1 718 231 2243
hdorfman@montefiore.org

Dr. Harry L. EVANS
Division of Anatomic Pathology
University of Texas MD Anderson Cancer
Center, 1515 Holcombe Boulevard
Houston, TX 77030
USA
Tel. +1 713 792 2143
Fax +1 713 792 5531
hevans@mdanderson.org

Dr. Julie C. FANBURG-SMITH*
Soft Tissue Pathology
Armed Forces Institute of Pathology
14th Street & Alaska Ave. NW
Washington, DC 20306-6000
USA
Tel. +1 202 782 2788
Fax +1 202 782 9182
fanburg@afip.osd.mil

Dr. Gelareh FARSHID
Tissue Pathology
Institute of Medical and
Veterinary Science
P.O. Box 14, Rundle Mall
Adelaide 5000
AUSTRALIA
Tel. +61 8 8222 3000
gelareh.farshid@imvs.sa.gov.au

Dr. John F. FETSCH
Soft Tissue Pathology
Armed Forces Institute of Pathology
14th Street & Alaska Ave. NW
Washington, DC 20306-6000
USA
Tel. +1 202 782 2790
Fax +1 202 782 9182

Dr. Cyril FISHER*
Histopathology/Cytopathology
Royal Marsden Hospital
Fulham Road
London SW3 6JJ
UNITED KINGDOM
Tel. +44 207 808 2630
Fax +44 207 351 5376
cfisher@icr.ac.uk

Dr. Christopher D.M. FLETCHER*
Dept. of Pathology
Brigham and Women's Hospital
75 Francis Street
Boston, MA 02115
USA
Tel. +1 617 732 8558
Fax +1 617 566 3897
cfletcher@partners.org

Dr. Jonathan A. FLETCHER
Dept. of Pathology
Brigham and Women's Hospital
75 Francis Street
Boston, MA 02115
USA
Tel. +1 617 732 51 52
Fax +1 617 278 69 13
jfletcher@partners.org

Dr. Andrew L. FOLPE*
Dept. of Pathology and Lab Medicine,
Emory University Hospital, H-180
1364 Clifton Road, NE
Atlanta, GA 30322
USA
Tel. +1 404 712 1265
Fax +1 404 712 4454
afolpe@bellsouth.net

Dr. Michel FOREST
Dept. of Pathology
Groupe Hospitalier Cochin
27, rue du Faubourg Saint-Jacques
75679 Paris, Cedex 14
FRANCE
Tel. +33 1 58 41 14 70
Fax +33 1 58 41 14 80

Dr. Victor FORNASIER
Dept. of Pathology
St. Michael's Hospital
30 Bond Street
Toronto, ON M5B 1W8
CANADA
Tel. +1 416 864 5851
Fax +1 416 864 5648
vfornasi@smh.toronto.on.ca

Dr. Anthony FREEMONT
University of Manchester
Stopford Building
Oxford Road
Manchester, M139PT
UNITED KINGDOM
Tel. +44 161 275 5268
Fax +44 161 275 5268
tony.freemont@man.ac.uk

Dr. William GERALD
Dept. of Pathology
Memorial Sloan-Kettering Cancer Center
1275 York Ave.
New York, NY 10021
USA
Tel. +1 212 639 5905
Fax +1 212 639 4559
geraldw@mskcc.org

Dr. Ad GEURTS VAN KESSEL
UMC St Radboud
Postbus 9101
417 Antropogenetica
6500 HB Nijmegen
THE NETHERLANDS
Tel. +31 24 361 41 07
Fax +31 24 354 04 88
a.geurtsvankessel@antrg.azn.nl

Dr. Bernard Ghelman
Dept. of Radiology and Imaging
Hospital for Special Surgery
535 East 70th Str.
New York, NY 10021
USA
Tel. +1 212 606 1129
Fax +1 212 734 7475
ghelmanbh@hss.edu

Dr. John R. GOLDBLUM
Dept. of Anatomic Pathology/L25
The Cleveland Clinic Foundation
9500 Euclid Avenue
Cleveland, OH 44195
USA
Tel. +1 216 444 8238
Fax +1 216 445 6967
goldblj@ccf.org

Dr. Louis GUILLOU*
Médecin Associé
Institut Universitaire de Pathologie
Rue du Bugnon 25
CH-1011 Lausanne
SWITZERLAND
Tel. +41 21 3147216
Fax +41 21 3147207
louis.guillou@chuv.hospvd.ch

Dr Theodora HADJISTILIANOU
Dept. of Ophtalmology
University of Siena
School of Medicine
Siena
ITALY
Tel. +39 0577 585 784
Fax +39 0577 233 358
hadjistilian@unisi.it

Dr. Hiroshi HASHIMOTO*
Dept of Pathology and Oncology
Univ. of Occupational and Environmental Health
1-1 Iseigaoka, Yahatanishi-ku
Kitakyushu 807-8555
JAPAN
Tel. +81 93 691 7239
Fax +81 93 692 0189
hiroshi@med.uoeh-u.ac.jp

Dr. Sverre HEIM
Dept. of Cancer Genetics
The Norwegian Radium Hospital
Montebello
N-0310 Oslo
NORWAY
Tel. +47 22 934 468
Fax +47 22 935 477
sverre.heim@labmed.uio.no

Dr. Pancras C. W. HOGENDOORN*
Dept. of Pathology
Leiden University Medical Center
P.O. Box 9600, I-L 1-Q
Leiden, 2300 RC
THE NETHERLANDS
Tel. +31 71 526 66 39
Fax +31 71 524 81 58
p.c.w.hogendoorn@lumc.nl

Dr. Carrie Y. INWARDS*
Dept. of Pathology
Mayo Clinic
200 First Avenue SW
Rochester, MN 55905
USA
Tel. +1 507 284 4526
Fax +1 507 284 1599
inwards.carrie@mayo.edu

Dr. Nirmala JAMBHEKAR*
Dept. of Pathology
Tata Memorial Hospital
Dr. Ernest Borges Road
Parel, Mumbai 400 012
INDIA
Tel. +91-22-414-6750
Fax +91-22-414-6937
najambhekar@rediffmail.com

Dr. Gernot JUNDT*
Institut fuer Pathologie
Universitaet Basel
Schoenbeinstrasse 40
CH-4003 Basel
SWITZERLAND
Tel. +41-61-2652867
Fax +41-61-2653194
gjundt@uhbs.ch

Dr. Leonard KAHN
Dept. of Pathology
Long Island Jewish Medical Center
270-05 76th Avenue
New Hyde Park, NY 11040
USA
Tel. +1 718 470 7491
Fax +1 718 347 9171

Dr. Ricardo K. KALIL*
Area de Patologia Cirurgica
Rede SARAH de Hospitals do Aparelho
Locomotor, SMHS Q 501 Conjunto A
70.335-901 Brasilia - DF
BRAZIL
Tel. +55-61-319-1375
Fax +55-61-319-1564
kalil@bsb.sarah.br

Dr. Yasuhiko KANEKO
Dept. of Cancer Chemotherapy
Saitama Cancer Center Hospital
818 Komuro
Ina, Saitama 362
JAPAN
Tel. +81 48 722 1111
Fax +81 48 723 5197
kaneko@cancer-c.pres.saitama.jp

Dr. Silloo B. KAPADIA
Division of Surgical Pathology
M.S. Hershey Medical Center, M.C. H179
500 University Drive, P.O. Box 850
Hershey, PA 17033-0850
USA
Tel. +1 717-531-8246
Fax +1 717-531-7741
skapadia@psu.edu

Dr. Jasvir KHURANA*
Dept. of Pathology, Founders-6
Hospital of the University of Pennsylvania
3400 Spruce Street
Philadelphia, PA 19104
USA
Tel. +1 215 662 6506
jkhurana@worldnet.att.net

Dr. Scott E. KILPATRICK
Dept. of Pathology
University of North Carolina
CB #7525, Brinkhous-Bullitt Building
Chapel Hill, NC 27599-7525
USA
Tel. +1 919-966-8312
Fax +1 919-966-6417
Scott_Kilpatrick@med.unc.edu

Dr. Lars-Gunnar KINDBLOM
Dept. of Pathology
Sahlgrenska University Hospital
S-413 45 Gothenburg
SWEDEN
Tel. +46 31 601000
Fax +46 31 827194

Dr. Alan KING
Dept. of Pathology
South Auckland Health
Middlemore Hospital, Private Bad 93311
Otahuhu, Auckland 6
NEW ZEALAND
Tel. +64 9 276 0154
Fax +64 9 270 4753
aking@middlemore.co.nz

Dr Paul KLEIHUES*
International Agency for
Research on Cancer (IARC)
150 Cours Albert Thomas
F-69008 Lyon
FRANCE
Tel. +33 4 7273 8577
Fax +33 4 7273 8564
kleihues@iarc.fr

Dr. Michael KLEIN
Dept. of Pathology
Mount Sinai Medical Center
One Gustave L. Levy Place
New York, NY 10029
USA
Tel. +1 212 241 3129
Michael.Klein@mssm.edu

Dr. Sakari KNUUTILA*
Dept. of Medical Genetics
Haartman Institute
Haartmaninkatu 3, 4th flr
FIN-00290 Helsinki
FINLAND
Tel. +358 9 191 26 527
Fax +358 9 191 26 788
sakari.knuutila@helsinki.fi

Dr. Paul KOMMINOTH
Institut für Pathologie
Departement Medizinische Dienste
Kantonsspital Baden
CH-5404 Baden
SWITZERLAND
Tel. +41 56 486 3901
Fax +41 56 486 3919
paul.komminoth@ksb.ch

Dr. Rainer KOTZ
Orthopädische Universitäts-Klinik
Garnisongasse 13
A-1097 Vienna
AUSTRIA
Tel. +43 1 40400 4084
Fax +43 1 40400 4029
rainer.kotz@univie.ac.at

Dr. Michael KYRIAKOS
Dept. of Pathology
Washington University
School of Medicine
Box 8118
St. Louis, MO 63110
USA
Tel. +1 314 362 0119
Fax +1 314 747 2040

Dr. Marc LADANYI
Dept. of Pathology
Memorial Sloan-Kettering Cancer Center
1275 York Avenue
New York, NY 10021
USA
Tel. +1 212 639 6369
Fax +1 212 717 3515
ladanyim@mskcc.org

Dr. Janez LAMOVEC*
Dept. of Pathology
Institute of Oncology
Zaloska 2
1105 Ljubljana
SLOVENIA
Tel. +386-1-4322099
Fax +386-1-4314180
jlamovec@onko-i.si

Dr. William B. LASKIN
Dept. of Pathology
Northwestern Memorial hospital
Feinberg Pavilion 7-325
251 East Huron St
Chicago, IL 60611-2908
USA
Tel. +1 312 926 3211
Fax +1 312 926 3127

Dr. Jerzy LASOTA
Dept. of Soft Tissue Pathology
Armed Forces Institute of Pathology
14th Street and Alaska Avenue
Washington, DC 20306-6000
USA
Tel. +1 202 782 2813
Fax +1 202 782 9182
lasota@afip.osd.mil

Dr. Janusz LIMON
Dept. of Biology and Genetics
Medical School
Debinki 1
80-211 Gdansk
POLAND
Tel. +48 58 349 1531
Fax +48 58 349 1535
jlimon@amg.gda.pl

Dr. Noralane LINDOR
Dept. of Medical Genetics
Mayo Clinic
200 First Street SW
Rochester, MN 55905
USA
Tel. +1 507 284 3750
Fax +1 507 284 1067
nlindor@mayo.edu

Dr. Juan LORENZO-ROLDAN
Hospital Universitan
"Germans Trias i Pujol"
Carretera del Canyet s/n
08916 Badalona
SPAIN
Tel. +43 3 418 2191
Fax +43 3 254 0215
4683jcl@comb.es

Dr. David R. LUCAS
Dept. of Pathology
Harper University Hospital
3990 John R
Detroit, MI 48201-2097
USA
Tel. +1 313 745 8555
Fax +1 313 745 9299
dlucas@dmc.org

Dr. Rikuo MACHINAMI
Dept. of Pathology
Kawakita General Hospital
Asagaya Kita 1-7-3, Suginami-ku
Tokyo 166-8588
JAPAN
Tel. +81 3 3339 2121
Fax +81 3 3339 8500
machinami-tky@unim.ac.jp

Dr. Archie J. MALCOLM
Dept. of Pathology
Royal Shrewsbury Hospital
Mytton Oak Road
Shrewsbury SY3 8XQ
UNITED KINGDOM
Tel. +44 174 3261 168
Fax +44 174 3355 963
AMJ@rshhis.demon.co.uk

Dr. Nils MANDAHL*
Dept. of Clinical Genetics
Lund University Hospital
SE-221 85 Lund
SWEDEN
Tel. +46 46 17 33 64
Fax +46 46 13 10 61
nils.mandahl@klingen.lu.se

Dr. Marcel MANNENS
Institute of Human Genetics
University of Amsterdam
Meibergdreef 15
NL-1105 AZ Amsterdam
THE NETHERLANDS
Tel. +31 20 566 5110
Fax +31 20 691 8626
m.a.mannens@amc.uva.nl

Dr. John A MARTIGNETTI
Dept of Human Genetics
Mount Sinai School of Medicine
Box 1498, 1425 Madison Avenue
New York, NY 10029
USA
Tel. +1 212 659 6744
Fax +1 212 849 2638
john.martignetti@mssm.edu

Dr. F.J. MARTINEZ-TELLO*
Dept. of Pathology
Hospital "12 de Octubre
Ctra. Andalucia km 5,400
28041 Madrid
SPAIN
Tel. +34 91 390 82 75
Fax +34 91 390 80 68
fmartinez@hdoc.insalud.es

Dr. Takeo MATSUNO
Dept. of Orthopaedics
Asahikawa Medical College
Midorigaoka-higashi 2-1, 1-1
Asahikawa 078-8510
JAPAN
Tel. +81 166 68 2510
Fax +81 166 68 2519
matsuno@asahikawa-med.ac.jp

Dr. Edward F. MCCARTHY*
Dept. of Pathology
John Hopkins Hospital
The Weinberg Bldg., Room 2242
Baltimore, MD 21231-2410
USA
Tel. +1 410 614 3653
Fax +1 410 614 3766
mccarthy@jhmi.edu

Dr. Mairin E. MCMENAMIN
Dept. of Pathology
St. James's Hospital
James's Street
Dublin 8
IRELAND
Tel. +353 141 62 992
Fax +353 141 03 466
mairinmcmenamin@hotmail.com

Dr. Jeanne M. MEIS-KINDBLOM
Dept. of Pathology
Sahlgrenska University Hospital
S-413 45 Gothenburg
SWEDEN
Tel. +46 31 601000
Fax +46 31 827194

Dr. Thomas MENTZEL*
Dermatohistopathologische
Gemeinschaftspraxis
Siemensstrasse 6/1, Postfach 16 46
D-88006 Friedrichshafen
GERMANY
Tel. +49 7541 604431
Fax +49 7541 604410
tmentzel@w-4.de

Dr. Fredrik MERTENS*
Dept. of Clinical Genetics
Lund University Hospital
SE-221 85 Lund
SWEDEN
Tel. +46 46 17 33 62
Fax +46 46 13 10 61
fredrik.mertens@klingen.lu.se

Dr. Michal MICHAL
Dept. of Anatomic Pathology
Charles University Medical Faculty
Dr. E. Benese 13
305 99 Plzen
CZECH REPUBLIK
Tel. +42 06 03 88 66 33
Fax +42 01 97 10 46 50
michal@fnplzen.cz

Dr. Markku M. MIETTINEN
Soft Tissue Pathology
Armed Forces Institute of Pathology
14th Street & Alaska Ave. NW
Washington, DC 20306-6000
USA
Tel. +1 202 782 2793
Fax +1 202 782 9182
miettinen@afip.osd.mil

Dr. Sara MILCHGRUB
Dept. of Pathology
UT Southwestern Medical Center
5323 Harry Hines Boulevard
Dallas, TX 75390-9073
USA
Tel. +1 214 590 6590
Fax +1 214 590 6586
sara.milchgrub@utsouthwestern.edu

Dr. Mary V. MILLER
Dept. of Pathology
South Auckland Health
Private Bag 93311
Otahuhu, Auckland 6
NEW ZEALAND
Tel. +64-9-276-0154
Fax +64-9-270-4753
mmiller@middlemore.co.nz

Dr. Joseph MIRRA
Dept. of Pathology
Orthopaedic Hospital
2400 S. Flower Street, Room 524
Los Angeles, CA 90007
USA
Tel. +1 213 742 1017
Fax +1 213 747 1077

Dr. W.M. MOLENAAR
Dept. of Medical Genetics
University of Groningen
Antonius Deusinglaan 4
9713 AW Groningen
THE NETHERLANDS
Tel. +31 50 363 2938
Fax +31 50 363 2947

Dr. Raymond J. MONNAT, JR
Dept. of Pathology Box 357705
University of Washington
1959 N.E. Pacific St. Room K-065 HSB
Seattle, WA 98195-7705
USA
Tel. +1 206 543 6585
Fax +1 206 543 3967
monnat@u.washington.edu

Dr. Elizabeth MONTGOMERY
Dept. of Pathology
Johns Hopkins Medical Institute
632 Ross Building, 720 Rutland Ave
Baltimore, MD 21205-2196
USA
Tel. +1 410 955 3511
Fax +1 410 614 0671
emontgom@jhmi.edu

Dr Yasuaki NAKASHIMA*
Laboratory of Anatomic Pathology
Kyoto University Hospital
54 Shogoin-Kawahara-cho
Sakyo-ku Kyoto 606-8507
JAPAN
Tel. +81 75 751 3488
Fax +81 75 751 3499
nakashim@kuhp.kyoto-u.ac.jp

Dr. Antonio G. NASCIMENTO*
Division of Surgical Pathology
Mayo Clinic
Mayo Graduate School of Medicine
200 First Street SW, Rochester, MN 55905
USA
Tel. +1 507 284 6956
Fax +1 507 284 1599
Nascimento.Antonio@mayo.edu

Dr. Simon NAYLER
Dept. of Anatomical Pathology
South African Institute for Medical
Research, P.O. Box 1038
Johannesburg 2000
SOUTH AFRICA
Tel. +27 11 489 8528
Fax +27 11 489 8512
simonn@mail.saimr.wits.ac.za

Dr. Scott D. NELSON
Dept. of Pathology
University of California, Los Angeles
10833 Le Conte Avenue
Los Angeles, CA 90095-1713
USA
Tel. +1 310 794 1489
Fax +1 310 267 2058
sdnelson@mednet.ucla.edu

Dr. Irene F. NEWSHAM
Dept. of Neurosurgery and Hermelin Brain
Tumor Center
Henry Ford Hospital
2799 West Grand Boulevard
Detroit, MI 48202, USA
Tel. +1 313 916 8640
Fax +1 313 916 9855
irene@bogler.net

Dr. G. Petur NIELSEN
Dept. of Pathology
Massachusetts General Hospital
55 Fruit Street, Warren 251C
Boston, MA 02114-2696
USA
Tel. +1 617 724 1469
Fax +1 617 726 7474
gnielsen@partners.org

Dr Mef NILBERT
Dept. of Oncology
Lund University Hospital
SE-221 85 LUND
Sweden
Tel: +46 46 177640
Fax: +46 46 147327
mef.nilbert@onk.lu.se

Dr. John X. O'CONNELL
Dept. of Pathology
Surrey Memorial Hospital
13750 96th Ave.
Surrey BC V3V 122
CANADA
Tel. +1 604 585 5953
Fax +1 604 585 5562
john.oconnell@southfraserhealth.com

Dr. Kyoji OKADA
Dept. of Orthopedic Surgery
Akita University
School of Medicine
1-1-1 Hondo
Akita 010
JAPAN
Fax +81-18-836-2617
cshokada@med.akita-u.ac.jp

Dr. Nelson G. ORDONEZ
Dept. of Pathology, Box 085
The University of Texas
1515 Holcombe Boulevard
Houston, TX 77030
USA
Tel. +1 713 792 3167
Fax +1 713 792 3696
nordonez@mdanderson.org

Dr. Mary L. OSTROWSKI
Dept. of Pathology
Baylor College of Medicine
One Baylor Plaza
Houston, TX 77030
USA
Tel. +1 713 394 6479
Fax +1 713 793 1603
maryo@bcm.tmc.edu

Dr. David M. PARHAM*
Dept. of Pathology
Arkansas Children's Research Hospital
800 Marshall Street
Little Rock, AR 72202-3591
USA
Tel. +1 501 320 1307
Fax +1 501 320 3912
parhamdavidm@uams.edu

Dr. May PARISIEN
Columbia University College Of Physicians
and Surgeons PHI5 W. Rm 1575
1630 West 168 St.
New York, NY 10032
USA
Tel. +1 212 305 6719
Fax +1 212 305 6595
mp11@columbia.edu

Dr. Yong-Koo PARK
Dept. of Pathology
Kyung Hee University Hospital
#1 Hoeki-dong, Dongdaemoon-ku
Seoul, 130-702
KOREA
Tel. +82 2 958 8742
Fax +82 2 957 0489
ykpark@khmc.or.kr

Dr. Florence PEDEUTOUR
Laboratoire de Génétique, Hôpital de Archet
151 Route St Antoine de Ginestiere
BP 3079
06202 Nice Cedex 3
FRANCE
Tel. +33 04 92 03 64 56
Fax +33 04 92 03 64 65
pedeutour.f@chu-nice.fr

Dr. Kenneth P.H. PRITZKER
Pathology and Laboratory Medicine
Mount Sinai Hospital
600 University Avenue, 6th Floor, Room 600-1
M5G 1X5 Toronto, Ontario
CANADA
Tel. +1 416 586 4453
Fax +1 416 586 8589
kpritzker@mtsinai.on.ca

Dr. Brad QUADE
Dept. of Pathology
Brigham and Women's
Hospital
75 Francis Street
Boston
MA 02115
USA
bquade@rics.bwh.harvard.edu

Dr. A. Kevin RAYMOND*
Dept. of Pathology
The University of Texas
M.D. Anderson Cancer Center
1515 Holcombe Boulevard
Houston, TX 77030-4095
USA
Tel. +1 713 794 5698
Fax +1 713 745 8610

Dr. Robin REID
Dept. of Pathology
University of Glasgow
Western Infirmary
Glasgow G12 6NT
SCOTLAND
Tel. +44 141 211 2062
Fax +44 141 337 2494
r.p.reid@clinmed.gla.ac.uk

Dr. Albert ROESSNER
Dept. of Pathology
Medical Faculty
D-39120 Magdeburg
GERMANY
Tel. +49 391 67 15817
Fax +49 391 67 15818
albert.roessner@medizin.uni-magdeburg.de

Dr. Andrew E. ROSENBERG*
Dept. of Pathology
Massachusetts General Hospital
Fruit Street
Boston, MA 02114
USA
Tel. +1 617 726 5127
Fax +1 617 726 9312
arosenberg@partners.org

Dr. Brian P. RUBIN*
Bone and Soft Tissue Pathology
University of Washington Medical Center
1959 N.E. Pacific Street, Room BB210E
Box 356100 Seattle, WA 98195-6100
USA
Tel. +1 206 598 5024
Fax +1 206 598 8697
bprubin@u.washington.edu

Dr. Anders RYDHOLM
Dept. of Orthopedic Surgery
University Hospital
S-221 85 Lund
SWEDEN
Tel. +46 46 171596
anders.rydholm@ort.lv.se

Dr. Eduardo SANTINI ARAUJO*
Dept. of Pathology
Central Army Hospital
"CIR MY Dr. Cosme Argerich"
Paraguay 2302 11 Floor OF 1
1121 ABL Buenos Aires
ARGENTINA
Tel. +54 11 4966 1224
Fax +54 11 4964 0379

Dr. Alan SCHILLER
Dept. of Pathology
Mount Sinai
Medical Center
One Gustave L. Levy Place
New York, NY 10029
USA
Tel. +1 212 241 8014
Alan.Schiller@mssm.edu

Dr. Regine SCHNEIDER-STOCK
Dept of Pathology
Otto-von-Guericke University
Leipziger Str. 44
D-39120 Magdeburg
GERMANY
Tel. +49 391 671 5060
Fax +49 391 671 5060
regine.schneider-stock@medizin.uni-magdeburg.de

Dr. Deborah SCHOFIELD
Dept. of Pathology
Children's Hospital of Los Angeles
4650 Sunset Boulevard, Mailstop 43
Los Angeles, CA 90027
USA
Tel. +1 323 669 5667
Fax +1 323 667 1123
schofiel@hsc.usc.edu

Dr. Raf SCIOT*
Dienst Pathologische Ontleedkunde
U.Z. St. Rafael
Minderbroedersstraat 12
B-3000 Leuven
BELGIUM
Tel. +32 16 336593
Fax +32 16 336548
Raf.Sciot@uz.kuleuven.ac.be

Dr. Janet SHIPLEY
Molecular Cytogenetics
The Institute of Cancer Research
15 Cotswold Road
Belmont, Sutton, Surrey SM2 5NG
UNITED KINGDOM
Tel. +44 20 8722 4273
Fax +44 20 8770 7290
shipley@icr.ac.uk

Dr. Gene SIEGAL
Dept. of Anatomic Pathology, KB 506
University of Alabama at Birmingham
619 South 19th Street
Birmingham, AL 35233
USA
Tel. +1 205 934 6608
Fax +1 205 975 7284
gsiegal@path.uab.edu

Dr. Samuel SINGER
Memorial Sloan-Kettering
Cancer Center
1275 York Avenue
New York, NY 10021
USA
Tel. +1 212 639 2940
singers@mskcc.org

Dr. Leslie H. SOBIN*
Division of Gastroenterology
Armed Forces
Institute of Pathology
Washington, DC 20306
USA
Tel. +1 202 782 2880
Fax +1 202 782 9020
sobin@afip.osd.mil

Dr. Poul SORENSEN
Dept. of Pathology and Laboratory Medicine
BC Research Institute for Children's and
Women's Health, 950 West 28th Avenue
Vancouver, BC V5Z 4H4
CANADA
Tel. +1 604 875 2936
Fax +1 604 875 3417
psor@interchange.ubc.ca

Dr. Frank SPELEMAN
Dept. of Medical Genetics
University Hospital
De Pintelaan 185
B-9000 Ghent
BELGIUM
Fax +32 9240 38 75
franki.speleman@rug.ac.be

Dr. Harlan SPJUT
Dept. of Pathology
Baylor College of Medicine
One Baylor Plaza
Houston, TX 77030
USA
Tel. +1 713 798 4661
Fax +1 713 798 5838

Dr. German C. STEINER
Dept. of Pathology
Hospital for Joint Diseases
Orthopedic Institute
301 East 17th Street, New York, NY 10003
USA
Tel. +1 212 598 6231
Fax +1 212 598 6057
german.steiner@med.nyu.edu

Dr. Göran STENMAN
Lundberg Laboratory for Cancer Research
Dept. of Pathology, Göteborg University
Sahlgrenska University Hospital
PSE-413 45 GÖTEBORG
SWEDEN
Tel. +46 31 3422 922

Fax +46 31 820 525
goran.stenman@ucr.med.gu.se
Dr. Isamu SUGANO
Dept. of Surgical Pathology
Teikyo University School of Medicine
Ichihara Hospital
3426-3 Anesaki, Ichihara
JAPAN
Tel. +81 436 62 1211
Fax +81 436 62 0412
i-sugano@med.teikyo-u.ac.jp

Dr. Murali SUNDARAM
Dept. of Radiology
Mayo Clinic
200 First Street SW
Rochester MN 55905
USA
Tel. +1 507 266 1207
Fax +1 507 266 1657
sundaram.murali@mayo.edu

Dr. Donald SWEET
Armed Forces Institute of Pathology
Alaska Avenue 14th Str NW
Washington, DC 20306-600
USA
Tel. +1 202 782 2850
Fax +1 202 782 3149
sweet@afip.osd.mil

Dr. William Y.W. TSANG
Institute of Pathology
Queen Elizabeth Hospital
30 Gascoigne Road,
Kowloon
HONG KONG
Tel. +852-2958-6834
Fax +852-2385-2455
tsangyw@ha.org.hk

Dr. K. Krishnan UNNI*
Dept. of Surgical Pathology
Mayo Clinic
Rochester, MN 55905
USA
Tel. +1 507 284 1193
Fax +1 507 284 1599
balzum.debbie@mayo.edu

Dr. Shinichiro USHIGOME
Dept. of Pathology
Jikei University School of Medicine
3-25-8 Nishi-shinbashi
Tokyo 105, Minato-ku
JAPAN

Tel. +81 3 3362 0732
Fax +81 3 3362 0732
shin-ichiro@mvd.biglobe.ne.jp
Dr. Eva VAN DEN BERG
Dept. of Medical Genetics
University of Groningen
Antonius Deusinglaan 4
9713 AW GRONINGEN
THE NETHERLANDS
Tel. +31 50 363 2938
Fax +31 50 363 2947
e.van.den.berg-de.ruiter@medgen.azg.nl

Dr. Daniel VANEL*
Dept. of Radiology
Institut Gustave Roussy
39 rue Camille Desmoulins
94805 Villejuif Cedex
FRANCE
Tel. +33 1 42114825
Fax +33 1 42 11 5279
vanel@igr.fr

Dr. Vincent VIGORITA
Lutheran Medical Center
150-55 Street
Brooklyn, NY 11220
USA
Tel. +1 718 630 7380
Fax +1 718 630 6330
vvigorita@lmcmc.com

Dr. Tuyethoa N. VINH
Armed Forces Institute of Pathology
Orthopedic Division, R#2059 Bldg 54
14th st Alaska Avenue NW
Washington, DC 20306-6000
USA
Tel. +1 202 782 2855
Fax +1 202 782 3149
vinh@afip.osd.mil

Dr. Sharon W. WEISS*
Dept. of Pathology and Lab Medicine
Emory University Hospital, H-180
1364 Clifton Road, NE
Atlanta, GA 30322
USA
Tel. +1 404 712 0708
Fax +1 404 712 4454
sharon_weiss@emory.org

Dr. Lester WOLD*
Dept. Laboratory Medicine and Pathology
Mayo Medical Center
200 First Street SW HI 530
Rochester, MN 55905

Source of charts and photographs

Soft Tissue Tumours

01.

00.01	Dr. J.M. Coindre
01.01–01.05B	Dr. G.P. Nielsen
01.06 A,B	Dr. F. Mertens
01.07–01.08	Dr. J. Fanburg-Smith
01.09–01.11B	Dr. G.P. Nielsen
01.12A–01.14B	Dr. R. Sciot
01.15–01.16B	Dr. J.M. Meis-Kindblom
01.17A–01.18	Dr. L.G. Kindblom
01.19 A, B	Dr. C.D.M. Fletcher
01.20	Dr. M.M. Miettinen
01.21A	Dr. C.D.M. Fletcher
01.21B	Dr. J. Fanburg-Smith
01.21C	Dr. C.D.M. Fletcher
01.22	Dr. C.D.M. Fletcher
01.23–01.27	Dr. M.M. Miettinen
01.28	Dr. F. Mertens
01.29–01.31B	Dr. A.P. Dei Tos
01.31C	Dr. C.D.M. Fletcher
01.32A	Dr. J.M. Coindre
01.32B	Dr. A.P. Dei Tos
01.33	Dr. F. Mertens
01.34	Dr. A.G Nascimento
01.35A–01.36C	Dr. A.P. Dei Tos
01.37- 01.42	Dr. C.R. Antonescu
01.43	Dr. F. Mertens
01.44	Dr. C.R. Antonescu
01.45–01.50B	Dr. T. Mentzel

02.

02.01A–02.05A	Dr. R.L. Kempson Dept. of Pathology Stanford University Medical Center Stanford, CA, USA
02.05B	Dr. J. Fanburg-Smith
02.06- 02.07B	Dr. A.E. Rosenberg
02.08A	Dr. J. Lamovec
02.08B	Dr. C.D.M. Fletcher
02.09A–02.10B	Dr. A.E. Rosenberg
02.11A	Dr. J. Fanburg-Smith
02.11B	Dr. A.G Nascimento
02.11 C, D	Dr. M. Michal
02.12	Dr. J. Fanburg-Smith

The copyright remains with the authors. Requests for permission to reproduce figures or charts should be directed to the respective contributor. For address see Contributors List.

02.13A–02.16B	Dr. H. Hashimoto
02.17- 02.18A	Dr. B.P. Rubin
02.18B–02.19A	Dr. C.M. Coffin
02.19B–02.20A	Dr. B.P. Rubin
02.20B–02.21	Dr. C.M. Coffin
02.22 A, B	Dr. C.D.M. Fletcher
02.23	Dr. Dr. V.J. Ojeda
	Dr. C.D.M. Fletcher
02.24	Dr. C.D.M. Fletcher
02.25A–02.27B	Dr. J.X O'Connell
02.28	Dr. C.D.M. Fletcher
02.29	Dr. J.X O'Connell
02.30 A-C	Dr. G. Farshid
02.31–02.34	Dr. M.M. Miettinen
02.35A–02.36C	Dr. M.E. Mc Menamin
02.37A	Dr. J. Fanburg-Smith
02.37B–02.39A	Dr. G. Farshid
02.39B	Dr. J. Fanburg-Smith
02.40A–02.41D	Dr. C.D.M. Fletcher
02.42–02.43B	Dr. W.B. Laskin
02.44 A, B	Dr. C.D.M. Fletcher
02.45 A, B	Dr. M. Michal
02.46A	Dr. C.D.M. Fletcher
02.46B–02.46D	Dr. C.M. Coffin
02.47–02.49	Dr. E. Montgomery
02.50A–02.51	Dr. L. Guillou
02.52A–02.53B	Dr. C.D.M. Fletcher
02.53C	Dr. J.R. Goldblum
02.53D	Dr. C.D.M. Fletcher
02.54A	Dr. A.G Nascimento
02.54 B-D	Dr. J.R. Goldblum
02.55	Dr. J. Fanburg-Smith
02.56A	Dr. A.G Nascimento
02.56 B, C	Dr. J.R. Goldblum
02.57A–02.58A	Dr. C.D.M. Fletcher
02.58B	Dr. M.M. Miettinen
02.58C	Dr. C.D.M. Fletcher
02.59- 02.62C	Dr. L. Guillou
02.63A–02.63F	Dr. C.D.M. Fletcher
02.64A–02.65C	Dr. L. Guillou
02.66–02.68B	Dr. C.M. Coffin
02.69A	Dr. C.D.M. Fletcher
02.69B–02.70C	Dr. C.M. Coffin
02.71–02.73B	Dr. T. Mentzel
02.74–02.77B	Dr. L.G. Kindblom
02.78A–02.81B	Dr. C.M. Coffin
02.82	Dr. C.D.M. Fletcher
02.83 A-C	Dr. C. Fisher
02.84–02.85F	Dr. T. Mentzel
02.86A	Dr. C.R. Antonescu
02.86 B-D	Dr. T. Mentzel
02.87A–02.89A	Dr. A.L. Folpe
02.89B	Dr. J. Fanburg-Smith
02.90–02.94	Dr. J.M. Meis-Kindblom

03.

03.01 A,B	Dr. A.L. Folpe
03.02A–03.03A	Dr. N. de St. Aubain Somerhausen
03.03B	Dr. A.L. Folpe
03.04	Dr. F. Mertens
03.05A–03.07B	Dr. N. de St. Aubain Somerhausen
03.08 A,B	Dr. A.L. Folpe
03.09 A,B	Dr. J. Fanburg-Smith
03.10–03.12B	Dr. J.M. Coindre
03.13A–03.20B	Dr. A.G. Nascimento
03.21–03.28	Dr. C.D.M. Fletcher
03.29A–03.30B	Dr. J.M. Coindre

04.

04.01–04.03B	Dr. H. Hashimoto
04.04	Dr. C.D.M. Fletcher
04.05–04.08C	Dr. H.L. Evans
04.09	Dr. C.D.M. Fletcher
04.10–04.11	Dr. Rubin Wang, Molecular Cytogenetics Institute Cancer Research, UK

05.

05.01–05.04A	Dr. C.D.M. Fletcher
05.04B	Dr. C.R. Antonescu
05.05–05.06B	Dr. A.L. Folpe
05.07A–05.10	Dr. M.E. Mc Menamin

06.

06.01A–06.06C	Dr. S.B. Kapadia
06.07A–06.10B	Dr. D.M. Parham
06.11 A,B	Dr. C.D.M. Fletcher
06.12A–06.13	Dr. D.M. Parham
06.14	Dr. C.R. Antonescu
06.15–06.18B	Dr. D.M. Parham
06.19	Dr. J.A. Bridge
06.20	Dr. F.G. Barr
06.21A–06.24A	Dr. E. Montgomery
06.24B	Dr. C. Fisher

07.

07.01	Dr. E. Calonje
07.02A	Dr. C.D.M. Fletcher
07.02B–07.05C	Dr. E. Calonje

07.06–07.08	Dr. J.F. Fetsch
07.09 A,B	Dr. S.W. Weiss
07.10A–07.12C	Dr. A. Beham
07.13 A,B	Dr. C.D.M. Fletcher
07.13C–07.14C	Dr. W.Y.W. Tsang
07.15–07.17C	Dr. E. Calonje
07.18	Dr. B. Azadeh Dept. of Pathology Hamad General Hospital, Doha, Qatar Dr. C.D.M. Fletcher
07.19–07.21B	Dr. B.P. Rubin
07.22–07.26A	Dr. J. Lamovec
07.26B	Dr. E. Calonje
07.26C–07.27A	Dr. J. Lamovec
07.27B	Dr. E. Calonje
07.28	Dr. C.D.M. Fletcher
07.29 A,B	Dr. S.W. Weiss
07.30	Dr. J.A. Bridge
07.31 A,B	Dr. S.W. Weiss
07.32	Dr. C.R. Antonescu
07.33A–07.35B	Dr. S.W. Weiss
07.36	Dr. C.R. Antonescu

08.

08.01A	Dr. J. Fanburg-Smith
08.01B–08.02A	Dr. S. Nayler
08.02B–08.03B	Dr. C.D.M. Fletcher
08.04–08.07A	Dr. A.E. Rosenberg
08.07B	Dr. J. Fanburg-Smith

09.

09.01–09.07C	Dr. G.P. Nielsen
09.08–09.11C	Dr. J.F. Fetsch
09.12 A-C	Dr. S.W. Weiss
09.13A–09.15B	Dr. J.K.C. Chan
09.16–09.19D	Dr. J. Fanburg-Smith
09.20A–09.23	Dr. B.P. Rubin
09.24A	Dr. S.E. Kilpatrick
09.24B	Dr. C.D.M. Fletcher
09.25 A,B	Dr. S.E. Kilpatrick
09.26A	Dr. C.D.M. Fletcher
09.26B	Dr. S.E. Kilpatrick
09.27A–09.28B	Dr. C.D.M. Fletcher
09.29 A,B	Dr. C.R. Antonescu
09.30A–09.33A	Dr. C. Fisher
09.33B	Dr. C.D.M. Fletcher
09.34 A,B	Dr. C. Fisher
09.35 A,B	Dr. C.R. Antonescu
09.36A	Dr. C. Fisher
09.36B	Dr. C.D.M. Fletcher

09.37	Dr. F. Mertens
09.38 A,B	Dr. A. Geurts van Kessel
09.39A–09.42B	Dr. L. Guillou
09.43A–09.44C	Dr. N.G. Ordonez
09.45	Dr. D.M. Parham
09.46	Dr. C. R. Antonescu
09.47–09.48B	Dr. N.G. Ordonez
09.49	Dr. C.D.M. Fletcher
09.50A–09.50D	Dr. R. Sciot
09.51	Dr. C. R. Antonescu
09.52	Dr. J.A. Bridge
09.53–09.57C	Dr. D.R. Lucas
09.58 A,B	Dr. S. Heim
09.59–09.67	Dr. C.R. Antonescu
09.68	Dr. T. Boyd, Dept of Pathology Children's Hospital Boston, MA, USA
09.69A–09.70	Dr. D. Parham
09.71A	Dr. J. Fanburg-Smith
09.71B	Dr. D.M. Parham
09.72	Dr. F. Mertens
09.73 A,B	Dr. C.D.M. Fletcher
09.74A–09.75B	Dr. A.L. Folpe
09.76–09.77	Dr. C.D.M. Fletcher
09.78A–09.81	Dr. B. Bode-Lesniewska

Bone Tumours

B.01	Dr. H. Dorfman
B.02–B.04	Dr. R. Kotz
B.05	Dr. D. Vanel

10.

10.01–10.05B	Dr. J. Khurana
10.06A	Dr. J. A. Bridge
10.06B	Dr. J.V.M.G. Bovee
10.07–10.16	Dr. D.R. Lucas
10.17–10.19B	Dr. S.E. Kilpatrick
10.20	Dr. J.A. Bridge
10.21–10.26C	Dr. M.L. Ostrowski
10.27	Dr. J.A. Bridge

10.28A–10.29B	Dr. M.V. Miller
	Dr. A. King
10.30–10.51B	Dr. F. Bertoni
10.52	Dr. J.V.M.G. Bovee
10.53A–10.55B	Dr. K.K. Unni
10.56A	Dr. Y. Nakashima
10.56 B-D	Dr. K.K. Unni
10.57	Dr. P.C.W. Hogendoorn
10.58 A,B	Dr. K.K. Unni
10.59–10.62B	Dr. Y. Nakashima
10.63–10.65B	Dr. E.F. McCarthy

11.

11.01A–11.03D	Dr. M.J. Klein
11.04A–11.08B	Dr. A.J. Malcolm
11.09–11.25	Dr. A.K. Raymond
11.26	Dr. S. Knuutila
11.27–11.30	Dr. T. Matsuno
11.31–11.34B	Dr. R.K. Kalil
11.35–11.38B	Dr. C.Y. Inwards
11.39	Dr. M. Forest
11.40–11.48	Dr. K. K. Unni
11.49	Dr. S. Knuutila
11.50–11.54A	Dr. A. Ayala
11.54B	Dr. K.K. Unni
11.55–11.58B	Dr. L. Wold

12.

12.01–12.02	Dr. K. K. Unni
12.03	Dr. H. Dorfman
12.04	Dr. L.B. Kahn Dr. V. Vigorita
12.05 A,B	Dr. H. Dorfman
12.05 C,D	Dr. Sam Liu, Manhattan, NY

13.

13.01–13.04B	Dr. M. Kyriakos
13.05–13.10	Dr. G.C. Steiner
13.11	Dr. J.A.Martignetti

14.

14.01 A,B	Dr. R. Machinami
14.02A–14.03	Dr. S. Ushigome
14.04A	Dr. R. Machinami
14.04B	Dr. S. Ushigome
14.05A	Dr. F. Mertens
14.05B	Dr. P. Sorensen

15.

15.01A–15.06C	Dr. F.J. Martinez-Tello
15.07	Dr. K.K. Unni
15.08 A,B	Dr. A. Hopkovitz, Dallas, Texas, USA
15.09 A-C	Dr. K. K. Unni
15.09D	Dr. A. Hopkovitz, Dallas, Texas, USA
15.10	Dr. K. K. Unni

16.

16.01	Dr. R. Reid
16.02	Dr. K. K. Unni
16.03–16.05	Dr. R. Reid
16.06	Dr. R. Sciot
16.07	Dr. H. Dorfman

17.

17.01–17.03D	Dr. J. Mirra
17.04	Dr. F. Mertens

18.

18.01A–18.04	Dr. C.P. Adler
18.05–18.08B	Dr. K.K. Unni

19.

19.01–19.05B	Dr. E.F. McCarthy
19.06–19.11B	Dr. A.E. Rosenberg

19.12	Dr. Sam Dachs, Great Falls, Montana, USA
19.13A–19.14	Dr. K.K. Unni
19.15–19.18B	Dr. P.C.W. Hogendoorn
19.19–19.21	Dr. N. Jambhekar

20.

20.01A–20.04	Dr. A.E. Rosenberg
20.05–20.07	Dr. R.K. Kalil
20.08–20.10	Dr. G. Siegal
20.11 A,B	Dr. K. K. Unni
20.12	Dr. V. Vigorita
20.13–20.14	Dr. K. K. Unni
20.15–20.16B	Dr. B.R. De Young
20.17–20.19	Dr. T.N. Vinh
20.20–20.22C	Dr. E.F. McCarthy

Congenital and inherited tumour syndromes

21.

21.01–21.02B	Dr. I. C. Talbot Dept. of Pathology St Mark's Hospital Academic Institute Middlesex, UK
21.03	Dr. C.M. Coffin
21.04	Dr. M. Mannens
21.05	Committee on Bone Tumors, The Nether-lands
21.06	Dr. P.C.W. Hogendoorn
21.07	Dr. G. Siegal
21.08–21.10	Dr. M.M. Cohen Jr.
21.11	Dr. P.C.W. Hogendoorn
21.12–21.13	Dr. J.V.M.G. Bovee
21.14–21.15	Dr. W.K. Cavenee
21.16	Dr. P.C.W. Hogendoorn

References

1. Anon. (1988). Age and dose of chemotherapy as major prognostic factors in a trial of adjuvant therapy of osteosarcoma combining two alternating drug combinations and early prophylactic lung irradiation. French Bone Tumor Study Group. *Cancer* 61: 1304-1311.

2. Anon. (1994). Case records of the Massachusetts General Hospital. Weekly clinicopathological exercises. Case 38-1994. A 55-year-old man with a paraspinal mass and a history of radiation treatment of a testicular tumor. *N Engl J Med* 331: 1079-1084.

3. Anon. (1997). Adjuvant chemotherapy for localised resectable soft-tissue sarcoma: meta-analysis of individual data. Sarcoma Meta-analysis Collaboration. *Lancet* 350: 1647-1654.

4. Anon. (1997). *Polichlorinated Dibenzo-para-Dioxins and Polychlorinated Dibenzo-furans*. In: IARC Monographs Vol. 69. IARC Press: Lyon.

5. Anon. (1998). Recommendations for the reporting of soft tissue sarcomas. Association of Directors of Anatomic and Surgical Pathology. *Mod Pathol* 11: 1257-1261.

6. Anon. (1999). Surgical implants and other foreign bodies. In: *IARC monographs on the evaluation of carcinogenic risks to humans*, Vol. 74. IARC Press: Lyon.

7. Abdul-Karim FW, el Naggar AK, Joyce MJ, Makley JT, Carter JR (1992). Diffuse and localized tenosynovial giant cell tumor and pigmented villonodular synovitis: a clinicopathologic and flow cytometric DNA analysis. *Hum Pathol* 23: 729-735.

8. Abraham SC, Montgomery EA, Giardiello FM, Wu TT (2001). Frequent beta-catenin mutations in juvenile nasopharyngeal angiofibromas. *Am J Pathol* 158: 1073-1078.

9. Abraham SC, Reynolds C, Lee JH, Montgomery EA, Baisden BL, Krasinskas AM, Wu TT (2002). Fibromatosis of the breast and mutations involving the APC/beta-catenin pathway. *Hum Pathol* 33: 39-46.

10. Abraham SC, Wu TT (2001). Nasopharyngeal angiofibroma. *Hum Pathol* 32: 455.

11. Abraham Z, Rozenbaum M, Rosner I, Naschitz Y, Boss Y, Rosenmann E (1997). Nuchal fibroma. *J Dermatol* 24: 262-265.

12. Abramson DH, Ellsworth RM, Kitchin FD, Tung G (1984). Second nonocular tumors in retinoblastoma survivors. Are they radiation-induced? *Ophthalmology* 91: 1351-1355.

13. Ackerman LV (1958). Extra-osseous localized non-neoplastic bone and cartilage formation (so-called myositis ossificans). *J Bone Joint Surg* 40A: 279-298.

14. Adamicova K, Fetisovova Z, Mellova Y, Statelova D, Hutka Z (1998). [Microstructure of subcutaneous lesions in juvenile hyaline fibromatosis]. *Cesk Patol* 34: 99-104.

15. Addison AK, Payne SR (1982). Primary liposarcoma of bone. Case report. *J Bone Joint Surg Am* 64: 301-304.

16. Adem C, Gisselsson D, Dal Cin P, Nascimento AG (2001). ETV6 rearrangements in patients with infantile fibrosarcomas and congenital mesoblastic nephromas by fluorescence in situ hybridization. *Mod Pathol* 14: 1246-1251.

17. Adickes ED, Goodrich P, AuchMoedy J, Bickers G, Bowden B, Koh J, Nelson RM, Shuman RM, Wilson RB (1985). Central nervous system involvement in congenital visceral fibromatosis. *Pediatr Pathol* 3: 329-340.

18. Adler CP (2000). Hemangioma of the Bone. In: *Bone Diseases*. Springer: Berlin, pp. 370-375.

19. Ahn C, Harvey JC (1990). Mediastinal hibernoma, a rare tumor. *Ann Thorac Surg* 50: 828-830.

20. Ahn J, Lüdecke HJ, Lindow S, Horton WA, Lee B, Wagner MJ, Horsthemke B, Wells DE (1995). Cloning of the putative tumour suppressor gene for hereditary multiple exostoses (EXT1). *Nat Genet* 11: 137-143.

21. Aiba M, Hirayama A, Kuramochi S (1988). Glomangiosarcoma in a glomus tumor. An immunohistochemical and ultrastructural study. *Cancer* 61: 1467-1471.

22. Aigner T, Dertinger S, Vornehm SI, Dudhia J, von der Mark K, Kirchner T (1997). Phenotypic diversity of neoplastic chondrocytes and extracellular matrix gene expression in cartilaginous neoplasms. *Am J Pathol* 150: 2133-2141.

23. Aigner T, Unni KK (1999). Is dedifferentiated chondrosarcoma a 'de-differentiated' chondrosarcoma? *J Pathol* 189: 445-447.

24. Aisen AM, Martel W, Braunstein EM, McMillin KI, Phillips WA, Kling TF (1986). MRI and CT evaluation of primary bone and soft-tissue tumors. *AJR Am J Roentgenol* 146: 749-756.

25. Akbarnia BA, Wirth CR, Colman N (1976). Fibrosarcoma arising from chronic osteomyelitis. Case report and review of the literature. *J Bone Joint Surg Am* 58: 123-125.

26. Alam M, Morehead RS, Weinstein MH (2000). Dermatomyositis as a presentation of pulmonary inflammatory pseudotumor (Myofibroblastic tumor). *Chest* 117: 1793-1795.

27. Alawi F, Stratton D, Freedman PD (2001). Solitary fibrous tumor of the oral soft tissues: a clinicopathologic and immunohistochemical study of 16 cases. *Am J Surg Pathol* 25: 900-910.

28. Albert DM, Lahav M, Lesser R, Craft J (1974). Recent observations regarding retinoblastoma. I. Ultrastructure, tissue culture growth, incidence, and animal models. *Trans Ophthalmol Soc U K* 94: 909-928.

29. Albert DM, McGhee CN, Seddon JM, Weichselbaum RR (1984). Development of additional primary tumors after 62 years in the first patient with retinoblastoma cured by radiation therapy. *Am J Ophthalmol* 97: 189-196.

30. Albores-Saavedra J, Manivel JC, Essenfeld H, Dehner LP, Drut R, Gould E, Rosai J (1990). Pseudosarcomatous myofibroblastic proliferations in the urinary bladder of children. *Cancer* 66: 1234-1241.

31. Albright F, Butler AM, Hampton AO, Smith P (1937). Syndrome characterized by osteitis fibrosa disseminata, areas of pigmentation and endocrine dysfunction, with precocious puberty in females: report of five cases. *N Engl J Med* 216: 727-746.

32. Albright F, Reifenstein EC, Jr. (1948). *The Parathyroid Glands and Metabolic Bone Disease: Selected Studies*. Wiliams and Wilkins: Baltimore.

33. Albright F, Scoville B, Sulkowitch HW (1938). Syndrome characterized by osteitis fibrosa disseminata, areas of pigmentation, and a gonadal dysfunction: further observations including the report of two more cases. *Endocrinology* 22: 411-421.

34. Alders M, Ryan A, Hodges M, Bliek J, Feinberg AP, Privitera O, Westerveld A, Little PF, Mannens M (2000). Disruption of a novel imprinted zinc-finger gene, ZNF215, in Beckwith-Wiedemann syndrome. *Am J Hum Genet* 66: 1473-1484.

35. Alguacil-Garcia A, Unni KK, Goellner JR (1978). Giant cell tumor of tendon sheath and pigmented villonodular synovitis: an ultrastructural study. *Am J Clin Pathol* 69: 6-17.

36. Alho A, Skjeldal S, Pettersen EO, Melvik JE, Larsen TE (1994). Aneuploidy in benign tumors and nonneoplastic lesions of musculoskeletal tissues. *Cancer* 73: 1200-1205.

37. Ali SZ, Smilari TF, Teichberg S, Hajdu SI (1995). Pleomorphic rhabdomyosarcoma of the heart metastatic to bone. Report of a case with fine needle aspiration biopsy findings. *Acta Cytol* 39: 555-558.

38. Allderdice PW, Davis JG, Miller OJ, Klinger HP, Warburton D, Miller DA, Allen FH, Jr., Abrams CA, McGilvray E (1969). The 13q-deletion syndrome. *Am J Hum Genet* 21: 499-512.

39. Allen PW (1972). Nodular fasciitis. *Pathology* 4: 9-26.

40. Allen PW (1977). The fibromatoses: a clinicopathologic classification based on 140 cases. *Am J Surg Pathol* 1: 255-270.

41. Allen PW (2000). Myxoma is not a single entity: a review of the concept of myxoma. *Ann Diagn Pathol* 4: 99-123.

42. Allen PW (2001). Nuchal-type fibroma appearance in a desmoid fibromatosis. *Am J Surg Pathol* 25: 828-829.

43. Allen PW, Enzinger FM (1970). Juvenile aponeurotic fibroma. *Cancer* 26: 857-867.

44. Allen PW, Enzinger FM (1972). Hemangioma of skeletal muscle. An analysis of 89 cases. *Cancer* 29: 8-22.

45. Allen RA, Woolner LB, Ghormley RK (1955). Soft tissue tumors of the sole: with special reference to plantar fibromatosis. *J Bone Joint Surg Am* 37: 14.

46. Alman BA, Li C, Pajerski ME, Diaz-Cano S, Wolfe HJ (1997). Increased beta-catenin protein and somatic APC mutations in sporadic aggressive fibromatoses (desmoid tumors). *Am J Pathol* 151: 329-334.

47. Alqahtani A, Nguyen LT, Flageole H, Shaw K, Laberge JM (1999). 25 years' experience with lymphangiomas in children. *J Pediatr Surg* 34: 1164-1168.

48. Altemani AM, Amstalden EI, Martins FJ (1985). Congenital generalized fibromatosis causing spinal cord compression. *Hum Pathol* 16: 1063-1065.

49. Aluisio FV, Mair SD, Hall RL (1996). Plantar fibromatosis: treatment of primary and recurrent lesions and factors associated with recurrence. *Foot Ankle Int* 17: 672-678.

50. Alvegård TA, Berg NO, Baldetorp B, Ferno M, Killander D, Ranstam J, Rydholm A, Åkerman M (1990). Cellular DNA content and prognosis of high-grade soft tissue sarcoma: the Scandinavian Sarcoma Group experience. *J Clin Oncol* 8: 538-547.

51. Alvegård TA, Sigurdsson H, Mouridsen H, Solheim O, Unsgaard B, Ringborg U, Dahl O, Nordentoft AM, Blomqvist C, Rydholm A, . (1989). Adjuvant chemotherapy with doxorubicin in high-grade soft tissue sarcoma: a randomized trial of the Scandinavian Sarcoma Group. *J Clin Oncol* 7: 1504-1513.

52. Ambacher T, Maurer F, Weise K (1999). [Spontaneous healing of a juvenile bone cyst of the tibia after pathological fracture]. *Unfallchirurg* 102: 972-974.

53. Amir G, Mogle P, Sucher E (1992). Case report 729. Myositis ossificans and aneurysmal bone cyst. *Skeletal Radiol* 21: 257-259.

54. Anagnostou GD, Papademetriou DG, Toumazani MN (1973). Subcutaneous glomus tumors. *Surg Gynecol Obstet* 136: 945-950.

55. Anderson MW, Temple HT, Dussault RG, Kaplan PA (1999). Compartmental anatomy: relevance to staging and biopsy of musculoskeletal tumors. *AJR Am J Roentgenol* 173: 1663-1671.

56. Anderson RL, Jr., Popowitz L, Li JK (1969). An unusual sarcoma arising in a solitary osteochondroma. *J Bone Joint Surg Am* 51: 1199-1204.

57. Ando K, Goto Y, Hirabayashi N, Matsumoto Y, Ohashi M (1995). Cutaneous cartilaginous tumor. *Dermatol Surg* 21: 339-341.

58. Andreassen A, Oyjord T, Hovig E, Holm R, Florenes VA, Nesland JM, Myklebost O, Hoie J, Bruland OS, Borresen AL, . (1993). p53 abnormalities in different subtypes of human sarcomas. *Cancer Res* 53: 468-471.

59. Andriko JW, Kaldjian EP, Tsokos M, Abbondanzo SL, Jaffe ES (1998). Reticulum cell neoplasms of lymph nodes: a clinicopathologic study of 11 cases with recognition of a new subtype derived from fibroblastic reticular cells. *Am J Surg Pathol* 22: 1048-1058.

60. Angervall L, Dahl I, Kindblom LG, Save S (1976). Spindle cell lipoma. *Acta Pathol Microbiol Scand [A]* 84: 477-487.

61. Angervall L, Hagmar B, Kindblom LG, Merck C (1981). Malignant giant cell tumor of soft tissues: a clinicopathologic, cytologic, ultrastructural, angiographic, and microangiographic study. *Cancer* 47: 736-747.

62. Angervall L, Kindblom LG, Lindholm E, Eriksson S (1992). Plexiform fibrohistiocytic tumor. Report of a case involving preoperative aspiration cytology and immunohistochemical and ultrastructural analysis of surgical specimens. *Pathol Res Pract* 188: 350-356.

63. Angervall L, Nielsen JM, Stener B, Svendsen P (1979). Concomitant arteriovenous vascular malformation in skeletal muscle: a clinical, angiographic and histologic study. *Cancer* 44: 232-238.

64. Antman K, Ryan L, Borden E (1990). *Pooled results from three randomized adjuvant studies of doxorubicin versus observation in soft tissue sarcoma : 10-year results and review of the literature.* WB Saunders Company: Philadelphia.

65. Antonescu CR, Argani P, Erlandson RA, Healey JH, Ladanyi M, Huvos AG (1998). Skeletal and extraskeletal myxoid chondrosarcoma: a comparative clinicopathologic, ultrastructural, and molecular study. *Cancer* 83: 1504-1521.

66. Antonescu CR, Elahi A, Healey JH, Brennan MF, Lui MY, Lewis J, Jhanwar SC, Woodruff JM, Ladanyi M (2000). Monoclonality of multifocal myxoid liposarcoma: confirmation by analysis of TLS-CHOP or EWS-CHOP rearrangements. *Clin Cancer Res* 6: 2788-2793.

67. Antonescu CR, Elahi A, Humphrey M, Lui MY, Healey JH, Brennan MF, Woodruff JM, Jhanwar SC, Ladanyi M (2000). Specificity of TLS-CHOP rearrangement for classic myxoid/round cell liposarcoma: absence in predominantly myxoid well-differentiated liposarcomas. *J Mol Diagn* 2: 132-138.

68. Antonescu CR, Erlandson RA, Huvos AG (1997). Primary leiomyosarcoma of bone: a clinicopathologic, immunohistochemical, and ultrastructural study of 33 patients and a literature review. *Am J Surg Pathol* 21: 1281-1294.

69. Antonescu CR, Erlandson RA, Huvos AG (2000). Primary fibrosarcoma and malignant fibrous histiocytoma of bone – a comparative ultrastructural study: evidence of a spectrum of fibroblastic differentiation. *Ultrastruct Pathol* 24: 83-91.

70. Antonescu CR, Gerald WL, Magid MS, Ladanyi M (1998). Molecular variants of the EWS-WT1 gene fusion in desmoplastic small round cell tumor. *Diagn Mol Pathol* 7: 24-28.

71. Antonescu CR, Kawai A, Leung DH, Lonardo F, Woodruff JM, Healey JH, Ladanyi M (2000). Strong association of SYT-SSX fusion type and morphologic epithelial differentiation in synovial sarcoma. *Diagn Mol Pathol* 9: 1-8.

72. Antonescu CR, Rosenblum MK, Pereira P, Nascimento AG, Woodruff JM (2001). Sclerosing epithelioid fibrosarcoma: a study of 16 cases and confirmation of a clinicopathologically distinct tumor. *Am J Surg Pathol* 25: 699-709.

73. Antonescu CR, Tschernyavsky SJ, Decuseara R, Leung DH, Woodruff JM, Brennan MF, Bridge JA, Neff JR, Goldblum JR, Ladanyi M (2001). Prognostic impact of P53 status, TLS-CHOP fusion transcript structure, and histological grade in myxoid liposarcoma: a molecular and clinicopathologic study of 82 cases. *Clin Cancer Res* 7: 3977-3987.

74. Antonescu CR, Tschernyavsky SJ, Woodruff JM, Jungbluth AA, Brennan MF, Ladanyi M (2002). Molecular diagnosis of clear cell sarcoma: detection of EWS-ATF1 and MITF-M transcripts and histopathological and ultrastructural analysis of 12 cases. *J Mol Diagn* 4: 44-52.

75. Araki N, Uchida A, Kimura T, Yoshikawa H, Aoki Y, Ueda T, Takai S, Miki T, Ono K (1991). Involvement of the retinoblastoma gene in primary osteosarcomas and other bone and soft-tissue tumors. *Clin Orthop* 271-277.

76. Arden RL, Bahu SJ, Lucas DR (1997). Mandibular aneurysmal bone cyst associated with fibrous dysplasia. *Otolaryngol Head Neck Surg* 117: S153-S156.

77. Argani P, Antonescu CR, Illei PB, Lui MY, Timmons CF, Newbury R, Reuter VE, Garvin AJ, Perez-Atayde AR, Fletcher JA, Beckwith JB, Bridge JA, Ladanyi M (2001). Primary renal neoplasms with the ASPL-TFE3 gene fusion of alveolar soft part sarcoma: a distinctive tumor entity previously included among renal cell carcinomas of children and adolescents. *Am J Pathol* 159: 179-192.

78. Argani P, Facchetti F, Inghirami G, Rosai J (1997). Lymphocyte-rich well-differentiated liposarcoma: report of nine cases. *Am J Surg Pathol* 21: 884-895.

79. Argani P, Faria PA, Epstein JI, Reuter VE, Perlman EJ, Beckwith JB, Ladanyi M (2000). Primary renal synovial sarcoma: molecular and morphologic delineation of an entity previously included among embryonal sarcomas of the kidney. *Am J Surg Pathol* 24: 1087-1096.

80. Argani P, Fritsch MK, Shuster AE, Perlman EJ, Coffin CM (2001). Reduced sensitivity of paraffin-based RT-PCR assays for ETV6-NTRK3 fusion transcripts in morphologically defined infantile fibrosarcoma. *Am J Surg Pathol* 25: 1461-1464.

81. Argenyi ZB, Van Rybroek JJ, Kemp JD, Soper RT (1988). Congenital angiomatoid malignant fibrous histiocytoma. A light-microscopic, immunopathologic, and electron-microscopic study. *Am J Dermatopathol* 10: 59-67.

82. Argyle JC, Tomlinson GE, Stewart D, Schneider NR (1992). Ultrastructural, immunocytochemical, and cytogenetic characterization of a large congenital fibrosarcoma. *Arch Pathol Lab Med* 116: 972-975.

83. Armour A, Williamson JM (1993). Ectopic cervical hamartomatous thymoma showing extensive myoid differentiation. *J Laryngol Otol* 107: 155-158.

84. Armstrong SJ, Duncan AW, Mott MG (1991). Rhabdomyosarcoma associated with familial adenomatous polyposis. *Pediatr Radiol* 21: 445-446.

85. Arnold WH (1973). Hereditary bone dysplasia with sarcomatous degeneration. Study of a family. *Ann Intern Med* 78: 902-906.

86. Arnould L, Jouannelle C, Mege F, Maillefert F, Fargeot P, Devillebichot C, Collin F (2000). [Sclerosing epithelioid fibrosarcoma: a fibrosarcoma with a very long course]. *Ann Pathol* 20: 154-157.

87. Arthaud JB (1972). Pigmented nodular synovitis: report of 11 lesions in non-articular locations. *Am J Clin Pathol* 58: 511-517.

88. Arvand A, Bastians H, Welford SM, Thompson AD, Ruderman JV, Denny CT (1998). EWS/FLI1 up regulates mE2-C, a cyclin-selective ubiquitin conjugating enzyme involved in cyclin B destruction. *Oncogene* 17: 2039-2045.

89. Arvand A, Denny CT (2001). Biology of EWS/ETS fusions in Ewing's family tumors. *Oncogene* 20: 5747-5754.

90. Ashar HR, Schoenberg Fejzo M, Tkachenko A, Zhou X, Fletcher JA, Weremowicz S, Morton CC, Chada K (1995). Disruption of the architectural factor HMGI-C: DNA-binding AT hook motifs fused in lipomas to distinct transcriptional regulatory domains. *Cell* 82: 57-65.

91. Asp J, Sangiorgi L, Inerot SE, Lindahl A, Molendini L, Benassi MS, Picci P (2000). Changes of the p16 gene but not the p53 gene in human chondrosarcoma tissues. *Int J Cancer* 85: 782-786.

92. Aspberg F, Mertens F, Bauer HC, Lindholm J, Mitelman F, Mandahl N (1995). Near-haploidy in two malignant fibrous histiocytomas. *Cancer Genet Cytogenet* 79: 119-122.

93. Assoun J, Richardi G, Railhac JJ, Baunin C, Fajadet P, Giron J, Maquin P, Haddad J, Bonnevialle P (1994). Osteoid osteoma: MR imaging versus CT. *Radiology* 191: 217-223.

94. Athale UH, Shurtleff SA, Jenkins JJ, Poquette CA, Tan M, Downing JR, Pappo AS (2001). Use of reverse transcriptase polymerase chain reaction for diagnosis and staging of alveolar rhabdomyosarcoma, Ewing sarcoma family of tumors, and desmoplastic small round cell tumor. *Am J Pediatr Hematol Oncol* 23: 99-104.

95. Auerbach HE, Brooks JJ (1987). Alveolar soft part sarcoma. A clinicopathologic and immunohistochemical study. *Cancer* 60: 66-73.

96. Aurias A, Rimbaut C, Buffe D, Dubousset J, Mazabraud A (1983). Chromosomal translocations in Ewing's sarcoma. *N Engl J Med* 309: 496-497.

97. Ayala AG, Ro JY, Bolio-Solis A, Hernandez-Batres F, Eftekhari F, Edeiken J (1993). Mesenchymal hamartoma of the chest wall in infants and children: a clinicopathological study of five patients. *Skeletal Radiol* 22: 569-576.

98. Ayala AG, Ro JY, Raymond AK, Jaffe N, Chawla S, Carrasco H, Link M, Jimenez J, Edeiken J, Wallace S, . (1989). Small cell osteosarcoma. A clinicopathologic study of 27 cases. *Cancer* 64: 2162-2173.

99. Aymard B, Boman-Ferrand F, Vernhes L, Floquet A, Floquet J, Morel O, Merle M, Delagoutte JP (1987). [Fibrolipomatous hamartoma of the peripheral nerves. Anatomico-clinical study of 5 cases, including 2 with ultrastructural study]. *Ann Pathol* 7: 320-324.

100. Azouz EM (1995). Benign fibrous histiocytoma of the proximal tibial epiphysis in a 12-year-old girl. *Skeletal Radiol* 24: 375-378.

101. Azumi N, Curtis J, Kempson RL, Hendrickson MR (1987). Atypical and malignant neoplasms showing lipomatous differentiation. A study of 111 cases. *Am J Surg Pathol* 11: 161-183.

102. Azzopardi JG, Iocco J, Salm R (1983). Pleomorphic lipoma: a tumour simulating liposarcoma. *Histopathology* 7: 511-523.

103. Azzopardi JG, Tanda F, Salm R (1983). Tenosynovial fibroma. *Diagn Histopathol* 6: 69-76.

104. Åman P, Ron D, Mandahl N, Fioretos T, Heim S, Arheden K, Willén H, Rydholm A, Mitelman F (1992). Rearrangement of the transcription factor gene CHOP in myxoid liposarcomas with t(12;16)(q13;p11). *Genes Chromosomes Cancer* 5: 278-285.

105. Åström A, d'Amore ES, Sainati L, Panarello C, Morerio C, Mark J, Stenman G (2000). Evidence of involvement of the PLAG1 gene in lipoblastomas. *Int J Oncol* 16: 1107-1110.

106. Bacci G, Ferrari S, Ruggieri P, Biagini R, Fabbri N, Campanacci L, Bacchini P, Longhi A, Forni C, Bertoni F (2001). Telangiectatic osteosarcoma of the extremity: neoadjuvant chemotherapy in 24 cases. *Acta Orthop Scand* 72: 167-172.

107. Bacci G, Picci P, Ferrari S, Ruggieri P, Casadei R, Tienghi A, Brach dP, Gherlinzoni F, Mercuri M, Monti C (1993). Primary chemotherapy and delayed surgery for nonmetastatic osteosarcoma of the extremities. Results in 164 patients preoperatively treated with high doses of methotrexate followed by cisplatin and doxorubicin. *Cancer* 72: 3227-3238.

108. Bae DK, Park YK, Chi SG, Lee CW, Unni KK (2000). Mutational alterations of the p16CDKN2A tumor suppressor gene have low incidence in mesenchymal chondrosarcoma. *Oncol Res* 12: 5-10.

109. Bahk WJ, Mirra JM, Sohn KR, Shin DS (1998). Pseudoanaplastic chondromyxoid fibroma. *Ann Diagn Pathol* 2: 241-246.

110. Bailey JS, Nikitakis NG, Lopes M, Ord RA (2001). Nonossifying fibroma of the mandible in a 6-year-old girl: a case report and review of the literature. *J Oral Maxillofac Surg* 59: 815-818.

111. Bailly RA, Bosselut R, Zucman J, Cormier F, Delattre O, Roussel M, Thomas G, Ghysdael J (1994). DNA-binding and transcriptional activation properties of the EWS-FLI-1 fusion protein resulting from the t(11;22) translocation in Ewing sarcoma. *Mol Cell Biol* 14: 3230-3241.

112. Baker PL, Dockerty MB, Coventry MB (1954). Adamantinoma (so-called) of the long bones. Review of the literature and a report of three new cases. *J Bone Joint Surg Am* 36A: 704-720.

113. Balachandran K, Allen PW, MacCormac LB (1995). Nuchal fibroma. A clinicopathological study of nine cases. *Am J Surg Pathol* 19: 313-317.

114. Baldassano MF, Rosenberg AE, Flotte TJ (1998). Atypical decubital fibroplasia: a series of three cases. *J Cutan Pathol* 25: 149-152.

115. Baldini EH, Goldberg J, Jenner C, Manola JB, Demetri GD, Fletcher CD, Singer S (1999). Long-term outcomes after function-sparing surgery without radiotherapy for soft tissue sarcoma of the extremities and trunk. *J Clin Oncol* 17: 3252-3259.

116. Ballance WA, Jr., Mendelsohn G, Carter JR, Abdul-Karim FW, Jacobs G, Makley JT (1988). Osteogenic sarcoma. Malignant fibrous histiocytoma subtype. *Cancer* 62: 763-771.

117. Balsaver AM, Butler JJ, Martin RG (1967). Congenital fibrosarcoma. *Cancer* 20: 1607-1616.

118. Bancroft LW, Berquist TH (1998). Erdheim-Chester disease: radiographic findings in five patients. *Skeletal Radiol* 27: 127-132.

119. Bane BL, Evans HL, Ro JY, Carrasco CH, Grignon DJ, Benjamin RS, Ayala AG (1990). Extraskeletal osteosarcoma. A clinicopathologic review of 26 cases. *Cancer* 65: 2762-2770.

120. Bansal M, Goldman AB, DiCarlo EF, McCormack R (1993). Soft tissue chondromas: diagnosis and differential diagnosis. *Skeletal Radiol* 22: 309-315.

121. Barcelo M, Pathria MN, Abdul-Karim FW (1992). Intraosseous lipoma. A clinicopathologic study of four cases. *Arch Pathol Lab Med* 116: 947-950.

122. Bardwick PA, Zvaifler NJ, Gill GN, Newman D, Greenway GD, Resnick DL (1980). Plasma cell dyscrasia with polyneuropathy, organomegaly, endocrinopathy, M protein, and skin changes: the POEMS syndrome. Report on two cases and a review of the literature. *Medicine (Baltimore)* 59: 311-322.

123. Barlogie B, Epstein J, Selvanayagam P, Alexanian R (1989). Plasma cell myeloma – new biological insights and advances in therapy. *Blood* 73: 865-879.

124. Barnoud R, Sabourin JC, Pasquier D, Ranchere D, Bailly C, Terrier-Lacombe MJ, Pasquier B (2000). Immunohistochemical expression of WT1 by desmoplastic small round cell tumor: a comparative study with other small round cell tumors. *Am J Surg Pathol* 24: 830-836.

125. Barr FG (1997). Molecular genetics and pathogenesis of rhabdomyosarcoma. *J Pediatr Hematol Oncol* 19: 483-491.

126. Barr FG, Chatten J, D'Cruz CM, Wilson AE, Nauta LE, Nycum LM, Biegel JA, Womer RB (1995). Molecular assays for chromosomal translocations in the diagnosis of pediatric soft tissue sarcomas. *JAMA* 273: 553-557.

127. Barr FG, Galili N, Holick J, Biegel JA, Rovera G, Emanuel BS (1993). Rearrangement of the PAX3 paired box gene in the paediatric solid tumour alveolar rhabdomyosarcoma. *Nat Genet* 3: 113-117.

128. Barr FG, Nauta LE, Davis RJ, Schafer BW, Nycum LM, Biegel JA (1996). In vivo amplification of the PAX3-FKHR and PAX7-FKHR fusion genes in alveolar rhabdomyosarcoma. *Hum Mol Genet* 5: 15-21.

129. Barr FG, Qualman SJ, Macris MH, Melnyk N, Lawlor ER, Strzelecki DM, Triche TJ, Bridge JA, Sorensen PH (2002). Genetic heterogeneity in the alveolar rhabdomyosarcoma subset without typical gene fusions. *Cancer Res* 62: 4704-4710.

130. Barrios C, Castresana JS, Ruiz J, Kreicbergs A (1993). Amplification of c-myc oncogene and absence of c-Ha-ras point mutation in human bone sarcoma. *J Orthop Res* 11: 556-563.

131. Barros Filho TE, Oliveira RP, Taricco MA, Gonzalez CH (1995). Hereditary multiple exostoses and cervical ventral protuberance causing dysphagia. A case report. *Spine* 20: 1640-1642.

132. Barry HC (1969). *Paget's Disease of Bone*. Livingstone: Edinburgh.

133. Bartl R, Frisch B, Burkhardt R, Fateh-Moghadam A, Mahl G, Gierster P, Sund M, Kettner G (1982). Bone marrow histology in myeloma: its importance in diagnosis, prognosis, classification and staging. *Br J Haematol* 51: 361-375.

134. Bartsch O, Wuyts W, Van Hul W, Hecht JT, Meinecke P, Hogue D, Werner W, Zabel B, Hinkel GK, Powell CM, Shaffer LG, Willems PJ (1996). Delineation of a contiguous gene syndrome with multiple exostoses, enlarged parietal foramina, craniofacial dysostosis, and mental retardation, caused by deletions in the short arm of chromosome 11. *Am J Hum Genet* 58: 734-742.

135. Baruffi MR, Neto JB, Barbieri CH, Casartelli C (2001). Aneurysmal bone cyst with chromosomal changes involving 7q and 16p. *Cancer Genet Cytogenet* 129: 177-180.

136. Baruffi MR, Volpon JB, Neto JB, Casartelli C (2001). Osteoid osteomas with chromosome alterations involving 22q. *Cancer Genet Cytogenet* 124: 127-131.

137. Bataille R (1982). Localized Plasmacytomas. *Clin Haematol* 11: 113-122.

138. Bataille R, Sany J (1981). Solitary myeloma: clinical and prognostic features of a review of 114 cases. *Cancer* 48: 845-851.

139. Bathurst N, Sanerkin N, Watt I (1986). Osteoclast-rich osteosarcoma. *Br J Radiol* 59: 667-673.

140. Batson OV (1940). The function of the vertebral veins and their role in the spread of metastases. *Ann Surg* 112: 138-149.

141. Batstone P, Forsyth L, Goodlad J (2001). Clonal chromosome aberrations secondary to chromosome instability in an elastofibroma. *Cancer Genet Cytogenet* 128: 46-47.

142. Battifora HA, Eisenstein R, Schild JA (1969). Rhabdomyoma of larynx. Ultrastructural study and comparison with granular cell tumors (myoblastomas). *Cancer* 23: 183-190.

143. Bauer HC, Trovik CS, Alvegård TA, Berlin O, Erlanson M, Gustafson P, Klepp R, Moller TR, Rydholm A, Saeter G, Wahlström O, Wiklund T (2001). Monitoring referral and treatment in soft tissue sarcoma: study based on 1,851 patients from the Scandinavian Sarcoma Group Register. *Acta Orthop Scand* 72: 150-159.

144. Bauer TW, Dorfman HD, Latham JT, Jr. (1982). Periosteal chondroma. A clinicopathologic study of 23 cases. *Am J Surg Pathol* 6: 631-637.

145. Bechler JR, Robertson WW, Jr., Meadows AT, Womer RB (1992). Osteosarcoma as a second malignant neoplasm in children. *J Bone Joint Surg Am* 74: 1079-1083.

146. Beck JC, Devaney KO, Weatherly RA, Koopmann CF, Jr., Lesperance MM (1999). Pediatric myofibromatosis of the head and neck. *Arch Otolaryngol Head Neck Surg* 125: 39-44.

147. Beck K, Jensen OA (1961). Bilateral retinoblastoma in Denmark. *Arch Ophthalmol* 39: 561-568.

148. Beckett JH, Jacobs AH (1977). Recurring digital fibrous tumors of childhood: a review. *Pediatrics* 59: 401-406.

149. Beckwith J (1963). Extreme cytomegaly of the adrenal cortex, omphalocele, hyperplasia of kidneys and pancreas, and Leydig-cell hyperplasia: Another syndrome? *West Soc Ped Res (Los Angeles)* Nov 11.

150. Begin LR, Clement PB, Kirk ME, Jothy S, McCaughey WT, Ferenczy A (1985). Aggressive angiomyxoma of pelvic soft parts: a clinicopathologic study of nine cases. *Hum Pathol* 16: 621-628.

151. Beham A, Badve S, Suster S, Fletcher CD (1993). Solitary myofibroma in adults: clinicopathological analysis of a series. *Histopathology* 22: 335-341.

152. Beham A, Fletcher CD (1991). Intramuscular angioma: a clinicopathological analysis of 74 cases. *Histopathology* 18: 53-59.

153. Behrens GM, Stoll M, Schmidt RE (2000). Lipodystrophy syndrome in HIV infection: what is it, what causes it and how can it be managed? *Drug Saf* 23: 57-76.

154. Belec L, Mohamed AS, Authier FJ, Hallouin MC, Soe AM, Cotigny S, Gaulard P, Gherardi RK (1999). Human herpesvirus 8 infection in patients with POEMS syndrome-associated multicentric Castleman's disease. *Blood* 93: 3643-3653.

155. Bell RS, O'Sullivan B, Liu FF, Powell J, Langer F, Fornasier VL, Cummings B, Miceli PN, Hawkins N, Quirt I. (1989). The surgical margin in soft-tissue sarcoma. *J Bone Joint Surg Am* 71: 370-375.

156. Bellaiche Y, The I, Perrimon N (1998). Tout-velu is a Drosophila homologue of the putative tumour suppressor EXT-1 and is needed for Hh diffusion. *Nature* 394: 85-88.

157. Ben Izhak O, Itin L, Feuchtwanger Z, Lifschitz-Mercer B, Czernobilsky B (2001). Calcifying fibrous pseudotumor of mesentery presenting with acute peritonitis: case report with immunohistochemical study and review of literature. *Int J Surg Pathol* 9: 249-253.

158. Bendl BJ, Asano K, Lewis RJ (1977). Nodular angioblastic hyperplasia with eosinophilia and lymphofolliculosis. *Cutis* 19: 327-329.

159. Benisch B, Peison B, Marquet E, Sobel HJ (1983). Pre-elastofibroma and elastofibroma (the continuum of elastic-producing fibrous tumors). A light and ultrastructural study. *Am J Clin Pathol* 80: 88-92.

160. Benjamin RS, Patel SR, Armen T, Carrasco CH, Raymond AK, Ayala A, Chawla SP, Yasko AW, Murray JA (1995). The value of ifosfamide in postoperative neoadjuvant chemotherapy of osteosarcoma. *Am Soc Clin Oncol* 14: 516.

161. Benjamin SP, Mercer RD, Hawk WA (1977). Myofibroblastic contraction in spontaneous regression of multiple congenital mesenchymal hamartomas. *Cancer* 40: 2343-2352.

162. Bennicelli JL, Advani S, Schafer BW, Barr FG (1999). PAX3 and PAX7 exhibit conserved cis-acting transcription repression domains and utilize a common gain of function mechanism in alveolar rhabdomyosarcoma. *Oncogene* 18: 4348-4356.

163. Bennicelli JL, Edwards RH, Barr FG (1996). Mechanism for transcriptional gain of function resulting from chromosomal translocation in alveolar rhabdomyosarcoma. *Proc Natl Acad Sci U S A* 93: 5455-5459.

164. Berger H, Hundeiker M (1967). [Multiple glomus tumors as a phakomatosis]. *Dermatol Wochenschr* 153: 673-678.

165. Berlin O, Angervall L, Kindblom LG, Berlin IC, Stener B (1987). Primary leiomyosarcoma of bone. A clinical, radiographic, pathologic-anatomic, and prognostic study of 16 cases. *Skeletal Radiol* 16: 364-376.

166. Berlin O, Stener B, Kindblom LG, Angervall L (1984). Leiomyosarcomas of venous origin in the extremities. A correlated clinical, roentgenologic, and morphologic study with diagnostic and surgical implications. *Cancer* 54: 2147-2159.

167. Bernado L, Admella C, Lucaya J, Sanchez dT, Bosch J (1987). Infantile fibrosarcoma of femur. *Pediatr Pathol* 7: 201-207.

168. Bernard MA, Hall CE, Hogue DA, Cole WG, Scott A, Snuggs MB, Clines GA, Lüdecke HJ, Lovett M, Van Winkle WB, Hecht JT (2001). Diminished levels of the putative tumor suppressor proteins EXT1 and EXT2 in exostosis chondrocytes. *Cell Motil Cytoskeleton* 48: 149-162.

169. Bernard MA, Hogue DA, Cole WG, Sanford T, Snuggs MB, Montufar-Solis D, Duke PJ, Carson DD, Scott A, Van Winkle WB, Hecht JT (2000). Cytoskeletal abnormalities in chondrocytes with EXT1 and EXT2 mutations. *J Bone Miner Res* 15: 442-450.

170. Bernasconi M, Remppis A, Fredericks WJ, Rauscher FJ, III, Schafer BW (1996). Induction of apoptosis in rhabdomyosarcoma cells through down-regulation of PAX proteins. *Proc Natl Acad Sci U S A* 93: 13164-13169.

171. Berner JM, Forus A, Elkahloun A, Meltzer PS, Fodstad O, Myklebost O (1996). Separate amplified regions encompassing CDK4 and MDM2 in human sarcomas. *Genes Chromosomes Cancer* 17: 254-259.

172. Berner JM, Meza-Zepeda LA, Kools PF, Forus A, Schoenmakers EF, Van de Ven WJ, Fodstad O, Myklebost O (1997). HMGIC, the gene for an architectural transcription factor, is amplified and rearranged in a subset of human sarcomas. *Oncogene* 14: 2935-2941.

173. Bernstein KE, Lattes R (1982). Nodular (pseudosarcomatous) fasciitis, a nonrecurrent lesion: clinicopathologic study of 134 cases. *Cancer* 49: 1668-1678.

174. Berrettoni BA, Carter JR (1986). Mechanisms of cancer metastasis to bone. *J Bone Joint Surg Am* 68: 308-312.

175. Bertario L, Russo A, Sala P, Eboli M, Giarola M, D'amico F, Gismondi V, Varesco L, Pierotti MA, Radice P (2001). Genotype and phenotype factors as determinants of desmoid tumors in patients with familial adenomatous polyposis. *Int J Cancer* 95: 102-107.

176. Berti E, Roncaroli F (1994). Fibrolipomatous hamartoma of a cranial nerve. *Histopathology* 24: 391-392.

177. Bertoni F, Bacchini P, Capanna R, Ruggieri P, Biagini R, Ferruzzi A, Bettelli G, Picci P, Campanacci M (1993). Solid variant of aneurysmal bone cyst. *Cancer* 71: 729-734.

178. Bertoni F, Bacchini P, Fabbri N, Mercuri M, Picci P, Ruggieri P, Campanacci M (1993). Osteosarcoma. Low-grade intraosseous-type osteosarcoma, histologically resembling parosteal osteosarcoma, fibrous dysplasia, and desmoplastic fibroma. *Cancer* 71: 338-345.

179. Bertoni F, Boriani S, Laus M, Campanacci M (1982). Periosteal chondrosarcoma and periosteal osteosarcoma. Two distinct entities. *J Bone Joint Surg Br* 64: 370-376.

180. Bertoni F, Calderoni P, Bacchini P, Sudanese A, Baldini N, Present D, Campanacci M (1986). Benign fibrous histiocytoma of bone. *J Bone Joint Surg Am* 68: 1225-1230.

181. Bertoni F, Capanna R, Calderoni P, Patrizia B, Campanacci M (1984). Primary central (medullary) fibrosarcoma of bone. *Semin Diagn Pathol* 1: 185-198.

182. Bertoni F, Picci P, Bacchini P, Capanna R, Innao V, Bacci G, Campanacci M (1983). Mesenchymal chondrosarcoma of bone and soft tissues. *Cancer* 52: 533-541.

183. Bertoni F, Present D, Bacchini P, Picci P, Pignatti G, Gherlinzoni F, Campanacci M (1989). Dedifferentiated peripheral chondrosarcomas. A report of seven cases. *Cancer* 63: 2054-2059.

184. Bertoni F, Present D, Bacchini P, Pignatti G, Picci P, Campanacci M (1989). The Istituto Rizzoli experience with small cell osteosarcoma. *Cancer* 64: 2591-2599.

185. Bertoni F, Present D, Hudson T, Enneking WF (1985). The meaning of radiolucencies in parosteal osteosarcoma. *J Bone Joint Surg Am* 67: 901-910.

186. Bertoni F, Unni KK, Beabout JW, Harner SG, Dahlin DC (1987). Chondroblastoma of the skull and facial bones. *Am J Clin Pathol* 88: 1-9.

187. Bertoni F, Unni KK, Beabout JW, Sim FH (1997). Malignant giant cell tumor of the tendon sheaths and joints (malignant pigmented villonodular synovitis). *Am J Surg Pathol* 21: 153-163.

188. Bessler W, Eich G, Stuckmann G, Zollikofer C (1997). Kissing osteochondromata leading to synostoses. *Eur Radiol* 7: 480-485.

189. Bibbo C, Warren AM (1994). Fibrolipomatous hamartoma of nerve. *J Foot Ankle Surg* 33: 64-71.

190. Biegel JA, Conard K, Brooks JJ (1993). Translocation (11;22)(p13;q12): primary change in intra-abdominal desmoplastic small round cell tumor. *Genes Chromosomes Cancer* 7: 119-121.

191. Biegel JA, Womer RB, Emanuel BS (1989). Complex karyotypes in a series of pediatric osteosarcomas. *Cancer Genet Cytogenet* 38: 89-100.

192. Biegel JA, Zhou JY, Rorke LB, Stenstrom C, Wainwright LM, Fogelgren B (1999). Germ-line and acquired mutations of INI1 in atypical teratoid and rhabdoid tumors. *Cancer Res* 59: 74-79.

193. Bielack SS, Schroeders A, Fuchs N, Bacci G, Bauer HC, Mapeli S, Tomeno B, Winkler K (1999). Malignant fibrous histiocytoma of bone: a retrospective EMSOS study of 125 cases. European Musculo-Skeletal Oncology Society. *Acta Orthop Scand* 70: 353-360.

194. Biggar RJ (2001). AIDS-related cancers in the era of highly active antiretroviral therapy. *Oncology (Huntingt)* 15: 439-448.

195. Billig R, Baker R, Immergut M, Maxted W (1975). Peyronie's disease. *Urology* 6: 409-418.

196. Billings SD, Folpe AL, Weiss SW (2001). Do leiomyomas of deep soft tissue exist? An analysis of highly differentiated smooth muscle tumors of deep soft tissue supporting two distinct subtypes. *Am J Surg Pathol* 25: 1134-1142.

197. Billings SD, Meisner LF, Cummings OW, Tejada E (2000). Synovial sarcoma of the upper digestive tract: a report of two cases with demonstration of the X;18 translocation by fluorescence in situ hybridization. *Mod Pathol* 13: 68-76.

198. Binder H, Eng GD, Gaiser JF, Koch B (1987). Congenital muscular torticollis: results of conservative management with long-term follow-up in 85 cases. *Arch Phys Med Rehabil* 68: 222-225.

199. Birdsall SH, Shipley JM, Summersgill BM, Black AJ, Jackson P, Kissin MW, Gusterson BA (1995). Cytogenetic findings in a case of nodular fasciitis of the breast. *Cancer Genet Cytogenet* 81: 166-168.

200. Biscaglia R, Bacchini P, Bertoni F (2000). Giant cell tumor of the bones of the hand and foot. *Cancer* 88: 2022-2032.

201. Bisceglia M, Magro G (1999). Low-grade myofibroblastic sarcoma of the salivary gland. *Am J Surg Pathol* 23: 1435-1436.

202. Biselli R, Boldrini R, Ferlini C, Boglino C, Inserra A, Bosman C (1999). Myofibroblastic tumours: neoplasias with divergent behaviour. Ultrastructural and flow cytometric analysis. *Pathol Res Pract* 195: 619-632.

203. Biselli R, Ferlini C, Fattorossi A, Boldrini R, Bosman C (1996). Inflammatory myofibroblastic tumor (inflammatory pseudotumor): DNA flow cytometric analysis of nine pediatric cases. *Cancer* 77: 778-784.

204. Bisgaard ML, Fenger K, Bulow S, Niebuhr E, Mohr J (1994). Familial adenomatous polyposis (FAP): frequency, penetrance, and mutation rate. *Hum Mutat* 3: 121-125.

205. Bjerkehagen B, Dietrich C, Reed W, Micci F, Saeter G, Berner A, Nesland JM, Heim S (1999). Extraskeletal myxoid chondrosarcoma: multimodal diagnosis and identification of a new cytogenetic subgroup characterized by t(9;17)(q22;q11). *Virchows Arch* 435: 524-530.

206. Bjerregaard P, Hagen K, Daugaard S, Kofoed H (1989). Intramuscular lipoma of the lower limb. Long-term follow-up after local resection. *J Bone Joint Surg Br* 71: 812-815.

207. Bjornsson J, Inwards CY, Wold LE, Sim FH, Taylor WF (1993). Prognostic significance of spontaneous tumour necrosis in osteosarcoma. *Virchows Arch A Pathol Anat Histopathol* 423: 195-199.

208. Bjornsson J, McLeod RA, Unni KK, Ilstrup DM, Pritchard DJ (1998). Primary chondrosarcoma of long bones and limb girdles. *Cancer* 83: 2105-2119.

209. Bjornsson J, Unni KK, Dahlin DC, Beabout JW, Sim FH (1984). Clear cell chondrosarcoma of bone. Observations in 47 cases. *Am J Surg Pathol* 8: 223-230.

210. Bjornsson J, Wold LE, Ebersold MJ, Laws ER (1993). Chordoma of the mobile spine. A clinicopathologic analysis of 40 patients. *Cancer* 71: 735-740.

211. Black B, Dooley J, Pyper A, Reed M (1993). Multiple hereditary exostoses. An epidemiologic study of an isolated community in Manitoba. *Clin Orthop* 212-217.

212. Blanco P, Schaeverbeke T, Baillet L, Lequen L, Bannwarth B, Dehais J (1999). Chondrosarcoma in a patient with McCune-Albright syndrome. Report of a case. *Rev Rhum Engl Ed* 66: 177-179.

213. Bleiweiss IJ, Klein MJ (1990). Chondromyxoid fibroma: report of six cases with immunohistochemical studies. *Mod Pathol* 3: 664-666.

214. Blocker S, Koenig J, Ternberg J (1987). Congenital fibrosarcoma. *J Pediatr Surg* 22: 665-670.

215. Bloem JL, Mulder JD (1985). Chondroblastoma: a clinical and radiological study of 104 cases. *Skeletal Radiol* 14: 1-9.

216. Bloem JL, Taminiau AH, Eulderink F, Hermans J, Pauwels EK (1988). Radiologic staging of primary bone sarcoma: MR imaging, scintigraphy, angiography, and CT correlated with pathologic examination. *Radiology* 169: 805-810.

217. Bloem JL, van der Heul RO, Schuttevaer HM, Kuipers D (1991). Fibrous dysplasia vs adamantinoma of the tibia: differentiation based on discriminant analysis of clinical and plain film findings. *AJR Am J Roentgenol* 156: 1017-1023.

218. Blum MR, Danford M, Speight PM (1993). Soft tissue chondroma of the cheek. *J Oral Pathol Med* 22: 334-336.

219. Bode-Lesniewska B, Zhao J, Speel EJ, Biraima AM, Turina M, Komminoth P, Heitz PU (2001). Gains of 12q13-14 and overexpression of mdm2 are frequent findings in intimal sarcomas of the pulmonary artery. *Virchows Arch* 438: 57-65.

220. Boehm AK, Neff JR, Squire JA, Bayani J, Nelson M, Bridge JA (2000). Cytogenetic findings in 36 osteosarcoma specimens and a review of the literature. *Ped Pathol Mol Med* 19: 359-376.

221. Bohle RM, Brettreich S, Repp R, Borkhardt A, Kosmehl H, Altmannsberger HM (1996). Single somatic ras gene point mutation in soft tissue malignant fibrous histiocytomas. *Am J Pathol* 148: 731-738.

222. Bohndorf K, Reiser M, Lochner B, Feaux dL, Steinbrich W (1986). Magnetic resonance imaging of primary tumours and tumour-like lesions of bone. *Skeletal Radiol* 15: 511-517.

223. Bolen JW, Thorning D (1980). Benign lipoblastoma and myxoid liposarcoma: a comparative light- and electron-microscopic study. *Am J Surg Pathol* 4: 163-174.

224. Boman F, Foliguet B, Metaizeau JP, Olive D, Rauber G (1984). [Myofibromatosis in children. Histopathologic and ultrastructural study of a localized form with a spontaneously regressive course]. *Ann Pathol* 4: 211-216.

225. Bonetti F, Martignoni G, Colato C, Manfrin E, Gambacorta M, Faleri M, Bacchi C, Sin VC, Wong NL, Coady M, Chan JK (2001). Abdominopelvic sarcoma of perivascular epithelioid cells. Report of four cases in young women, one with tuberous sclerosis. *Mod Pathol* 14: 563-568.

226. Bonetti F, Pea M, Martignoni G, Doglioni C, Zamboni G, Capelli P, Rimondi P, Andrion A (1994). Clear cell ("sugar") tumor of the lung is a lesion strictly related to angiomyolipoma – the concept of a family of lesions characterized by the presence of the perivascular epithelioid cells (PEC). *Pathology* 26: 230-236.

227. Bonetti F, Pea M, Martignoni G, Zamboni G (1992). PEC and sugar. *Am J Surg Pathol* 16: 307-308.

228. Bookstein R, Lee EY, To H, Young LJ, Sery TW, Hayes RC, Friedmann T, Lee WH (1988). Human retinoblastoma susceptibility gene: genomic organization and analysis of heterozygous intragenic deletion mutants. *Proc Natl Acad Sci U S A* 85: 2210-2214.

229. Boon LM, Brouillard P, Irrthum A, Karttunen L, Warman ML, Rudolph R, Mulliken JB, Olsen BR, Vikkula M (1999). A gene for inherited cutaneous venous anomalies ("glomangiomas") localizes to chromosome 1p21-22. *Am J Hum Genet* 65: 125-133.

230. Bordet R, Ghawche F, Destee A (1991). [Epidural angiolipoma and multiple familial lipomatosis]. *Rev Neurol (Paris)* 147: 740-742.

231. Bos GD, Pritchard DJ, Reiman HM, Dobyns JH, Ilstrup DM, Landon GC (1988). Epithelioid sarcoma. An analysis of fifty-one cases. *J Bone Joint Surg Am* 70: 862-870.

232. Boudousquie AC, Lawce HJ, Sherman R, Olson S, Magenis RE, Corless CL (1996). Complex translocation [7;22] identified in an epithelioid hemangioendothelioma. *Cancer Genet Cytogenet* 92: 116-121.

233. Boudova L, Michal M (1999). Atypical decubital fibroplasia associated with bizarre parosteal osteochondromatous proliferation (Nora's reaction). *Pathol Res Pract* 195: 99-103.

234. Boufassa F, Dulioust A, Lascaux AS, Meyer L, Boue F, Delfraissy JF, Sobel A, Goujard C (2001). Lipodystrophy in 685 HIV-1-treated patients: influence of antiretroviral treatment and immunovirological response. *HIV Clin Trials* 2: 339-345.

235. Bourgeois JM, Knezevich SR, Mathers JA, Sorensen PH (2000). Molecular detection of the ETV6-NTRK3 gene fusion differentiates congenital fibrosarcoma from other childhood spindle cell tumors. *Am J Surg Pathol* 24: 937-946.

236. Bovée JV, Cleton-Jansen AM, Kuipers-Dijkshoorn NJ, Van den Broek LJ, Taminiau AH, Cornelisse CJ, Hogendoorn PC (1999). Loss of heterozygosity and DNA ploidy point to a diverging genetic mechanism in the origin of peripheral and central chondrosarcoma. *Genes Chromosomes Cancer* 26: 237-246.

237. Bovée JV, Cleton-Jansen AM, Rosenberg C, Taminiau AH, Cornelisse CJ, Hogendoorn PC (1999). Molecular genetic characterization of both components of a dedifferentiated chondrosarcoma, with implications for its histogenesis. *J Pathol* 189: 454-462.

238. Bovée JV, Cleton-Jansen AM, Wuyts W, Caethoven G, Taminiau AH, Bakker E, Van Hul W, Cornelisse CJ, Hogendoorn PC (1999). EXT-mutation analysis and loss of heterozygosity in sporadic and hereditary osteochondromas and secondary chondrosarcomas. *Am J Hum Genet* 65: 689-698.

239. Bovée JV, Sakkers RJ, Geirnaerdt MJ, Taminiau AH, Hogendoorn PC (2002). Intermediate grade osteosarcoma and chondrosarcoma arising in a osteochondroma. A case report of a patient with hereditary multiple exostoses. *J Clin Pathol* 55: 246-249.

240. Bovée JV, Sciot R, Dal Cin P, Debiec-Rychter M, van Zelderen-Bhola SL, Cornelisse CJ, Hogendoorn PC (2001). Chromosome 9 alterations and trisomy 22 in central chondrosarcoma: a cytogenetic and DNA flow cytometric analysis of chondrosarcoma subtypes. *Diagn Mol Pathol* 10: 228-235.

241. Bovée JV, Van den Broek LJ, Cleton-Jansen AM, Hogendoorn PC (2000). Up-regulation of PTHrP and Bcl-2 expression characterizes the progression of osteochondroma towards peripheral chondrosarcoma and is a late event in central chondrosarcoma. *Lab Invest* 80: 1925-1934.

242. Bovée JV, Van den Broek LJ, de Boer WI, Hogendoorn PC (1998). Expression of growth factors and their receptors in adamantinoma of long bones and the implication for its histogenesis. *J Pathol* 184: 24-30.

243. Bovée JV, van Roggen JF, Cleton-Jansen AM, Taminiau AH, van der Woude HJ, Hogendoorn PC (2000). Malignant progression in multiple enchondromatosis (Ollier's disease): an autopsy-based molecular genetic study. *Hum Pathol* 31: 1299-1303.

244. Bracko M, Cindro L, Golouh R (1992). Familial occurrence of infantile myofibromatosis. *Cancer* 69: 1294-1299.

245. Bramwell V, Rouesse J, Steward W, Santoro A, Schraffordt-Koops H, Buesa J, Ruka W, Priario J, Wagener T, Burgers M (1994). Adjuvant CYVADIC chemotherapy for adult soft tissue sarcoma – reduced local recurrence but no improvement in survival: a study of the European Organization for Research and Treatment of Cancer Soft Tissue and Bone Sarcoma Group. *J Clin Oncol* 12: 1137-1149.

246. Bramwell VH, Steward WP, Nooij J, Whelan J, Craft AW, Grimer RJ, Taminiau AH, Cannon SR, Malcolm AJ, Hogendoorn PC, Uscinska B, Kirkpatrick AL, Machin D, Van Glabbeke MM (1999). Neoadjuvant chemotherapy with doxorubicin and cisplatin in malignant fibrous histiocytoma of bone: A European Osteosarcoma Intergroup study. *J Clin Oncol* 17: 3260-3269.

247. Brathwaite CD, Poppiti RJ, Jr. (1996). Malignant glomus tumor. A case report of widespread metastases in a patient with multiple glomus body hamartomas. *Am J Surg Pathol* 20: 233-238.

248. Braun BS, Frieden R, Lessnick SL, May WA, Denny CT (1995). Identification of target genes for the Ewing's sarcoma EWS/FLI fusion protein by representational difference analysis. *Mol Cell Biol* 15: 4623-4630.

249. Braunstein EM, White SJ (1980). Non-Hodgkin lymphoma of bone. *Radiology* 135: 59-63.

250. Breier F, Fang-Kircher S, Wolff K, Jurecka W (1997). Juvenile hyaline fibromatosis: impaired collagen metabolism in human skin fibroblasts. *Arch Dis Child* 77: 436-440.

251. Breiner JA, Nelson M, Bredthauer BD, Neff JR, Bridge JA (1999). Trisomy 8 and trisomy 14 in plantar fibromatosis. *Cancer Genet Cytogenet* 108: 176-177.

252. Brett D, Whitehouse S, Antonson P, Shipley J, Cooper C, Goodwin G (1997). The SYT protein involved in the t(X;18) synovial sarcoma translocation is a transcriptional activator localised in nuclear bodies. *Hum Mol Genet* 6: 1559-1564.

253. Bridge JA, Bhatia PS, Anderson JR, Neff JR (1993). Biologic and clinical significance of cytogenetic and molecular cytogenetic abnormalities in benign and malignant cartilaginous lesions. *Cancer Genet Cytogenet* 69: 79-90.

254. Bridge JA, DeBoer J, Travis J, Johansson SL, Elmberger G, Noel SM, Neff JR (1994). Simultaneous interphase cytogenetic analysis and fluorescence immunophenotyping of dedifferentiated chondrosarcoma. Implications for histopathogenesis. *Am J Pathol* 144: 215-220.

255. Bridge JA, DeBoer J, Walker CW, Neff JR (1995). Translocation t(3;12)(q28;q14) in parosteal lipoma. *Genes Chromosomes Cancer* 12: 70-72.

256. Bridge JA, Dembinski A, DeBoer J, Travis J, Neff JR (1994). Clonal chromosomal abnormalities in osteofibrous dysplasia. Implications for histopathogenesis and its relationship with adamantinoma. *Cancer* 73: 1746-1752.

257. Bridge JA, Fidler ME, Neff JR, Degenhardt J, Wang M, Walker C, Dorfman HD, Baker KS, Seemayer TA (1999). Adamantinoma-like Ewing's sarcoma: genomic confirmation, phenotypic drift. *Am J Surg Pathol* 23: 159-165.

258. Bridge JA, Kanamori M, Ma Z, Pickering D, Hill DA, Lydiatt W, Lui MY, Colleoni GW, Antonescu CR, Ladanyi M, Morris SW (2001). Fusion of the ALK gene to the clathrin heavy chain gene, CLTC, in inflammatory myofibroblastic tumor. *Am J Pathol* 159: 411-415.

259. Bridge JA, Liu J, Qualman SJ, Suijkerbuijk R, Wenger G, Zhang J, Wan X, Baker KS, Sorensen P, Barr FG (2002). Genomic gains and losses are similar in genetic and histologic subsets of rhabdomyosarcoma, whereas amplification predominates in embryonal with anaplasia and alveolar subtypes. *Genes Chromosomes Cancer* 33: 310-321.

260. Bridge JA, Liu J, Weibolt V, Baker KS, Perry D, Kruger R, Qualman S, Barr F, Sorensen P, Triche T, Suijkerbuijk R (2000). Novel genomic imbalances in embryonal rhabdomyosarcoma revealed by comparative genomic hybridization and fluorescence in situ hybridization: an intergroup rhabdomyosarcoma study. *Genes Chromosomes Cancer* 27: 337-344.

261. Bridge JA, Meloni AM, Neff JR, DeBoer J, Pickering D, Dalence C, Jeffrey B, Sandberg AA (1996). Deletion 5q in desmoid tumor and fluorescence in situ hybridization for chromosome 8 and/or 20 copy number. *Cancer Genet Cytogenet* 92: 150-151.

262. Bridge JA, Neff JR, Mouron BJ (1992). Giant cell tumor of bone. Chromosomal analysis of 48 specimens and review of the literature. *Cancer Genet Cytogenet* 58: 2-13.

263. Bridge JA, Nelson M, McComb E, McGuire MH, Rosenthal H, Vergara G, Maale GE, Spanier S, Neff JR (1997). Cytogenetic findings in 73 osteosarcoma specimens and a review of the literature. *Cancer Genet Cytogenet* 95: 74-87.

264. Bridge JA, Nelson M, Örndal C, Bhatia P, Neff JR (1998). Clonal karyotypic abnormalities of the hereditary multiple exostoses chromosomal loci 8q24.1 (EXT1) and 11p11-12 (EXT2) in patients with sporadic and hereditary osteochondromas. *Cancer* 82: 1657-1663.

265. Bridge JA, Persons DL, Neff JR, Bhatia P (1992). Clonal karyotypic aberrations in enchondromas. *Cancer Detect Prev* 16: 215-219.

266. Bridge JA, Sanger WG, Neff JR (1989). Translocations involving chromosomes 2 and 13 in benign and malignant cartilaginous neoplasms. *Cancer Genet Cytogenet* 38: 83-88.

267. Bridge JA, Swarts SJ, Buresh C, Nelson M, Degenhardt JM, Spanier S, Maale G, Meloni A, Lynch JC, Neff JR (1999). Trisomies 8 and 20 characterize a subgroup of benign fibrous lesions arising in both soft tissue and bone. *Am J Pathol* 154: 729-733.

268. Brien EW, Mirra JM, Ippolito V, Vaughan L (1996). Clear-cell chondrosarcoma with elevated alkaline phosphatase, mistaken for osteosarcoma on biopsy. *Skeletal Radiol* 25: 770-774.

269. Brien EW, Mirra JM, Kerr R (1997). Benign and malignant cartilage tumors of bone and joint: their anatomic and theoretical basis with an emphasis on radiology, pathology and clinical biology. I. The intramedullary cartilage tumors. *Skeletal Radiol* 26: 325-353.

270. Brien EW, Mirra JM, Luck JV, Jr. (1999). Benign and malignant cartilage tumors of bone and joint: their anatomic and theoretical basis with an emphasis on radiology, pathology and clinical biology. II. Juxtacortical cartilage tumors. *Skeletal Radiol* 28: 1-20.

271. Brien WW, Salvati EA, Healey JH, Bansal M, Ghelman B, Betts F (1990). Osteogenic sarcoma arising in the area of a total hip replacement. A case report. *J Bone Joint Surg Am* 72: 1097-1099.

272. Broders AC (1920). Squamous cell epithelioma of the lip: a study of 537 cases. *JAMA* 74: 656-664.

273. Broeders A, Smet MH, Breysem L, Marchal G (2000). Lipoblastoma: a rare mediastinal tumour in a child. *Pediatr Radiol* 30: 580.

274. Brostrom LA, Strander H, Nilsonne U (1982). Survival in osteosarcoma in relation to tumor size and location. *Clin Orthop* 250-254.

275. Brotherston TM, Balakrishnan C, Milner RH, Brown HG (1994). Long term follow-up of dermofasciectomy for Dupuytren's contracture. *Br J Plast Surg* 47: 440-443.

276. Brower AC, Worsham GF, Dudley AH (1984). Erdheim-Chester disease: a distinct lipoidosis or part of the spectrum of histiocytosis? *Radiology* 151: 35-38.

277. Brown G, Shaw DG (1995). Inflammatory pseudotumours in children: CT and ultrasound appearances with histopathological correlation. *Clin Radiol* 50: 782-786.

278. Brown HK, Healey JH (2001). Metastatic cancer to the bone. In: *Cancer Principles and Practice of Oncology*, DeVita VT, Hellman S, Rosenberg SA, eds. 6th ed. Lippincott, Williams & Wilkins: Philadelphia, pp. 2713-2729.

279. Brown KT, Kattapuram SV, Rosenthal DI (1986). Computed tomography analysis of bone tumors: patterns of cortical destruction and soft tissue extension. *Skeletal Radiol* 15: 448-451.

280. Brown MJ, Logan PM, O'Connell JX, Janzen DL, Connell DG (1996). Diaphyseal telangiectatic osteosarcoma as a second tumor after bilateral retinoblastomas. *Skeletal Radiol* 25: 685-688.

281. Brownlee RD, Sevick RJ, Rewcastle NB, Tranmer BI (1997). Intracranial chondroma. *AJNR Am J Neuroradiol* 18: 889-893.

282. Bruder E, Zanetti M, Boos N, von Hochstetter AR (1999). Chondromyxoid fibroma of two thoracic vertebrae. *Skeletal Radiol* 28: 286-289.

283. Brunnemann RB, Ro JY, Ordonez NG, Mooney J, el Naggar AK, Ayala AG (1999). Extrapleural solitary fibrous tumor: a clinicopathologic study of 24 cases. *Mod Pathol* 12: 1034-1042.

284. Buchkovich K, Duffy LA, Harlow E (1989). The retinoblastoma protein is phosphorylated during specific phases of the cell cycle. *Cell* 58: 1097-1105.

285. Bulow S, Sondergaard JO, Witt I, Larsen E, Tetens G (1984). Mandibular osteomas in familial polyposis coli. *Dis Colon Rectum* 27: 105-108.

286. Burke A, Virami R (1996). Tumors of the great vessels. In: *AFIP Atlas of Tumor Pathology. Tumors of the Heart and Great Vessels*, Burke A, Virami R, eds. AFIP: Washington, DC, pp. 211-227.

287. Burke AP, Virmani R (1993). Sarcomas of the great vessels. A clinicopathologic study. *Cancer* 71: 1761-1773.

288. Busam KJ, Jungbluth AA (1999). Melan-A, a new melanocytic differentiation marker. *Adv Anat Pathol* 6: 12-18.

289. Byrne J, Blanc WA, Warburton D, Wigger J (1984). The significance of cystic hygroma in fetuses. *Hum Pathol* 15: 61-67.

290. Cai YC, McMenamin ME, Rose G, Sandy CJ, Cree IA, Fletcher CD (2001). Primary liposarcoma of the orbit: A clinicopathological study of seven cases. *Ann Diagn Pathol* 5: 255-266.

291. Caillaud JM, Gerard-Marchant R, Marsden HB, van Unnik AJ, Rodary C, Rey A, Flamant F (1989). Histopathological classification of childhood rhabdomyosarcoma: a report from the International Society of Pediatric Oncology pathology panel. *Med Pediatr Oncol* 17: 391-400.

292. Callister MD, Ballo MT, Pisters PW, Patel SR, Feig BW, Pollock RE, Benjamin RS, Zagars GK (2001). Epithelioid sarcoma: results of conservative surgery and radiotherapy. *Int J Radiat Oncol Biol Phys* 51: 384-391.

293. Calonje E, Fletcher CD (1995). Cutaneous intraneural glomus tumor. *Am J Dermatopathol* 17: 395-398.

294. Calonje E, Fletcher CD (2000). Hemangiopericytoma. In: *Diagnostic Histopathology of Tumors*, Fletcher CD, ed. 2nd ed. Churchill Livingstone: London, pp. 77-80.

295. Calonje E, Fletcher CD (2000). Tumors of blood vessels and lymphatics. In: *Diagnostic Histopathology of Tumors*, Fletcher CD, ed. 2nd ed. Churchill Livingstone: London, pp. 77-80.

296. Calonje E, Fletcher CD, Wilson-Jones E, Rosai J (1994). Retiform hemangioendothelioma. A distinctive form of low-grade angiosarcoma delineated in a series of 15 cases. *Am J Surg Pathol* 18: 115-125.

297. Calvert JT, Burns S, Riney TJ, Sahoo T, Orlow SJ, Nevin NC, Haisley-Royster C, Prose N, Simpson SA, Speer MC, Marchuk DA (2001). Additional glomangioma families link to chromosome 1p: no evidence for genetic heterogeneity. *Hum Hered* 51: 180-182.

298. Campanacci M (1999). *Bone and Soft Tissue Tumors*. Springer-Verlag: New York.

299. Campanacci M, Baldini N, Boriani S, Sudanese A (1987). Giant-cell tumor of bone. *J Bone Joint Surg Am* 69: 106-114.

300. Campanacci M, Boriani S, Giunti A (1980). Hemangioendothelioma of bone: a study of 29 cases. *Cancer* 46: 804-814.

301. Campanacci M, Laus M (1981). Osteofibrous dysplasia of the tibia and fibula. *J Bone Joint Surg Am* 63: 367-375.

302. Candeliere GA, Glorieux FH, Prud'homme J, St Arnaud R (1995). Increased expression of the c-fos proto-oncogene in bone from patients with fibrous dysplasia. *N Engl J Med* 332: 1546-1551.

303. Cannon SR, Sweetnam DR (1985). Multiple chondrosarcomas in dyschondroplasia (Ollier's disease). *Cancer* 55: 836-840.

304. Canpolat C, Evans HL, Corpron C, Andrassy RJ, Chan K, Eifel P, Elidemir O, Raney B (1996). Fibromyxoid sarcoma in a four-year-old child: case report and review of the literature. *Med Pediatr Oncol* 27: 561-564.

305. Capanna R, Bertoni F, Bacchini P, Bacci G, Guerra A, Campanacci M (1984). Malignant fibrous histiocytoma of bone. The experience at the Rizzoli Institute: report of 90 cases. *Cancer* 54: 177-187.

306. Caparros-Lefebvre D, Pruvo JP, Remy M, Wallaert B, Petit H (1995). Neuroradiologic aspects of Erdheim-Chester disease. *Am J Neuroradiol* 16: 735-740.

307. Carla TG, Filotico R, Filotico M (1991). Bizarre angiomyomas of superficial soft tissues. *Pathologica* 83: 237-242.

308. Carrasco CH, Charnsangavej C, Raymond AK, Richli WR, Wallace S, Chawla SP, Ayala AG, Murray JA, Benjamin RS (1989). Osteosarcoma: angiographic assessment of response to preoperative chemotherapy. *Radiology* 170: 839-842.

309. Carroll KL, Yandow SM, Ward K, Carey JC (1999). Clinical correlation to genetic variations of hereditary multiple exostosis. *J Pediatr Orthop* 19: 785-791.

310. Casadei R, Ricci M, Ruggieri P, Biagini R, Benassi S, Picci P, Campanacci M (1991). Chondrosarcoma of the soft tissues. Two different sub-groups. *J Bone Joint Surg Br* 73: 162-168.

311. Casalone R, Albini A, Righi R, Granata P, Toniolo A (2001). Nonrandom chromosome changes in Kaposi sarcoma: cytogenetic and FISH results in a new cell line (KS-IMM) and literature review. *Cancer Genet Cytogenet* 124: 16-19.

312. Caspari R, Olschwang S, Friedl W, Mandl M, Boisson C, Boker T, Augustin A, Kadmon M, Moslein G, Thomas G, Propping P (1995). Familial adenomatous polyposis: desmoid tumours and lack of ophthalmic lesions (CHRPE) associated with APC mutations beyond codon 1444. *Hum Mol Genet* 4: 337-340.

313. Castresana JS, Rubio MP, Gomez L, Kreicbergs A, Zetterberg A, Barrios C (1995). Detection of TP53 gene mutations in human sarcomas. *Eur J Cancer* 31A: 735-738.

314. Castro C, Winkelmann RK (1974). Angiolymphoid hyperplasia with eosinophilia in the skin. *Cancer* 34: 1696-1705.

315. Cates JM, Rosenberg AE, O'Connell JX, Nielsen GP (2001). Chondroblastoma-like chondroma of soft tissue: an underrecognized variant and its differential diagnosis. *Am J Surg Pathol* 25: 661-666.

316. Cavazzana AO, Schmidt D, Ninfo V, Harms D, Tollot M, Carli M, Treuner J, Betto R, Salviati G (1992). Spindle cell rhabdomyosarcoma. A prognostically favorable variant of rhabdomyosarcoma. *Am J Surg Pathol* 16: 229-235.

317. Cavenee WK, Dryja TP, Phillips RA, Benedict WF, Godbout R, Gallie BL, Murphree AL, Strong LC, White RL (1983). Expression of recessive alleles by chromosomal mechanisms in retinoblastoma. *Nature* 305: 779-784.

318. Cavenee WK, Hansen MF, Nordenskjöld M, Kock E, Maumenee I, Squire JA, Phillips RA, Gallie BL (1985). Genetic origin of mutations predisposing to retinoblastoma. *Science* 228: 501-503.

319. Cavenee WK, Murphree AL, Shull MM, Benedict WF, Sparkes RS, Kock E, Nordenskjöld M (1986). Prediction of familial predisposition to retinoblastoma. *N Engl J Med* 314: 1201-1207.

320. Cerilli LA, Huffman HT, Anand A (1998). Primary renal angiosarcoma: a case report with immunohistochemical, ultrastructural, and cytogenetic features and review of the literature. *Arch Pathol Lab Med* 122: 929-935.

321. Cessna MH, Zhou H, Perkins SL, Tripp SR, Layfield L, Daines C, Coffin CM (2001). Are myogenin and myoD1 expression specific for rhabdomyosarcoma? A study of 150 cases, with emphasis on spindle cell mimics. *Am J Surg Pathol* 25: 1150-1157.

322. Chabrel CM, Beilby JO (1980). Vaginal rhabdomyoma. *Histopathology* 4: 645-651.

323. Chadwick EG, Connor EJ, Hanson IC, Joshi VV, Abu-Farsakh H, Yogev R, McSherry G, McClain K, Murphy SB (1990). Tumors of smooth-muscle origin in HIV-infected children. *JAMA* 263: 3182-3184.

324. Chaljub G, Johnson PR (1996). In vivo MRI characteristics of lipoma arborescens utilizing fat suppression and contrast administration. *J Comput Assist Tomogr* 20: 85-87.

325. Chan CW, Kung TM, Ma L (1986). Telangiectatic osteosarcoma of the mandible. *Cancer* 58: 2110-2115.

326. Chan JK, Cheuk W, Shimizu M (2001). Anaplastic lymphoma kinase expression in inflammatory pseudotumors. *Am J Surg Pathol* 25: 761-768.

327. Chan JK, Frizzera G, Fletcher CD, Rosai J (1992). Primary vascular tumors of lymph nodes other than Kaposi's sarcoma. Analysis of 39 cases and delineation of two new entities. *Am J Surg Pathol* 16: 335-350.

328. Chan JK, Rosai J (1991). Tumors of the neck showing thymic or related branchial pouch differentiation: a unifying concept. *Hum Pathol* 22: 349-367.

329. Chan JK, Tsang WY, Pau MY, Tang MC, Pang SW, Fletcher CD (1993). Lymphangiomyomatosis and angiomyolipoma: closely related entities characterized by hamartomatous proliferation of HMB-45-positive smooth muscle. *Histopathology* 22: 445-455.

330. Chan YM, Hon E, Ngai SW, Ng TY, Wong LC, Chan IM (2000). Aggressive angiomyxoma in females: is radical resection the only option? *Acta Obstet Gynecol Scand* 79: 216-220.

331. Chang CH, Piatt ED, Thomas KE, Watne AL (1968). Bone abnormalities in Gardner's syndrome. *Am J Roentgenol Radium Ther Nucl Med* 103: 645-652.

332. Chang Y, Cesarman E, Pessin MS, Lee F, Culpepper J, Knowles DM, Moore PS (1994). Identification of herpesvirus-like DNA sequences in AIDS-associated Kaposi's sarcoma. *Science* 266: 1865-1869.

333. Chapurlat RD, Meunier PJ (2000). Fibrous dysplasia of bone. *Baillieres Best Pract Res Clin Rheumatol* 14: 385-398.

334. Chase DR (1990). Rhabdoid versus epithelioid sarcoma. *Am J Surg Pathol* 14: 792-794.

335. Chase DR (1997). Do "rhabdoid features" impart a poorer prognosis to proximal-type epithelioid sarcoma? *Adv Anat Pathol* 4: 293-299.

336. Chase DR, Enzinger FM (1985). Epithelioid sarcoma. Diagnosis, prognostic indicators, and treatment. *Am J Surg Pathol* 9: 241-263.

336a. Chauveinc L, Mosseri V, Quintana E, Desjardins L, Schlienger P, Doz F, Dutrillaux B (2001). Osteosarcoma following retinoblastoma: age at onset and latency period. *Ophthalmic Genet* 22: 77-88.

337. Chen K (1996). Intraabdominal calcifying fibrous pseudotumor. *Int J Surg Pathol* 4: 9-12.

338. Chen KT, Hoffman KD, Hendricks EJ (1979). Angiosarcoma following therapeutic irradiation. *Cancer* 44: 2044-2048.

339. Chervenak FA, Isaacson G, Blakemore KJ, Breg WR, Hobbins JC, Berkowitz RL, Tortora M, Mayden K, Mahoney MJ (1983). Fetal cystic hygroma. Cause and natural history. *N Engl J Med* 309: 822-825.

340. Cheung PK, McCormick C, Crawford BE, Esko JD, Tufaro F, Duncan G (2001). Etiological point mutations in the hereditary multiple exostoses gene EXT1: a functional analysis of heparan sulfate polymerase activity. *Am J Hum Genet* 69: 55-66.

341. Chibon F, Mairal A, Freneaux P, Terrier P, Coindre JM, Sastre X, Aurias A (2000). The RB1 gene is the target of chromosome 13 deletions in malignant fibrous histiocytoma. *Cancer Res* 60: 6339-6345.

342. Chigira M, Maehara S, Arita S, Udagawa E (1983). The aetiology and treatment of simple bone cysts. *J Bone Joint Surg Br* 65: 633-637.

343. Chilosi M, Facchettti F, Dei Tos AP, Lestani M, Morassi ML, Martignoni G, Sorio C, Benedetti A, Morelli L, Doglioni C, Barberis M, Menestrina F, Viale G (1997). bcl-2 expression in pleural and extrapleural solitary fibrous tumours. *J Pathol* 181: 362-367.

344. Choi KC, Hashimoto K, Setoyama M, Kagetsu N, Tronnier M, Sturman S (1990). Infantile digital fibromatosis. Immunohistochemical and immunoelectron microscopic studies. *J Cutan Pathol* 17: 225-232.

345. Choong PF, Pritchard DJ, Rock MG, Sim FH, McLeod RA, Unni KK (1996). Low grade central osteogenic sarcoma. A long-term followup of 20 patients. *Clin Orthop* 198-206.

346. Chow LT, Lee KC (1992). Intraosseous lipoma. A clinicopathologic study of nine cases. *Am J Surg Pathol* 16: 401-410.

347. Christensen DR, Ramsamooj R, Gilbert TJ (1997). Sclerosing epithelioid fibrosarcoma: short T2 on MR imaging. *Skeletal Radiol* 26: 619-621.

348. Chung EB, Enzinger FM (1973). Benign lipoblastomatosis. An analysis of 35 cases. *Cancer* 32: 482-492.

349. Chung EB, Enzinger FM (1975). Proliferative fasciitis. *Cancer* 36: 1450-1458.

350. Chung EB, Enzinger FM (1976). Infantile fibrosarcoma. *Cancer* 38: 729-739.

351. Chung EB, Enzinger FM (1978). Chondroma of soft parts. *Cancer* 41: 1414-1424.

352. Chung EB, Enzinger FM (1979). Fibroma of tendon sheath. *Cancer* 44: 1945-1954.

353. Chung EB, Enzinger FM (1981). Infantile myofibromatosis. *Cancer* 48: 1807-1818.

354. Chung EB, Enzinger FM (1983). Malignant melanoma of soft parts. A reassessment of clear cell sarcoma. *Am J Surg Pathol* 7: 405-413.

355. Chung EB, Enzinger FM (1987). Extraskeletal osteosarcoma. *Cancer* 60: 1132-1142.

356. Cibas ES, Goss GA, Kulke MH, Demetri GD, Fletcher CD (2001). Malignant epithelioid angiomyolipoma ('sarcoma ex angiomyolipoma') of the kidney: a case report and review of the literature. *Am J Surg Pathol* 25: 121-126.

357. Cina SJ, Radentz SS, Smialek JE (1999). A case of familial angiolipomatosis with Lisch nodules. *Arch Pathol Lab Med* 123: 946-948.

358. Clapton WK, James CL, Morris LL, Davey RB, Peacock MJ, Byard RW (1992). Myositis ossificans in childhood. *Pathology* 24: 311-314.

359. Clark J, Benjamin H, Gill S, Sidhar S, Goodwin G, Crew J, Gusterson BA, Shipley J, Cooper CS (1996). Fusion of the EWS gene to CHN, a member of the steroid/thyroid receptor gene superfamily, in a human myxoid chondrosarcoma. *Oncogene* 12: 229-235.

360. Clark J, Rocques PJ, Crew AJ, Gill S, Shipley J, Chan AM, Gusterson BA, Cooper CS (1994). Identification of novel genes, SYT and SSX, involved in the t(X;18)(p11.2;q11.2) translocation found in human synovial sarcoma. *Nat Genet* 7: 502-508.

361. Clark SK, Pack K, Pritchard J, Hodgson SV (1997). Familial adenomatous polyposis presenting with childhood desmoids. *Lancet* 349: 471-472.

362. Clark SK, Phillips RK (1996). Desmoids in familial adenomatous polyposis. *Br J Surg* 83: 1494-1504.

363. Clark SK, Smith TG, Katz DE, Reznek RH, Phillips RK (1998). Identification and progression of a desmoid precursor lesion in patients with familial adenomatous polyposis. *Br J Surg* 85: 970-973.

364. Clark TD, Stelling CB, Fechner RE (1985). Benign fibrous histiocytoma of the left 8th rib. Case report 328. *Skeletal Radiol* 14: 149-151.

365. Clarke BE, Xipell JM, Thomas DP (1985). Benign fibrous histiocytoma of bone. *Am J Surg Pathol* 9: 806-815.

366. Classen DA, Hurst LN (1992). Plantar fibromatosis and bilateral flexion contractures: a review of the literature. *Ann Plast Surg* 28: 475-478.

367. Clatch RJ, Drake WK, Gonzalez JG (1993). Aggressive angiomyxoma in men. A report of two cases associated with inguinal hernias. *Arch Pathol Lab Med* 117: 911-913.

368. Cleveland DB, Chen SY, Allen CM, Ahing SI, Svirsky JA (1994). Adult rhabdomyoma. A light microscopic, ultrastructural, virologic, and immunologic analysis. *Oral Surg Oral Med Oral Pathol* 77: 147-153.

369. Clines GA, Ashley JA, Shah S, Lovett M (1997). The structure of the human multiple exostoses 2 gene and characterization of homologs in mouse and Caenorhabditis elegans. *Genome Res* 7: 359-367.

370. Cody JD, Singer FR, Roodman GD, Otterund B, Lewis TB, Leppert M, Leach RJ (1997). Genetic linkage of Paget disease of the bone to chromosome 18q. *Am J Hum Genet* 61: 1117-1122.

371. Cofer BR, Vescio PJ, Wiener ES (1996). Infantile fibrosarcoma: complete excision is the appropriate treatment. *Ann Surg Oncol* 3: 159-161.

372. Coffin CM, Dehner LP (1991). Fibroblastic-myofibroblastic tumors in children and adolescents: a clinicopathologic study of 108 examples in 103 patients. *Pediatr Pathol* 11: 569-588.

373. Coffin CM, Dehner LP (1993). Vascular tumors in children and adolescents: a clinicopathologic study of 228 tumors in 222 patients. *Pathol Annu* 28 Pt 1: 97-120.

374. Coffin CM, Dehner LP, Meis-Kindblom JM (1998). Inflammatory myofibroblastic tumor, inflammatory fibrosarcoma, and related lesions: a historical review with differential diagnostic considerations. *Semin Diagn Pathol* 15: 102-110.

375. Coffin CM, Dehner LP, O'Shea PA (1997). Pediatric Soft Tissue Tumors. Williams & Wilkins.

376. Coffin CM, Humphrey PA, Dehner LP (1998). Extrapulmonary inflammatory myofibroblastic tumor: a clinical and pathological survey. *Semin Diagn Pathol* 15: 85-101.

377. Coffin CM, Jaszcz W, O'Shea PA, Dehner LP (1994). So-called congenital-infantile fibrosarcoma: does it exist and what is it? *Pediatr Pathol* 14: 133-150.

378. Coffin CM, Patel A, Perkins S, Elenitoba-Johnson KS, Perlman E, Griffin CA (2001). ALK1 and p80 expression and chromosomal rearrangements involving 2p23 in inflammatory myofibroblastic tumor. *Mod Pathol* 14: 569-576.

379. Coffin CM, Rulon J, Smith L, Bruggers C, White FV (1997). Pathologic features of rhabdomyosarcoma before and after treatment: a clinicopathologic and immunohistochemical analysis. *Mod Pathol* 10: 1175-1187.

380. Coffin CM, Watterson J, Priest JR, Dehner LP (1995). Extrapulmonary inflammatory myofibroblastic tumor (inflammatory pseudotumor). A clinicopathologic and immunohistochemical study of 84 cases. *Am J Surg Pathol* 19: 859-872.

381. Cohen DM, Dahlin DC, Pugh DG (1962). Fibrous dysplasia associated with adamantinoma of the long bones. *Cancer* 15: 515-521.

382. Cohen MM, Jr. (2001). Fibrous dysplasia is a neoplasm. *Am J Med Genet* 98: 290-293.

383. Cohen MM, Jr., Howell RE (1999). Etiology of fibrous dysplasia and McCune-Albright syndrome. *Int J Oral Maxillofac Surg* 28: 366-371.

384. Coindre JM, de Mascarel A, Trojani M, de Mascarel I, Pages A (1988). Immunohistochemical study of rhabdomyosarcoma. Unexpected staining with S100 protein and cytokeratin. *J Pathol* 155: 127-132.

385. Coindre JM, Terrier P, Bui NB, Bonichon F, Collin F, Le D, V, Mandard AM, Vilain MO, Jacquemier J, Duplay H, Sastre X, Barlier C, Henry-Amar M, Mace-Lesech J, Contesso G (1996). Prognostic factors in adult patients with locally controlled soft tissue sarcoma. A study of 546 patients from the French Federation of Cancer Centers Sarcoma Group. *J Clin Oncol* 14: 869-877.

386. Coindre JM, Terrier P, Guillou L, Le D, V, Collin F, Ranchere D, Sastre X, Vilain MO, Bonichon F, N'Guyen BB (2001). Predictive value of grade for metastasis development in the main histologic types of adult soft tissue sarcomas: a study of 1240 patients from the French Federation of Cancer Centers Sarcoma Group. *Cancer* 91: 1914-1926.

387. Coindre JM, Trojani M, Contesso G, David M, Rouesse J, Bui NB, Bodaert A, de Mascarel I, de Mascarel A, Goussot JF (1986). Reproducibility of a histopathologic grading system for adult soft tissue sarcoma. *Cancer* 58: 306-309.

388. Coley BL (1960). *Neoplasms of Bone and Related Conditions.* 2nd ed. Hoeber: London.

389. Colin D, Lazure T, Fabre M, De Watteville JC, Bedossa P (2001). Pleomorphic rhabdomyosarcoma of the uterine corpus: a case report. *Eur J Gynaecol Oncol* 22: 116-117.

390. Collins DH (1956). Paget's disease of bone: incidence and subclinical forms. *Lancet* 2: 51.

391. Collins MH, Chatten J (1997). Lipoblastoma/lipoblastomatosis: a clinicopathologic study of 25 tumors. *Am J Surg Pathol* 21: 1131-1137.

392. Collins MT, Shenker A (1999). McCune-Albright syndrome: new insights. *Endocrinol Diabetes* 6: 119-125.

393. Colombat M, Liard-Meillon ME, Saint-Maur P, Sevestre H, Gontier MF (2001). [Cellular angiofibroma. A rare vulvar tumor. Report of a case]. *Ann Pathol* 21: 145-148.

394. Comtesse PP, Simons A, Siepman A, Stellink F, Suijkerbuijk RF, Hulsbergen-van de Kaa CA, Van Haelst UG, van Kessel AG, Wobbes T (1999). Isochromosome (12p) and peritriploidy in a highly malignant extrarenal rhabdoid tumor. *Cancer Genet Cytogenet* 109: 175-177.

395. Cook A, Raskind W, Blanton SH, Pauli RM, Gregg RG, Francomano CA, Puffenberger E, Conrad EU, Schmale G, Schellenberg G, Wijsman E, Hecht JT, Wells D, Wagner MJ (1993). Genetic heterogeneity in families with hereditary multiple exostoses. *Am J Hum Genet* 53: 71-79.

396. Cook JR, Dehner LP, Collins MH, Ma Z, Morris SW, Coffin CM, Hill DA (2001). Anaplastic lymphoma kinase (ALK) expression in the inflammatory myofibroblastic tumor: a comparative immunohistochemical study. *Am J Surg Pathol* 25: 1364-1371.

397. Cooper KL, Beabout JW, Dahlin DC (1984). Giant cell tumor: ossification in soft-tissue implants. *Radiology* 153: 597-602.

398. Cordoba JC, Parham DM, Meyer WH, Douglass EC (1994). A new cytogenetic finding in an epithelioid sarcoma, t(8;22)(q22;q11). *Cancer Genet Cytogenet* 72: 151-154.

399. Cordon-Cardo C, Latres E, Drobnjak M, Oliva MR, Pollack D, Woodruff JM, Marechal V, Chen J, Brennan MF, Levine AJ (1994). Molecular abnormalities of mdm2 and p53 genes in adult soft tissue sarcomas. *Cancer Res* 54: 794-799.

400. Cossarizza A, Mussini C, Vigano A (2001). Mitochondria in the pathogenesis of lipodystrophy induced by anti-HIV antiretroviral drugs: actors or bystanders? *Bioessays* 23: 1070-1080.

401. Costa J (1990). The grading and staging of soft tissue sarcomas. In: *Pathobiology of Soft Tissue Tumors,* Fletcher CD, McKee PH, eds. Churchill Livingstone: Edinburgh, pp. 221-238.

402. Costa J, Wesley RA, Glatstein E, Rosenberg SA (1984). The grading of soft tissue sarcomas. Results of a clinicohistopathologic correlation in a series of 163 cases. *Cancer* 53: 530-541.

403. Costa MJ, McGlothlen L, Pierce M, Munn R, Vogt PJ (1995). Angiomatoid features in fibrohistiocytic sarcomas. Immunohistochemical, ultrastructural, and clinical distinction from vascular neoplasms. *Arch Pathol Lab Med* 119: 1065-1071.

404. Costa MJ, Weiss SW (1990). Angiomatoid malignant fibrous histiocytoma. A follow-up study of 108 cases with evaluation of possible histologic predictors of outcome. *Am J Surg Pathol* 14: 1126-1132.

405. Costes V, Magen V, Legouffe E, Durand L, Baldet P, Rossi JF, Klein B, Brochier J (1999). The Mi15 monoclonal antibody (anti-syndecan-1) is a reliable marker for quantifying plasma cells in paraffin-embedded bone marrow biopsy specimens. *Hum Pathol* 30: 1405-1411.

406. Costes V, Medioni D, Durand L, Sarran N, Marguerite G, Baldet P (1997). [Undifferentiated soft tissue tumor with rhabdoid phenotype (extra-renal rhabdoid tumor). Report of a congenital case associated with medulloblastoma in a brother]. *Ann Pathol* 17: 41-43.

407. Crawford SC, Harnsberger HR, Johnson L, Aoki JR, Giley J (1988). Fibromatosis colli of infancy: CT and sonographic findings. *AJR Am J Roentgenol* 151: 1183-1184.

408. Crew AJ, Clark J, Fisher C, Gill S, Grimer R, Chand A, Shipley J, Gusterson BA, Cooper CS (1995). Fusion of SYT to two genes, SSX1 and SSX2, encoding proteins with homology to the Kruppel-associated box in human synovial sarcoma. *EMBO J* 14: 2333-2340.

409. Crotty PL, Nakhleh RE, Dehner LP (1993). Juvenile rhabdomyoma. An intermediate form of skeletal muscle tumor in children. *Arch Pathol Lab Med* 117: 43-47.

410. Crozat A, Åman P, Mandahl N, Ron D (1993). Fusion of CHOP to a novel RNA-binding protein in human myxoid liposarcoma. *Nature* 363: 640-644.

411. Culver JE, Jr., Sweet DE, McCue FC (1975). Chondrosarcoma of the hand arising from a pre-existent benign solitary enchondroma. *Clin Orthop* 128-131.

412. Cummings OW, Ulbright TM, Young RH, Del Tos AP, Fletcher CD, Hull MT (1997). Desmoplastic small round cell tumors of the paratesticular region. A report of six cases. *Am J Surg Pathol* 21: 219-225.

413. Curry JL, Olejnik JL, Wojcik EM (2001). Cellular angiofibroma of the vulva with DNA ploidy analysis. *Int J Gynecol Pathol* 20: 200-203.

414. Cuvelier CA, Roels HJ (1979). Cytophotometric studies of the nuclear DNA content in cartilaginous tumors. *Cancer* 44: 1363-1374.

415. D'Ambrosia R, Ferguson AB, Jr. (1968). The formation of osteochondroma by epiphyseal cartilage transplantation. *Clin Orthop* 61: 103-115.

416. d'Amore ES, Ninfo V (1997). Clear cell tumors of the somatic soft tissues. *Semin Diagn Pathol* 14: 270-280.

417. D'Andrea V, Lippolis G, Biancari F, Ruco LP, Marzullo A, Wedard BM, Di Matteo FM, Sarmiento R, Dibra A, De Antoni E (1999). [A uterine pecoma: a case report]. *G Chir* 20: 163-164.

418. D'Haen B, De Jaegere T, Goffin J, Dom R, Demaerel P, Plets C (1995). Chordoma of the lower cervical spine. *Clin Neurol Neurosurg* 97: 245-248.

419. Dabska M (1969). Malignant endovascular papillary angioendothelioma of the skin in childhood. Clinicopathologic study of 6 cases. *Cancer* 24: 503-510.

420. Dabska M (1977). Parachordoma: a new clinicopathologic entity. *Cancer* 40: 1586-1592.

421. Dabska M, Huvos AG (1983). Mesenchymal chondrosarcoma in the young. *Virchows Arch A Pathol Anat Histopathol* 399: 89-104.

422. Daffner RH, Kirks DR, Gehweiler JA, Jr., Heaston DK (1982). Computed tomography of fibrous dysplasia. *AJR Am J Roentgenol* 139: 943-948.

423. Dahl I, Angervall L (1974). Cutaneous and subcutaneous leiomyosarcoma. A clinicopathologic study of 47 patients. *Pathol Eur* 9: 307-315.

424. Dahl I, Save-Soderbergh J, Angervall L (1973). Fibrosarcoma in early infancy. *Pathol Eur* 8: 193-209.

425. Dahlin DC (1982). Case report 189. Infantile fibrosarcoma (congenital fibrosarcoma-like fibromatosis). *Skeletal Radiol* 8: 77-78.

426. Dahlin DC, Coventry MB (1967). Osteogenic sarcoma. A study of six hundred cases. *J Bone Joint Surg Am* 49: 101-110.

427. Dahlin DC, Johnson EW, Jr. (1954). Giant osteoid osteoma. *J Bone Joint Surg Am* 36: 559-572.

428. Dahlin DC, Salvador AH (1974). Cartilaginous tumors of the soft tissues of the hands and feet. *Mayo Clin Proc* 49: 721-726.

429. Dahlin DC, Unni KK (1973). *Bone Tumors: General Aspects and Data on 3,987 Cases.* 2nd ed. Charles C. Thomas: Springfield.

430. Dahlin DC, Unni KK (1977). Osteosarcoma of bone and its important recognizable varieties. *Am J Surg Pathol* 1: 61-72.

431. Daimaru Y, Hashimoto H, Enjoji M (1989). Myofibromatosis in adults (adult counterpart of infantile myofibromatosis). *Am J Surg Pathol* 13: 859-865.

432. Daimaru Y, Hashimoto H, Tsuneyoshi M, Enjoji M (1987). Epithelial profile of epithelioid sarcoma. An immunohistochemical analysis of eight cases. *Cancer* 59: 134-141.

433. Dal Cin P, De Smet L, Sciot R, Van Damme B, van den Berghe H (1999). Trisomy 7 and trisomy 8 in dividing and non-dividing tumor cells in Dupuytren's disease. *Cancer Genet Cytogenet* 108: 137-140.

434. Dal Cin P, Kools P, Sciot R, de Wever I, Van Damme B, van de Ven W, van den Berghe H (1993). Cytogenetic and fluorescence in situ hybridization investigation of ring chromosomes characterizing a specific pathologic subgroup of adipose tissue tumors. *Cancer Genet Cytogenet* 68: 85-90.

435. Dal Cin P, Kozakewich HP, Goumnerova L, Mankin HJ, Rosenberg AE, Fletcher JA (2000). Variant translocations involving 16q22 and 17p13 in solid variant and extraosseous forms of aneurysmal bone cyst. *Genes Chromosomes Cancer* 28: 233-234.

436. Dal Cin P, Pauwels P, Sciot R, van den Berghe H (1996). Multiple chromosome rearrangements in a fibrosarcoma. *Cancer Genet Cytogenet* 87: 176-178.

437. Dal Cin P, Qi H, Sciot R, van den Berghe H (1997). Involvement of chromosomes 6 and 11 in a soft tissue chondroma. *Cancer Genet Cytogenet* 93: 177-178.

438. Dal Cin P, Sciot R, Aly MS, Delabie J, Stas M, de Wever I, Van Damme B, van den Berghe H (1994). Some desmoid tumors are characterized by trisomy 8. *Genes Chromosomes Cancer* 10: 131-135.

439. Dal Cin P, Sciot R, Brys P, de Wever I, Dorfman H, Fletcher CD, Jonsson K, Mandahl N, Mertens F, Mitelman F, Rosai J, Rydholm A, Samson I, Tallini G, Van den Berghe H., Vanni R, Willén H (2000). Recurrent chromosome aberrations in fibrous dysplasia of the bone: a report of the CHAMP study group. *Cancer Genet Cytogenet* 122: 30-32.

440. Dal Cin P, Sciot R, De Smet L, van den Berghe H (1998). Translocation 2;11 in a fibroma of tendon sheath. *Histopathology* 32: 433-435.

441. Dal Cin P, Sciot R, Fletcher CD, Hilliker C, de Wever I, Van Damme B, van den Berghe H (1996). Trisomy 21 in solitary fibrous tumor. *Cancer Genet Cytogenet* 86: 58-60.

442. Dal Cin P, Sciot R, Polito P, Stas M, de Wever I, Cornelis A, van den Berghe H (1997). Lesions of 13q may occur independently of deletion of 16q in spindle cell/pleomorphic lipomas. *Histopathology* 31: 222-225.

443. Dal Cin P, Sciot R, Samson I, de Wever I, van den Berghe H (1998). Osteoid osteoma and osteoblastoma with clonal chromosome changes. *Br J Cancer* 78: 344-348.

444. Dal Cin P, Sciot R, Van Damme B, de Wever I, van den Berghe H (1995). Trisomy 20 characterizes a second group of desmoid tumors. *Cancer Genet Cytogenet* 79: 189.

445. Dal Cin P, van den Berghe H, Pauwels P (1999). Epithelioid sarcoma of the proximal type with complex karyotype including i(8q). *Cancer Genet Cytogenet* 114: 80-82.

446. Daluiski A, Seeger LL, Dobrneck SA, Finerman GA, Eckardt JJ (1995). A case of juxta-articular myxoma of the knee. *Skeletal Radiol* 24: 389-391.

447. Dangel A, Meloni AM, Lynch HT, Sandberg AA (1994). Deletion (5q) in a desmoid tumor of a patient with Gardner's syndrome. *Cancer Genet Cytogenet* 78: 94-98.

448. Dargent JL, Delplace J, Roufosse C, Laget JP, Lespagnard L (1999). Development of a calcifying fibrous pseudotumour within a lesion of Castleman disease, hyaline-vascular subtype. *J Clin Pathol* 52: 547-549.

449. Darling JM, Goldring SR, Harada Y, Handel ML, Glowacki J, Gravallese EM (1997). Multinucleated cells in pigmented villonodular synovitis and giant cell tumor of tendon sheath express features of osteoclasts. *Am J Pathol* 150: 1383-1393.

450. Daroca PJ, Jr., Pulitzer DR, LoCicero J, III (1982). Ossifying fasciitis. *Arch Pathol Lab Med* 106: 682-685.

451. Davies DR, Armstrong JG, Thakker N, Horner K, Guy SP, Clancy T, Sloan P, Blair V, Dodd C, Warnes TW, Harris R, Evans DG (1995). Severe Gardner syndrome in families with mutations restricted to a specific region of the APC gene. *Am J Hum Genet* 57: 1151-1158.

452. Davies JD, Rees GJ, Mera SL (1983). Angiosarcoma in irradiated post-mastectomy chest wall. *Histopathology* 7: 947-956.

453. Davis AM, Bell RS, Goodwin PJ (1994). Prognostic factors in osteosarcoma: a critical review. *J Clin Oncol* 12: 423-431.

454. Davis RI, Hamilton A, Biggart JD (1998). Primary synovial chondromatosis: a clinico-pathological review and assessment of malignant potential. *Hum Pathol* 29: 683-688.

455. Davis RJ, Barr FG (1997). Fusion genes resulting from alternative chromosomal translocations are overexpressed by gene-specific mechanisms in alveolar rhabdomyosarcoma. *Proc Natl Acad Sci U S A* 94: 8047-8051.

456. Davis RJ, D'Cruz CM, Lovell MA, Biegel JA, Barr FG (1994). Fusion of PAX7 to FKHR by the variant t(1;13)(p36;q14) translocation in alveolar rhabdomyosarcoma. *Cancer Res* 54: 2869-2872.

457. Dawson EK (1955). Liposarcoma of bone. *J Pathol Bacteriol* 70: 513-520.

458. Day DL, Sane S, Dehner LP (1986). Inflammatory pseudotumor of the mesentery and small intestine. *Pediatr Radiol* 16: 210-215.

459. Day SJ, Nelson M, Rosenthal H, Vergara GG, Bridge JA (1997). Der(16)t(1;16)(q21;q13) as a secondary structural aberration in yet a third sarcoma, extraskeletal myxoid chondrosarcoma. *Genes Chromosomes Cancer* 20: 425-427.

460. de Alava E, Kawai A, Healey JH, Fligman I, Meyers PA, Huvos AG, Gerald WL, Jhanwar SC, Argani P, Antonescu CR, Pardo-Mindan FJ, Ginsberg J, Womer R, Lawlor ER, Wunder J, Andrulis I, Sorensen PH, Barr FG, Ladanyi M (1998). EWS-FLI1 fusion transcript structure is an independent determinant of prognosis in Ewing's sarcoma. *J Clin Oncol* 16: 1248-1255.

461. de Alava E, Ladanyi M, Rosai J, Gerald WL (1995). Detection of chimeric transcripts in desmoplastic small round cell tumor and related developmental tumors by reverse transcriptase polymerase chain reaction. A specific diagnostic assay. *Am J Pathol* 147: 1584-1591.

462. de Alava E, Lozano MD, Patino A, Sierrasesumaga L, Pardo-Mindan FJ (1998). Ewing family tumors: potential prognostic value of reverse-transcriptase polymerase chain reaction detection of minimal residual disease in peripheral blood samples. *Diagn Mol Pathol* 7: 152-157.

463. de Baere T, Vanel D, Shapeero LG, Charpentier A, Terrier P, di Paola M (1992). Osteosarcoma after chemotherapy: evaluation with contrast material-enhanced subtraction MR imaging. *Radiology* 185: 587-592.

464. De Beuckeleer LH, De Schepper AM, Ramon F (1996). Magnetic resonance imaging of cartilaginous tumors: is it useful or necessary? *Skeletal Radiol* 25: 137-141.

465. De Beuckeleer LH, De Schepper AM, Vandevenne JE, Bloem JL, Davies AM, Oudkerk M, Hauben E, Van Marck E, Somville J, Vanel D, Steinbach LS, Guinebretiere JM, Hogendoorn PC, Mooi WJ, Verstraete K, Zaloudek C, Jones H (2000). MR imaging of clear cell sarcoma (malignant melanoma of the soft parts): a multicenter correlative MRI-pathology study of 21 cases and literature review. *Skeletal Radiol* 29: 187-195.

466. de Bruijn DR, Baats E, Zechner U, de Leeuw B, Balemans M, Olde Weghuis DE, Hirning-Folz U, van Kessel AG (1996). Isolation and characterization of the mouse homolog of SYT, a gene implicated in the development of human synovial sarcomas. *Oncogene* 13: 643-648.

467. de Bruijn DR, don Santos NR, Kater-Baats E, Thijssen J, van den Berk L, Stap J, Balemans M, Schepens M, Merkx G, Geurts van Kessel AG (2002). The cancer-related protein SSX2 interacts with the human homologue of a RAS-like GTPase interactor, RAB3IP, and a novel nuclear protein, SSX2IP. *Genes Chromosomes Cancer* 34: 285-298.

468. de Bruijn DR, dos Santos NR, Thijssen J, Balemans M, Debernardi S, Linder B, Young BD, Geurts van Kessel AG (2001). The synovial sarcoma associated protein SYT interacts with the acute leukemia associated protein AF10. *Oncogene* 20: 3281-3289.

469. de Bruijn DR, Kater-Baats E, Eleveld M, Merkx G, Geurts van Kessel AG (2001). Mapping and characterization of the mouse and human SS18 genes, two human SS18-like genes and a mouse Ss18 pseudo-gene. *Cytogenet Cell Genet* 92: 310-319.

470. de Gauzy JS, Kany J, Darodes P, Dequae P, Cahuzac JP (1999). Kienbock's disease and multiple hereditary osteochondromata: a case report. *J Hand Surg [Am]* 24: 642-646.

471. de Leeuw B, Balemans M, Olde Weghuis DE, van Kessel AG (1995). Identification of two alternative fusion genes, SYT-SSX1 and SYT-SSX2, in t(X;18)(p11.2;q11.2)-positive synovial sarcomas. *Hum Mol Genet* 4: 1097-1099.

472. de Leeuw B, Balemans M, Weghuis DO, Seruca R, Janz M, Geraghty MT, Gilgenkrantz S, Ropers HH, Geurts van Kessel AG (1994). Molecular cloning of the synovial sarcoma-specific translocation (X;18)(p11.2;q11.2) breakpoint. *Hum Mol Genet* 3: 745-749.

473. de Leeuw B, Suijkerbuijk RF, Olde Weghuis DE, Meloni AM, Stenman G, Kindblom LG, Balemans M, van den Berg E, Molenaar WM, Sandberg AA, Geurts van Kessel AG (1994). Distinct Xp11.2 breakpoint regions in synovial sarcoma revealed by metaphase and interphase FISH: relationship to histologic subtypes. *Cancer Genet Cytogenet* 73: 89-94.

474. De Maeseneer M, Jaovisidha S, Lenchik L, Witte D, Schweitzer ME, Sartoris DJ, Resnick D (1997). Fibrolipomatous hamartoma: MR imaging findings. *Skeletal Radiol* 26: 155-160.

475. de Pinieux G, Beabout JW, Unni KK, Sim FH (2001). Primary mixed tumor of bone. *Skeletal Radiol* 30: 534-536.

476. de Wever I, Dal Cin P, Fletcher CD, Mandahl N, Mertens F, Mitelman F, Rosai J, Rydholm A, Sciot R, Tallini G, van den Berghe H, Vanni R, Willén H (2000). Cytogenetic, clinical, and morphologic correlations in 78 cases of fibromatosis: a report from the CHAMP Study Group. CHromosomes And Morphology. *Mod Pathol* 13: 1080-1085.

477. De Young BR, Frierson HF, Jr., Ly MN, Smith D, Swanson PE (1998). CD31 immunoreactivity in carcinomas and mesotheliomas. *Am J Clin Pathol* 110: 374-377.

478. De Zen L, Sommaggio A, d'Amore ES, Masiero L, di Montezemolo LC, Linari A, Madon E, Dominici C, Bosco S, Bisogno G, Carli M, Ninfo V, Basso G (1997). Clinical relevance of DNA ploidy and proliferative activity in childhood rhabdomyosarcoma: a retrospective analysis of patients enrolled onto the Italian Cooperative Rhabdomyosarcoma Study RMS88. *J Clin Oncol* 15: 1198-1205.

479. DeBaun MR, Tucker MA (1998). Risk of cancer during the first four years of life in children from The Beckwith-Wiedemann Syndrome Registry. *J Pediatr* 132: 398-400.

480. Debiec-Rychter M, Sciot R, Hagemeijer A (2000). Common chromosome aberrations in the proximal type of epithelioid sarcoma. *Cancer Genet Cytogenet* 123: 133-136.

481. DeCaprio JA, Ludlow JW, Figge J, Shew JY, Huang CM, Lee WH, Marsilio E, Paucha E, Livingston DM (1988). SV40 large tumor antigen forms a specific complex with the product of the retinoblastoma susceptibility gene. *Cell* 54: 275-283.

482. DeCaprio JA, Ludlow JW, Lynch D, Furukawa Y, Griffin J, Piwnica-Worms H, Huang CM, Livingston DM (1989). The product of the retinoblastoma susceptibility gene has properties of a cell cycle regulatory element. *Cell* 58: 1085-1095.

483. DeCristofaro MF, Betz BL, Wang W, Weissman BE (1999). Alteration of hSNF5/INI1/BAF47 detected in rhabdoid cell lines and primary rhabdomyosarcomas but not Wilms' tumors. *Oncogene* 18: 7559-7565.

484. Deenik W, Mooi WJ, Rutgers EJ, Peterse JL, Hart AA, Kroon BB (1999). Clear cell sarcoma (malignant melanoma) of soft parts: A clinicopathologic study of 30 cases. *Cancer* 86: 969-975.

485. Dehner LP, Enzinger FM, Font RL (1972). Fetal rhabdomyoma. An analysis of nine cases. *Cancer* 30: 160-166.

486. Dei Tos AP (2000). Liposarcoma: new entities and evolving concepts. *Ann Diagn Pathol* 4: 252-266.

487. Dei Tos AP, Doglioni C, Piccinin S, Maestro R, Mentzel T, Barbareschi M, Boiocchi M, Fletcher CD (1997). Molecular abnormalities of the p53 pathway in dedifferentiated liposarcoma. *J Pathol* 181: 8-13.

488. Dei Tos AP, Maestro R, Doglioni C, Piccinin S, Libera DD, Boiocchi M, Fletcher CD (1996). Tumor suppressor genes and related molecules in leiomyosarcoma. *Am J Pathol* 148: 1037-1045.

489. Dei Tos AP, Mentzel T, Fletcher CD (1998). Primary liposarcoma of the skin: a rare neoplasm with unusual high grade features. *Am J Dermatopathol* 20: 332-338.

490. Dei Tos AP, Mentzel T, Newman PL, Fletcher CD (1994). Spindle cell liposarcoma, a hitherto unrecognized variant of liposarcoma. Analysis of six cases. *Am J Surg Pathol* 18: 913-921.

491. Dei Tos AP, Seregard S, Calonje E, Chan JK, Fletcher CD (1995). Giant cell angiofibroma. A distinctive orbital tumor in adults. *Am J Surg Pathol* 19: 1286-1293.

492. Dei Tos AP, Wadden C, Calonje E, Sciot R, Pauwels P, Knight JC, Dal Cin P, Fletcher CD (1995). Immunohistochemical demonstration of glycoprotein p30/32mic2 (CD99) in synovial sarcoma. A potential cause of diagnostic confusion. *Appl Immunohistochem* 3: 168-173.

493. Dei Tos AP, Wadden C, Fletcher CD (1996). S-100 protein staining in liposarcoma. Its diagnostic utility in the high grade myxoid (round cell) variant. *Appl Immunohistochem* 4: 95-101.

494. Dei Tos AP, Wadden C, Fletcher CD (1997). Extraskeletal myxoid chondrosarcoma: an immunohistochemical reappraisal of 39 cases. *Appl Immunohistochem* 5: 73-77.

495. del Peso L, Gonzalez VM, Hernandez R, Barr FG, Nunez G (1999). Regulation of the forkhead transcription factor FKHR, but not the PAX3-FKHR fusion protein, by the serine/threonine kinase Akt. *Oncogene* 18: 7328-7333.

496. Delattre O, Zucman J, Melot T, Garau XS, Zucker JM, Lenoir GM, Ambros PF, Sheer D, Turc-Carel C, Triche TJ, Aurias A, Thomas G (1994). The Ewing family of tumors – a subgroup of small-round-cell tumors defined by specific chimeric transcripts. *N Engl J Med* 331: 294-299.

497. Delattre O, Zucman J, Plougastel B, Desmaze C, Melot T, Peter M, Kovar H, Joubert I, de Jong P, Rouleau G, Aurias A, Thomas G (1992). Gene fusion with an ETS DNA-binding domain caused by chromosome translocation in human tumours. *Nature* 359: 162-165.

498. Delsol G, Gatter KC, Stein H, Erber WN, Pulford KA, Zinne K, Mason DY (1984). Human lymphoid cells express epithelial membrane antigen. Implications for diagnosis of human neoplasms. *Lancet* 2: 1124-1129.

499. Dembinski A, Bridge JA, Neff JR, Berger C, Sandberg AA (1992). Trisomy 2 in proliferative fasciitis. *Cancer Genet Cytogenet* 60: 27-30.

500. Demircan M, Sayan A, Erikci V, Bayol U, Arikan A (1998). An hourglass type of intrathoracic lipoblastoma manifested by edema in right upper limb. *J Pak Med Assoc* 48: 108-110.

501. Deneen B, Denny CT (2001). Loss of p16 pathways stabilizes EWS/FLI1 expression and complements EWS/FLI1 mediated transformation. *Oncogene* 20: 6731-6741.

502. Derkinderen DJ, Koten JW, Wolterbeek R, Beemer FA, Tan KE, Den Otter W (1987). Non-ocular cancer in hereditary retinoblastoma survivors and relatives. *Ophthalmic Paediatr Genet* 8: 23-25.

503. Desai P, Perino G, Present D, Steiner GC (1996). Sarcoma in association with bone infarcts. Report of five cases. *Arch Pathol Lab Med* 120: 482-489.

504. Desai S, Jambhekar N (1995). Clinicopathological evaluation of metastatic carcinomas of bone: a retrospective analysis of 114 cases over 10 years. *Indian J Pathol Microbiol* 38: 49-54.

505. deSantos LA, Edeiken B (1982). Purely lytic osteosarcoma. *Skeletal Radiol* 9: 1-7.

506. Destouet JM, Kyriakos M, Gilula LA (1980). Fibrous histiocytoma (fibroxanthoma) of a cervical vertebra. A report with a review of the literature. *Skeletal Radiol* 5: 241-246.

507. Devaney DM, Dervan P, O'Neill S, Carney D, Leader M (1990). Low-grade fibromyxoid sarcoma. *Histopathology* 17: 463-465.

508. Devaney K, Vinh TN, Sweet DE (1993). Small cell osteosarcoma of bone: an immunohistochemical study with differential diagnostic considerations. *Hum Pathol* 24: 1211-1225.

509. Devaney K, Vinh TN, Sweet DE (1993). Synovial hemangioma: a report of 20 cases with differential diagnostic considerations. *Hum Pathol* 24: 737-745.

510. Devaney K, Vinh TN, Sweet DE (1994). Skeletal-extraskeletal angiomatosis. A clinicopathological study of fourteen patients and nosologic considerations. *J Bone Joint Surg Am* 76: 878-891.

511. Devesa SS (1975). The incidence of retinoblastoma. *Am J Ophthalmol* 80: 263-265.

512. Devesa SS, Silverman DT, Young JL, Jr., Pollack ES, Brown CC, Horm JW, Percy CL, Myers MH, McKay FW, Fraumeni JF, Jr. (1987). Cancer incidence and mortality trends among whites in the United States, 1947-84. *J Natl Cancer Inst* 79: 701-770.

513. Devoe K, Weidner N (2000). Immunohistochemistry of small round-cell tumors. *Semin Diagn Pathol* 17: 216-224.

514. DeYoung BR, Wick MR (2000). Immunohistologic evaluation of metastatic carcinomas of unknown origin: an algorithmic approach. *Semin Diagn Pathol* 17: 184-193.

515. di Sant'Agnese PA, Knowles DM (1980). Extracardiac rhabdomyoma: a clinicopathologic study and review of the literature. *Cancer* 46: 780-789.

516. Dias P, Chen B, Dilday B, Palmer H, Hosoi H, Singh S, Wu C, Li X, Thompson J, Parham D, Qualman S, Houghton P (2000). Strong immunostaining for myogenin in rhabdomyosarcoma is significantly associated with tumors of the alveolar subclass. *Am J Pathol* 156: 399-408.

517. Dias P, Parham DM, Shapiro DN, Webber BL, Houghton PJ (1990). Myogenic regulatory protein (MyoD1) expression in childhood solid tumors: diagnostic utility in rhabdomyosarcoma. *Am J Pathol* 137: 1283-1291.

518. Dickersin GR, Rosenberg AE (1991). The ultrastructure of small-cell osteosarcoma, with a review of the light microscopy and differential diagnosis. *Hum Pathol* 22: 267-275.

519. Dickey GE, Sotelo-Avila C (1999). Fibrous hamartoma of infancy: current review. *Pediatr Dev Pathol* 2: 236-243.

520. Dickman PS, Triche TJ (1986). Extraosseous Ewing's sarcoma versus primitive rhabdomyosarcoma: diagnostic criteria and clinical correlation. *Hum Pathol* 17: 881-893.

521. Dictor M, Ferno M, Baldetorp B (1991). Flow cytometric DNA content in Kaposi's sarcoma by histologic stage. Comparison with angiosarcoma. *Anal Quant Cytol Histol* 13: 201-208.

522. Dimitrakopoulou-Strauss A, Strauss LG, Schwarzbach M, Burger C, Heichel T, Willeke F, Mechtersheimer G, Lehnert T (2001). Dynamic PET 18F-FDG studies in patients with primary and recurrent soft-tissue sarcomas: impact on diagnosis and correlation with grading. *J Nucl Med* 42: 713-720.

523. Dimmick JE, Wood WS (1983). Congenital multiple fibromatosis. *Am J Dermatopathol* 5: 289-295.

524. DiSanto S, Abt AB, Boal DK, Krummel TM (1992). Fetal rhabdomyoma and nevoid basal cell carcinoma syndrome. *Pediatr Pathol* 12: 441-447.

525. Dishop MK, O'Connor WN, Abraham S, Cottrill CM (2001). Primary cardiac lipoblastoma. *Pediatr Dev Pathol* 4: 276-280.

526. Diwan AH, Graves ED, King JA, Horenstein MG (2000). Nuchal-type fibroma in two related patients with Gardner's syndrome. *Am J Surg Pathol* 24: 1563-1567.

527. Dixon AY, McGregor DH, Lee SH (1981). Angiolipomas: an ultrastructural and clinicopathological study. *Hum Pathol* 12: 739-747.

528. Djindjian R, Cophignon J, Theron J, Merland JJ, Houdart R (1973). Embolization by superselective arteriography from the femoral route in neuroradiology. Review of 60 cases. 1. Technique, indications, complications. *Neuroradiology* 6: 20-26.

529. Dobin SM, Donner LR, Speights VO, Jr. (1995). Mesenchymal chondrosarcoma. A cytogenetic, immunohistochemical and ultrastructural study. *Cancer Genet Cytogenet* 83: 56-60.

530. Dobson L (1956). Spontaneous regression of malignant tumors. *Am J Surg* 92: 162-173.

531. Donahoo JS, Miller JA, Lal B, Rosario PG (1996). Chest wall hamartoma in an adult: an unusual chest wall tumor. *Thorac Cardiovasc Surg* 44: 110-111.

532. Donato G, Lavano A, Volpentesta G, Chirchiglia D, Veraldi A, De Rose F, Iannello AN, Stroscio C, Signorelli CD (1997). Telangiectatic osteosarcoma of the skull. A post-Paget case. *Clin Neuropathol* 16: 201-203.

533. Donner LR (1992). Ossifying fibromyxoid tumor of soft parts: evidence supporting Schwann cell origin. *Hum Pathol* 23: 200-202.

534. Donner LR, Clawson K, Dobin SM (2000). Sclerosing epithelioid fibrosarcoma: a cytogenetic, immunohistochemical, and ultrastructural study of an unusual histological variant. *Cancer Genet Cytogenet* 119: 127-131.

535. Donner LR, Trompler RA, Dobin S (1998). Clear cell sarcoma of the ileum: the crucial role of cytogenetics for the diagnosis. *Am J Surg Pathol* 22: 121-124.

536. Donner LR, Trompler RA, White RR (1996). Progression of inflammatory myofibroblastic tumor (inflammatory pseudotumor) of soft tissue into sarcoma after several recurrences. *Hum Pathol* 27: 1095-1098.

537. Dorfman HD, Czerniak B (1995). Bone cancers. *Cancer* 75: 203-210.

538. Dorfman HD, Czerniak B (1998). *Bone Tumors*. Mosby: St.Louis.

539. Dorfman HD, Czerniak B (1998). Vascular lesions. In: *Bone Tumors*. Mosby: St.Louis, pp. 729-814.

540. Dorfman HD, Habermann ET (1988). The risk of bone sarcoma in patients with bone infarction. *Proc Am Acad Orthop Surg* February (abstract).

541. Dorfman HD, Weiss SW (1984). Borderline osteoblastic tumors: problems in the differential diagnosis of aggressive osteoblastoma and low-grade osteosarcoma. *Semin Diagn Pathol* 1: 215-234.

542. Dorwart RH, Genant HK, Johnston WH, Morris JM (1984). Pigmented villonodular synovitis of synovial joints: clinical, pathologic, and radiologic features. *AJR Am J Roentgenol* 143: 877-885.

543. dos Santos NR, de Bruijn DR, Balemans M, Janssen B, Gartner F, Lopes JM, de Leeuw B, van Kessel AG (1997). Nuclear localization of SYT, SSX and the synovial sarcoma-associated SYT-SSX fusion proteins. *Hum Mol Genet* 6: 1549-1558.

543a. dos Santos NR, de Bruijn DR, van Kessel AG (2001). Molecular mechanisms underlying human synovial sarcoma development. *Genes Chromosomes Cancer* 30: 1-14.

544. Dosoretz DE, Raymond AK, Murphy GF, Doppke KP, Schiller AL, Wang CC, Suit HD (1982). Primary lymphoma of bone: the relationship of morphologic diversity to clinical behavior. *Cancer* 50: 1009-1014.

545. Dotan ZA, Mor Y, Olchovsky D, Aviel-Ronen S, Engelberg S, Pinthus J, Shefi S, Leibovitch I, Ramon J (1999). Solitary fibrous tumor presenting as perirenal mass associated with hypoglycemia. *J Urol* 162: 2087-2088.

546. Douglass EC, Valentine M, Rowe ST, Parham DM, Wilimas JA, Sanders JM, Houghton PJ (1990). Malignant rhabdoid tumor: a highly malignant childhood tumor with minimal karyotypic changes. *Genes Chromosomes Cancer* 2: 210-216.

547. Dowler JG, Sanders MD, Brown PM (1995). Bilateral sudden visual loss due to sphenoid mucocele in Albright's syndrome. *Br J Ophthalmol* 79: 503-504.

548. Downes KA, Goldblum JR, Montgomery EA, Fisher C (2001). Pleomorphic liposarcoma: a clinicopathologic analysis of 19 cases. *Mod Pathol* 14: 179-184.

549. Downing JR, Head DR, Parham DM, Douglass EC, Hulshof MG, Link MP, Motroni TA, Grier HE, Curcio-Brint AM, Shapiro DN (1993). Detection of the (11;22)(q24;q12) translocation of Ewing's sarcoma and peripheral neuroectodermal tumor by reverse transcription polymerase chain reaction. *Am J Pathol* 143: 1294-1300.

550. Draper GJ, Sanders BM, Kingston JE (1986). Second primary neoplasms in patients with retinoblastoma. *Br J Cancer* 53: 661-671.

551. Drut R (1988). Ossifying fibrolipomatous hamartoma of the ulnar nerve. *Pediatr Pathol* 8: 179-184.

552. Dryja TP, Cavenee W, White R, Rapaport JM, Petersen R, Albert DM, Bruns GA (1984). Homozygosity of chromosome 13 in retinoblastoma. *N Engl J Med* 310: 550-553.

553. Dubus P, Coindre JM, Groppi A, Jouan H, Ferrer J, Cohen C, Rivel J, Copin MC, Leroy JP, de Muret A, Merlio JP (2001). The detection of Tel-TrkC chimeric transcripts is more specific than TrkC immunoreactivity for the diagnosis of congenital fibrosarcoma. *J Pathol* 193: 88-94.

554. Dudgeon J, Lee WR (1983). The trilateral retinoblastoma syndrome. *Trans Ophthalmol Soc U K* 103 (Pt 5): 523-529.

555. Duhig JT, Ayer JP (1959). Vascular leiomyoma: a study of sixty-one cases. *Arch Pathol Lab Med* 68: 424-430.

556. Duke D, Dvorak A, Harris TJ, Cohen LM (1996). Multiple retiform hemangioendotheliomas. A low-grade angiosarcoma. *Am J Dermatopathol* 18: 606-610.

557. Dumont P, de Muret A, Skrobala D, Robin P, Toumieux B (1997). Calcifying fibrous pseudotumor of the mediastinum. *Ann Thorac Surg* 63: 543-544.

558. Dunn JM, Phillips RA, Zhu X, Becker A, Gallie BL (1989). Mutations in the RB1 gene and their effects on transcription. *Mol Cell Biol* 9: 4596-4604.

559. Dupree WB, Enzinger FM (1986). Fibroosseous pseudotumor of the digits. *Cancer* 58: 2103-2109.

560. Durie BG (1986). Staging and kinetics of multiple myeloma. *Semin Oncol* 13: 300-309.

561. Durie BG, Salmon SE (1975). A clinical staging system for multiple myeloma. Correlation of measured myeloma cell mass with presenting clinical features, response to treatment, and survival. *Cancer* 36: 842-854.

562. Durroux R, Ducoin H, Gaubert J (1993). [Adamantinoma of the tibia and osteofibrodysplasia. Report of a case]. *Ann Pathol* 13: 336-340.

563. Dvornik G, Barbareschi M, Gallotta P, Dalla PP (1997). Low grade fibromyxoid sarcoma. *Histopathology* 30: 274-276.

564. Dyson N, Howley PM, Munger K, Harlow E (1989). The human papilloma virus-16 E7 oncoprotein is able to bind to the retinoblastoma gene product. *Science* 243: 934-937.

565. Eary JF, Conrad EU, Bruckner JD, Folpe A, Hunt KJ, Mankoff DA, Howlett AT (1998). Quantitative [F-18]fluorodeoxyglucose positron emission tomography in pretreatment and grading of sarcoma. *Clin Cancer Res* 4: 1215-1220.

566. Eccles DM, Lunt PW, Wallis Y, Griffiths M, Sandhu B, McKay S, Morton D, Shea-Simonds J, Macdonald F (1997). An unusually severe phenotype for familial adenomatous polyposis. *Arch Dis Child* 77: 431-435.

567. Eckardt JJ, Pritchard DJ, Soule EH (1983). Clear cell sarcoma. A clinicopathologic study of 27 cases. *Cancer* 52: 1482-1488.

568. Edeiken J, Raymond AK, Ayala AG, Benjamin RS, Murray JA, Carrasco HC (1987). Small-cell osteosarcoma. *Skeletal Radiol* 16: 621-628.

569. Edel G, Ueda Y, Nakanishi J, Brinker KH, Roessner A, Blasius S, Vestring T, Muller-Miny H, Erlemann R, Wuisman P (1992). Chondroblastoma of bone. A clinical, radiological, light and immunohistochemical study. *Virchows Arch A Pathol Anat Histopathol* 421: 355-366.

570. Efem SE, Ekpo MD (1993). Clinicopathological features of untreated fibrous hamartoma of infancy. *J Clin Pathol* 46: 522-524.

571. Eftekhari F, Ater JL, Ayala AG, Czerniak BA (2001). Case report: Calcifying fibrous pseudotumour of the adrenal gland. *Br J Radiol* 74: 452-454.

572. Eich GF, Hoeffel JC, Tschappeler H, Gassner I, Willi UV (1998). Fibrous tumours in children: imaging features of a heterogeneous group of disorders. *Pediatr Radiol* 28: 500-509.

573. Ekfors TO, Kujari H, Isomaki M (1993). Clear cell sarcoma of tendons and aponeuroses (malignant melanoma of soft parts) in the duodenum: the first visceral case. *Histopathology* 22: 255-259.

574. el Jabbour JN, Bennett MH, Burke MM, Lessells A, O'Halloran A (1991). Proliferative myositis. An immunohistochemical and ultrastructural study. *Am J Surg Pathol* 15: 654-659.

575. el Jabbour JN, Wilson GD, Bennett MH, Burke MM, Davey AT, Eames K (1991). Flow cytometric study of nodular fasciitis, proliferative fasciitis, and proliferative myositis. *Hum Pathol* 22: 1146-1149.

576. el Naggar AK, Hurr K, Tu ZN, Teague K, Raymond KA, Ayala AG, Murray J (1995). DNA and RNA content analysis by flow cytometry in the pathobiologic assessment of bone tumors. *Cytometry* 19: 256-262.

577. el Rifai W, Sarlomo-Rikala M, Knuutila S, Miettinen M (1998). DNA copy number changes in development and progression in leiomyosarcomas of soft tissues. *Am J Pathol* 153: 985-990.

578. Elgar F, Goldblum JR (1997). Well-differentiated liposarcoma of the retroperitoneum: a clinicopathologic analysis of 20 cases, with particular attention to the extent of low-grade dedifferentiation. *Mod Pathol* 10: 113-120.

579. Elkahloun AG, Bittner M, Hoskins K, Gemmill R, Meltzer PS (1996). Molecular cytogenetic characterization and physical mapping of 12q13-15 amplification in human cancers. *Genes Chromosomes Cancer* 17: 205-214.

580. Elliott M, Bayly R, Cole T, Temple IK, Maher ER (1994). Clinical features and natural history of Beckwith-Wiedemann syndrome: presentation of 74 new cases. *Clin Genet* 46: 168-174.

581. Ellis JH, Siegel CL, Martel W, Weatherbee L, Dorfman H (1988). Radiologic features of well-differentiated osteosarcoma. *AJR Am J Roentgenol* 151: 739-742.

582. Ellsworth RM (1969). The practical management of retinoblastoma. *Trans Am Ophthalmol Soc* 67: 462-534.

583. Elzay RP, Mills S, Kay S (1984). Fibrous defect (nonossifying fibroma) of the mandible. *Oral Surg Oral Med Oral Pathol* 58: 402-407.

584. Emile JF, Wechsler J, Brousse N, Boulland ML, Cologon R, Fraitag S, Voisin MC, Gaulard P, Boumsell L, Zafrani ES (1995). Langerhans' cell histiocytosis. Definitive diagnosis with the use of monoclonal antibody O10 on routinely paraffin-embedded samples. *Am J Surg Pathol* 19: 636-641.

585. Enjoji M, Sumiyoshi K, Sueyoshi K (1985). Elastofibromatous lesion of the stomach in a patient with elastofibroma dorsi. *Am J Surg Pathol* 9: 233-237.

586. Enneking WF, Kagan A (1975). "Skip" metastases in osteosarcoma. *Cancer* 36: 2192-2205.

587. Ensoli B, Sgadari C, Barillari G, Sirianni MC, Sturzl M, Monini P (2001). Biology of Kaposi's sarcoma. *Eur J Cancer* 37: 1251-1269.

588. Enzinger FM (1962). Liposarcoma. A study of 103 cases. *Virchows Arch Pathol Anat* 335: 367-388.

589. Enzinger FM (1965). Clear cell sarcoma of tendons and aponeuroses. An analysis of 21 cases. *Cancer* 18: 1163-1174.

590. Enzinger FM (1965). Fibrous hamartoma of infancy. *Cancer* 18: 241-248.

591. Enzinger FM (1965). Intramuscular myxoma. A review and follow-up study of 34 cases. *Am J Clin Pathol* 43: 104-113.

592. Enzinger FM (1970). Epithelioid sarcoma. A sarcoma simulating a granuloma or a carcinoma. *Cancer* 26: 1029-1041.

593. Enzinger FM (1979). Angiomatoid malignant fibrous histiocytoma: a distinct fibrohistiocytic tumor of children and young adults simulating a vascular neoplasm. *Cancer* 44: 2147-2157.

594. Enzinger FM, Dulcey F (1967). Proliferative myositis. Report of thirty-three cases. *Cancer* 20: 2213-2223.

595. Enzinger FM, Harvey DA (1975). Spindle cell lipoma. *Cancer* 36: 1852-1859.

596. Enzinger FM, Shiraki M (1969). Alveolar rhabdomyosarcoma. An analysis of 110 cases. *Cancer* 24: 18-31.

597. Enzinger FM, Shiraki M (1972). Extraskeletal myxoid chondrosarcoma. An analysis of 34 cases. *Hum Pathol* 3: 421-435.

598. Enzinger FM, Smith BH (1976). Hemangiopericytoma. An analysis of 106 cases. *Hum Pathol* 7: 61-82.

599. Enzinger FM, Weiss SW (1983). Malignant fibrohistiocytic tumors. In: *Soft Tissue Tumors*. 1st ed. C.V.Mosby: St.Louis, pp. 166-198.

600. Enzinger FM, Weiss SW (1988). Benign tumors and tumorlike lesions of fibrous tissue. In: *Soft Tissue Tumors*. 2nd ed. C.V.Mosby: St.Louis.

601. Enzinger FM, Weiss SW (1988). *Soft Tissue Tumors*. 2nd ed. C.V.Mosby: St.Louis.

602. Enzinger FM, Weiss SW, Liang CY (1989). Ossifying fibromyxoid tumor of soft parts. A clinicopathological analysis of 59 cases. *Am J Surg Pathol* 13: 817-827.

603. Enzinger FM, Zhang RY (1988). Plexiform fibrohistiocytic tumor presenting in children and young adults. An analysis of 65 cases. *Am J Surg Pathol* 12: 818-826.

604. Epstein CJ, Martin GM, Schultz AL, Motulsky AG (1966). Werner's syndrome a review of its symptomatology, natural history, pathologic features, genetics and relationship to the natural aging process. *Medicine (Baltimore)* 45: 177-221.

605. Epstein JA, Lam P, Jepeal L, Maas RL, Shapiro DN (1995). Pax3 inhibits myogenic differentiation of cultured myoblast cells. *J Biol Chem* 270: 11719-11722.

606. Erasmus JJ, McAdams HP, Patz EF, Jr., Murray JG, Pinkard NB (1996). Calcifying fibrous pseudotumor of pleura: radiologic features in three cases. *J Comput Assist Tomogr* 20: 763-765.

607. Eriksson M, Hardell L, Adami HO (1990). Exposure to dioxins as a risk factor for soft tissue sarcoma: a population-based case-control study. *J Natl Cancer Inst* 82: 486-490.

608. Eriksson M, Hardell L, Berg NO, Möller T, Axelson O (1981). Soft-tissue sarcomas and exposure to chemical substances: a case-referent study. *Br J Ind Med* 38: 27-33.

609. Erlandson RA (1987). The ultrastructural distinction between rhabdomyosarcoma and other undifferentiated "sarcomas". *Ultrastruct Pathol* 11: 83-101.

610. Esnaola NF, Rubin BP, Baldini EH, Vasudevan N, Demetri GD, Fletcher CD, Singer S (2001). Response to chemotherapy and predictors of survival in adult rhabdomyosarcoma. *Ann Surg* 234: 215-223.

611. Esparza J, Castro S, Portillo JM, Roger R (1978). Vertebral hemangiomas: spinal angiography and preoperative embolization. *Surg Neurol* 10: 171-173.

612. Essner R, Selch M, Eilber FR (1990). Reirradiation for extremity soft tissue sarcomas: local control and complications (meeting abstract). *Proc 72 Ann Am Radium Soc Meeting* April, 1990.

613. Etcubanas E, Peiper S, Stass S, Green A (1989). Rhabdomyosarcoma, presenting as disseminated malignancy from an unknown primary site: a retrospective study of ten pediatric cases. *Med Pediatr Oncol* 17: 39-44.

614. Eto H, Toriyama K, Tsuda N, Tagawa Y, Itakura H (1992). Flow cytometric DNA analysis of vascular soft tissue tumors, including African endemic-type Kaposi's sarcoma. *Hum Pathol* 23: 1055-1060.

615. Eulderink F, de Graaf PW (1998). Ectopic hamartomatous thymoma located presternally. *Eur J Surg* 164: 629-630.

616. Eusebi V, Ceccarelli C, Daniele E, Collina G, Viale G, Mancini AM (1988). Extracardiac rhabdomyoma: An immunocytochemical study and review of the literature. *Appl Pathol* 6: 197-207.

617. Evans HL (1979). Liposarcoma: a study of 55 cases with a reassessment of its classification. *Am J Surg Pathol* 3: 507-523.

618. Evans HL (1985). Alveolar soft-part sarcoma. A study of 13 typical examples and one with a histologically atypical component. *Cancer* 55: 912-917.

619. Evans HL (1987). Low-grade fibromyxoid sarcoma. A report of two metastasizing neoplasms having a deceptively benign appearance. *Am J Clin Pathol* 88: 615-619.

620. Evans HL (1988). Liposarcoma and atypical lipomatous tumors: a study of 66 cases followed for a minimum of 10 years. *Surg Pathol* 1: 41-54.

621. Evans HL (1993). Low-grade fibromyxoid sarcoma. A report of 12 cases. *Am J Surg Pathol* 17: 595-600.

622. Evans HL (1995). Desmoplastic fibroblastoma. A report of seven cases. *Am J Surg Pathol* 19: 1077-1081.

623. Evans HL (2002). Multinucleated giant cells in plantar fibromatosis. *Am J Surg Pathol* 26: 244-248.

624. Evans HL, Ayala AG, Romsdahl MM (1977). Prognostic factors in chondrosarcoma of bone: a clinicopathologic analysis with emphasis on histologic grading. *Cancer* 40: 818-831.

625. Evans HL, Baer SC (1993). Epithelioid sarcoma: a clinicopathologic and prognostic study of 26 cases. *Semin Diagn Pathol* 10: 286-291.

626. Evans HL, Soule EH, Winkelmann RK (1979). Atypical lipoma, atypical intramuscular lipoma, and well differentiated retroperitoneal liposarcoma: a reappraisal of 30 cases formerly classified as well differentiated liposarcoma. *Cancer* 43: 574-584.

627. Evans S, Williams F (1986). Case report: Erdheim-Chester disease: polyostotic sclerosing histiocytosis. *Clin Radiol* 37: 93-96.

628. Exelby PR, Knapper WH, Huvos AG, Beattie EJ, Jr. (1973). Soft-tissue fibrosarcoma in children. *J Pediatr Surg* 8: 415-420.

629. Eyden BP, Manson C, Banerjee SS, Roberts IS, Harris M (1998). Sclerosing epithelioid fibrosarcoma: a study of five cases emphasizing diagnostic criteria. *Histopathology* 33: 354-360.

630. Faivre L, Nivelon-Chevallier A, Kottler ML, Robinet C, Van Kien PK, Lorcerie B, Munnich A, Maroteaux P, Cormier-Daire V, LeMerrer M (2001). Mazabraud syndrome in two patients: clinical overlap with McCune-Albright syndrome. *Am J Med Genet* 99: 132-136.

631. Falk S, Schmidts HL, Muller H, Berger K, Schneider M, Schlote W, Helm EB, Stille W, Hubner K, Stutte HJ (1987). Autopsy findings in AIDS – a histopathological analysis of fifty cases. *Klin Wochenschr* 65: 654-663.

632. Fanburg-Smith JC, Bratthauer GL, Miettinen M (1999). Osteocalcin and osteonectin immunoreactivity in extraskeletal osteosarcoma: a study of 28 cases. *Hum Pathol* 30: 32-38.

633. Fanburg-Smith JC, Devaney KO, Miettinen M, Weiss SW (1998). Multiple spindle cell lipomas: a report of 7 familial and 11 nonfamilial cases. *Am J Surg Pathol* 22: 40-48.

634. Fanburg-Smith JC, Hengge M, Hengge UR, Smith JS, Jr., Miettinen M (1998). Extrarenal rhabdoid tumors of soft tissue: a clinicopathologic and immunohistochemical study of 18 cases. *Ann Diagn Pathol* 2: 351-362.

635. Fanburg-Smith JC, Michal M, Partanen TA, Alitalo K, Miettinen M (1999). Papillary intralymphatic angioendothelioma (PILA): a report of twelve cases of a distinctive vascular tumor with phenotypic features of lymphatic vessels. *Am J Surg Pathol* 23: 1004-1010.

636. Fanburg-Smith JC, Miettinen M (1998). Liposarcoma with meningothelial-like whorls: a study of 17 cases of a distinctive histological pattern associated with dedifferentiated liposarcoma. *Histopathology* 33: 414-424.

637. Fanburg-Smith JC, Miettinen M (1998). Malignant giant cell tumors of the tendon sheath: histologic classification with clinical correlation. *Clin Exp Pathol* 46: 16A.

638. Fanburg-Smith JC, Miettinen M (1999). Angiomatoid "malignant" fibrous histiocytoma: a clinicopathologic study of 158 cases and further exploration of the myoid phenotype. *Hum Pathol* 30: 1336-1343.

639. Fanburg JC, Meis-Kindblom JM, Rosenberg AE (1995). Multiple enchondromas associated with spindle-cell hemangioendotheliomas. An overlooked variant of Maffucci's syndrome. *Am J Surg Pathol* 19: 1029-1038.

640. Fanburg JC, Rosenberg AE, Weaver DL, Leslie KO, Mann KG, Taatjes DJ, Tracy RP (1997). Osteocalcin and osteonectin immunoreactivity in the diagnosis of osteosarcoma. *Am J Clin Pathol* 108: 464-473.

641. Faria SL, Schlupp WR, Chiminazzo H, Jr. (1985). Radiotherapy in the treatment of vertebral hemangiomas. *Int J Radiat Oncol Biol Phys* 11: 387-390.

642. Farshid G, Pradhan M, Goldblum J, Weiss SW (2002). Leiomyosarcoma of somatic soft tissues: a tumor of vascular origin with multivariate analysis of outcome in 42 cases. *Am J Surg Pathol* 26: 14-24.

643. Fechner RE, Mills SE (1993). Lesions of the synovium. In: *Tumours of the Bones and Joints. Atlas of Tumour Pathology*. AFIP: Washington DC, pp. 279-282.

644. Fechner RE, Mills SE (1993). *Tumors of the Bones and Joints. Atlas of Tumor Pathology*. AFIP: Washington,D.C.

645. Feely MG, Boehm AK, Bridge RS, Krallman PM, Neff JR, Nelson M, Bridge JA (2002). Cytogenetic and molecular cytogenetic evidence of recurrent 8q24.1 loss in osteochondroma. *Hum Pathol* (in press).

646. Feely MG, Fidler ME, Nelson M, Neff JR, Bridge JA (2000). Cytogenetic findings in a case of epithelioid sarcoma and a review of the literature. *Cancer Genet Cytogenet* 119: 155-157.

647. Feldman F, Norman D (1972). Intra- and extraosseous malignant histiocytoma (malignant fibrous xanthoma). *Radiology* 104: 497-508.

648. Felix CA, Kappel CC, Mitsudomi T, Nau MM, Tsokos M, Crouch GD, Nisen PD, Winick NJ, Helman LJ (1992). Frequency and diversity of p53 mutations in childhood rhabdomyosarcoma. *Cancer Res* 52: 2243-2247.

649. Ferber L, Lampe I (1942). Hemangioma of vertebra associated with compression of the cord: response to radiation therapy. *Arch Neurol* 47: 19.

650. Ferguson RJ, Yunis EJ (1978). The ultrastructure of human osteosarcoma: a study of nine cases. *Clin Orthop* 234-246.

651. Fergusson IL (1972). Haemangiomata of skeletal muscle. *Br J Surg* 59: 634-637.

652. Ferracini R, Di Renzo MF, Scotlandi K, Baldini N, Olivero M, Lollini P, Cremona O, Campanacci M, Comoglio PM (1995). The Met/HGF receptor is over-expressed in human osteosarcomas and is activated by either a paracrine or an autocrine circuit. *Oncogene* 10: 739-749.

653. Ferracini R, Scotlandi K, Cagliero E, Acquarone F, Olivero M, Wunder J, Baldini N (2000). The expression of Met/hepatocyte growth factor receptor gene in giant cell tumors of bone and other benign musculoskeletal tumors. *J Cell Physiol* 184: 191-196.

654. Ferreiro JA, Nascimento AG (1995). Hyaline-cell rich chondroid syringoma. A tumor mimicking malignancy. *Am J Surg Pathol* 19: 912-917.

655. Ferry JA, Malt RA, Young RH (1991). Renal angiomyolipoma with sarcomatous transformation and pulmonary metastases. *Am J Surg Pathol* 15: 1083-1088.

656. Fetsch JF, Laskin WB, Lefkowitz M, Kindblom LG, Meis-Kindblom JM (1996). Aggressive angiomyxoma: a clinicopathologic study of 29 female patients. *Cancer* 78: 79-90.

657. Fetsch JF, Miettinen M (1998). Calcifying aponeurotic fibroma: a clinicopathologic study of 22 cases arising in uncommon sites. *Hum Pathol* 29: 1504-1510.

658. Fetsch JF, Miettinen M, Laskin WB, Michal M, Enzinger FM (2000). A clinicopathologic study of 45 pediatric soft tissue tumors with an admixture of adipose tissue and fibroblastic elements, and a proposal for classification as lipofibromatosis. *Am J Surg Pathol* 24: 1491-1500.

659. Fetsch JF, Montgomery EA, Meis JM (1993). Calcifying fibrous pseudotumor. *Am J Surg Pathol* 17: 502-508.

660. Fetsch JF, Weiss SW (1990). Ectopic hamartomatous thymoma: clinicopathologic, immunohistochemical, and histogenetic considerations in four new cases. *Hum Pathol* 21: 662-668.

661. Fetsch JF, Weiss SW (1991). Observations concerning the pathogenesis of epithelioid hemangioma (angiolymphoid hyperplasia). *Mod Pathol* 4: 449-455.

662. Feugeas O, Guriec N, Babin-Boilletot A, Marcellin L, Simon P, Babin S, Thyss A, Hofman P, Terrier P, Kalifa C, Brunat-Mentigny M, Patricot LM, Oberling F (1996). Loss of heterozygosity of the RB gene is a poor prognostic factor in patients with osteosarcoma. *J Clin Oncol* 14: 467-472.

663. Fine G, Stout AP (1956). Osteogenic sarcoma of the extraskeletal soft tissues. *Cancer* 9: 1027-1043.

664. Fink MG, Levinson DJ, Brown NL, Sreekanth S, Sobel GW (1991). Erdheim-Chester disease. Case report with autopsy findings. *Arch Pathol Lab Med* 115: 619-623.

665. Fisher C (1986). Synovial sarcoma: ultrastructural and immunohistochemical features of epithelial differentiation in monophasic and biphasic tumors. *Hum Pathol* 17: 996-1008.

666. Fisher C (1988). Epithelioid sarcoma: the spectrum of ultrastructural differentiation in seven immunohistochemically defined cases. *Hum Pathol* 19: 265-275.

667. Fisher C (1990). The value of electronmicroscopy and immunohistochemistry in the diagnosis of soft tissue sarcomas: a study of 200 cases. *Histopathology* 16: 441-454.

668. Fisher C (1998). Synovial sarcoma. *Ann Diagn Pathol* 2: 401-421.

669. Fisher C, Hedges M, Weiss SW (1994). Ossifying fibromyxoid tumor of soft parts with stromal cyst formation and ribosome-lamella complexes. *Ultrastruct Pathol* 18: 593-600.

670. Fitzgerald RH, Jr., Dahlin DC, Sim FH (1973). Multiple metachronous osteogenic sarcoma. Report of twelve cases with two long-term survivors. *J Bone Joint Surg Am* 55: 595-605.

671. Flanagan BP, Helwig EB (1977). Cutaneous lymphangioma. *Arch Dermatol* 113: 24-30.

672. Fleming ID, Cooper JS, Henson GE, et al. (1997). *AJCC Cancer Staging Manual*. 5th ed. Lippincott-Raven: Philadelphia.

673. Fletcher CD (1990). Benign fibrous histiocytoma of subcutaneous and deep soft tissue: a clinicopathologic analysis of 21 cases. *Am J Surg Pathol* 14: 801-809.

674. Fletcher CD (1991). Angiomatoid "malignant fibrous histiocytoma": an immunohistochemical study indicative of myoid differentiation. *Hum Pathol* 22: 563-568.

675. Fletcher CD (1992). Pleomorphic malignant fibrous histiocytoma: fact or fiction? A critical reappraisal based on 159 tumors diagnosed as pleomorphic sarcoma. *Am J Surg Pathol* 16: 213-228.

676. Fletcher CD (1994). Haemangiopericytoma – a dying breed? Reappraisal of an 'entity' and its variants. *Curr Diagn Pathol* 1: 19-23.

677. Fletcher CD (1997). Will we ever reliably predict prognosis in a patient with myxoid and round cell liposarcoma? *Adv Anat Pathol* 4: 108-113.

678. Fletcher CD (2000). Soft tissue tumours. In: *Diagnostic Histopathology of Tumors*, Fletcher CD, ed. 2nd ed. Churchill Livingstone: London.

679. Fletcher CD, Achu P, van Noorden S, McKee PH (1987). Infantile myofibromatosis: a light microscopic, histochemical and immunohistochemical study suggesting true smooth muscle differentiation. *Histopathology* 11: 245-258.

680. Fletcher CD, Åkerman M, Dal Cin P, de Wever I, Mandahl N, Mertens F, Mitelman F, Rosai J, Rydholm A, Sciot R, Tallini G, van den Berghe H, van de Ven W, Vanni R, Willén H (1996). Correlation between clinicopathological features and karyotype in lipomatous tumors. A report of 178 cases from the chromosomes and morphology (CHAMP) collaborative study group. *Am J Pathol* 148: 623-630.

681. Fletcher CD, Beham A, Bekir S, Clarke AM, Marley NJ (1991). Epithelioid angiosarcoma of deep soft tissue: a distinctive tumor readily mistaken for an epithelial neoplasm. *Am J Surg Pathol* 15: 915-924.

682. Fletcher CD, Dal Cin P, de Wever I, Mandahl N, Mertens F, Mitelman F, Rosai J, Rydholm A, Sciot R, Tallini G, van den Berghe H, Vanni R, Willén H (1999). Correlation between clinicopathological features and karyotype in spindle cell sarcomas. A report of 130 cases from the CHAMP study group. *Am J Pathol* 154: 1841-1847.

683. Fletcher CD, Gustafson P, Rydholm A, Willén H, Åkerman M (2001). Clinicopathologic re-evaluation of 100 malignant fibrous histiocytomas: prognostic relevance of subclassification. *J Clin Oncol* 19: 3045-3050.

684. Fletcher CD, Martin-Bates E (1987). Spindle cell lipoma: a clinicopathological study with some original observations. *Histopathology* 11: 803-817.

685. Fletcher CD, Martin-Bates E (1988). Intramuscular and intermuscular lipoma: neglected diagnoses. *Histopathology* 12: 275-287.

686. Fletcher CD, Powell G, van Noorden S, McKee PH (1988). Fibrous hamartoma of infancy: a histochemical and immunohistochemical study. *Histopathology* 12: 65-74.

687. Fletcher CD, Tsang WY, Fisher C, Lee KC, Chan JK (1992). Angiomyofibroblastoma of the vulva. A benign neoplasm distinct from aggressive angiomyxoma. *Am J Surg Pathol* 16: 373-382.

688. Fletcher JA, Gebhardt MC, Kozakewich HP (1994). Cytogenetic aberrations in osteosarcomas. Nonrandom deletions, rings, and double-minute chromosomes. *Cancer Genet Cytogenet* 77: 81-88.

689. Fletcher JA, Naeem R, Xiao S, Corson JM (1995). Chromosome aberrations in desmoid tumors. Trisomy 8 may be a predictor of recurrence. *Cancer Genet Cytogenet* 79: 139-143.

690. Flieder DB, Moran CA (1998). Primary cutaneous synovial sarcoma: a case report. *Am J Dermatopathol* 20: 509-512.

691. Flieder DB, Moran CA, Suster S (1997). Primary alveolar soft-part sarcoma of the mediastinum: a clinicopathological and immunohistochemical study of two cases. *Histopathology* 31: 469-473.

692. Florenes VA, Maelandsmo GM, Forus A, Andreassen A, Myklebost O, Fodstad O (1994). MDM2 gene amplification and transcript levels in human sarcomas: relationship to TP53 gene status. *J Natl Cancer Inst* 86: 1297-1302.

693. Fodde R, Smits R, Clevers H (2001). APC, signal transduction and genetic instability in colorectal cancer. *Nature Rev Cancer* 1: 55-67.

694. Folpe AL, Agoff SN, Willis J, Weiss SW (1999). Parachordoma is immunohistochemically and cytogenetically distinct from axial chordoma and extraskeletal myxoid chondrosarcoma. *Am J Surg Pathol* 23: 1059-1067.

695. Folpe AL, Chand EM, Goldblum JR, Weiss SW (2001). Expression of Fli-1, a nuclear transcription factor, distinguishes vascular neoplasms from potential mimics. *Am J Surg Pathol* 25: 1061-1066.

696. Folpe AL, Devaney K, Weiss SW (1999). Lipomatous hemangiopericytoma: a rare variant of hemangiopericytoma that may be confused with liposarcoma. *Am J Surg Pathol* 23: 1201-1207.

697. Folpe AL, Fanburg-Smith JC, Miettinen M, Weiss SW (2001). Atypical and malignant glomus tumors: analysis of 52 cases, with a proposal for the reclassification of glomus tumors. *Am J Surg Pathol* 25: 1-12.

698. Folpe AL, Goodman ZD, Ishak KG, Paulino AF, Taboada EM, Meehan SA, Weiss SW (2000). Clear cell myomelanocytic tumor of the falciform ligament/ligamentum teres: a novel member of the perivascular epithelioid clear cell family of tumors with a predilection for children and young adults. *Am J Surg Pathol* 24: 1239-1246.

699. Folpe AL, Lane KL, Paull G, Weiss SW (2000). Low-grade fibromyxoid sarcoma and hyalinizing spindle cell tumor with giant rosettes: a clinicopathologic study of 73 cases supporting their identity and assessing the impact of high-grade areas. *Am J Surg Pathol* 24: 1353-1360.

700. Folpe AL, Lyles RH, Sprouse JT, Conrad EU, III, Eary JF (2000). (F-18) fluorodeoxyglucose positron emission tomography as a predictor of pathologic grade and other prognostic variables in bone and soft tissue sarcoma. *Clin Cancer Res* 6: 1279-1287.

701. Folpe AL, McKenney JK, Li Z, Smith SJ, Weiss SW (2002). Clear cell myomelanocytic tumor of the thigh: report of a unique case. *Am J Surg Pathol* 26: 809-812.

702. Folpe AL, Morris RJ, Weiss SW (1999). Soft tissue giant cell tumor of low malignant potential: a proposal for the reclassification of malignant giant cell tumor of soft parts. *Mod Pathol* 12: 894-902.

703. Folpe AL, Schmidt RA, Chapman D, Gown AM (1998). Poorly differentiated synovial sarcoma: immunohistochemical distinction from primitive neuroectodermal tumors and high-grade malignant peripheral nerve sheath tumors. *Am J Surg Pathol* 22: 673-682.

704. Folpe AL, Veikkola T, Valtola R, Weiss SW (2000). Vascular endothelial growth factor receptor-3 (VEGFR-3): a marker of vascular tumors with presumed lymphatic differentiation, including Kaposi's sarcoma, kaposiform and Dabska-type hemangioendotheliomas, and a subset of angiosarcomas. *Mod Pathol* 13: 180-185.

705. Folpe AL, Weiss SW, Fletcher CD, Gown AM (1998). Tenosynovial giant cell tumors: evidence for a desmin-positive dendritic cell subpopulation. *Mod Pathol* 11: 939-944.

706. Font RL, Hidayat AA (1982). Fibrous histiocytoma of the orbit. A clinicopathologic study of 150 cases. *Hum Pathol* 13: 199-209.

707. Fornasier VL, Horne JG (1975). Metastases to the vertebral column. *Cancer* 36: 590-594.

708. Forus A, Berner JM, Meza-Zepeda LA, Saeter G, Mischke D, Fodstad O, Myklebost O (1998). Molecular characterization of a novel amplicon at 1q21-q22 frequently observed in human sarcomas. *Br J Cancer* 78: 495-503.

709. Forus A, D'Angelo A, Henriksen J, Merla G, Maelandsmo GM, Florenes VA, Olivieri S, Bjerkehagen B, Meza-Zepeda LA, del Vecchio BF, Muller C, Sanvito F, Kononen J, Nesland J, Fodstad O, Reymond A, Kallioniemi OP, Arrigoni G, Ballabio A, Myklebost O, Zollo M (2001). Amplification and overexpression of PRUNE in human sarcomas and breast carcinomas-a possible mechanism for altering the nm23-H1 activity. *Oncogene* 20: 6881-6890.

710. Forus A, Florenes VA, Maelandsmo GM, Fodstad O, Myklebost O (1994). 12q13-14 amplica in human sarcomas without MDM2 include CDK4, SAS and GADD153/CHOP. *Cancer Genet Cytogenet* 77: 200.

711. Forus A, Florenes VA, Maelandsmo GM, Fodstad O, Myklebost O (1994). The protooncogene CHOP/GADD153, involved in growth arrest and DNA damage response, is amplified in a subset of human sarcomas. *Cancer Genet Cytogenet* 78: 165-171.

712. Forus A, Florenes VA, Maelandsmo GM, Meltzer PS, Fodstad O, Myklebost O (1993). Mapping of amplification units in the q13-14 region of chromosome 12 in human sarcomas: some amplica do not include MDM2. *Cell Growth Differ* 4: 1065-1070.

713. Foschini MP, Eusebi V (1994). Alveolar soft-part sarcoma: a new type of rhabdomyosarcoma? *Semin Diagn Pathol* 11: 58-68.

714. Francannet C, Cohen-Tanugi A, Le Merrer M, Munnich A, Bonaventure J, Legeai-Mallet L (2001). Genotype-phenotype correlation in hereditary multiple exostoses. *J Med Genet* 38: 430-434.

715. Franceschina MJ, Hankin RC, Irwin RB (1997). Low-grade central osteosarcoma resembling fibrous dysplasia. A report of two cases. *Am J Orthop* 26: 432-440.

716. Francke U (1976). Retinoblastoma and chromosome 13. *Cytogenet Cell Genet* 16: 131-134.

717. Francke U, Kung F (1976). Sporadic bilateral retinoblastoma and 13q- chromosomal deletion. *Med Pediatr Oncol* 2: 379-385.

718. Francois J (1978). Differential diagnosis of leukocoria in children. *Ann Ophtalmol* 10: 1375-1378.

719. Frassica DA, Frassica FJ, Schray MF, Sim FH, Kyle RA (1989). Solitary plasmacytoma of bone: Mayo Clinic experience. *Int J Radiat Oncol Biol Phys* 16: 43-48.

720. Frassica FJ, Waltrip RL, Sponseller PD, Ma LD, McCarthy EF, Jr. (1996). Clinicopathologic features and treatment of osteoid osteoma and osteoblastoma in children and adolescents. *Orthop Clin North Am* 27: 559-574.

721. Freeburn AM, McAloon J (2001). Infantile chest hamartoma – case outcome aged 11. *Arch Dis Child* 85: 244-245.

722. Freud E, Bilik R, Yaniv I, Horev G, Cohen D, Mimouni M, Zer M (1991). Inflammatory pseudotumor in childhood. A diagnostic and therapeutic dilemma. *Arch Surg* 126: 653-655.

723. Friedman L, Patel M, Lew E, Silberberg P (1989). Benign histiocytic fibroma of rib with CT correlation. *Can Assoc Radiol J* 40: 114-116.

724. Friend SH, Bernards R, Rogelj S, Weinberg RA, Rapaport JM, Albert DM, Dryja TP (1986). A human DNA segment with properties of the gene that predisposes to retinoblastoma and osteosarcoma. *Nature* 323: 643-646.

725. Frierson HF, Jr., Fechner RE, Stallings RG, Wang GJ (1987). Malignant fibrous histiocytoma in bone infarct. Association with sickle cell trait and alcohol abuse. *Cancer* 59: 496-500.

726. Fritz A, Percy C, Jack A, Shanmugaratnam K, Sobin LH, Parkin DM, Whelan S (2000). *International Classification of Diseases for Oncology*. 3rd ed. World Health Organization: Geneva.

727. Fu YS, Kay S (1974). A comparative ultrastructural study of mesenchymal chondrosarcoma and myxoid chondrosarcoma. *Cancer* 33: 1531-1542.

728. Fujimura Y, Ohno T, Siddique H, Lee L, Rao VN, Reddy ES (1996). The EWS-ATF-1 gene involved in malignant melanoma of soft parts with t(12;22) chromosome translocation, encodes a constitutive transcriptional activator. *Oncogene* 12: 159-167.

729. Fujimura Y, Siddique H, Lee L, Rao VN, Reddy ES (2001). EWS-ATF-1 chimeric protein in soft tissue clear cell sarcoma associates with CREB-binding protein and interferes with p53-mediated trans-activation function. *Oncogene* 20: 6653-6659.

730. Fukuda T, Ishikawa H, Ohnishi Y, Tachikawa S, Onizuka S, Sakashita I (1986). Extraskeletal myxoid chondrosarcoma arising from the retroperitoneum. *Am J Clin Pathol* 85: 514-519.

731. Fukuda T, Kakihara T, Baba K, Yamaki T, Yamaguchi T, Suzuki T (2000). Clear cell sarcoma arising in the transverse colon. *Pathol Int* 50: 412-416.

732. Fukuda T, Tsuneyoshi M, Enjoji M (1988). Malignant fibrous histiocytoma of soft parts: an ultrastructural quantitative study. *Ultrastruct Pathol* 12: 117-129.

733. Fukuda Y, Miyake H, Masuda Y, Masugi Y (1987). Histogenesis of unique elastinophilic fibers of elastofibroma: ultrastructural and immunohistochemical studies. *Hum Pathol* 18: 424-429.

734. Fukunaga M, Endo Y, Masui F, Yoshikawa T, Ishikawa E, Ushigome S (1996). Retiform haemangioendothelioma. *Virchows Arch* 428: 301-304.

735. Fukunaga M, Endo Y, Ushigome S (1999). Radiation-induced inflammatory malignant fibrous histiocytoma of the ileum. *APMIS* 107: 837-842.

736. Fukunaga M, Naganuma H, Nikaido T, Harada T, Ushigome S (1997). Extrapleural solitary fibrous tumor: a report of seven cases. *Mod Pathol* 10: 443-450.

737. Fukunaga M, Naganuma H, Ushigome S, Endo Y, Ishikawa E (1996). Malignant solitary fibrous tumour of the peritoneum. *Histopathology* 28: 463-466.

738. Fukunaga M, Nomura K, Matsumoto K, Doi K, Endo Y, Ushigome S (1997). Vulval angiomyofibroblastoma. Clinicopathologic analysis of six cases. *Am J Clin Pathol* 107: 45-51.

739. Fukunaga M, Shimoda T, Nikaido T, Ushigome S, Ishikawa E (1993). Soft tissue vascular tumors. A flow cytometric DNA analysis. *Cancer* 71: 2233-2241.

740. Fukunaga M, Ushigome S (1998). Giant cell angiofibroma of the mediastinum. *Histopathology* 32: 187-189.

741. Fukunaga M, Ushigome S (1998). Periosteal Ewing-like adamantinoma. *Virchows Arch* 433: 385-389.

742. Fukunaga M, Ushigome S, Fukunaga N (1996). Low-grade fibromyxoid sarcoma. *Virchows Arch* 429: 301-303.

743. Fuller CE, Pfeifer J, Humphrey P, Bruch LA, Dehner LP, Perry A (2001). Chromosome 22q dosage in composite extrarenal rhabdoid tumors: clonal evolution or a phenotypic mimic? *Hum Pathol* 32: 1102-1108.

744. Fung YK, Murphree AL, T'Ang A, Qian J, Hinrichs SH, Benedict WF (1987). Structural evidence for the authenticity of the human retinoblastoma gene. *Science* 236: 1657-1661.

745. Furin MM, Eisele DW, Carson BS (1997). McCune-Albright syndrome (polyostotic fibrous dysplasia) with intracranial frontoethmoid mucocele. *Otolaryngol Head Neck Surg* 116: 559-562.

746. Furlong MA, Fanburg-Smith JC (2001). Pleomorphic rhabdomyosarcoma in children: four cases in the pediatric age group. *Ann Diagn Pathol* 5: 199-206.

747. Furlong MA, Fanburg-Smith JC, Miettinen M (2001). The morphologic spectrum of hibernoma: a clinicopathologic study of 170 cases. *Am J Surg Pathol* 25: 809-814.

748. Furlong MA, Mentzel T, Fanburg-Smith JC (2001). Pleomorphic rhabdomyosarcoma in adults: a clinicopathologic study of 38 cases with emphasis on morphologic variants and recent skeletal muscle-specific markers. *Mod Pathol* 14: 595-603.

749. Furuichi Y (2001). Premature aging and predisposition to cancers caused by mutations in RecQ family helicases. *Ann N Y Acad Sci* 928: 121-131.

750. Gad A, Eusebi V (1975). Rhabdomyoma of the vagina. *J Pathol* 115: 179-181.

751. Gaertner EM, Steinberg DM, Huber M, Hayashi T, Tsuda N, Askin FB, Bell SW, Nguyen B, Colby TV, Nishimura SL, Miettinen M, Travis WD (2000). Pulmonary and mediastinal glomus tumors – report of five cases including a pulmonary glomangiosarcoma: a clinicopathologic study with literature review. *Am J Surg Pathol* 24: 1105-1114.

752. Gaffey MJ, Mills SE, Askin FB, Ross GW, Sale GE, Kulander BG, Visscher DW, Yousem SA, Colby TV (1990). Clear cell tumor of the lung. A clinicopathologic, immunohistochemical, and ultrastructural study of eight cases. *Am J Surg Pathol* 14: 248-259.

753. Gaffney EF, Dervan PA, Fletcher CD (1993). Pleomorphic rhabdomyosarcoma in adulthood. Analysis of 11 cases with definition of diagnostic criteria. *Am J Surg Pathol* 17: 601-609.

754. Gaffney EF, Hargreaves HK, Semple E, Vellios F (1983). Hibernoma: distinctive light and electron microscopic features and relationship to brown adipose tissue. *Hum Pathol* 14: 677-687.

755. Gailani MR, Bale SJ, Leffell DJ, DiGiovanna JJ, Peck GL, Poliak S, Drum MA, Pastakia B, McBride OW, Kase R, Greene M, Mulvihill JJ, Bale AE (1992). Developmental defects in Gorlin syndrome related to a putative tumor suppressor gene on chromosome 9. *Cell* 69: 111-117.

756. Galasko CS (1982). Mechanisms of lytic and blastic metastatic disease of bone. *Clin Orthop* 20-27.

757. Galasko CSB (1986). Incidence and distribution of skeletal metastases. In: *Skeletal Metastases*. Butterworth & Co: 17.

758. Galed-Placed I, Garcia-Ureta E, Sanchez-Blas M, Lago-Novoa M (1998). Giant-cell tumor in soft parts in a patient with osseous Paget's disease: diagnosis by fine-needle aspiration. *Diagn Cytopathol* 19: 352-354.

759. Galili N, Davis RJ, Fredericks WJ, Mukhopadhyay S, Rauscher FJ, III, Emanuel BS, Rovera G, Barr FG (1993). Fusion of a fork head domain gene to PAX3 in the solid tumour alveolar rhabdomyosarcoma. *Nat Genet* 5: 230-235.

760. Galli SJ, Weintraub HP, Proppe KH (1978). Malignant fibrous histiocytoma and pleomorphic sarcoma in association with medullary bone infarcts. *Cancer* 41: 607-619.

761. Gamberi G, Benassi MS, Böhling T, Ragazzini P, Molendini L, Sollazzo MR, Pompetti F, Merli M, Magagnoli G, Balladelli A, Picci P (1998). C-myc and c-fos in human osteosarcoma: prognostic value of mRNA and protein expression. *Oncology* 55: 556-563.

762. Gangopadhyay AN, Khurana SK, Rastogi BL, Kulshrestha S (1991). Soft tissue chondroma in an infant. *J Indian Med Assoc* 89: 315.

763. Gao SJ, Kingsley L, Hoover DR, Spira TJ, Rinaldo CR, Saah A, Phair J, Detels R, Parry P, Chang Y, Moore PS (1996). Seroconversion to antibodies against Kaposi's sarcoma-associated herpesvirus-related latent nuclear antigens before the development of Kaposi's sarcoma. *N Engl J Med* 335: 233-241.

764. Garcia-Bustinduy M, Alvarez-Arguelles H, Guimera F, Garcia-Castro C, Sanchez-Gonzalez R, Hernandez N, Diaz-Flores L, Garcia-Montelongo R (1999). Malignant rhabdoid tumor beside benign skin mesenchymal neoplasm with myofibromatous features. *J Cutan Pathol* 26: 509-515.

765. Gardiner GA, Linda L (1974). Clavicular nonosteogenic fibroma. An old tumor in a new location. *Am J Dis Child* 127: 734-735.

766. Gardner EJ (1950). Cancer of the lower digestive tract in one family group. *Am J Hum Genet* 2: 41-48.

767. Gardner EJ (1951). A genetic and clinical study of intestinal polyposis, a predisposing factor for carcinoma of the colon and rectum. *Am J Hum Genet* 3: 167-176.

768. Gardner EJ (1960). Follow-up study of a family group exhibiting dominant inheritance for a syndrome including intestinal polyps, osteomas, fibromas, and epidermal cysts. *Am J Hum Genet* 14: 376-390.

769. Gardner EJ, Richards RC (1953). Multiple cutaneous and subcutaneous lesions occurring simultaneously with hereditary polyposis and osteomatosis. *Am J Hum Genet* 5: 139-147.

770. Garijo MF, Val-Bernal JF (1998). Extravulvar subcutaneous cellular angiofibroma. *J Cutan Pathol* 25: 327-332.

771. Gaumann A, Petrow P, Mentzel T, Mayer E, Dahm M, Otto M, Kirkpatrick CJ, Kriegsmann J (2001). Osteopontin expression in primary sarcomas of the pulmonary artery. *Virchows Arch* 439: 668-674.

772. Gaumann A, Tews DS, Mayer E, Dahm M, Petrow PK, Otto M, James C, Kriegsmann J (2001). Expression of apoptosis-related proteins, p53, and DNA fragmentation in sarcomas of the pulmonary artery. *Cancer* 92: 1237-1244.

773. Gaynor JJ, Tan CC, Casper ES, Collin CF, Friedrich C, Shiu M, Hajdu SI, Brennan MF (1992). Refinement of clinicopathologic staging for localized soft tissue sarcoma of the extremity: a study of 423 adults. *J Clin Oncol* 10: 1317-1329.

774. Gebhard S, Coindre JM, Michels JJ, Terrier P, Bertrand G, Trassard M, Taylor S, Chateau MC, Marques B, Picot V, Guillou L (2002). Pleomorphic liposarcoma. Clinicopathologic and immunohistochemical study of 63 cases. A study of the French Sarcoma Group. *Am J Surg Pathol* 26; 601-616.

775. Geirnaerdt MJ, Hogendoorn PC, Bloem JL, Taminiau AH, van der Woude HJ (2000). Cartilaginous tumors: fast contrast-enhanced MR imaging. *Radiology* 214: 539-546.

776. Gerald WL, Ladanyi M, de Alava E, Cuatrecasas M, Kushner BH, LaQuaglia MP, Rosai J (1998). Clinical, pathologic, and molecular spectrum of tumors associated with t(11;22)(p13;q12): desmoplastic small round-cell tumor and its variants. *J Clin Oncol* 16: 3028-3036.

777. Gerald WL, Miller HK, Battifora H, Miettinen M, Silva EG, Rosai J (1991). Intra-abdominal desmoplastic small round-cell tumor. Report of 19 cases of a distinctive type of high-grade polyphenotypic malignancy affecting young individuals. *Am J Surg Pathol* 15: 499-513.

778. Gerald WL, Rosai J (1989). Case 2. Desmoplastic small cell tumor with divergent differentiation. *Pediatr Pathol* 9: 177-183.

779. Gerald WL, Rosai J (1993). Desmoplastic small cell tumor with multiphenotypic differentiation. *Zentralbl Pathol* 139: 141-151.

780. Gerald WL, Rosai J, Ladanyi M (1995). Characterization of the genomic breakpoint and chimeric transcripts in the EWS-WT1 gene fusion of desmoplastic small round cell tumor. *Proc Natl Acad Sci U S A* 92: 1028-1032.

781. Gherlinzoni F, Rock M, Picci P (1983). Chondromyxoid fibroma. The experience at the Istituto Ortopedico Rizzoli. *J Bone Joint Surg Am* 65: 198-204.

782. Giannini C, Scheithauer BW, Wenger DE, Unni KK (1996). Pigmented villonodular synovitis of the spine: a clinical, radiological, and morphological study of 12 cases. *J Neurosurg* 84: 592-597.

783. Giard F, Bonneau R, Raymond GP (1991). Plexiform fibrohistiocytic tumor. *Dermatologica* 183: 290-293.

784. Giardiello FM, Hamilton SR, Krush AJ, Offerhaus JA, Booker SV, Petersen GM (1993). Nasopharyngeal angiofibroma in patients with familial adenomatous polyposis. *Gastroenterology* 105: 1550-1552.

785. Giarola M, Wells D, Mondini P, Pilotti S, Sala P, Azzarelli A, Bertario L, Pierotti MA, Delhanty JD, Radice P (1998). Mutations of adenomatous polyposis coli (APC) gene are uncommon in sporadic desmoid tumours. *Br J Cancer* 78: 582-587.

786. Giebel GD, Bierhoff E, Vogel J (1996). Elastofibroma and pre-elastofibroma – a biopsy and autopsy study. *Eur J Surg Oncol* 22: 93-96.

787. Gil-Benso R, Lopez-Gines C, Soriano P, Almenar S, Vazquez C, Llombart-Bosch A (1994). Cytogenetic study of angiosarcoma of the breast. *Genes Chromosomes Cancer* 10: 210-212.

788. Gillespie WJ, Frampton CM, Henderson RJ, Ryan PM (1988). The incidence of cancer following total hip replacement. *J Bone Joint Surg Br* 70: 539-542.

789. Gillespy T, III, Manfrini M, Ruggieri P, Spanier SS, Pettersson H, Springfield DS (1988). Staging of intraosseous extent of osteosarcoma: correlation of preoperative CT and MR imaging with pathologic macroslides. *Radiology* 167: 765-767.

790. Giovannini M, Biegel JA, Serra M, Wang JY, Wei YH, Nycum L, Emanuel BS, Evans GA (1994). EWS-erg and EWS-Fli1 fusion transcripts in Ewing's sarcoma and primitive neuroectodermal tumors with variant translocations. *J Clin Invest* 94: 489-496.

791. Gisselsson D, Andreasson P, Meis-Kindblom JM, Kindblom LG, Mertens F, Mandahl N (1998). Amplification of 12q13 and 12q15 sequences in a sclerosing epithelioid fibrosarcoma. *Cancer Genet Cytogenet* 107: 102-106.

792. Gisselsson D, Hibbard MK, Dal Cin P, Sciot R, Hsi BL, Kozakewich HP, Fletcher JA (2001). PLAG1 alterations in lipoblastoma: involvement in varied mesenchymal cell types and evidence for alternative oncogenic mechanisms. *Am J Pathol* 159: 955-962.

793. Gisselsson D, Höglund M, Mertens F, Dal Cin P, Mandahl N (1999). Hibernomas are characterized by homozygous deletions in the multiple endocrine neoplasia type I region. Metaphase fluorescence in situ hybridization reveals complex rearrangements not detected by conventional cytogenetics. *Am J Pathol* 155: 61-66.

794. Gisselsson D, Höglund M, Mertens F, Johansson B, Dal Cin P, van den Berghe H, Earnshaw WC, Mitelman F, Mandahl N (1999). The structure and dynamics of ring chromosomes in human neoplastic and non-neoplastic cells. *Hum Genet* 104: 315-325.

795. Gisselsson D, Höglund M, Mertens F, Mitelman F, Mandahl N (1998). Chromosomal organization of amplified chromosome 12 sequences in mesenchymal tumors detected by fluorescence in situ hybridization. *Genes Chromosomes Cancer* 23: 203-212.

796. Gisselsson D, Pålsson E, Höglund M, Domanski H, Mertens F, Pandis N, Sciot R, Dal Cin P, Bridge JA, Mandahl N (2002). Differentially amplified chromosome 12 sequences in low- and high-grade osteosarcoma. *Genes Chromosomes Cancer* 33: 133-140.

797. Giunti A, Laus M (1978). Malignant tumours in chronic osteomyelitis. (A report of thirty nine cases, twenty six with long term follow up). *Ital J Orthop Traumatol* 4: 171-182.

798. Glass RB, Poznanski AK, Fisher MR, Shkolnik A, Dias L (1986). MR imaging of osteoid osteoma. *J Comput Assist Tomogr* 10: 1065-1067.

799. Godette GA, O'Sullivan M, Menelaus MB (1997). Plantar fibromatosis of the heel in children: a report of 14 cases. *J Pediatr Orthop* 17: 16-17.

800. Goedert JJ (2000). The epidemiology of acquired immunodeficiency syndrome malignancies. *Semin Oncol* 27: 390-401.

801. Goetz SP, Robinson RA, Landas SK (1992). Extraskeletal myxoid chondrosarcoma of the pleura. Report of a case clinically simulating mesothelioma. *Am J Clin Pathol* 97: 498-502.

802. Goh SG, Ho JM, Chuah KL, Tan PH, Poh WT, Riddell RH (2001). Leiomyomatosis-like lymphangioleiomyomatosis of the colon in a female with tuberous sclerosis. *Mod Pathol* 14: 1141-1146.

803. Gold JH, Bossen EH (1976). Benign vaginal rhabdomyoma: a light and electron microscopic study. *Cancer* 37: 2283-2294.

804. Goldblum JR, Rice TW (1995). Epithelioid angiosarcoma of the pulmonary artery. *Hum Pathol* 26: 1275-1277.

805. Goldman AB (1976). Myositis ossificans circumscripta: a benign lesion with a malignant differential diagnosis. *Am J Roentgenol* 126: 32-40.

806. Gomez-Roman JJ, Ocejo-Vinyals G, Sanchez-Velasco P, Nieto EH, Leyva-Cobian F, Val-Bernal JF (2000). Presence of human herpesvirus-8 DNA sequences and overexpression of human IL-6 and cyclin D1 in inflammatory myofibroblastic tumor (inflammatory pseudotumor). *Lab Invest* 80: 1121-1126.

807. Gonzalez-Crussi F, Campbell RJ (1970). Juvenile xanthogranuloma: ultrastructural study. *Arch Pathol* 89: 65-72.

808. Gonzalez-Crussi F, Chou P, Crawford SE (1991). Congenital, infiltrating giant-cell angioblastoma. A new entity? *Am J Surg Pathol* 15: 175-183.

809. Gonzalez-Crussi F, deMello DE, Sotelo-Avila C (1983). Omental-mesenteric myxoid hamartomas. Infantile lesions simulating malignant tumors. *Am J Surg Pathol* 7: 567-578.

810. Gonzalez-Crussi F, Wiederhold MD, Sotelo-Avila C (1980). Congenital fibrosarcoma: presence of a histiocytic component. *Cancer* 46: 77-86.

811. Good DA, Busfield F, Fletcher BH, Duffy DL, Kesting JB, Andersen J, Shaw JT (2002). Linkage of Paget disease of bone to a novel region on human chromosome 18q23. *Am J Hum Genet* 70: 517-525.

812. Goodlad JR, Fletcher CD (1990). Intradermal variant of nodular 'fasciitis'. *Histopathology* 17: 569-571.

813. Goodlad JR, Mentzel T, Fletcher CD (1995). Low grade fibromyxoid sarcoma: clinicopathological analysis of eleven new cases in support of a distinct entity. *Histopathology* 26: 229-237.

814. Gordon AT, Brinkschmidt C, Anderson J, Coleman N, Dockhorn-Dworniczak B, Pritchard-Jones K, Shipley J (2000). A novel and consistent amplicon at 13q31 associated with alveolar rhabdomyosarcoma. *Genes Chromosomes Cancer* 28: 220-226.

815. Gordon SL, Buchanan JR, Ladda RL (1981). Hereditary multiple exostoses: report of a kindred. *J Med Genet* 18: 428-430.

816. Gordon T, McManus A, Anderson J, Min T, Swansbury J, Pritchard-Jones K, Shipley J (2001). Cytogenetic abnormalities in 42 rhabdomyosarcoma: a United Kingdom Cancer Cytogenetics Group Study. *Med Pediatr Oncol* 36: 259-267.

817. Gorlick R, Huvos AG, Heller G, Aledo A, Beardsley GP, Healey JH, Meyers PA (1999). Expression of HER2/erbB-2 correlates with survival in osteosarcoma. *J Clin Oncol* 17: 2781-2788.

818. Gorlin RJ (1995). Nevoid basal cell carcinoma syndrome. *Dermatol Clin* 13: 113-125.

819. Goto M (1997). Hierarchical deterioration of body systems in Werner's syndrome: implications for normal ageing. *Mech Ageing Dev* 98: 239-254.

820. Goto M, Miller RW, Ishikawa Y, Sugano H (1996). Excess of rare cancers in Werner syndrome (adult progeria). *Cancer Epidemiol Biomarkers Prev* 5: 239-246.

821. Goto M, Yamabe Y, Shiratori M, Okada M, Kawabe T, Matsumoto T, Sugimoto M, Furuichi Y (1999). Immunological diagnosis of Werner syndrome by down-regulated and truncated gene products. *Hum Genet* 105: 301-307.

822. Goto T, Kojima T, Iijima T, Yokokura S, Motoi T, Kawano H, Yamamoto A, Matsuda K (2002). Intraosseous lipoma: a clinical study of 12 patients. *J Orthop Sci* 7: 274-280.

823. Gould EW, Manivel JC, Albores-Saavedra J, Monforte H (1990). Locally infiltrative glomus tumors and glomangiosarcomas. A clinical, ultrastructural, and immunohistochemical study. *Cancer* 65: 310-318.

824. Grace J, McCarthy S, Stankovic R, Marsden W (1993). Malignant transformation of osteoblastoma: study using image analysis microdensitometry. *J Clin Pathol* 46: 1024-1029.

825. Granter SR, Badizadegan K, Fletcher CD (1998). Myofibromatosis in adults, glomangiopericytoma, and myopericytoma: a spectrum of tumors showing perivascular myoid differentiation. *Am J Surg Pathol* 22: 513-525.

826. Granter SR, Nucci MR, Fletcher CD (1997). Aggressive angiomyxoma: reappraisal of its relationship to angiomyofibroblastoma in a series of 16 cases. *Histopathology* 30: 3-10.

827. Granter SR, Renshaw AA, Fletcher CD, Bhan AK, Rosenberg AE (1996). CD99 reactivity in mesenchymal chondrosarcoma. *Hum Pathol* 27: 1273-1276.

828. Granter SR, Renshaw AA, Kozakewich HP, Fletcher JA (1998). The pericentromeric inversion, inv (6)(p25q13), is a novel diagnostic marker in chondromyxoid fibroma. *Mod Pathol* 11: 1071-1074.

829. Granter SR, Weilbaecher KN, Quigley C, Fletcher CD, Fisher DE (2001). Clear cell sarcoma shows immunoreactivity for microphthalmia transcription factor: further evidence for melanocytic differentiation. *Mod Pathol* 14: 6-9.

830. Greco MA, Schinella RA, Vuletin JC (1984). Fibrous hamartoma of infancy: an ultrastructural study. *Hum Pathol* 15: 717-723.

831. Green FL, Page DL, Fleming ID, Fritz AG, Balch CM, Haller DG, Morrow M (2002). *AJCC Cancer Staging Manual*. 6th ed. Springer: New York.

832. Green MF, Sirikumara M (1987). Desmoplastic fibroma of the mandible. *Ann Plast Surg* 19: 284-290.

833. Green P, Whittaker RP (1975). Benign chondroblastoma. Case report with pulmonary metastasis. *J Bone Joint Surg Am* 57: 418-420.

834. Greenberg P, Parker RG, Fu YS, Abemayor E (1987). The treatment of solitary plasmacytoma of bone and extramedullary plasmacytoma. *Am J Clin Oncol* 10: 199-204.

835. Greenspan A, Azouz EM, Matthews J, Decarie JC (1995). Synovial hemangioma: imaging features in eight histologically proven cases, review of the literature, and differential diagnosis. *Skeletal Radiol* 24: 583-590.

836. Greiss ME, Williams DH (1991). Macrodystrophia lipomatosis in the foot. A case report and review of the literature. *Arch Orthop Trauma Surg* 110: 220-221.

837. Grieten M, Buckwalter KA, Cardinal E, Rougraff B (1994). Case report 873: Lipoma arborescens (villous lipomatous proliferation of the synovial membrane). *Skeletal Radiol* 23: 652-655.

838. Griffin CA, Hawkins AL, Dvorak C, Henkle C, Ellingham T, Perlman EJ (1999). Recurrent involvement of 2p23 in inflammatory myofibroblastic tumors. *Cancer Res* 59: 2776-2780.

839. Grimmett GM, Hall MG, Jr., Aird CC, Kurtz LH (1973). Pelvic lipomatosis. *Am J Surg* 125: 347-349.

840. Groden J, Thliveris A, Samowitz W, Carlson M, Gelbert L, Albertsen H, Joslyn G, Stevens J, Spirio L, Robertson M, . (1991). Identification and characterization of the familial adenomatous polyposis coli gene. *Cell* 66: 589-600.

841. Grogan TM, Durie BG, Lomen C, Spier C, Wirt DP, Nagle R, Wilson GS, Richter L, Vela E, Maxey V, . (1987). Delineation of a novel pre-B cell component in plasma cell myeloma: immunochemical, immunophenotypic, genotypic, cytologic, cell culture, and kinetic features. *Blood* 70: 932-942.

842. Grogan TM, Durie BG, Spier CM, Richter L, Vela E (1989). Myelomonocytic antigen positive multiple myeloma. *Blood* 73: 763-769.

843. Grogan TM, Spier CM (2001). The B cell immunoproliferative disorders, including multiple myeloma and amyloidosis. In: *Neoplastic Hematopathology*, Knowles DM, ed. 2nd ed. Lippincott Williams and Wilkins: Philadelphia.

844. Grogan TM, Van Camp B, Kyle RA, Muller-Hermelink HK, Harris NL (2001). Plasma cell neoplasms. In: *WHO Classification of Tumours. Pathology and Genetics of Tumours of Haematopoietic and Lymphoid Tissues*, Jaffe ES, Harris NL, Stein H, Vardiman JW, eds. IARC Press: Lyon, pp. 142-156.

845. Groisman G, Lichtig C (1991). Fibrous hamartoma of infancy: an immunohistochemical and ultrastructural study. *Hum Pathol* 22: 914-918.

846. Grovas A, Fremgen A, Rauck A, Ruymann FB, Hutchinson CL, Winchester DP, Menck HR (1997). The National Cancer Data Base report on patterns of childhood cancers in the United States. *Cancer* 80: 2321-2332.

847. Grubb RL, Jr., Dehner LP (1974). Congenital fibrosarcoma of the thoracolumbar region. *J Pediatr Surg* 9: 785-786.

848. Guccion JG, Enzinger FM (1972). Malignant giant cell tumor of soft parts. An analysis of 32 cases. *Cancer* 29: 1518-1529.

849. Guccion JG, Font RL, Enzinger FM, Zimmerman LE (1973). Extraskeletal mesenchymal chondrosarcoma. *Arch Pathol* 95: 336-340.

850. Guertl B, Beham A, Zechner R, Stammberger H, Hoefler G (2000). Nasopharyngeal angiofibroma: an APC-gene-associated tumor? *Hum Pathol* 31: 1411-1413.

851. Guillou L, Coindre JM, Bonichon F, Nguyen BB, Terrier P, Collin F, Vilain MO, Mandard AM, Le D, V, Leroux A, Jacquemier J, Duplay H, Sastre-Garau X, Costa J (1997). Comparative study of the National Cancer Institute and French Federation of Cancer Centers Sarcoma Group grading systems in a population of 410 adult patients with soft tissue sarcoma. *J Clin Oncol* 15: 350-362.

852. Guillou L, Gebhard S, Coindre JM (2000). Lipomatous hemangiopericytoma: a fat-containing variant of solitary fibrous tumor? Clinicopathologic, immunohistochemical, and ultrastructural analysis of a series in favor of a unifying concept. *Hum Pathol* 31: 1108-1115.

853. Guillou L, Gebhard S, Coindre JM (2000). Orbital and extraorbital giant cell angiofibroma: a giant cell-rich variant of solitary fibrous tumor? Clinicopathologic and immunohistochemical analysis of a series in favor of a unifying concept. *Am J Surg Pathol* 24: 971-979.

854. Guillou L, Kraus MD, Dei Tos AP, Fletcher CD (1996). S-100 protein reactivity in synovial sarcomas – a potentially frequent diagnostic pitfall. Immunohistochemical analysis of 100 cases. *Appl Immunohistochem* 4: 167-175.

855. Guillou L, Wadden C, Coindre JM, Krausz T, Fletcher CD (1997). "Proximal-type" epithelioid sarcoma, a distinctive aggressive neoplasm showing rhabdoid features. Clinicopathologic, immunohistochemical, and ultrastructural study of a series. *Am J Surg Pathol* 21: 130-146.

856. Gunawan B, Weber M, Bergmann F, Wildberger J, Niethard FU, Füzesi L (2000). Clonal chromosome abnormalities in enchondromas and chondrosarcomas. *Cancer Genet Cytogenet* 120: 127-130.

857. Gunawardena S, Chintagumpala M, Trautwein L, Brewer E, Gresik MV, Hicks MJ, Harrison WR, Morad A, Cooley LD (1999). Multifocal osteosarcoma: an unusual presentation. *J Pediatr Hematol Oncol* 21: 58-62.

858. Guo W, Gorlick R, Ladanyi M, Meyers PA, Huvos AG, Bertino JR, Healey JH (1999). Expression of bone morphogenetic proteins and receptors in sarcomas. *Clin Orthop* 175-183.

859. Gurbuz AK, Giardiello FM, Petersen GM, Krush AJ, Offerhaus GJ, Booker SV, Kerr MC, Hamilton SR (1994). Desmoid tumours in familial adenomatous polyposis. *Gut* 35: 377-381.

860. Gurney JG, Davis S, Severson RK, Fang JY, Ross JA, Robison LL (1996). Trends in cancer incidence among children in the U.S. *Cancer* 78: 532-541.

861. Gustafson P (1994). Soft tissue sarcoma. Epidemiology and prognosis in 508 patients. *Acta Orthop Scand Suppl* 259: 1-31.

862. Gustafson P, Dreinhofer KE, Rydholm A (1994). Soft tissue sarcoma should be treated at a tumor center. A comparison of quality of surgery in 375 patients. *Acta Orthop Scand* 65: 47-50.

863. Hachisuga T, Hashimoto H, Enjoji M (1984). Angioleiomyoma. A clinicopathologic reappraisal of 562 cases. *Cancer* 54: 126-130.

864. Hachitanda Y, Tsuneyoshi M, Daimaru Y, Enjoji M, Nakagawara A, Ikeda K, Sueishi K (1988). Extraskeletal myxoid chondrosarcoma in young children. *Cancer* 61: 2521-2526.

865. Hahm KB, Cho K, Lee C, Im YH, Chang J, Choi SG, Sorensen PH, Thiele CJ, Kim SJ (1999). Repression of the gene encoding the TGF-beta type II receptor is a major target of the EWS-FLI1 oncoprotein. *Nat Genet* 23: 222-227.

866. Hahn H, Wicking C, Zaphiropoulous PG, Gailani MR, Shanley S, Chidambaram A, Vorechovsky I, Holmberg E, Unden AB, Gillies S, Negus K, Smyth I, Pressman C, Leffell DJ, Gerrard B, Goldstein AM, Dean M, Toftgård R, Chenevix-Trench G, Wainwright B, Bale AE (1996). Mutations of the human homolog of Drosophila patched in the nevoid basal cell carcinoma syndrome. *Cell* 85: 841-851.

867. Haibach H, Farrell C, Dittrich FJ (1985). Neoplasms arising in Paget's disease of bone: a study of 82 cases. *Am J Clin Pathol* 83: 594-600.

868. Hainaut P, Lesage V, Weynand B, Coche E, Noirhomme P (1999). Calcifying fibrous pseudotumor (CFPT): a patient presenting with multiple pleural lesions. *Acta Clin Belg* 54: 162-164.

869. Hakimi M, Pai RP, Fine D, Davila JC (1975). Fibrous histiocytoma of the trachea. *Chest* 68: 367-368.

870. Halbert AR, Harrison WR, Hicks MJ, Davino N, Cooley LD (1998). Cytogenetic analysis of a scapular chondromyxoid fibroma. *Cancer Genet Cytogenet* 104: 52-56.

871. Hall FM, Gore SM (1988). Osteoscle-rotic myeloma variants. *Skeletal Radiol* 17: 101-105.

872. Hall MB, Sclar AG, Gardner DF (1984). Albright's syndrome with reactivation of fibrous dysplasia secondary to pituitary adenoma and further complicated by osteogenic sarcoma. Report of a case. *Oral Surg Oral Med Oral Pathol* 57: 616-619.

873. Hall PN, Fitzgerald A, Sterne GD, Logan AM (1997). Skin replacement in Dupuytren's disease. *J Hand Surg [Br]* 22: 193-197.

874. Hall RB, Robinson LH, Malawar MM, Dunham WK (1985). Periosteal osteosarcoma. *Cancer* 55: 165-171.

875. Hallel T, Lew S, Bansal M (1988). Villous lipomatous proliferation of the synovial membrane (lipoma arborescens). *J Bone Joint Surg Am* 70: 264-270.

876. Halling AC, Wollan PC, Pritchard DJ, Vlasak R, Nascimento AG (1996). Epithelioid sarcoma: a clinicopathologic review of 55 cases. *Mayo Clin Proc* 71: 636-642.

877. Hamada T, Ito H, Araki Y, Fujii K, Inoue M, Ishida O (1996). Benign fibrous histiocytoma of the femur: review of three cases. *Skeletal Radiol* 25: 25-29.

878. Hamakawa H, Hino H, Sumida T, Tanioka H (2000). Infiltrating angiolipoma of the cheek: a case report and a review of the literature. *J Oral Maxillofac Surg* 58: 674-677.

879. Hamblen DL, Carter RL (1984). Sarcoma and joint replacement. *J Bone Joint Surg Br* 66: 625-627.

880. Hamper K, Renninghoff J, Schafer H (1989). Rhabdomyoma of the larynx recurring after 12 years: immunocytochemistry and differential diagnosis. *Arch Otorhinolaryngol* 246: 222-226.

881. Handgretinger R, Kimmig A, Koscielnak E, Schmidt D, Rudolph G, Wolburg H, Paulus W, Schilbach-Stueckle K, Ottenlinger C, Menrad A (1990). Establishment and characterization of a cell line (Wa-2) derived from an extrarenal rhabdoid tumor. *Cancer Res* 50: 2177-2182.

882. Hansen MF, Koufos A, Gallie BL, Phillips RA, Fodstad O, Brogger A, Gedde-Dahl T, Cavenee WK (1985). Osteosarcoma and retinoblastoma: a shared chromosomal mechanism revealing recessive predisposition. *Proc Natl Acad Sci U S A* 82: 6216-6220.

883. Hansen MF, Nellissery MJ, Bhatia P (1999). Common mechanisms of osteosarcoma and Paget's disease. *J Bone Miner Res* 14 Suppl 2: 39-44.

884. Happle R, Konig A (1999). Type 2 segmental manifestation of multiple glomus tumors: A review and reclassification of 5 case reports. *Dermatology* 198: 270-272.

885. Haque S, Modlin IM, West AB (1992). Multiple glomus tumors of the stomach with intravascular spread. *Am J Surg Pathol* 16: 291-299.

886. Hardcastle P, Nade S, Arnold W (1986). Hereditary bone dysplasia with malignant change. Report of three families. *J Bone Joint Surg Am* 68: 1079-1089.

887. Harms D (1995). Alveolar rhabdomyosarcoma: a prognostically unfavorable rhabdomyosarcoma type and its necessary distinction from embryonal rhabdomyosarcoma. *Curr Top Pathol* 89: 273-296.

888. Harms D (1995). New entities, concepts, and questions in childhood tumor pathology. *Gen Diagn Pathol* 141: 1-14.

889. Harris M, Coyne J, Tariq M, Eyden BP, Atkinson M, Freemont AJ, Varley J, Attwooll C, Telford N (2000). Extraskeletal myxoid chondrosarcoma with neuroendocrine differentiation: a pathologic, cytogenetic, and molecular study of a case with a novel translocation t(9;17)(q22;q11.2). *Am J Surg Pathol* 24: 1020-1026.

890. Harris WH, Dudley HR, Barry RJ (1962). The natural history of fibrous dysplasia. *J Bone Joint Surg Am* 44: 207-233.

891. Harwood AR, Krajbich JI, Fornasier VL (1981). Mesenchymal chondrosarcoma: a report of 17 cases. *Clin Orthop* 144-148.

892. Hasegawa T, Dorfman H, Habermann ET (1988). Sarcoma associated with bone infarction: a clinicopathologic and immunohistochemical study of 22 cases (in press).

893. Hasegawa T, Hirose T, Kudo E, Hizawa K, Usui M, Ishii S (1991). Immunophenotypic heterogeneity in osteosarcomas. *Hum Pathol* 22: 583-590.

894. Hasegawa T, Hirose T, Seki K, Hizawa K, Okada J, Nakanishi H (1993). Solitary infantile myofibromatosis of bone. An immunohistochemical and ultrastructural study. *Am J Surg Pathol* 17: 308-313.

895. Hasegawa T, Hirose T, Seki K, Yang P, Sano T (1996). Solitary fibrous tumor of the soft tissue. An immunohistochemical and ultrastructural study. *Am J Clin Pathol* 106: 325-331.

896. Hasegawa T, Matsuno Y, Shimoda T, Hasegawa F, Sano T, Hirohashi S (1999). Extrathoracic solitary fibrous tumors: their histological variability and potentially aggressive behavior. *Hum Pathol* 30: 1464-1473.

897. Hasegawa T, Matsuno Y, Shimoda T, Umeda T, Yokoyama R, Hirohashi S (2001). Proximal-type epithelioid sarcoma: a clinicopathologic study of 20 cases. *Mod Pathol* 14: 655-663.

898. Hasegawa T, Seki K, Ono K, Hirohashi S (2000). Angiomatoid (malignant) fibrous histiocytoma: a peculiar low-grade tumor showing immunophenotypic heterogeneity and ultrastructural variations. *Pathol Int* 50: 731-738.

899. Hasegawa T, Seki K, Yang P, Hirose T, Hizawa K (1994). Mechanism of pain and cytoskeletal properties in angioleiomyomas: an immunohistochemical study. *Pathol Int* 44: 66-72.

900. Hasegawa T, Shimoda T, Hirohashi S, Hizawa K, Sano T (1998). Collagenous fibroma (desmoplastic fibroblastoma): report of four cases and review of the literature. *Arch Pathol Lab Med* 122: 455-460.

901. Hashimoto H (1995). Incidence of soft tissue sarcomas in adults. *Curr Top Pathol* 89: 1-16.

902. Hashimoto H, Daimaru Y, Takeshita S, Tsuneyoshi M, Enjoji M (1992). Prognostic significance of histologic parameters of soft tissue sarcomas. *Cancer* 70: 2816-2822.

903. Hashimoto H, Daimaru Y, Tsuneyoshi M, Enjoji M (1986). Leiomyosarcoma of the external soft tissues. A clinicopathologic, immunohistochemical, and electron microscopic study. *Cancer* 57: 2077-2088.

904. Hashimoto H, Tsuneyoshi M, Daimaru Y, Enjoji M, Shinohara N (1986). Intramuscular myxoma. A clinicopathologic, immunohistochemical, and electron microscopic study. *Cancer* 58: 740-747.

905. Hashimoto H, Tsuneyoshi M, Daimaru Y, Ushijima M, Enjoji M (1985). Fibroma of tendon sheath: a tumor of myofibroblasts. A clinicopathologic study of 18 cases. *Acta Pathol Jpn* 35: 1099-1107.

906. Hashimoto H, Tsuneyoshi M, Enjoji M (1985). Malignant smooth muscle tumors of the retroperitoneum and mesentery: a clinicopathologic analysis of 44 cases. *J Surg Oncol* 28: 177-186.

907. Hassel B (1992). Calcifying aponeurotic fibroma. A case of multiple primary tumours. Case report. *Scand J Plast Reconstr Surg Hand Surg* 26: 115-116.

908. Hauben E, van den Broek LC, Van Marck E, Hogendoorn PC (2001). Adamantinoma-like Ewing's sarcoma and Ewing's-like adamantinoma. The t(11; 22), t(21; 22) status. *J Pathol* 195: 218-221.

909. Hauben EI, Weeden S, Pringle J, Van Marck EA, Hogendoorn PCW (2002). Does the histological subtype of high-grade central osteosarcoma influence the response to treatment with chemotherapy and does it affect overall survival? A study on 570 patients of two consecutive trials of the European Osteosarcoma Intergroup. *Eur J Cancer* 38: 1218-1225.

910. Hawkins WG, Hoos A, Antonescu CR, Urist MJ, Leung DH, Gold JS, Woodruff JM, Lewis JJ, Brennan MF (2001). Clinicopathologic analysis of patients with adult rhabdomyosarcoma. *Cancer* 91: 794-803.

911. Hawley IC, Krausz T, Evans DJ, Fletcher CD (1994). Spindle cell lipoma – a pseudoangiomatous variant. *Histopathology* 24: 565-569.

912. Hayashi N, Borodic G, Karesh JW, Tolentino MJ, Remulla HD, Van Wesep RA, Grossniklaus HE, Jakobiec FA, Green WR (1999). Giant cell angiofibroma of the orbit and eyelid. *Ophthalmology* 106: 1223-1229.

913. Hayashi T, Tsuda N, Chowdhury PR, Anami M, Kishikawa M, Iseki M, Kobayashi K (1995). Infantile digital fibromatosis: a study of the development and regression of cytoplasmic inclusion bodies. *Mod Pathol* 8: 548-552.

914. Hayry P, Reitamo JJ, Totterman S, Hopfner-Hallikainen D, Sivula A (1982). The desmoid tumor. II. Analysis of factors possibly contributing to the etiology and growth behavior. *Am J Clin Pathol* 77: 674-680.

915. Hays DM, Mirabal VQ, Karlan MS, Patel HR, Landing BH (1970). Fibrosarcomas in infants and children. *J Pediatr Surg* 5: 176-183.

916. Hazelbag HM, Fleuren GJ, Cornelisse CJ, Van den Broek LJ, Taminiau AH, Hogendoorn PC (1995). DNA aberrations in the epithelial cell component of adamantinoma of long bones. *Am J Pathol* 147: 1770-1779.

917. Hazelbag HM, Fleuren GJ, Van den Broek LJ, Taminiau AH, Hogendoorn PC (1993). Adamantinoma of the long bones: keratin subclass immunoreactivity pattern with reference to its histogenesis. *Am J Surg Pathol* 17: 1225-1233.

918. Hazelbag HM, Taminiau AH, Fleuren GJ, Hogendoorn PC (1994). Adamantinoma of the long bones. A clinicopathological study of thirty-two patients with emphasis on histological subtype, precursor lesion, and biological behavior. *J Bone Joint Surg Am* 76: 1482-1499.

919. Hazelbag HM, Van den Broek LJ, Fleuren GJ, Taminiau AH, Hogendoorn PC (1997). Distribution of extracellular matrix components in adamantinoma of long bones suggests fibrous-to-epithelial transformation. *Hum Pathol* 28: 183-188.

920. Hazelbag HM, Wessels JW, Mollevangers P, van den Berg E, Molenaar WM, Hogendoorn PC (1997). Cytogenetic analysis of adamantinoma of long bones: further indications for a common histogenesis with osteofibrous dysplasia. *Cancer Genet Cytogenet* 97: 5-11.

921. He TC, Sparks AB, Rago C, Hermeking H, Zawel L, da Costa LT, Morin PJ, Vogelstein B, Kinzler KW (1998). Identification of c-MYC as a target of the APC pathway. *Science* 281: 1509-1512.

922. Healey JH, Ghelman B (1986). Osteoid osteoma and osteoblastoma. Current concepts and recent advances. *Clin Orthop* 76-85.

923. Healey JH, Turnbull AD, Miedema B, Lane JM (1986). Acrometastases. A study of twenty-nine patients with osseous involvement of the hands and feet. *J Bone Joint Surg Am* 68: 743-746.

924. Hecht JT, Hogue D, Strong LC, Hansen MF, Blanton SH, Wagner M (1995). Hereditary multiple exostosis and chondrosarcoma: linkage to chromosome II and loss of heterozygosity for EXT-linked markers on chromosomes II and 8. *Am J Hum Genet* 56: 1125-1131.

925. Heffelfinger MJ, Dahlin DC, MacCarty CS, Beabout JW (1973). Chordomas and cartilaginous tumors at the skull base. *Cancer* 32: 410-420.

926. Heim S, Mandahl N, Kristoffersson U, Mitelman F, Rööser B, Rydholm A, Willén H (1986). Structural chromosome aberrations in a case of angioleiomyoma. *Cancer Genet Cytogenet* 20: 325-330.

927. Heimann P, Devalck C, Debusscher C, Sariban E, Vamos E (1998). Alveolar soft-part sarcoma: further evidence by FISH for the involvement of chromosome band 17q25. *Genes Chromosomes Cancer* 23: 194-197.

928. Heimann P, El Housni H, Ogur G, Weterman MA, Petty EM, Vassart G (2001). Fusion of a novel gene, RCC17, to the TFE3 gene in t(X;17)(p11.2;q25.3)-bearing papillary renal cell carcinomas. *Cancer Res* 61: 4130-4135.

929. Heimann P, Ogur G, Debusscher C, Devalck C, Sariban F, Vamos E (1993). Multiple complex chromosome aberrations in a case of childhood hepatic angiosarcoma. *Cancer Genet Cytogenet* 63: 171.

930. Heise HW, Myers MH, Russell WO, Suit HD, Enzinger FM, Edmonson JH, Cohen J, Martin RG, Miller WT, Hajdu SI (1986). Recurrence-free survival time for surgically treated soft tissue sarcoma patients. Multivariate analysis of five prognostic factors. *Cancer* 57: 172-177.

931. Heiskanen I, Jarvinen HJ (1996). Occurrence of desmoid tumours in familial adenomatous polyposis and results of treatment. *Int J Colorectal Dis* 11: 157-162.

932. Heller AJ, DiNardo LJ, Massey D (2001). Fibrous dysplasia, chondrosarcoma, and McCune-Albright syndrome. *Am J Otolaryngol* 22: 297-301.

933. Helliwell TR, Sissons MC, Stoney PJ, Ashworth MT (1988). Immunochemistry and electron microscopy of head and neck rhabdomyoma. *J Clin Pathol* 41: 1058-1063.

934. Helson C, Melamed M, Braverman S, Traganos F, Preti RA, Helson L (1995). VA-ES-BJ: an epithelioid sarcoma cell line. *Int J Oncol* 7: 51-56.

935. Henderson CJ, Gupta L (2000). Ectopic hamartomatous thymoma: a case study and review of the literature. *Pathology* 32: 142-146.

936. Hennig Y, Caselitz J, Stern C, Bartnitzke S, Bullerdiek J (1999). Karyotype evolution in a case of uterine angioleiomyoma. *Cancer Genet Cytogenet* 108: 79-80.

937. Henricks WH, Chu YC, Goldblum JR, Weiss SW (1997). Dedifferentiated liposarcoma: a clinicopathological analysis of 155 cases with a proposal for an expanded definition of dedifferentiation. *Am J Surg Pathol* 21: 271-281.

938. Herens C, Thiry A, Dresse MF, Born J, Flagothier C, Vanstraelen G, Allington N, Bex V (2001). Translocation (16;17)(q22;p13) is a recurrent anomaly of aneurysmal bone cysts. *Cancer Genet Cytogenet* 127: 83-84.

939. Hermann G, Steiner GC, Sherry HH (1988). Case report 465: Benign fibrous histiocytoma (BFH). *Skeletal Radiol* 17: 195-198.

940. Herrera L, Kakati S, Gibas L, Pietrzak E, Sandberg AA (1986). Gardner syndrome in a man with an interstitial deletion of 5q. *Am J Med Genet* 25: 473-476.

941. Hethcote HW, Knudson AG, Jr. (1978). Model for the incidence of embryonal cancers: application to retinoblastoma. *Proc Natl Acad Sci U S A* 75: 2453-2457.

942. Heymann WR, Fiorillo A, Simons J (1988). Eruptive familial angiolipomas occurring during pregnancy. *Cutis* 42: 525-526.

943. Heyning FH, Hogendoorn PC, Kramer MH, Hermans J, Kluin-Nelemans JC, Noordijk EM, Kluin PM (1999). Primary non-Hodgkin's lymphoma of bone: a clinicopathological investigation of 60 cases. *Leukemia* 13: 2094-2098.

944. Heyns CF (1991). Pelvic lipomatosis: a review of its diagnosis and management. *J Urol* 146: 267-273.

945. Hibbard MK, Kozakewich HP, Dal Cin P, Sciot R, Tan X, Xiao S, Fletcher JA (2000). PLAG1 fusion oncogenes in lipoblastoma. *Cancer Res* 60: 4869-4872.

946. Higginson J, Muir CS, Munoz N (1992). Bone. In: *Human cancer: epidemiology and environmental causes*. University Press: Cambridge, pp. 353-357.

947. Hill DA, Pfeifer JD, Marley EF, Dehner LP, Humphrey PA, Zhu X, Swanson PE (2000). WT1 staining reliably differentiates desmoplastic small round cell tumor from Ewing sarcoma/primitive neuroectodermal tumor. An immunohistochemical and molecular diagnostic study. *Am J Clin Pathol* 114: 345-353.

948. Hill KA, Gonzalez-Crussi F, Chou PM (2001). Calcifying fibrous pseudotumor versus inflammatory myofibroblastic tumor: a histological and immunohistochemical comparison. *Mod Pathol* 14: 784-790.

949. Hinrichs SH, Jaramillo MA, Gumerlock PH, Gardner MB, Lewis JP, Freeman AE (1985). Myxoid chondrosarcoma with a translocation involving chromosomes 9 and 22. *Cancer Genet Cytogenet* 14: 219-226.

950. Hirabayashi Y, Ishida T, Yoshida MA, Kojima T, Ebihara Y, Machinami R, Ikeuchi T (1995). Translocation (9;22)(q22;q12). A recurrent chromosome abnormality in extraskeletal myxoid chondrosarcoma. *Cancer Genet Cytogenet* 81: 33-37.

951. Hirata M, Kusuzaki K, Hirasawa Y (2001). Eleven cases of intraosseous lipoma of the calcaneus. *Anticancer Res* 21: 4099-4103.

952. Hirose T, Hasegawa T, Seki K, Yang P, Sano T, Morizumi H, Tsuyuguchi M (1996). Atypical glomus tumor in the mediastinum: a case report with immunohistochemical and ultrastructural studies. *Ultrastruct Pathol* 20: 451-456.

953. Hiruta N, Kameda N, Tokudome T, Tsuchiya K, Nonaka H, Hatori T, Akima M, Miura M (1997). Malignant glomus tumor: a case report and review of the literature. *Am J Surg Pathol* 21: 1096-1103.

954. Hisada M, Garber JE, Fung CY, Fraumeni JF, Jr., Li FP (1998). Multiple primary cancers in families with Li-Fraumeni syndrome. *J Natl Cancer Inst* 90: 606-611.

955. Hisaoka M, Morimitsu Y, Hashimoto H, Ishida T, Mukai H, Satoh H, Motoi T, Machinami R (1999). Retroperitoneal liposarcoma with combined well-differentiated and myxoid malignant fibrous histiocytoma-like myxoid areas. *Am J Surg Pathol* 23: 1480-1492.

956. Hisaoka M, Tsuji S, Hashimoto H, Aoki T, Uriu K (1997). Dedifferentiated liposarcoma with an inflammatory malignant fibrous histiocytoma-like component presenting a leukemoid reaction. *Pathol Int* 47: 642-646.

957. Hizawa K, Iida M, Mibu R, Aoyagi K, Yao T, Fujishima M (1997). Desmoid tumors in familial adenomatous polyposis / Gardner's syndrome. *J Clin Gastroenterol* 25: 334-337.

958. Hoang MP, Suarez PA, Donner LR, Ro Y, Ordonez NG, Ayala AG, Czerniak B (2000). Mesenchymal Chondrosarcoma: A Small Cell Neoplasm with Polyphenotypic Differentiation. *Int J Surg Pathol* 8: 291-301.

959. Hoeffel JC, Boman-Ferrand F, Tachet F, Lascombes P, Czorny A, Bernard C (1992). So-called benign fibrous histiocytoma: report of a case. *J Pediatr Surg* 27: 672-674.

960. Hojo H, Newton WA, Jr., Hamoudi AB, Qualman SJ, Wakasa H, Suzuki S, Jaynes F (1995). Pseudosarcomatous myofibroblastic tumor of the urinary bladder in children: a study of 11 cases with review of the literature. An Intergroup Rhabdomyosarcoma Study. *Am J Surg Pathol* 19: 1224-1236.

961. Hollowood K, Fletcher CD (1995). Malignant fibrous histiocytoma: morphologic pattern or pathologic entity? *Semin Diagn Pathol* 12: 210-220.

962. Hollowood K, Holley MP, Fletcher CD (1991). Plexiform fibrohistiocytic tumour: clinicopathological, immunohistochemical and ultrastructural analysis in favour of a myofibroblastic lesion. *Histopathology* 19: 503-513.

963. Hollstein M, Marion MJ, Lehman T, Welsh J, Harris CC, Martel-Planche G, Kusters I, Montesano R (1994). p53 mutations at A:T base pairs in angiosarcomas of vinyl chloride-exposed factory workers. *Carcinogenesis* 15: 1-3.

964. Holscher HC, Bloem JL, Vanel D, Hermans J, Nooy MA, Taminiau AH, Henry-Amar M (1992). Osteosarcoma: chemotherapy-induced changes at MR imaging. *Radiology* 182: 839-844.

965. Hoogerwerf WA, Hawkins AL, Perlman EJ, Griffin CA (1994). Chromosome analysis of nine osteosarcomas. *Genes Chromosomes Cancer* 9: 88-92.

966. Hoos A, Lewis JJ, Antonescu CR, Dudas ME, Leon L, Woodruff JM, Brennan MF, Cordon-Cardo C (2001). Characterization of molecular abnormalities in human fibroblastic neoplasms: a model for genotype-phenotype association in soft tissue tumors. *Cancer Res* 61: 3171-3175.

967. Hoovers JM, Kalikin LM, Johnson LA, Alders M, Redeker B, Law DJ, Bliek J, Steenman M, Benedict M, Wiegant J, Cremer C, Taillon-Miller P, Schlessinger D, Ivens A, Westerveld A, Little PF, Mannens M, Feinberg AP (1995). Multiple genetic loci within 11p15 defined by Beckwith-Wiedemann syndrome rearrangement breakpoints and subchromosomal transferable fragments. *Proc Natl Acad Sci U S A* 92: 12456-12460.

968. Hopyan S, Gokgoz N, Poon R, Gensure RC, Yu C, Cole WG, Bell RS, Juppner H, Andrulis IL, Wunder JS, Alman BA (2002). A mutant PTH/PTHrP type I receptor in enchondromatosis. *Nat Genet* 30: 306-310.

969. Horowitz JM, Park SH, Bogenmann E, Cheng JC, Yandell DW, Kaye FJ, Minna JD, Dryja TP, Weinberg RA (1990). Frequent inactivation of the retinoblastoma antioncogene is restricted to a subset of human tumor cells. *Proc Natl Acad Sci U S A* 87: 2775-2779.

970. Horsthemke B, Barnert HJ, Greger V, Passarge E, Hopping W (1987). Early diagnosis in hereditary retinoblastoma by detection of molecular deletions at gene locus. *Lancet* 1: 511-512.

971. Hosaka T, Kanoe H, Nakayama T, Murakami H, Yamamoto H, Nakamata T, Tsuboyama T, Oka M, Kasai M, Sasaki MS, Nakamura T, Toguchida J (2000). Translin binds to the sequences adjacent to the breakpoints of the TLS and CHOP genes in liposarcomas with translocation t(12;6). *Oncogene* 19: 5821-5825.

972. Hosli I, Holzgreve W, Danzer E, Tercanli S (2001). Two case reports of rare fetal tumors: an indication for surface rendering? *Ultrasound Obstet Gynecol* 17: 522-526.

973. Hostein I, Menard A, Bui BN, Lussan C, Wafflart J, Delattre O, Peter M, Benhattar J, Guillou L, Coindre JM (2002). Molecular detection of the synovial sarcoma translocation t(X;18) by real-time polymerase chain reaction in paraffin-embedded material. *Diagn Mol Pathol* 11: 16-21.

974. Hottenrott G, Mentzel T, Peters A, Schroder A, Katenkamp D (1999). Intravascular ("intimal") epithelioid angiosarcoma: clinicopathological and immunohistochemical analysis of three cases. *Virchows Arch* 435: 473-478.

975. Hou J, Parrish J, Lüdecke HJ, Sapru M, Wang Y, Chen W, Hill A, Siegel-Bartelt J, Northrup H, Elder FF, Chinault C, Horsthemke B, Wagner MJ, Wells DE (1995). A 4-megabase YAC contig that spans the Langer-Giedion syndrome region on human chromosome 8q24.1: use in refining the location of the trichorhinophalangeal syndrome and multiple exostoses genes (TRPS1 and EXT1). *Genomics* 29: 87-97.

976. Howard GM, Ellsworth RM (1965). Differential diagnosis of retinoblastoma: a statistical study of 500 children. *Am J Ophthalmol* 60: 610-621.

977. Howard WR, Helwig EB (1960). Angiolipoma. *Arch Dermatol* 82: 924-931.

978. Howat AJ, Campbell PE (1987). Angiomatosis: a vascular malformation of infancy and childhood. Report of 17 cases. *Pathology* 19: 377-382.

979. Howat AJ, Dickens DR, Boldt DW, Waters KD, Campbell PE (1986). Bilateral metachronous periosteal osteosarcoma. *Cancer* 58: 1139-1143.

980. Hsueh C, Kuo TT (1998). Congenital malignant rhabdoid tumor presenting as a cutaneous nodule: report of 2 cases with review of the literature. *Arch Pathol Lab Med* 122: 1099-1102.

981. Humphreys S, McKee PH, Fletcher CD (1986). Fibroma of tendon sheath: a clinicopathologic study. *J Cutan Pathol* 13: 331-338.

982. Humphreys S, Pambakian H, McKee PH, Fletcher CD (1986). Soft tissue chondroma – a study of 15 tumours. *Histopathology* 10: 147-159.

983. Hunt SJ, Santa Cruz DJ, Barr RJ (1990). Cellular angiolipoma. *Am J Surg Pathol* 14: 75-81.

984. Hussong JW, Brown M, Perkins SL, Dehner LP, Coffin CM (1999). Comparison of DNA ploidy, histologic, and immunohistochemical findings with clinical outcome in inflammatory myofibroblastic tumors. *Mod Pathol* 12: 279-286.

985. Hutter RVP, Stewart FW, Foote FW (1962). Fasciitis: a report of 70 cases with follow-up proving the benignity of the lesion. *Cancer* 15: 992-1003.

986. Huvos AG (1986). Osteogenic sarcoma of bones and soft tissues in older persons. A clinicopathologic analysis of 117 patients older than 60 years. *Cancer* 57: 1442-1449.

987. Huvos AG (1991). Adamantinoma of extragnathic bones. In: *Bone Tumors. Diagnosis, Treatment, and Prognosis*, Huvos AG, ed. W.B. Saunders Company: Philadelphia, pp. 677-693.

988. Huvos AG (1999). *Bone Tumors: Diagnosis, Treatment and Prognosis*. 2nd ed. W.B. Saunders Company.

989. Huvos AG, Butler A, Bretsky SS (1983). Osteogenic sarcoma associated with Paget's disease of bone. A clinicopathologic study of 65 patients. *Cancer* 52: 1489-1495.

990. Huvos AG, Heilweil M, Bretsky SS (1985). The pathology of malignant fibrous histiocytoma of bone. A study of 130 patients. *Am J Surg Pathol* 9: 853-871.

991. Huvos AG, Higinbotham NL (1975). Primary fibrosarcoma of bone. A clinicopathologic study of 130 patients. *Cancer* 35: 837-847.

992. Huvos AG, Higinbotham NL, Miller TR (1972). Bone sarcomas arising in fibrous dysplasia. *J Bone Joint Surg Am* 54: 1047-1056.

993. Huvos AG, Marcove RC, Erlandson RA, Mike V (1972). Chondroblastoma of bone. A clinicopathologic and electron microscopic study. *Cancer* 29: 760-771.

994. Huvos AG, Rosen G, Dabska M, Marcove RC (1983). Mesenchymal chondrosarcoma. A clinicopathologic analysis of 35 patients with emphasis on treatment. *Cancer* 51: 1230-1237.

995. Huvos AG, Sundaresan N, Bretsky SS, Butler A (1985). Osteogenic sarcoma of the skull. A clinicopathologic study of 19 patients. *Cancer* 56: 1214-1221.

996. Huvos AG, Woodard HQ, Cahan WG, Higinbotham NL, Stewart FW, Butler A, Bretsky SS (1985). Postradiation osteogenic sarcoma of bone and soft tissues. A clinicopathologic study of 66 patients. *Cancer* 55: 1244-1255.

997. Huvos AG, Woodard HQ, Heilweil M (1986). Postradiation malignant fibrous histiocytoma of bone. A clinicopathologic study of 20 patients. *Am J Surg Pathol* 10: 9-18.

998. Iczkowski KA, Shanks JH, Gadaleanu V, Cheng L, Jones EC, Neumann R, Nascimento AG, Bostwick DG (2001). Inflammatory pseudotumor and sarcoma of urinary bladder: differential diagnosis and outcome in thirty-eight spindle cell neoplasms. *Mod Pathol* 14: 1043-1051.

999. Iemoto Y, Ushigome S, Fukunaga M, Nikaido T, Asanuma K (1991). Case report 679. Central low-grade osteosarcoma with foci of dedifferentiation. *Skeletal Radiol* 20: 379-382.

1000. Iezzoni JC, Fechner RE, Wong LS, Rosai J (1995). Aggressive angiomyxoma in males. A report of four cases. *Am J Clin Pathol* 104: 391-396.

1001. Ihara C, Shimatsu A, Murabe H, Kataoka K, Kondo C, Nakao K (1996). Growth hormone-secreting pituitary adenoma associated with multiple bone cysts, skin pigmentation and aortitis syndrome. *J Endocrinol Invest* 19: 753-757.

1002. Ilhan H, Tokar B, Isiksoy S, Koku N, Pasaoglu O (1999). Giant mesenteric lipoma. *J Pediatr Surg* 34: 639-640.

1003. Im YH, Kim HT, Lee C, Poulin D, Welford S, Sorensen PH, Denny CT, Kim SJ (2000). EWS-FLI1, EWS-ERG, and EWS-ETV1 oncoproteins of Ewing tumor family all suppress transcription of transforming growth factor beta type II receptor gene. *Cancer Res* 60: 1536-1540.

1004. Inagaki H, Murase T, Otsuka T, Eimoto T (1999). Detection of SYT-SSX fusion transcript in synovial sarcoma using archival cytologic specimens. *Am J Clin Pathol* 111: 528-533.

1005. Inoue YZ, Frassica FJ, Sim FH, Unni KK, Petersen IA, McLeod RA (2000). Clinicopathologic features and treatment of postirradiation sarcoma of bone and soft tissue. *J Surg Oncol* 75: 42-50.

1006. Inwards CY, Unni KK (1995). Classification and grading of bone sarcomas. *Hematol Oncol Clin North Am* 9: 545-569.

1007. Inwards CY, Unni KK, Beabout JW, Shives TC (1991). Solitary congenital fibromatosis (infantile myofibromatosis) of bone. *Am J Surg Pathol* 15: 935-941.

1008. Ioachim HL, Adsay V, Giancotti FR, Dorsett B, Melamed J (1995). Kaposi's sarcoma of internal organs. A multiparameter study of 86 cases. *Cancer* 75: 1376-1385.

1009. Iolascon A, Faienza MF, Coppola B, Rosolen A, Basso G, Della Ragione F, Schettini F (1996). Analysis of cyclin-dependent kinase inhibitor genes (CDKN2A, CDKN2B, and CDKN2C) in childhood rhabdomyosarcoma. *Genes Chromosomes Cancer* 15: 217-222.

1010. Irgau I, McNicholas KW (1998). Mediastinal lipoblastoma involving the left innominate vein and the left phrenic nerve. *J Pediatr Surg* 33: 1540-1542.

1011. Isaacs H, Jr. (1985). Perinatal (congenital and neonatal) neoplasms: a report of 110 cases. *Pediatr Pathol* 3: 165-216.

1012. Isayama T, Iwasaki H, Kikuchi M (1991). Chondroblastomalike extraskeletal chondroma. *Clin Orthop* 214-217.

1013. Ishida T, Iijima T, Kikuchi F, Kitagawa T, Tanida T, Imamura T, Machinami R (1992). A clinicopathological and immunohistochemical study of osteofibrous dysplasia, differentiated adamantinoma, and adamantinoma of long bones. *Skeletal Radiol* 21: 493-502.

1014. Ishida T, Yamamoto M, Goto T, Kawano H, Yamamoto A, Machinami R (1999). Clear cell chondrosarcoma of the pelvis in a skeletally immature patient. *Skeletal Radiol* 28: 290-293.

1015. Iwama T, Mishima Y, Utsunomiya J (1993). The impact of familial adenomatous polyposis on the tumorigenesis and mortality at the several organs. Its rational treatment. *Ann Surg* 217: 101-108.

1016. Iwasaki H, Enjoji M (1974). Fibrous hamartoma of infancy: report of two cases. *Jpn J Cancer Clin* 20: 216-220.

1017. Iwasaki H, Enjoji M (1979). Infantile and adult fibrosarcomas of the soft tissues. *Acta Pathol Jpn* 29: 377-388.

1018. Iwasaki H, Ishiguro M, Ohjimi Y, Ikegami H, Takeuchi T, Kikuchi M, Kaneko Y, Ariyoshi A (1999). Synovial sarcoma of the prostate with t(X;18)(p11.2;q11.2). *Am J Surg Pathol* 23: 220-226.

1019. Iwasaki H, Kikuchi M, Eimoto T, Enjoji M, Yoh S, Sakurai H (1983). Juvenile aponeurotic fibroma: an ultrastructural study. *Ultrastruct Pathol* 4: 75-83.

1020. Iwasaki H, Kikuchi M, Mori R, Miyazono J, Enjoji M, Shinohara N, Matsuzaki A (1980). Infantile digital fibromatosis. Ultrastructural, histochemical, and tissue culture observations. *Cancer* 46: 2238-2247.

1021. Iwasaki H, Ohjimi Y, Ishiguro M, Isayama T, Kaneko Y, Yoh S, Emoto G, Kikuchi M (1996). Epithelioid sarcoma with an 18q aberration. *Cancer Genet Cytogenet* 91: 46-52.

1022. Jackson RP, Reckling FW, Mants FA (1977). Osteoid osteoma and osteoblastoma. Similar histologic lesions with different natural histories. *Clin Orthop* 303-313.

1023. Jacobs JL, Merriam JC, Chadburn A, Garvin J, Housepian E, Hilal SK (1994). Mesenchymal chondrosarcoma of the orbit. Report of three new cases and review of the literature. *Cancer* 73: 399-405.

1024. Jaffe HL (1935). Osteoid osteoma: a benign osteoblastic tumor composed of osteoid and atypical bone. *Arch Surg* 31: 709.

1025. Jaffe HL (1958). *Tumors and tumorous conditions of the bones and joints*. Lea & Febiger: Philadelphia.

1026. Jaffe HL, Lichtenstein L (1944). Eosinophilic granuloma of bone: a condition affecting one, several or many bones, but apparently limited to the skeleton and representing the mildest clinical expression of the peculiar inflammatory histiocytosis also underlying Letterer-Siwe disease and Schuller-Christian disease. *Arch Pathol* 37: 99.

1027. Jaffe HL, Lichtenstein L, Sutro CJ (1941). Pigmented villonodular synovitis, bursitis and tenosynovitis: a discussion of the synovial and bursal equivalents of the tenosynovial lesion commonly denoted as xanthoma, xanthogranuloma, giant cell tumor or myeloplaxoma of the tendon sheath, with some consideration of this tendon sheath lesion itself. *Arch Pathol* 31: 731-765.

1028. Jambhekar NA, Baraniya J, Barush R, Joshi U, Badhwar R (1997). Extraskeletal myxoid chondrosarcoma: a clinicopathologic, histochemical, and immunohistochemical study of 10 cases. *Int J Surg Pathol* 5: 77-82.

1029. Janoyer M, Reau AF, Pontallier JR, Zipoli B, Colombani JF (1999). Congenital fibrous hamartoma of the hand: a case report. *J Pediatr Orthop B* 8: 129-131.

1030. Jarvi OH, Lansimies PH (1975). Subclinical elastofibromas in the scapular region in an autopsy series. *Acta Pathol Microbiol Scand [A]* 83: 87-108.

1031. Jarvi OH, Saxen AE, Hopsu-Havu VK, Wartiovaara JJ, Vaissalo VT (1969). Elastofibroma – a degenerative pseudotumor. *Cancer* 23: 42-63.

1032. Jarvinen HJ (1987). Desmoid disease as a part of familial adenomatous polyposis coli. *Acta Chir Scand* 153: 379-383.

1033. Jarvinen HJ (1992). Epidemiology of familial adenomatous polyposis in Finland: impact of family screening on the colorectal cancer rate and survival. *Gut* 33: 357-360.

1034. Jebson PJ, Louis DS (1997). Fibrous hamartoma of infancy in the hand: a case report. *J Hand Surg [Am]* 22: 740-742.

1035. Jee WH, Choi KH, Choe BY, Park JM, Shinn KS (1996). Fibrous dysplasia: MR imaging characteristics with radiopathologic correlation. *AJR Am J Roentgenol* 167: 1523-1527.

1036. Jelinek JS, Kransdorf MJ, Shmookler BM, Aboulafia AA, Malawer MM (1994). Giant cell tumor of the tendon sheath: MR findings in nine cases. *AJR Am J Roentgenol* 162: 919-922.

1037. Jennings TA, Duray PH, Collins FS, Sabetta J, Enzinger FM (1984). Infantile myofibromatosis. Evidence for an autosomal-dominant disorder. *Am J Surg Pathol* 8: 529-538.

1038. Jeon IS, Davis JN, Braun BS, Sublett JE, Roussel MF, Denny CT, Shapiro DN (1995). A variant Ewing's sarcoma translocation (7;22) fuses the EWS gene to the ETS gene ETV1. *Oncogene* 10: 1229-1234.

1039. Johansson L, Carlen B (1994). Sarcoma of the pulmonary artery: report of four cases with electron microscopic and immunohistochemical examinations, and review of the literature. *Virchows Arch* 424: 217-224.

1040. Johnson DB, McGrath F, Ryan MJ (1995). Laryngeal chondroma: an unusual cause of upper airway obstruction. *Clin Radiol* 50: 412-413.

1041. Johnson L (1972). Congenital pseudoarthrosis, adamantinoma of long bone and intracortical fibrous dysplasia of the tibia. *J Bone Joint Surg Am* 54A: 1355.

1042. Johnson LL, Kempson RL (1965). Epidermoid carcinoma in chronic osteomyelitis: diagnostic problems and management. *J Bone Joint Surg* 47A: 133-144.

1043. Johnson RL, Rothman AL, Xie J, Goodrich LV, Bare JW, Bonifas JM, Quinn AG, Myers RM, Cox DR, Epstein EH, Jr., Scott MP (1996). Human homolog of patched, a candidate gene for the basal cell nevus syndrome. *Science* 272: 1668-1671.

1044. Jones EC, Clement PB, Young RH (1993). Inflammatory pseudotumor of the urinary bladder. A clinicopathological, immunohistochemical, ultrastructural, and flow cytometric study of 13 cases. *Am J Surg Pathol* 17: 264-274.

1045. Jones EW, Winkelmann RK, Zachary CB, Reda AM (1990). Benign lymphangioendothelioma. *J Am Acad Dermatol* 23: 229-235.

1046. Jones FE, Soule EH, Coventry MB (1969). Fibrous xanthoma of synovium (giant-cell tumor of tendon sheath, pigmented nodular synovitis). A study of one hundred and eighteen cases. *J Bone Joint Surg Am* 51: 76-86.

1047. Jones IT, Jagelman DG, Fazio VW, Lavery IC, Weakley FL, McGannon E (1986). Desmoid tumors in familial polyposis coli. *Ann Surg* 204: 94-97.

1048. Joyama S, Ueda T, Shimizu K, Kudawara I, Mano M, Funai H, Takemura K, Yoshikawa H (1999). Chromosome rearrangement at 17q25 and xp11.2 in alveolar soft-part sarcoma: A case report and review of the literature. *Cancer* 86: 1246-1250.

1049. Jundt G, Moll C, Nidecker A, Schilt R, Remagen W (1994). Primary leiomyosarcoma of bone: report of eight cases. *Hum Pathol* 25: 1205-1212.

1050. Jundt G, Remberger K, Roessner A, Schulz A, Bohndorf K (1995). Adamantinoma of long bones. A histopathological and immunohistochemical study of 23 cases. *Pathol Res Pract* 191: 112-120.

1051. Kaiser TE, Pritchard DJ, Unni KK (1984). Clinicopathologic study of sacrococcygeal chordoma. *Cancer* 53: 2574-2578.

1052. Kaiserling E, Ruck P, Handgretinger R, Leipoldt M, Hipfel R (1996). Immunohistochemical and cytogenetic findings in malignant rhabdoid tumor. *Gen Diagn Pathol* 141: 327-337.

1053. Kaji M, Konishi K, Funaki K, Nukui A, Goka T, Arakawa G, Onishi I, Kimura H, Maeda K, Yabushita K, Tsuji M, Yamashita H, Miwa A (1999). [A case of low-grade fibromyxoid sarcoma of the small bowel mesentery]. *Nippon Shokakibyo Gakkai Zasshi* 96: 670-674.

1054. Kalil RK, Inwards CY, Unni KK, Bertoni F, Bacchini P, Wenger DE, Sim FH (2000). Dedifferentiated clear cell chondrosarcoma. *Am J Surg Pathol* 24: 1079-1086.

1055. Kamineni S, Briggs TW, Saifuddin A, Sandison A (2001). Osteofibrous dysplasia of the ulna. *J Bone Joint Surg Br* 83: 1178-1180.

1056. Kamysz JW, Zawin JK, Gonzalez-Crussi F (1996). Soft tissue chondroma of the neck: a case report and review of the literature. *Pediatr Radiol* 26: 145-147.

1057. Kan AE, Rogers M (1989). Juvenile hyaline fibromatosis: an expanded clinicopathologic spectrum. *Pediatr Dermatol* 6: 68-75.

1058. Kanamori M, Antonescu CR, Scott M, Bridge RS, Jr., Neff JR, Spanier SS, Scarborough MT, Vergara G, Rosenthal HG, Bridge JA (2001). Extra copies of chromosomes 7, 8, 12, 19, and 21 are recurrent in adamantinoma. *J Mol Diagn* 3: 16-21.

1059. Kandii E (1970). Dermal angiolymphoid hyperplasia with eosinophilia versus pseudopyogenic granuloma. *Br J Dermatol* 83: 405-408.

1060. Kaneko Y, Yoshida K, Handa M, Toyoda Y, Nishihira H, Tanaka Y, Sasaki Y, Ishida S, Higashino F, Fujinaga K (1996). Fusion of an ETS-family gene, EIAF, to EWS by t(17;22)(q12;q12) chromosome translocation in an undifferentiated sarcoma of infancy. *Genes Chromosomes Cancer* 15: 115-121.

1061. Kanoe H, Nakayama T, Hosaka T, Murakami H, Yamamoto H, Nakashima Y, Tsuboyama T, Nakamura T, Ron D, Sasaki MS, Toguchida J (1999). Characteristics of genomic breakpoints in TLS-CHOP translocations in liposarcomas suggest the involvement of Translin and topoisomerase II in the process of translocation. *Oncogene* 18: 721-729.

1062. Kanter WR, Wolfort FG (1988). Multiple familial angiolipomatosis: treatment of liposuction. *Ann Plast Surg* 20: 277-279.

1063. Kapadia SB, Barnes L (1996). Muscle Tissue Neoplasms. In: *Surgical Pathology of Laryngeal Neoplasms*, Ferlito A, ed. Chapman & Hall: London, pp. 321-340.

1064. Kapadia SB, Meis JM, Frisman DM, Ellis GL, Heffner DK (1993). Fetal rhabdomyoma of the head and neck: a clinicopathologic and immunophenotypic study of 24 cases. *Hum Pathol* 24: 754-765.

1065. Kapadia SB, Meis JM, Frisman DM, Ellis GL, Heffner DK, Hyams VJ (1993). Adult rhabdomyoma of the head and neck: a clinicopathologic and immunophenotypic study. *Hum Pathol* 24: 608-617.

1066. Kapadia SB, Norris HJ (1993). Rhabdomyoma of the vagina. *Mod Pathol* 6: 75A.

1067. Kaplan RP, Wang JT, Amron DM, Kaplan L (1993). Maffucci's syndrome: two case reports with a literature review. *J Am Acad Dermatol* 29: 894-899.

1068. Karakousis CP, Berjian RA, Lopez R, Rao U (1978). Mesenteric fibromatosis in Gardner's syndrome. *Arch Surg* 113: 998-1000.

1069. Karlis V, Glickman RS, Zaslow M (1998). Synovial chondromatosis of the temporomandibular joint with intracranial extension. *Oral Surg Oral Med Oral Pathol Oral Radiol Endod* 86: 664-666.

1070. Karlsson P, Holmberg E, Samuelsson A, Johansson KA, Wallgren A (1998). Soft tissue sarcoma after treatment for breast cancer – a Swedish population-based study. *Eur J Cancer* 34: 2068-2075.

1071. Karnak I, Senocak ME, Ciftci AO, Caglar M, Bingol-Kologlu M, Tanyel FC, Buyukpamukcu N (2001). Inflammatory myofibroblastic tumor in children: diagnosis and treatment. *J Pediatr Surg* 36: 908-912.

1072. Karras SC, Wolford LM, Cottrell DA (1996). Concurrent osteochondroma of the mandibular condyle and ipsilateral cranial base resulting in temporomandibular joint ankylosis: report of a case and review of the literature. *J Oral Maxillofac Surg* 54: 640-646.

1073. Katagiri K, Takasaki S, Fujiwara S, Kayashima K, Ono T, Shinkai H (1996). Purification and structural analysis of extracellular matrix of a skin tumor from a patient with juvenile hyaline fibromatosis. *J Dermatol Sci* 13: 37-48.

1074. Kataoka Y, Matsuda M, Katsura T, Tanaka K, Ebara H, Yoshida F, Takaba E, Takimoto M (1997). [Case of low-grade fibromyxoid sarcoma]. *Nippon Naika Gakkai Zasshi* 86: 1458-1460.

1075. Katou F, Motegi K, Baba S (1989). Mandibular lesions in patients with adenomatosis coli. *J Craniomaxillofac Surg* 17: 354-358.

1076. Kawagishi N, Kashiwagi T, Ibe M, Manabe A, Ishida-Yamamoto A, Hashimoto Y, Iizuka H (2000). Pleomorphic angioleiomyoma. *Am J Dermatopathol* 22: 268-271.

1077. Kawai A, Woodruff J, Healey JH, Brennan MF, Antonescu CR, Ladanyi M (1998). SYT-SSX gene fusion as a determinant of morphology and prognosis in synovial sarcoma. *N Engl J Med* 338: 153-160.

1078. Kawasaki G, Yanamoto S, Mizuno A, Fujita S (2001). Juvenile hyaline fibromatosis complicated with oral squamous cell carcinoma: a case report. *Oral Surg Oral Med Oral Pathol Oral Radiol Endod* 91: 200-204.

1079. Kawashima A, Magid D, Fishman EK, Hruban RH, Ney DR (1993). Parosteal ossifying lipoma: CT and MR findings. *J Comput Assist Tomogr* 17: 147-150.

1080. Kazmierczak B, Dal Cin P, Sciot R, van den Berghe H, Bullerdiek J (1999). Inflammatory myofibroblastic tumor with HMGIC rearrangement. *Cancer Genet Cytogenet* 112: 156-160.

1081. Kazmierczak B, Dal Cin P, Wanschura S, Bartnitzke S, van den Berghe H, Bullerdiek J (1998). Cloning and molecular characterization of part of a new gene fused to HMGIC in mesenchymal tumors. *Am J Pathol* 152: 431-435.

1082. Kazmierczak B, Dal Cin P, Wanschura S, Borrmann L, Fusco A, van den Berghe H, Bullerdiek J (1998). HMGIY is the target of 6p21.3 rearrangements in various benign mesenchymal tumors. *Genes Chromosomes Cancer* 23: 279-285.

1083. Keel SB, Jaffe KA, Petur NG, Rosenberg AE (2001). Orthopaedic implant-related sarcoma: a study of twelve cases. *Mod Pathol* 14: 969-977.

1084. Keeney GL, Unni KK, Beabout JW, Pritchard DJ (1989). Adamantinoma of long bones. A clinicopathologic study of 85 cases. *Cancer* 64: 730-737.

1085. Kelly KM, Womer RB, Sorensen PH, Xiong QB, Barr FG (1997). Common and variant gene fusions predict distinct clinical phenotypes in rhabdomyosarcoma. *J Clin Oncol* 15: 1831-1836.

1086. Kempson RL, Fletcher CD, Evans HL, Hendrickson MR, Sibley RK (2001). *Atlas of Tumor Pathology. Tumors of Soft Tissues.* AFIP: Washington, DC.

1087. Kempson RL, Fletcher CD, Evans HL, Hendrickson MR, Sibley RK (2001). Cartilagineous and osseous tumors. In: *Atlas of Tumor Pathology. Tumors of Soft Tissues.* AFIP: Washington, DC.

1088. Kempson RL, Kyriakos M (1972). Fibroxanthosarcoma of the soft tissues. A type of malignant fibrous histiocytoma. *Cancer* 29: 961-976.

1089. Kenan S, Floman Y, Robin GC, Laufer A (1985). Aggressive osteoblastoma. A case report and review of the literature. *Clin Orthop* 294-298.

1090. Kenan S, Lewis MM, Abdelwahab IF, Hermann G, Klein MJ (1991). Case report 652: Primary intraosseous low grade myxoid sarcoma of the scapula (myxoid liposarcoma). *Skeletal Radiol* 20: 73-75.

1091. Kenn W, Stabler A, Zachoval R, Zietz C, Raum W, Wittenberg G (1999). Erdheim-Chester disease: a case report and literature overview. *Eur Radiol* 9: 153-158.

1092. Kenney PJ, Gilula LA, Murphy WA (1981). The use of computed tomography to distinguish osteochondroma and chondrosarcoma. *Radiology* 139: 129-137.

1093. Kern WH (1960). Proliferative myositis: a pseudosarcomatous reaction to injury: a report of seven cases. *Arch Pathol* 69: 209-215.

1094. Keser G, Karabulut B, Oksel F, Calli C, Ustun EE, Akalin T, Kocanaogullari H, Gumudis G, Doganavsargil E (1999). Two siblings with juvenile hyaline fibromatosis: case reports and review of the literature. *Clin Rheumatol* 18: 248-252.

1095. Kevorkian J, Cento DP (1973). Leiomyosarcoma of large arteries and veins. *Surgery* 73: 390-400.

1096. Khalidi HS, Singleton TP, Weiss SW (1997). Inflammatory malignant fibrous histiocytoma: distinction from Hodgkin's disease and non-Hodgkin's lymphoma by a panel of leukocyte markers. *Mod Pathol* 10: 438-442.

1097. Khan J, Bittner ML, Saal LH, Teichmann U, Azorsa DO, Gooden GC, Pavan WJ, Trent JM, Meltzer PS (1999). cDNA microarrays detect activation of a myogenic transcription program by the PAX3-FKHR fusion oncogene. *Proc Natl Acad Sci U S A* 96: 13264-13269.

1098. Khatib ZA, Matsushime H, Valentine M, Shapiro DN, Sherr CJ, Look AT (1993). Coamplification of the CDK4 gene with MDM2 and GLI in human sarcomas. *Cancer Res* 53: 5535-5541.

1099. Khoddami M, Bedard YC, Bell RS, Kandel RA (1996). Primary leiomyosarcoma of bone: report of seven cases and review of the literature. *Arch Pathol Lab Med* 120: 671-675.

1100. Kido A, Schneider-Stock R, Hauptmann K, Roessner A (1999). Telomerase activity in benign bone tumors and tumor-like lesions. *Pathol Res Pract* 195: 753-757.

1101. Kihara S, Nehlsen-Cannarella N, Kirsch WM, Chase D, Garvin AJ (1996). A comparative study of apoptosis and cell proliferation in infantile and adult fibrosarcomas. *Am J Clin Pathol* 106: 493-497.

1102. Kilpatrick SE (1999). Histologic prognostication in soft tissue sarcomas: grading versus subtyping or both? A comprehensive review of the literature with proposed practical guidelines. *Ann Diagn Pathol* 3: 48-61.

1103. Kilpatrick SE, Doyon J, Choong PF, Sim FH, Nascimento AG (1996). The clinicopathologic spectrum of myxoid and round cell liposarcoma. A study of 95 cases. *Cancer* 77: 1450-1458.

1104. Kilpatrick SE, Hitchcock MG, Kraus MD, Calonje E, Fletcher CD (1997). Mixed tumors and myoepitheliomas of soft tissue: a clinicopathologic study of 19 cases with a unifying concept. *Am J Surg Pathol* 21: 13-22.

1105. Kilpatrick SE, Inwards CY, Fletcher CD, Smith MA, Gitelis S (1997). Myxoid chondrosarcoma (chordoid sarcoma) of bone: a report of two cases and review of the literature. *Cancer* 79: 1903-1910.

1106. Kilpatrick SE, Mentzel T, Fletcher CD (1994). Leiomyoma of deep soft tissue. Clinicopathologic analysis of a series. *Am J Surg Pathol* 18: 576-582.

1107. Kilpatrick SE, Teot LA, Geisinger KR, Martin PL, Shumate DK, Zbieranski N, Russell GB, Fletcher CD (1994). Relationship of DNA ploidy to histology and prognosis in rhabdomyosarcoma. Comparison of flow cytometry and image analysis. *Cancer* 74: 3227-3233.

1108. Kim BT, Kitagawa H, Tamura J, Saito T, Kusche-Gullberg M, Lindahl U, Sugahara K (2001). Human tumor suppressor EXT gene family members EXTL1 and EXTL3 encode alpha 1,4- N-acetylglucosaminyltransferases that likely are involved in heparan sulfate/heparin biosynthesis. *Proc Natl Acad Sci U S A* 98: 7176-7181.

1109. Kim YC (2000). An additional case of solitary subungual glomus tumor associated with neurofibromatosis 1. *J Dermatol* 27: 418-419.

1110. Kim YH, Reiner L (1982). Ultrastructure of lipoma. *Cancer* 50: 102-106.

1111. Kindblom LG, Angervall L (1978). Congenital solitary fibromatosis of the skeleton: case report of a variant of congenital generalized fibromatosis. *Cancer* 41: 636-640.

1112. Kindblom LG, Angervall L, Fassina AS (1982). Atypical lipoma. *Acta Pathol Microbiol Immunol Scand [A]* 90: 27-36.

1113. Kindblom LG, Angervall L, Stener B, Wickbom I (1974). Intermuscular and intramuscular lipomas and hibernomas. A clinical, roentgenologic, histologic, and prognostic study of 46 cases. *Cancer* 33: 754-762.

1114. Kindblom LG, Angervall L, Svendsen P (1975). Liposarcoma a clinicopathologic, radiographic and prognostic study. *Acta Pathol Microbiol Scand Suppl* 1-71.

1115. Kindblom LG, Lodding P, Angervall L (1983). Clear-cell sarcoma of tendons and aponeuroses. An immunohistochemical and electron microscopic analysis indicating neural crest origin. *Virchows Arch A Pathol Anat Histopathol* 401: 109-128.

1116. Kindblom LG, Meis-Kindblom JM (1995). Chondroid lipoma: an ultrastructural and immunohistochemical analysis with further observations regarding its differentiation. *Hum Pathol* 26: 706-715.

1117. Kindblom LG, Merck C, Angervall L (1979). The ultrastructure of myxofibrosarcoma. A study of 11 cases. *Virchows Arch A Pathol Anat Histol* 381: 121-139.

1118. Kindblom LG, Spicer SS (1982). Elastofibroma. A correlated light and electron microscopic study. *Virchows Arch A Pathol Anat Histol* 396: 127-140.

1119. Kindblom LG, Stener B, Angervall L (1974). Intramuscular myxoma. *Cancer* 34: 1737-1744.

1120. Kindblom LG, Stenman G, Angervall L (1991). Morphological and cytogenetic studies of angiosarcoma in Stewart-Treves syndrome. *Virchows Arch A Pathol Anat Histopathol* 419: 439-445.

1121. King DG, Saifuddin A, Preston HV, Hardy GJ, Reeves BF (1995). Magnetic resonance imaging of juxta-articular myxoma. *Skeletal Radiol* 24: 145-147.

1122. Kinoshita Y, Shiratsuchi H, Tamiya S, Oshiro Y, Hachitanda Y, Oda Y, Suita S, Tsuneyoshi M (2001). Mutations of the p53 gene in malignant rhabdoid tumors of soft tissue and the kidney: immunohistochemical and DNA direct sequencing analysis. *J Cancer Res Clin Oncol* 127: 351-358.

1123. Kinzler KW, Nilbert MC, Su LK, Vogelstein B, Bryan TM, Levy DB, Smith KJ, Preisinger AC, Hedge P, McKechnie D (1991). Identification of FAP locus genes from chromosome 5q21. *Science* 253: 661-665.

1124. Kinzler KW, Vogelstein B (1996). Lessons from hereditary colorectal cancer. *Cell* 87: 159-170.

1125. Kirkpatrick CJ, Alves A, Kohler H, Kriegsmann J, Bittinger F, Otto M, Williams DF, Eloy R (2000). Biomaterial-induced sarcoma: A novel model to study preneoplastic change. *Am J Pathol* 156: 1455-1467.

1126. Kirwan EO, Hutton PA, Pozo JL, Ransford AO (1984). Osteoid osteoma and benign osteoblastoma of the spine. Clinical presentation and treatment. *J Bone Joint Surg Br* 66: 21-26.

1127. Kitagawa H, Shimakawa H, Sugahara K (1999). The tumor suppressor EXT-like gene EXTL2 encodes an alpha1, 4-N-acetylhexosaminyltransferase that transfers N-acetylgalactosamine and N-acetylglucosamine to the common glycosaminoglycan-protein linkage region. The key enzyme for the chain initiation of heparan sulfate. *J Biol Chem* 274: 13933-13937.

1128. Kitao S, Shimoto A, Goto M, Miller RW, Smithson WA, Lindor NM, Furuichi Y (1999). Mutations in RECQL4 cause a subset of cases of Rothmund-Thomson syndrome. *Nat Genet* 22: 82-84.

1129. Kitoh H, Nogami H (1999). A simple bone cyst containing secretory cells in its lining membrane in a patient with polyostotic fibrous dysplasia. *Pediatr Radiol* 29: 481-483.

1130. Kiuru-Kuhlefelt S, Sarlomo-Rikala M, Larramendy ML, Soderlund M, Hedman K, Miettinen M, Knuutila S (2000). FGF4 and INT2 oncogenes are amplified and expressed in Kaposi's sarcoma. *Mod Pathol* 13: 433-437.

1131. Kivioja A, Ervasti H, Kinnunen J, Kaitila I, Wolf M, Böhling T (2000). Chondrosarcoma in a family with multiple hereditary exostoses. *J Bone Joint Surg Br* 82: 261-266.

1132. Kiyosawa T, Umebayashi Y, Nakayama Y, Soeda S (1995). Hereditary multiple glomus tumors involving the glans penis. A case report and review of the literature. *Dermatol Surg* 21: 895-899.

1133. Kjellman M, Larsson C, Backdahl M (2001). Genetic background of adrenocortical tumor development. *World J Surg* 25: 948-956.

1134. Kleer CG, Unni KK, McLeod RA (1996). Epithelioid hemangioendothelioma of bone. *Am J Surg Pathol* 20: 1301-1311.

1135. Klein FA, Smith MJ, Kasenetz I (1988). Pelvic lipomatosis: 35-year experience. *J Urol* 139: 998-1001.

1136. Kleinstiver BJ, Rodriguez HA (1968). Nodular fasciitis. A study of forty-five cases and review of the literature. *J Bone Joint Surg Am* 50: 1204-1212.

1137. Klemmer S, Pascoe L, DeCosse J (1987). Occurrence of desmoids in patients with familial adenomatous polyposis of the colon. *Am J Med Genet* 28: 385-392.

1138. Klieger MR, Schultz E, Elkowitz DE, Arlen M, Hajdu SI (2002). Erdheim-Chester Disease: A Unique Presentation with Multiple Osteolytic Lesions of the Spine and Pelvis that Spared the Appendicular Skeleton. *AJR Am J Roentgenol* 178: 429-432.

1139. Klimstra DS, Moran CA, Perino G, Koss MN, Rosai J (1995). Liposarcoma of the anterior mediastinum and thymus. A clinicopathologic study of 28 cases. *Am J Surg Pathol* 19: 782-791.

1140. Klopstock T, Naumann M, Seibel P, Shalke B, Reiners K, Reichmann H (1997). Mitochondrial DNA mutations in multiple symmetric lipomatosis. *Mol Cell Biochem* 174: 271-275.

1141. Knezevich SR, Garnett MJ, Pysher TJ, Beckwith JB, Grundy PE, Sorensen PH (1998). ETV6-NTRK3 gene fusions and trisomy 11 establish a histogenetic link between mesoblastic nephroma and congenital fibrosarcoma. *Cancer Res* 58: 5046-5048.

1142. Knezevich SR, McFadden DE, Tao W, Lim JF, Sorensen PH (1998). A novel ETV6-NTRK3 gene fusion in congenital fibrosarcoma. *Nat Genet* 18: 184-187.

1143. Knight JC, Renwick PJ, Dal Cin P, van den Berghe H, Fletcher CD (1995). Translocation t(12;16)(q13;p11) in myxoid liposarcoma and round cell liposarcoma: molecular and cytogenetic analysis. *Cancer Res* 55: 24-27.

1144. Knowles DM, Pirog EC (2001). Pathology of AIDS-related lymphomas and other AIDS-defining neoplasms. *Eur J Cancer* 37: 1236-1250.

1145. Knudson AG, Jr. (1971). Mutation and cancer: statistical study of retinoblastoma. *Proc Natl Acad Sci U S A* 68: 820-823.

1146. Knuutila S, Autio K, Aalto Y (2000). Online access to CGH data of DNA sequence copy number changes. *Am J Pathol* 157: 689.

1147. Kobayashi S, Yamadori I, Ohmori M, Akaeda T (1992). Benign fibrous histiocytoma of the renal capsule. *Acta Pathol Jpn* 42: 217-220.

1148. Kocova L, Michal M, Sulc M, Zamecnik M (1997). Calcifying fibrous pseudotumour of visceral peritoneum. *Histopathology* 31: 182-184.

1149. Kodet R, Newton WA, Jr., Hamoudi AB, Asmar L, Jacobs DL, Maurer HM (1993). Childhood rhabdomyosarcoma with anaplastic (pleomorphic) features. A report of the Intergroup Rhabdomyosarcoma Study. *Am J Surg Pathol* 17: 443-453.

1150. Kodet R, Newton WA, Jr., Sachs N, Hamoudi AB, Raney RB, Asmar L, Gehan EA (1991). Rhabdoid tumors of soft tissues: a clinicopathologic study of 26 cases enrolled on the Intergroup Rhabdomyosarcoma Study. *Hum Pathol* 22: 674-684.

1151. Kodet R, Stejskal J, Pilat D, Kocourkova M, Smelhaus V, Eckschlager T (1996). Congenital-infantile fibrosarcoma: a clinicopathological study of five patients entered on the Prague children's tumor registry. *Pathol Res Pract* 192: 845-853.

1152. Koi M, Johnson LA, Kalikin LM, Little PF, Nakamura Y, Feinberg AP (1993). Tumor cell growth arrest caused by subchromosomal transferable DNA fragments from chromosome 11. *Science* 260: 361-364.

1153. Kondo S, Yoshizaki T, Minato H, Horikawa I, Tatsumi A, Furukawa M (2001). Myofibrosarcoma of the nasal cavity and paranasal sinus. *Histopathology* 39: 216-217.

1154. Konigsberg R, Zojer N, Ackermann J, Kromer E, Kittler H, Fritz E, Kaufmann H, Nosslinger T, Riedl L, Gisslinger H, Jager U, Simonitsch I, Heinz R, Ludwig H, Huber H, Drach J (2000). Predictive role of interphase cytogenetics for survival of patients with multiple myeloma. *J Clin Oncol* 18: 804-812.

1155. Konrad EA, Meister P, Hubner G (1982). Extracardiac rhabdomyoma: report of different types with light microscopic and ultrastructural studies. *Cancer* 49: 898-907.

1156. Konwaler B, Keasbey L, Kaplan L (1955). Subcutaneous pseudosarcomatous fibromatosis (fasciitis). *Am J Clin Pathol* 25: 241-252.

1157. Kopelman JE, McLean IW, Rosenberg SH (1987). Multivariate analysis of risk factors for metastasis in retinoblastoma treated by enucleation. *Ophthalmology* 94: 371-377.

1158. Koscielniak E, Rodary C, Flamant F, Carli M, Treuner J, Pinkerton CR, Grotto P (1992). Metastatic rhabdomyosarcoma and histologically similar tumors in childhood: a retrospective European multi-center analysis. *Med Pediatr Oncol* 20: 209-214.

1159. Kotz R, Salzer-Kuntschik M, Lechner G, Immenkamp M, Kogelnik HD, Salzer M (1984). *Knochentumoren*. Georg Thieme Verlag: Stuttgart, New York.

1160. Koufos A, Hansen MF, Copeland NG, Jenkins NA, Lampkin BC, Cavenee WK (1985). Loss of heterozygosity in three embryonal tumours suggests a common pathogenetic mechanism. *Nature* 316: 330-334.

1161. Kouho H, Aoki T, Hisaoka M, Hashimoto H (1997). Clinicopathological and interphase cytogenetic analysis of desmoid tumours. *Histopathology* 31: 336-341.

1162. Kovar H, Jug G, Aryee DN, Zoubek A, Ambros P, Gruber B, Windhager R, Gadner H (1997). Among genes involved in the RB dependent cell cycle regulatory cascade, the p16 tumor suppressor gene is frequently lost in the Ewing family of tumors. *Oncogene* 15: 2225-2232.

1163. Kovarik P, et al. (1998). Ploidy, proliferative activity, and p53 as biologic markers in inflammatory myofibroblastic tumors. *Mod Pathol* 11: 43A.

1164. Kozlowski K, Scougall JS, Oates RK (1980). Osteosarcoma in a boy with Rothmund-Thomson syndrome. *Pediatr Radiol* 10: 42-45.

1165. Kragh LV, Dahlin DC, Erich JB (1958). Osteogenic sarcoma of the jaws and facial bones. *Am J Surg* 96: 496-505.

1166. Kramer K, Hicks DG, Palis J, Rosier RN, Oppenheimer J, Fallon MD, Cohen HJ (1993). Epithelioid osteosarcoma of bone. Immunocytochemical evidence suggesting divergent epithelial and mesenchymal differentiation in a primary osseous neoplasm. *Cancer* 71: 2977-2982.

1167. Krane JF, Bertoni F, Fletcher CD (1999). Myxoid synovial sarcoma: an underappreciated morphologic subset. *Mod Pathol* 12: 456-462.

1168. Kransdorf MJ (1995). Malignant soft-tissue tumors in a large referral population: distribution of diagnoses by age, sex, and location. *AJR Am J Roentgenol* 164: 129-134.

1169. Kransdorf MJ, Meis JM, Jelinek JS (1991). Myositis ossificans: MR appearance with radiologic-pathologic correlation. *AJR Am J Roentgenol* 157: 1243-1248.

1170. Kransdorf MJ, Meis JM, Montgomery E (1992). Elastofibroma: MR and CT appearance with radiologic-pathologic correlation. *AJR Am J Roentgenol* 159: 575-579.

1171. Kransdorf MJ, Moser RP, Jr., Jelinek JS, Weiss SW, Buetow PC, Berrey BH (1989). Intramuscular myxoma: MR features. *J Comput Assist Tomogr* 13: 836-839.

1172. Kransdorf MJ, Moser RP, Jr., Meis JM, Meyer CA (1991). Fat-containing soft-tissue masses of the extremities. *Radiographics* 11: 81-106.

1173. Kransdorf MJ, Sweet DE (1995). Aneurysmal bone cyst: concept, controversy, clinical presentation, and imaging. *AJR Am J Roentgenol* 164: 573-580.

1174. Kraus MD, Guillou L, Fletcher CD (1997). Well-differentiated inflammatory liposarcoma: an uncommon and easily overlooked variant of a common sarcoma. *Am J Surg Pathol* 21: 518-527.

1175. Kravcik S (2000). HIV lipodystrophy: a review. *HIV Clin Trials* 1: 37-50.

1176. Krawczak M, Cooper DN (1997). The human gene mutation database. *Trends Genet* 13: 121-122.

1177. Krempl GA, McGuff HS, Pulitzer DR, Otto RA (1997). Lipoblastoma in the parotid gland of an infant. *Otolaryngol Head Neck Surg* 117: S234-S237.

1178. Kronland R, Grogan T, Spier C, Wirt D, Rangel C, Richter L, Durie B, Greenberg B, Miller T, Jones S (1985). Immunotopographic assessment of lymphoid and plasma cell malignancies in the bone marrow. *Hum Pathol* 16: 1247-1254.

1179. Kruzelock RP, Murphy EC, Strong LC, Naylor SL, Hansen MF (1997). Localization of a novel tumor suppressor locus on human chromosome 3q important in osteosarcoma tumorigenesis. *Cancer Res* 57: 106-109.

1180. Kubo K, Miyatani H, Takenoshita Y, Abe K, Oka M, Iida M, Itoh H (1989). Widespread radiopacity of jaw bones in familial adenomatosis coli. *J Craniomaxillofac Surg* 17: 350-353.

1181. Kumar S, Pack S, Kumar D, Walker R, Quezado M, Zhuang Z, Meltzer P, Tsokos M (1999). Detection of EWS-FLI-1 fusion in Ewing's sarcoma/peripheral primitive neuroectodermal tumor by fluorescence in situ hybridization using formalin-fixed paraffin-embedded tissue. *Hum Pathol* 30: 324-330.

1182. Kumaratilake JS, Krishnan R, Lomax-Smith J, Cleary EG (1991). Elastofibroma: disturbed elastic fibrillogenesis by periosteal-derived cells? An immunoelectron microscopic and in situ hybridization study. *Hum Pathol* 22: 1017-1029.

1183. Kunisada T, Ozaki T, Kawai A, Sugihara S, Taguchi K, Inoue H (1999). Imaging assessment of the responses of osteosarcoma patients to preoperative chemotherapy: angiography compared with thallium-201 scintigraphy. *Cancer* 86: 949-956.

1184. Kunze E, Enderle A, Radig K, Schneider-Stock R (1996). Aggressive osteoblastoma with focal malignant transformation and development of pulmonary metastases. A case report with a review of literature. *Gen Diagn Pathol* 141: 377-392.

1185. Kurkchubasche AG, Halvorson EG, Forman EN, Terek RM, Ferguson WS (2000). The role of preoperative chemotherapy in the treatment of infantile fibrosarcoma. *J Pediatr Surg* 35: 880-883.

1186. Kurt AM, Unni KK, McLeod RA, Pritchard DJ (1990). Low-grade intraosseous osteosarcoma. *Cancer* 65: 1418-1428.

1187. Kurtycz DF, Logrono R, Hoerl HD, Heatley DG (2000). Diagnosis of fibromatosis colli by fine-needle aspiration. *Diagn Cytopathol* 23: 338-342.

1188. Kuruvilla G, Steiner GC (1998). Osteofibrous dysplasia-like adamantinoma of bone: a report of five cases with immunohistochemical and ultrastructural studies. *Hum Pathol* 29: 809-814.

1189. Kushner BH, LaQuaglia MP, Wollner N, Meyers PA, Lindsley KL, Ghavimi F, Merchant TE, Boulad F, Cheung NK, Bonilla MA, Crouch G, Kelleher JF, Jr., Steinherz PG, Gerald WL (1996). Desmoplastic small round-cell tumor: prolonged progression-free survival with aggressive multimodality therapy. *J Clin Oncol* 14: 1526-1531.

1190. Kusuzaki K, Murata H, Takeshita H, Hirata M, Hashiguchi S, Tsuji Y, Nakamura S, Ashihara T, Hirasawa Y (1999). Usefulness of cytofluorometric DNA ploidy analysis in distinguishing benign cartilaginous tumors from chondrosarcomas. *Mod Pathol* 12: 863-872.

1191. Kusuzaki K, Takeshita H, Murata H, Hirata M, Hashiguchi S, Ashihara T, Hirasawa Y (1999). Prognostic significance of DNA ploidy pattern in osteosarcomas in association with chemotherapy. *Cancer Lett* 137: 27-33.

1192. Kwak JY, Ha DH, Kim YA, Shim JY (1999). Lipoblastoma of the parietal pleura in a 7-month-old infant. *J Comput Assist Tomogr* 23: 952-954.

1193. Kwittken J, Branche M (1969). Fasciitis ossificans. *Am J Clin Pathol* 51: 251-255.

1194. Kyle RA (1978). Monoclonal gammopathy of undetermined significance. Natural history in 241 cases. *Am J Med* 64: 814-826.

1195. Kynaston JA, Malcolm AJ, Craft AW, Davies SM, Jones PH, King DJ, Mitchell CD, Oakhill A, Stiller CA (1993). Chemotherapy in the management of infantile fibrosarcoma. *Med Pediatr Oncol* 21: 488-493.

1196. Kyriakos M (1980). Intracortical osteosarcoma. *Cancer* 46: 2525-2533.

1197. Kyriakos M, Hardy D (1991). Malignant transformation of aneurysmal bone cyst, with an analysis of the literature. *Cancer* 68: 1770-1780.

1198. Kyriakos M, Kempson RL (1976). Inflammatory fibrous histiocytoma. An aggressive and lethal lesion. *Cancer* 37: 1584-1606.

1199. L'Hostis H, Deminiere C, Ferriere JM, Coindre JM (1999). Renal angiomyolipoma: a clinicopathologic, immunohistochemical, and follow-up study of 46 cases. *Am J Surg Pathol* 23: 1011-1020.

1200. La Quaglia MP, Heller G, Ghavimi F, Casper ES, Vlamis V, Hajdu S, Brennan MF (1994). The effect of age at diagnosis on outcome in rhabdomyosarcoma. *Cancer* 73: 109-117.

1201. Labelle Y, Zucman J, Stenman G, Kindblom LG, Knight J, Turc-Carel C, Dockhorn-Dworniczak B, Mandahl N, Desmaze C, Peter M, Aurias A, Delattre O, Thomas G (1995). Oncogenic conversion of a novel orphan nuclear receptor by chromosome translocation. *Hum Mol Genet* 4: 2219-2226.

1202. Ladanyi M, Antonescu CR, Drobnjak M, Baren A, Lui MY, Golde DW, Cordon-Cardo C (2002). The pre-crystalline cytoplasmic granules of alveolar soft part sarcoma contain MCT1 and CD147. *Am J Pathol* 160: 1215-1221.

1203. Ladanyi M, Argani P, Hutchinson B, Reuter VE (2002). Prominent nuclear immunoreactivity for TFE3 as a specific marker for alveolar soft part sarcoma and pediatric renal tumors containing TFE3 gene fusions. *Mod Pathol* 15: 312A.

1204. Ladanyi M, Bridge JA (2000). Contribution of molecular genetic data to the classification of sarcomas. *Hum Pathol* 31: 532-538.

1205. Ladanyi M, Cha C, Lewis R, Jhanwar SC, Huvos AG, Healey JH (1993). MDM2 gene amplification in metastatic osteosarcoma. *Cancer Res* 53: 16-18.

1206. Ladanyi M, Gerald W (1994). Fusion of the EWS and WT1 genes in the desmoplastic small round cell tumor. *Cancer Res* 54: 2837-2840.

1207. Ladanyi M, Lui MY, Antonescu CR, Krause-Boehm A, Meindl A, Argani P, Healey JH, Ueda T, Yoshikawa H, Meloni-Ehrig A, Sorensen PH, Mertens F, Mandahl N, van den Berghe H, Sciot R, Dal Cin P, Bridge J (2001). The der(17)t(X;17)(p11;q25) of human alveolar soft part sarcoma fuses the TFE3 transcription factor gene to ASPL, a novel gene at 17q25. *Oncogene* 20: 48-57.

1208. Ladanyi M, Park CK, Lewis R, Jhanwar SC, Healey JH, Huvos AG (1993). Sporadic amplification of the MYC gene in human osteosarcomas. *Diagn Mol Pathol* 2: 163-167.

1209. Lagace R, Delage C, Seemayer TA (1979). Myxoid variant of malignant fibrous histiocytoma: ultrastructural observations. *Cancer* 43: 526-534.

1210. Lagier R, Cox JN (1975). Pseudomalignant myositis ossificans. A pathological study of eight cases. *Hum Pathol* 6: 653-665.

1211. Lam PY, Sublett JE, Hollenbach AD, Roussel MF (1999). The oncogenic potential of the Pax3-FKHR fusion protein requires the Pax3 homeodomain recognition helix but not the Pax3 paired-box DNA binding domain. *Mol Cell Biol* 19: 594-601.

1212. Lamant L, Dastugue N, Pulford K, Delsol G, Mariame B (1999). A new fusion gene TPM3-ALK in anaplastic large cell lymphoma created by a (1;2)(q25;p23) translocation. *Blood* 93: 3088-3095.

1213. Lambert I, Debiec-Rychter M, Guelinckx P, Hagemeijer A, Sciot R (2001). Acral myxoinflammatory fibroblastic sarcoma with unique clonal chromosomal changes. *Virchows Arch* 438: 509-512.

1214. Lamovec J, Spiler M, Jevtic V (1999). Osteosarcoma arising in a solitary osteochondroma of the fibula. *Arch Pathol Lab Med* 123: 832-834.

1215. Lamovec J, Zidar A, Cucek-Plenicar M (1988). Synovial sarcoma associated with total hip replacement. A case report. *J Bone Joint Surg Am* 70: 1558-1560.

1216. Lane JE, Walker AN, Mullis EN, Jr., Etheridge JG (2001). Cellular angiofibroma of the vulva. *Gynecol Oncol* 81: 326-329.

1217. Lane KL, Shannon RJ, Weiss SW (1997). Hyalinizing spindle cell tumor with giant rosettes: a distinctive tumor closely resembling low-grade fibromyxoid sarcoma. *Am J Surg Pathol* 21: 1481-1488.

1218. Lantz B, Lange TA, Heiner J, Herring GF (1989). Erdheim-Chester disease. A report of three cases. *J Bone Joint Surg Am* 71: 456-464.

1219. Larramendy ML, Tarkkanen M, Blomqvist C, Virolainen M, Wiklund T, Asko-Seljavaara S, Elomaa I, Knuutila S (1997). Comparative genomic hybridization of malignant fibrous histiocytoma reveals a novel prognostic marker. *Am J Pathol* 151: 1153-1161.

1220. Larramendy ML, Tarkkanen M, Valle J, Kivioja AH, Ervasti H, Karaharju E, Salmivalli T, Elomaa I, Knuutila S (1997). Gains, losses, and amplifications of DNA sequences evaluated by comparative genomic hybridization in chondrosarcomas. *Am J Pathol* 150: 685-691.

1221. Larsson SE, Lorentzon R, Boquist L (1976). Fibrosarcoma of bone. A demographic, clinical and histopathological study of all cases recorded in the Swedish cancer registry from 1958 to 1968. *J Bone Joint Surg Br* 58-B: 412-417.

1222. Laskin WB, Fetsch JF, Mostofi FK (1998). Angiomyofibroblastomalike tumor of the male genital tract: analysis of 11 cases with comparison to female angiomyofibroblastoma and spindle cell lipoma. *Am J Surg Pathol* 22: 6-16.

1223. Laskin WB, Fetsch JF, Tavassoli FA (1997). Angiomyofibroblastoma of the female genital tract: analysis of 17 cases including a lipomatous variant. *Hum Pathol* 28: 1046-1055.

1224. Laskin WB, Silverman TA, Enzinger FM (1988). Postradiation soft tissue sarcomas. An analysis of 53 cases. *Cancer* 62: 2330-2340.

1225. Lauer DH, Enzinger FM (1980). Cranial fasciitis of childhood. *Cancer* 45: 401-406.

1226. Lawrence B, Perez-Atayde A, Hibbard MK, Rubin BP, Dal Cin P, Pinkus JL, Pinkus GS, Xiao S, Yi ES, Fletcher CD, Fletcher JA (2000). TPM3-ALK and TPM4-ALK oncogenes in inflammatory myofibroblastic tumors. *Am J Pathol* 157: 377-384.

1227. Lawrence W, Jr., Donegan WL, Natarajan N, Mettlin C, Beart R, Winchester D (1987). Adult soft tissue sarcomas. A pattern of care survey of the American College of Surgeons. *Ann Surg* 205: 349-359.

1228. Lawrence WT, Azizkhan RG (1989). Congenital muscular torticollis: a spectrum of pathology. *Ann Plast Surg* 23: 523-530.

1229. Le Merrer M, Legeai-Mallet L, Jeannin PM, Horsthemke B, Schinzel A, Plauchu H, Toutain A, Achard F, Munnich A, Maroteaux P (1994). A gene for hereditary multiple exostoses maps to chromosome 19p. *Hum Mol Genet* 3: 717-722.

1230. Lee FY, Mankin HJ, Fondren G, Gebhardt MC, Springfield DS, Rosenberg AE, Jennings LC (1999). Chondrosarcoma of bone: an assessment of outcome. *J Bone Joint Surg Am* 81: 326-338.

1231. Lee JS, Fetsch JF, Wasdhal DA, Lee BP, Pritchard DJ, Nascimento AG (1995). A review of 40 patients with extraskeletal osteosarcoma. *Cancer* 76: 2253-2259.

1232. Lee SP, Nicholson GI, Hitchcock G (1977). Familial abdominal chemodectomas with associated cutaneous angiolipomas. *Pathology* 9: 173-177.

1233. Lee WH, Bookstein R, Hong F, Young LJ, Shew JY, Lee EY (1987). Human retinoblastoma susceptibility gene: cloning, identification, and sequence. *Science* 235: 1394-1399.

1234. Lee WH, Shew JY, Hong FD, Sery TW, Donoso LA, Young LJ, Bookstein R, Lee EY (1987). The retinoblastoma susceptibility gene encodes a nuclear phosphoprotein associated with DNA binding activity. *Nature* 329: 642-645.

1235. Legeai-Mallet L, Margaritte-Jeannin P, Lemdani M, Le Merrer M, Plauchu H, Maroteaux P, Munnich A, Clerget-Darpoux F (1997). An extension of the admixture test for the study of genetic heterogeneity in hereditary multiple exostoses. *Hum Genet* 99: 298-302.

1236. Legeai-Mallet L, Munnich A, Maroteaux P, Le Merrer M (1997). Incomplete penetrance and expressivity skewing in hereditary multiple exostoses. *Clin Genet* 52: 12-16.

1237. Legeai-Mallet L, Rossi A, Benoist-Lasselin C, Piazza R, Mallet JF, Delezoide AL, Munnich A, Bonaventure J, Zylberberg L (2000). EXT 1 gene mutation induces chondrocyte cytoskeletal abnormalities and defective collagen expression in the exostoses. *J Bone Miner Res* 15: 1489-1500.

1238. Legier JF, Tauber LN (1968). Solitary metastasis of occult prostatic carcinoma simulating osteogenic sarcoma. *Cancer* 22: 168-172.

1239. Leithner A, Windhager R, Lang S, Haas OA, Kainberger F, Kotz R (1999). Aneurysmal bone cyst. A population based epidemiologic study and literature review. *Clin Orthop* 176-179.

1240. Leone PG, Taylor HB (1973). Ultrastructure of a benign polypoid rhabdomyoma of the vagina. *Cancer* 31: 1414-1417.

1241. Leppert M, Dobbs M, Scambler P, O'Connell P, Nakamura Y, Stauffer D, Woodward S, Burt R, Hughes J, Gardner E (1987). The gene for familial polyposis coli maps to the long arm of chromosome 5. *Science* 238: 1411-1413.

1242. Lessnick SL, Braun BS, Denny CT, May WA (1995). Multiple domains mediate transformation by the Ewing's sarcoma EWS/FLI-1 fusion gene. *Oncogene* 10: 423-431.

1243. Leu HJ, Makek M (1986). Intramural venous leiomyosarcomas. *Cancer* 57: 1395-1400.

1244. Lewis JE, Olsen KD, Inwards CY (1997). Cartilaginous tumors of the larynx: clinicopathologic review of 47 cases. *Ann Otol Rhinol Laryngol* 106: 94-100.

1245. Lewis JJ, Antonescu CR, Leung DH, Blumberg D, Healey JH, Woodruff JM, Brennan MF (2000). Synovial sarcoma: a multivariate analysis of prognostic factors in 112 patients with primary localized tumors of the extremity. *J Clin Oncol* 18: 2087-2094.

1246. Lewis JJ, Boland PJ, Leung DH, Woodruff JM, Brennan MF (1999). The enigma of desmoid tumors. *Ann Surg* 229: 866-872.

1247. Lewis JJ, Leung D, Woodruff JM, Brennan MF (1998). Retroperitoneal soft-tissue sarcoma: analysis of 500 patients treated and followed at a single institution. *Ann Surg* 228: 355-365.

1248. Lewis MM, Kenan S, Yabut SM, Norman A, Steiner G (1990). Periosteal chondroma. A report of ten cases and review of the literature. *Clin Orthop* 185-192.

1249. Li C, Bapat B, Alman BA (1998). Adenomatous polyposis coli gene mutation alters proliferation through its beta-catenin-regulatory function in aggressive fibromatosis (desmoid tumor). *Am J Pathol* 153: 709-714.

1250. Li JJ, Huang YQ, Moscatelli D, Nicolaides A, Zhang WC, Friedman-Kien AE (1993). Expression of fibroblast growth factors and their receptors in acquired immunodeficiency syndrome-associated Kaposi sarcoma tissue and derived cells. *Cancer* 72: 2253-2259.

1251. Li M, Squire JA, Weksberg R (1998). Molecular genetics of Wiedemann-Beckwith syndrome. *Am J Med Genet* 79: 253-259.

1252. Libson E, Bloom RA, Husband JE, Stoker DJ (1987). Metastatic tumours of bones of the hand and foot. A comparative review and report of 43 additional cases. *Skeletal Radiol* 16: 387-392.

1253. Lichtenstein L (1953). Histiocytosis X: integration of eosinophilic granuloma of bone, "Letterer-Siwe disease" and "Schuller-Christian disease" as related manifestations of a single nosologic entity. *Arch Pathol* 56: 84-102.

1254. Lichtenstein L (1972). *Bone Tumors*. 4th ed. Mosby: St.Louis.

1255. Lichtenstein L, Goldman RL (1964). Cartilage tumours in soft tissues, particularly in the hand and foot. *Cancer* 17: 1203-1208.

1256. Lichtenstein L, Hall JE (1952). Periosteal chondroma: a distinctive benign cartilage tumor. *J Bone Joint Surg* 34-A: 691-697.

1257. Lidang JM, Schumacher B, Myhre JO, Steen NO, Keller J (1998). Extraskeletal osteosarcomas: a clinicopathologic study of 25 cases. *Am J Surg Pathol* 22: 588-594.

1258. Lieberman PH, Brennan MF, Kimmel M, Erlandson RA, Garin-Chesa P, Flehinger BY (1989). Alveolar soft-part sarcoma. A clinico-pathologic study of half a century. *Cancer* 63: 1-13.

1259. Lieberman PH, Jones CR, Steinman RM, Erlandson RA, Smith J, Gee T, Huvos A, Garin-Chesa P, Filippa DA, Urmacher C, Gangi MD, Sperber M (1996). Langerhans cell (eosinophilic) granulomatosis. A clinicopathologic study encompassing 50 years. *Am J Surg Pathol* 20: 519-552.

1260. Liebross RH, Ha CS, Cox JD, Weber D, Delasalle K, Alexanian R (1998). Solitary bone plasmacytoma: outcome and prognostic factors following radiotherapy. *Int J Radiat Oncol Biol Phys* 41: 1063-1067.

1261. Lillehei KO, Kleinschmidt-DeMasters B, Mitchell DH, Spector E, Kruse CA (1993). Alveolar soft part sarcoma: an unusually long interval between presentation and brain metastasis. *Hum Pathol* 24: 1030-1034.

1262. Limon J, Debiec-Rychter M, Nedoszytko B, Liberski PP, Babinska M, Szadowska A (1994). Aberrations of chromosome 22 and polysomy of chromosome 8 as non-random changes in clear cell sarcoma. *Cancer Genet Cytogenet* 72: 141-145.

1263. Limon J, Szadowska A, Iliszko M, Babinska M, Mrozek K, Jaskiewicz J, Kopacz A, Roszkiewicz A, Debiec-Rychter M (1998). Recurrent chromosome changes in two adult fibrosarcomas. *Genes Chromosomes Cancer* 21: 119-123.

1264. Lin JJ, Lin F (1974). Two entities in angiolipoma. A study of 459 cases of lipoma with review of literature on infiltrating angiolipoma. *Cancer* 34: 720-727.

1265. Lin X, Gan L, Klein WH, Wells D (1998). Expression and functional analysis of mouse EXT1, a homolog of the human multiple exostoses type 1 gene. *Biochem Biophys Res Commun* 248: 738-743.

1266. Lin X, Wells D (1997). Isolation of the mouse cDNA homologous to the human EXT1 gene responsible for Hereditary Multiple Exostoses. *DNA Seq* 7: 199-202.

1267. Lind T, Tufaro F, McCormick C, Lindahl U, Lidholt K (1998). The putative tumor suppressors EXT1 and EXT2 are glycosyltransferases required for the biosynthesis of heparan sulfate. *J Biol Chem* 273: 26265-26268.

1268. Lindberg GM, Maitra A, Gokaslan ST, Saboorian MH, Albores-Saavedra J (1999). Low grade fibromyxoid sarcoma: fine-needle aspiration cytology with histologic, cytogenetic, immunohistochemical, and ultrastructural correlation. *Cancer* 87: 75-82.

1269. Lindor NM, Furuichi Y, Kitao S, Shimamoto A, Arndt C, Jalal S (2000). Rothmund-Thomson syndrome due to RECQ4 helicase mutations: report and clinical and molecular comparisons with Bloom syndrome and Werner syndrome. *Am J Med Genet* 90: 223-228.

1270. Ling NR, MacLennan IC, Mason DY (1987). B-cell and plasma cell antigens: new and previously defined clusters. In: *Leukocyte Typing III: White Cell Differentiation Antigens*, McMichael AJ, Beverly PCL, Cobbold S, et al, eds. Oxford University Press: Oxford, p. 302.

1271. Ling RSM (1963). The genetic factor in Dupuytren's disease. *J Bone Joint Surg Br* 45: 709.

1272. Link TM, Haeussler MD, Poppek S, Woertler K, Blasius S, Lindner N, Rummeny EJ (1998). Malignant fibrous histiocytoma of bone: conventional X-ray and MR imaging features. *Skeletal Radiol* 27: 552-558.

1273. Lipper S, Kahn LB (1983). Case report 235. Ewing-like adamantinoma of the left radial head and neck. *Skeletal Radiol* 10: 61-66.

1274. Liu J, Hudkins PG, Swee RG, Unni KK (1987). Bone sarcomas associated with Ollier's disease. *Cancer* 59: 1376-1385.

1275. Liu W, Litwack ED, Stanley MJ, Langford JK, Lander AD, Sanderson RD (1998). Heparan sulfate proteoglycans as adhesive and anti-invasive molecules. Syndecans and glypican have distinct functions. *J Biol Chem* 273: 22825-22832.

1276. Lockhart R, Menard P, Martin JP, Auriol M, Vaillant JM, Bertrand JC (1998). Mesenchymal chondrosarcoma of the jaws. Report of four cases. *Int J Oral Maxillofac Surg* 27: 358-362.

1277. Logan PM, Janzen DL, O'Connell JX, Munk PL, Connell DG (1996). Chondroid lipoma: MRI appearances with clinical and histologic correlation. *Skeletal Radiol* 25: 592-595.

1278. Loh WE, Jr., Scrable HJ, Livanos E, Arboleda MJ, Cavenee WK, Oshimura M, Weissman BE (1992). Human chromosome 11 contains two different growth suppressor genes for embryonal rhabdomyosarcoma. *Proc Natl Acad Sci U S A* 89: 1755-1759.

1279. Lohmann DR, Buiting K, Lüdecke HJ, Horsthemke B (1997). The murine Ext1 gene shows a high level of sequence similarity with its human homologue and is part of a conserved linkage group on chromosome 15. *Cytogenet Cell Genet* 76: 164-166.

1280. Lopez-Barea F, Hardisson D, Rodriguez-Peralto JL, Sanchez-Herrera S, Lamas M (1998). Intracortical hemangioma of bone. Report of two cases and review of the literature. *J Bone Joint Surg Am* 80: 1673-1678.

1281. Lopez-Barea F, Rodriguez-Peralto JL, Burgos-Lizaldez E, Alvarez-Linera J, Sanchez-Herrera S (1996). Primary aneurysmal cyst of soft tissue. Report of a case with ultrastructural and MRI studies. *Virchows Arch* 428: 125-129.

1282. Lopez-Ben R, Pitt MJ, Jaffe KA, Siegal GP (1999). Osteosarcoma in a patient with McCune-Albright syndrome and Mazabraud's syndrome. *Skeletal Radiol* 28: 522-526.

1283. Lopez VC, Lopez dlR, La Cruz PC (1994). Vaginal rhabdomyomas. *Int J Gynaecol Obstet* 47: 169-170.

1284. Lorentzon R, Larsson SE, Boquist L (1979). Extra-osseous osteosarcoma: a clinical and histopathological study of four cases. *J Bone Joint Surg Br* 61-B: 205-208.

1285. Lorigan JG, O'Keeffe FN, Evans HL, Wallace S (1989). The radiologic manifestations of alveolar soft-part sarcoma. *AJR Am J Roentgenol* 153: 335-339.

1286. Lotfi AM, Dozois RR, Gordon H, Hruska LS, Weiland LH, Carryer PW, Hurt RD (1989). Mesenteric fibromatosis complicating familial adenomatous polyposis: predisposing factors and results of treatment. *Int J Colorectal Dis* 4: 30-36.

1287. Lubin J, Rywlin AM (1971). Lymphoma-like lymph node changes in Kaposi's sarcoma. Two additional cases. *Arch Pathol* 92: 338-341.

1288. Lucarelli MJ, Bilyk JR, Shore JW, Rubin PA, Yaremchuk MJ (1995). Aneurysmal bone cyst of the orbit associated with fibrous dysplasia. *Plast Reconstr Surg* 96: 440-445.

1289. Lucas DR, Fletcher CD, Adsay NV, Zalupski MM (1999). High-grade extraskeletal myxoid chondrosarcoma: a high-grade epithelioid malignancy. *Histopathology* 35: 201-208.

1290. Lucas DR, Nascimento AG, Sanjay BK, Rock MG (1994). Well-differentiated liposarcoma. The Mayo Clinic experience with 58 cases. *Am J Clin Pathol* 102: 677-683.

1291. Lucas DR, Nascimento AG, Sim FH (1992). Clear cell sarcoma of soft tissues. Mayo Clinic experience with 35 cases. *Am J Surg Pathol* 16: 1197-1204.

1292. Lucas DR, Unni KK, McLeod RA, O'Connor MI, Sim FH (1994). Osteoblastoma: clinicopathologic study of 306 cases. *Hum Pathol* 25: 117-134.

1293. Lucas JD, O'Doherty MJ, Cronin BF, Marsden PK, Lodge MA, McKee PH, Smith MA (1999). Prospective evaluation of soft tissue masses and sarcomas using fluorodeoxyglucose positron emission tomography. *Br J Surg* 86: 550-556.

1294. Lumley JS, Stansfeld AG (1972). Infiltrating glomus tumour of lower limb. *Br Med J* 1: 484-485.

1295. Lundgren L, Kindblom LG, Willems J, Falkmer U, Angervall L (1992). Proliferative myositis and fasciitis. A light and electron microscopic, cytologic, DNA-cytometric and immunohistochemical study. *APMIS* 100: 437-448.

1296. Lüdecke HJ, Ahn J, Lin X, Hill A, Wagner MJ, Schomburg L, Horsthemke B, Wells DE (1997). Genomic organization and promoter structure of the human EXT1 gene. *Genomics* 40: 351-354.

1297. Lüdecke HJ, Johnson C, Wagner MJ, Wells DE, Turleau C, Tommerup N, Latos-Bielenska A, Sandig KR, Meinecke P, Zabel B, Horsthemke B (1991). Molecular definition of the shortest region of deletion overlap in the Langer-Giedion syndrome. *Am J Hum Genet* 49: 1197-1206.

1298. Lüdecke HJ, Wagner MJ, Nardmann J, La Pillo B, Parrish JE, Willems PJ, Haan EA, Frydman M, Hamers GJ, Wells DE, Horsthemke B (1995). Molecular dissection of a contiguous gene syndrome: localization of the genes involved in the Langer-Giedion syndrome. *Hum Mol Genet* 4: 31-36.

1299. Lynch HT, Ruma TA, Albano WA, Lynch JF, Lynch PM (1982). Phenotypic variation in hereditary adenomatosis: unusual tumor spectrum. *Dis Colon Rectum* 25: 235-238.

1300. Mac-Moune LF, To KF, Choi PC, Leung PC, Kumta SM, Yuen PP, Lam WY, Cheung AN, Allen PW (2001). Kaposiform hemangioendothelioma: five patients with cutaneous lesion and long follow-up. *Mod Pathol* 14: 1087-1092.

1301. Macdonald D, Fornasier V, Holtby R (2000). Chondromyxoid fibroma of the acromium with soft tissue extension. *Skeletal Radiol* 29: 168-170.

1302. Macdonald RL, Deck JH (1990). Immunohistochemistry of ecchordosis physaliphora and chordoma. *Can J Neurol Sci* 17: 420-423.

1303. Machen SK, Fisher C, Gautam RS, Tubbs RR, Goldblum JR (1998). Utility of cytokeratin subsets for distinguishing poorly differentiated synovial sarcoma from peripheral primitive neuroectodermal tumour. *Histopathology* 33: 501-507.

1304. Mack TM (1995). Sarcomas and other malignancies of soft tissue, retroperitoneum, peritoneum, pleura, heart, mediastinum, and spleen. *Cancer* 75: 211-244.

1305. Madden NP, Spicer RD, Allibone EB, Lewis IJ (1992). Spontaneous regression of neonatal fibrosarcoma. *Br J Cancer Suppl* 18: S72-S75.

1306. Maeda T, Hirose T, Furuya K, Kameoka K (1999). Calcifying fibrous pseudotumor: an ultrastructural study. *Ultrastruct Pathol* 23: 189-192.

1307. Maelandsmo GM, Berner JM, Florenes VA, Forus A, Hovig E, Fodstad O, Myklebost O (1995). Homozygous deletion frequency and expression levels of the CDKN2 gene in human sarcomas – relationship to amplification and mRNA levels of CDK4 and CCND1. *Br J Cancer* 72: 393-398.

1308. Magliato HJ, Nastasi A (1967). Non-osteogenic fibroma occurring in the ilium. Report of a case. *J Bone Joint Surg Am* 49: 384-386.

1309. Magner D, Hill DP (1961). Encapsulated angiomyoma of the skin and subcutaneous tissue. *Am J Clin Pathol* 35: 137-141.

1310. Mahoney JP, Spanier SS, Morris JL (1979). Multifocal osteosarcoma: a case report with review of the literature. *Cancer* 44: 1897-1907.

1311. Mairal A, Terrier P, Chibon F, Sastre X, Lecesne A, Aurias A (1999). Loss of chromosome 13 is the most frequent genomic imbalance in malignant fibrous histiocytomas. A comparative genomic hybridization analysis of a series of 30 cases. *Cancer Genet Cytogenet* 111: 134-138.

1312. Majeste RM, Beckman EN (1988). Synovial sarcoma with an overwhelming epithelial component. *Cancer* 61: 2527-2531.

1313. Mancini GM, Stojanov L, Willemsen R, Kleijer WJ, Huijmans JG, van Diggelen OP, de Klerk JB, Vuzevski VD, Oranje AP (1999). Juvenile hyaline fibromatosis: clinical heterogeneity in three patients. *Dermatology* 198: 18-25.

1314. Mandahl N, Fletcher CD, Dal Cin P, de Wever I, Mertens F, Mitelman F, Rosai J, Rydholm A, Sciot R, Tallini G, van den Berghe H, Vanni R, Willén H (2000). Comparative cytogenetic study of spindle cell and pleomorphic leiomyosarcomas of soft tissues: a report from the CHAMP study group. *Cancer Genet Cytogenet* 116: 66-73.

1315. Mandahl N, Gustafson P, Mertens F, Åkerman M, Baldetorp B, Gisselsson D, Knuutila S, Bauer HC, Larsson O (2002). Cytogenetic aberrations and their prognostic impact in chondrosarcoma. *Genes Chromosomes Cancer* 33: 188-200.

1316. Mandahl N, Heim S, Arheden K, Rydholm A, Willén H, Mitelman F (1990). Chromosomal rearrangements in chondromatous tumors. *Cancer* 65: 242-248.

1317. Mandahl N, Heim S, Kristoffersson U, Mitelman F, Rööser B, Rydholm A, Willén H (1985). Telomeric association in a malignant fibrous histiocytoma. *Hum Genet* 71: 321-324.

1318. Mandahl N, Heim S, Rydholm A, Willén H, Mitelman F (1989). Structural chromosome aberrations in an adamantinoma. *Cancer Genet Cytogenet* 42: 187-190.

1319. Mandahl N, Heim S, Willén H, Rydholm A, Eneroth M, Nilbert M, Kreicbergs A, Mitelman F (1989). Characteristic karyotypic anomalies identify subtypes of malignant fibrous histiocytoma. *Genes Chromosomes Cancer* 1: 9-14.

1320. Mandahl N, Höglund M, Mertens F, Rydholm A, Willén H, Brosjö O, Mitelman F (1994). Cytogenetic aberrations in 188 benign and borderline adipose tissue tumors. *Genes Chromosomes Cancer* 9: 207-215.

1321. Mandahl N, Jin YS, Heim S, Willén H, Wennerberg J, Biörklund A, Mitelman F (1990). Trisomy 5 and loss of the Y chromosome as the sole cytogenetic anomalies in a cavernous hemangioma/angiosarcoma. *Genes Chromosomes Cancer* 1: 315-316.

1322. Mandahl N, Mertens F, Willén H, Rydholm A, Kreicbergs A, Mitelman F (1998). Nonrandom pattern of telomeric associations in atypical lipomatous tumors with ring and giant marker chromosomes. *Cancer Genet Cytogenet* 103: 25-34.

1323. Mandahl N, Willén H, Rydholm A, Heim S, Mitelman F (1993). Rearrangement of band q13 on both chromosomes 12 in a periosteal chondroma. *Genes Chromosomes Cancer* 6: 121-123.

1324. Manivel JC, Wick MR, Dehner LP, Sibley RK (1987). Epithelioid sarcoma. An immunohistochemical study. *Am J Clin Pathol* 87: 319-326.

1325. Mannens M (2000). Beckwith-Wiedemann syndrome. *Atlas Genet Cytogenet Oncol Haematol*. November 2000. URL: http://www infobiogen fr/services/chromcancer/Kprones/BeckwithWiedemannID10037.html

1326. Mannens M (2001). BWS associated childhood tumours. In: *Cancer Research, an encyclopedic reference*, Schwab M, ed. Springer Verlag: 111-118.

1327. Marcove RC, Mike V, Hajek JV, Levin AG, Hutter RV (1970). Osteogenic sarcoma under the age of twenty-one. A review of one hundred and forty-five operative cases. *J Bone Joint Surg Am* 52: 411-423.

1328. Margau R, Babyn P, Cole W, Smith C, Lee F (2000). MR imaging of simple bone cysts in children: not so simple. *Pediatr Radiol* 30: 551-557.

1329. Marin C, Gallego C, Manjon P, Martinez-Tello FJ (1997). Juxtacortical chondromyxoid fibroma: imaging findings in three cases and a review of the literature. *Skeletal Radiol* 26: 642-649.

1330. Marion MJ, Boivin-Angele S (1999). Vinyl chloride-specific mutations in humans and animals. IARC Press, Lyon: 315-324.

1331. Marion MJ, Froment O, Trepo C (1991). Activation of Ki-ras gene by point mutation in human liver angiosarcoma associated with vinyl chloride exposure. *Mol Carcinog* 4: 450-454.

1332. Mark-Vendel E, Terrier P, Turc-Carel C (1991). Rearrangement of 9q22: a crucial event in extraskeletal myxoid chondrosarcoma? *Cancer Genet Cytogenet* 52: 267.

1333. Mark J, Wedell B, Dahlenfors R, Grepp C, Burian P (1992). Human benign chondroblastoma with a pseudodiploid stemline characterized by a complex and balanced translocation. *Cancer Genet Cytogenet* 58: 14-17.

1334. Mark RJ, Poen J, Tran LM, Fu YS, Selch MT, Parker RG (1994). Postirradiation sarcomas. A single-institution study and review of the literature. *Cancer* 73: 2653-2662.

1335. Markhede G, Angervall L, Stener B (1982). A multivariate analysis of the prognosis after surgical treatment of malignant soft-tissue tumors. *Cancer* 49: 1721-1733.

1336. Marom EM, Helms CA (1999). Fibrolipomatous hamartoma: pathognomonic on MR imaging. *Skeletal Radiol* 28: 260-264.

1337. Martignetti JA, Desnick RJ, Aliprandis E, Norton KI, Hardcastle P, Nade S, Gelb BD (1999). Diaphyseal medullary stenosis with malignant fibrous histiocytoma: a hereditary bone dysplasia/cancer syndrome maps to 9p21-22. *Am J Hum Genet* 64: 801-807.

1338. Martignetti JA, Gelb BD, Pierce H, Picci P, Desnick RJ (2000). Malignant fibrous histiocytoma: inherited and sporadic forms have loss of heterozygosity at chromosome bands 9p21-22-evidence for a common genetic defect. *Genes Chromosomes Cancer* 27: 191-195.

1339. Martignoni G, Pea M, Bonetti F, Zamboni G, Carbonara C, Longa L, Zancanaro C, Maran M, Brisigotti M, Mariuzzi GM (1998). Carcinomalike monotypic epithelioid angiomyolipoma in patients without evidence of tuberous sclerosis: a clinicopathologic and genetic study. *Am J Surg Pathol* 22: 663-672.

1340. Martin SE, Dwyer A, Kissane JM, Costa J (1982). Small-cell osteosarcoma. *Cancer* 50: 990-996.

1341. Martinez-Tello FJ, Navas-Palacios JJ (1982). The ultrastructure of conventional, parosteal, and periosteal osteosarcomas. *Cancer* 50: 949-961.

1342. Martinez-Tello FJ, Navas-Palacios JJ (1982). Ultrastructural study of conventional chondrosarcomas and myxoid- and mesenchymal-chondrosarcomas. *Virchows Arch A Pathol Anat Histol* 396: 197-211.

1343. Martinez D, Millner PA, Coral A, Newman RJ, Hardy GJ, Butt WP (1992). Case report 745: Synovial lipoma arborescens. *Skeletal Radiol* 21: 393-395.

1344. Martinez JA, Quecedo E, Fortea JM, Oliver V, Aliaga A (1996). Pleomorphic angioleiomyoma. *Am J Dermatopathol* 18: 409-412.

1345. Martinez V, Sissons HA (1988). Aneurysmal bone cyst. A review of 123 cases including primary lesions and those secondary to other bone pathology. *Cancer* 61: 2291-2304.

1346. Marui T, Yamamoto T, Yoshihara H, Kurosaka M, Mizuno K, Akamatsu T (2001). De novo malignant transformation of giant cell tumor of bone. *Skeletal Radiol* 30: 104-108.

1347. Maruyama R, Nakano M, Yamashita S, Morooka K, Daimon Y, Tsuchimochi T, Ochiai T, Koono M (1992). Fine needle aspiration cytology of clear cell sarcoma. Report of a case with immunocytochemical, immunohistochemical and ultrastructural studies. *Acta Cytol* 36: 937-942.

1348. Mascarello JT, Krous HF, Carpenter PM (1993). Unbalanced translocation resulting in the loss of the chromosome 17 short arm in an osteoblastoma. *Cancer Genet Cytogenet* 69: 65-67.

1349. Masuda H, Miller C, Koeffler HP, Battifora H, Cline MJ (1987). Rearrangement of the p53 gene in human osteogenic sarcomas. *Proc Natl Acad Sci U S A* 84: 7716-7719.

1350. Masui F, Ushigome S, Fujii K (1998). Giant cell tumor of bone: a clinicopathologic study of prognostic factors. *Pathol Int* 48: 723-729.

1351. Masuzaki H, Masuzaki M, Ishimaru T, Yamabe T (1996). Chest wall hamartoma diagnosed prenatally using ultrasonography and computed tomography. *J Clin Ultrasound* 24: 83-85.

1352. Mathew J, Sen S, Chandi SM, Kumar NK, Zachariah N, Chacko J, Thomas G (2001). Pulmonary lipoblastoma: a case report. *Pediatr Surg Int* 17: 543-544.

1353. Matsubara O, Tan-Liu NS, Kenney RM, Mark EJ (1988). Inflammatory pseudo-tumors of the lung: progression from organizing pneumonia to fibrous histiocytoma or to plasma cell granuloma in 32 cases. *Hum Pathol* 19: 807-814.

1354. Matsumoto K, Ishizawa M, Okabe H, Taniguchi I (2000). Hemangioma of bone arising in the ulna: imaging findings with emphasis on MR. *Skeletal Radiol* 29: 231-234.

1355. Matsuno T (1990). Benign fibrous histiocytoma involving the ends of long bone. *Skeletal Radiol* 19: 561-566.

1356. Matsuno T, Ichioka Y, Yagi T, Ishii S (1988). Spindle-cell sarcoma in patients who have osteochondromatosis. A report of two cases. *J Bone Joint Surg Am* 70: 137-141.

1357. Matsuno T, Unni KK, McLeod RA, Dahlin DC (1976). Telangiectatic osteogenic sarcoma. *Cancer* 38: 2538-2547.

1358. Mawad JK, Mackay B, Raymond AK, Ayala AG (1994). Electron microscopy in the diagnosis of small round cell tumors of bone. *Ultrastruct Pathol* 18: 263-268.

1359. May WA, Arvand A, Thompson AD, Braun BS, Wright M, Denny CT (1997). EWS/FLI1-induced manic fringe renders NIH 3T3 cells tumorigenic. *Nat Genet* 17: 495-497.

1360. May WA, Gishizky ML, Lessnick SL, Lunsford LB, Lewis BC, Delattre O, Zucman J, Thomas G, Denny CT (1993). Ewing sarcoma 11;22 translocation produces a chimeric transcription factor that requires the DNA-binding domain encoded by FLI1 for transformation. *Proc Natl Acad Sci U S A* 90: 5752-5756.

1361. May WA, Lessnick SL, Braun BS, Klemsz M, Lewis BC, Lunsford LB, Hromas R, Denny CT (1993). The Ewing's sarcoma EWS/FLI-1 fusion gene encodes a more potent transcriptional activator and is a more powerful transforming gene than FLI-1. *Mol Cell Biol* 13: 7393-7398.

1362. Mayer-da-Silva A, Poiares-Baptista A, Guerra RF, Teresa-Lopes M (1988). Juvenile hyaline fibromatosis. A histologic and histochemical study. *Arch Pathol Lab Med* 112: 928-931.

1363. Mayr-Kanhauser S, Behmel A, Aberer W (2001). Multiple glomus tumors of the skin with male-to-male transmission over four generations. *J Invest Dermatol* 116: 475-476.

1364. Mazabraud A (1974). [Mesenchymatous chondrosarcoma. Apropos of 6 cases]. *Rev Chir Orthop Reparatrice Appar Mot* 60: 197-203.

1365. McCarthy DM, Dorr CA, Mackintosh CE (1969). Unilateral localised gigantism of the extremities with lipomatosis, arthropathy and psoriasis. *J Bone Joint Surg Br* 51: 348-353.

1366. McCarthy EF (1996). Osteochondroma vs. Surface Chondrosarcoma vs Periosteal Chondroma. In: *Differential Diagnosis in Pathology: Bone and Joint Disorders*, McCarthy EF, ed. Igaku-Shoin: New York, pp. 48-51.

1367. McCarthy EF, Matsuno T, Dorfman HD (1979). Malignant fibrous histiocytoma of bone: a study of 35 cases. *Hum Pathol* 10: 57-70.

1368. McClain KL, Leach CT, Jenson HB, Joshi VV, Pollock BH, Parmley RT, DiCarlo FJ, Chadwick EG, Murphy SB (1995). Association of Epstein-Barr virus with leiomyosarcomas in children with AIDS. *N Engl J Med* 332: 12-18.

1369. McCluggage WG, Patterson A, Maxwell P (2000). Aggressive angiomyoma of pelvic parts exhibits oestrogen and progesterone receptor positivity. *J Clin Pathol* 53: 603-605.

1370. McComb EN, Feely MG, Neff JR, Johansson SL, Nelson M, Bridge JA (2001). Cytogenetic instability, predominantly involving chromosome 1, is characteristic of elastofibroma. *Cancer Genet Cytogenet* 126: 68-72.

1371. McComb EN, Neff JR, Johansson SL, Nelson M, Bridge JA (1997). Chromosomal anomalies in a case of proliferative myositis. *Cancer Genet Cytogenet* 98: 142-144.

1372. McCormick C, Duncan G, Goutsos KT, Tufaro F (2000). The putative tumor suppressors EXT1 and EXT2 form a stable complex that accumulates in the Golgi apparatus and catalyzes the synthesis of heparan sulfate. *Proc Natl Acad Sci U S A* 97: 668-673.

1373. McCormick C, Leduc Y, Martindale D, Mattison K, Esford LE, Dyer AP, Tufaro F (1998). The putative tumour suppressor EXT1 alters the expression of cell-surface heparan sulfate. *Nat Genet* 19: 158-161.

1374. McCormick D, Mentzel T, Beham A, Fletcher CD (1994). Dedifferentiated liposarcoma. Clinicopathologic analysis of 32 cases suggesting a better prognostic subgroup among pleomorphic sarcomas. *Am J Surg Pathol* 18: 1213-1223.

1375. McCune DJ, Bruch H (1937). Progress in pediatrics: ostedystrophia fibrosa. *Am J Dis Child* 54: 806-848.

1376. McKusick VA (1998). Mendelian inheritance in Man. *Catalogs of Human Genes and Genetic Disorders*. 12th ed. Johns Hopkins University Press: Baltimore.

1377. McKusick VA (2000). *Online Mendelian Inheritance in Man, OMIM (TM)*. McKusick-Nathans Institute for Genetic Medicine, Johns Hopkins University (Baltimore, MD) and National Center for Biotechnology Information, World Wide Web URL: http://www ncbi nlm nih gov/omim

1378. McLeod RA, Berquist TH (1988). Bone tumor imaging: contribution of CT and MRI. *Contemp Issues Surg Pathol* 11: 1-34.

1379. McLeod RA, Dahlin DC (1979). Hamartoma (mesenchymoma) of the chest wall in infancy. *Radiology* 131: 657-661.

1380. McManus AP, Gusterson BA, Pinkerton CR, Shipley JM (1995). Diagnosis of Ewing's sarcoma and related tumours by detection of chromosome 22q12 translocations using fluorescence in situ hybridization on tumour touch imprints. *J Pathol* 176: 137-142.

1381. McMenamin ME, DeSchryver K, Fletcher CD (2000). Fibrous lesions of the breast. A review. *Int J Surg Pathol* 8: 99-108.

1382. McMenamin ME, Fletcher CD (2001). Mammary-type myofibroblastoma of soft tissue: a tumor closely related to spindle cell lipoma. *Am J Surg Pathol* 25: 1022-1029.

1383. McMenamin ME, Fletcher CDM (2002). Malignant myopericytoma: expanding the spectrum of tumours with myopericytic differentiation. *Histopathology* (in press).

1384. Mehregan AH, Shapiro L (1971). Angiolymphoid hyperplasia with eosinophilia. *Arch Dermatol* 103: 50-57.

1385. Meis-Kindblom JM, Bergh P, Gunterberg B, Kindblom LG (1999). Extraskeletal myxoid chondrosarcoma: a reappraisal of its morphologic spectrum and prognostic factors based on 117 cases. *Am J Surg Pathol* 23: 636-650.

1386. Meis-Kindblom JM, Kindblom LG (1998). Acral myxoinflammatory fibroblastic sarcoma: a low-grade tumor of the hands and feet. *Am J Surg Pathol* 22: 911-924.

1387. Meis-Kindblom JM, Kindblom LG (1998). Angiosarcoma of soft tissue: a study of 80 cases. *Am J Surg Pathol* 22: 683-697.

1388. Meis-Kindblom JM, Kindblom LG, Enzinger FM (1995). Sclerosing epithelioid fibrosarcoma. A variant of fibrosarcoma simulating carcinoma. *Am J Surg Pathol* 19: 979-993.

1389. Meis-Kindblom JM, Sjögren H, Kindblom LG, Peydro-Mellquist A, Roijer E, Åman P, Stenman G (2001). Cytogenetic and molecular genetic analyses of liposarcoma and its soft tissue simulators: recognition of new variants and differential diagnosis. *Virchows Arch* 439: 141-151.

1390. Meis JM, Butler JJ, Osborne BM, Manning JT (1986). Granulocytic sarcoma in nonleukemic patients. *Cancer* 58: 2697-2709.

1391. Meis JM, Butler JJ, Osborne BM, Ordonez NG (1987). Solitary plasmacytomas of bone and extramedullary plasmacytomas. A clinicopathologic and immunohistochemical study. *Cancer* 59: 1475-1485.

1392. Meis JM, Enzinger FM (1991). Inflammatory fibrosarcoma of the mesentery and retroperitoneum. A tumor closely simulating inflammatory pseudotumor. *Am J Surg Pathol* 15: 1146-1156.

1393. Meis JM, Enzinger FM (1991). Myolipoma of soft tissue. *Am J Surg Pathol* 15: 121-125.

1394. Meis JM, Enzinger FM (1992). Juxta-articular myxoma: a clinical and pathologic study of 65 cases. *Hum Pathol* 23: 639-646.

1395. Meis JM, Enzinger FM (1992). Proliferative fasciitis and myositis of childhood. *Am J Surg Pathol* 16: 364-372.

1396. Meis JM, Enzinger FM (1993). Chondroid lipoma. A unique tumor simulating liposarcoma and myxoid chondrosarcoma. *Am J Surg Pathol* 17: 1103-1112.

1397. Meis JM, Mackay B, Ordonez NG (1988). Epithelioid sarcoma: an immunohistochemical and ultrastructural study. *Surg Pathol* 1: 13-31.

1398. Meis JM, Raymond AK, Evans HL, Charles RE, Giraldo AA (1987). "Dedifferentiated" chordoma. A clinicopathologic and immunohistochemical study of three cases. *Am J Surg Pathol* 11: 516-525.

1399. Meister P, Buckmann FW, Konrad E (1978). Nodular fasciitis (analysis of 100 cases and review of the literature). *Pathol Res Pract* 162: 133-165.

1400. Meister P, Konrad E, Hubner G (1979). Malignant tumor of humerus with features of "adamantinoma" and Ewing's sarcoma. *Pathol Res Pract* 166: 112-122.

1401. Melhem MF, Meisler AI, Saito R, Finley GG, Hockman HR, Koski RA (1993). Cytokines in inflammatory malignant fibrous histiocytoma presenting with leukemoid reaction. *Blood* 82: 2038-2044.

1402. Meloni-Ehrig AM, Chen Z, Guan XY, Notohamiprodjo M, Shepard RR, Spanier SS, Trent JM, Sandberg AA (1999). Identification of a ring chromosome in a myxoid malignant fibrous histiocytoma with chromosome microdissection and fluorescence in situ hybridization. *Cancer Genet Cytogenet* 109: 81-85.

1403. Mendlick MR, Nelson M, Pickering D, Johansson SL, Seemayer TA, Neff JR, Vergara G, Rosenthal H, Bridge JA (2001). Translocation t(1;3)(p36.3;q25) is a nonrandom aberration in epithelioid hemangioendothelioma. *Am J Surg Pathol* 25: 684-687.

1404. Menghi-Sartorio S, Mandahl N, Mertens F, Picci P, Knuutila S (2001). DNA copy number amplifications in sarcomas with homogeneously staining regions and double minutes. *Cytometry* 46: 79-84.

1405. Mentzel T (2001). Myofibroblastic sarcomas: a brief review of sarcomas showing a myofibroblastic line of differentiation and discussion of the differential diagnosis. *Curr Diagn Pathol* 7: 17-24.

1406. Mentzel T, Bainbridge TC, Katenkamp D (1997). Solitary fibrous tumour: clinicopathological, immunohistochemical, and ultrastructural analysis of 12 cases arising in soft tissues, nasal cavity and nasopharynx, urinary bladder and prostate. *Virchows Arch* 430: 445-453.

1407. Mentzel T, Beham A, Calonje E, Katenkamp D, Fletcher CD (1997). Epithelioid hemangioendothelioma of skin and soft tissues: clinicopathologic and immunohistochemical study of 30 cases. *Am J Surg Pathol* 21: 363-374.

1408. Mentzel T, Bosenberg M, Fletcher CD (1999). Pleomorphic liposarcoma. Clinicopathologic and prognostic study of 31 cases. *Mod Pathol* 12: 13A.

1409. Mentzel T, Brown LF, Dvorak HF, Kuhnen C, Stiller KJ, Katenkamp D, Fletcher CD (2001). The association between tumour progression and vascularity in myxofibrosarcoma and myxoid/round cell liposarcoma. *Virchows Arch* 438: 13-22.

1410. Mentzel T, Calonje E, Fletcher CD (1993). Lipoblastoma and lipoblastomatosis: a clinicopathological study of 14 cases. *Histopathology* 23: 527-533.

1411. Mentzel T, Calonje E, Fletcher CD (1994). Leiomyosarcoma with prominent osteoclast-like giant cells. Analysis of eight cases closely mimicking the so-called giant cell variant of malignant fibrous histiocytoma. *Am J Surg Pathol* 18: 258-265.

1412. Mentzel T, Calonje E, Nascimento AG, Fletcher CD (1994). Infantile hemangiopericytoma versus infantile myofibromatosis. Study of a series suggesting a continuous spectrum of infantile myofibroblastic lesions. *Am J Surg Pathol* 18: 922-930.

1413. Mentzel T, Calonje E, Wadden C, Camplejohn RS, Beham A, Smith MA, Fletcher CD (1996). Myxofibrosarcoma. Clinicopathologic analysis of 75 cases with emphasis on the low-grade variant. *Am J Surg Pathol* 20: 391-405.

1414. Mentzel T, Dry S, Katenkamp D, Fletcher CD (1998). Low-grade myofibroblastic sarcoma: analysis of 18 cases in the spectrum of myofibroblastic tumors. *Am J Surg Pathol* 22: 1228-1238.

1415. Mentzel T, Fletcher CD (1994). Malignant mesenchymomas of soft tissue associated with numerous osteoclast-like giant cells mimicking the so-called giant cell variant of "malignant fibrous histiocytoma". *Virchows Arch* 424: 539-545.

1416. Mentzel T, Fletcher CD (1997). Dedifferentiated myxoid liposarcoma: a clinicopathological study suggesting a closer relationship between myxoid and well-differentiated liposarcoma. *Histopathology* 30: 457-463.

1417. Mentzel T, Katenkamp D, Fletcher CD (1996). [Low malignancy myxofibrosarcoma versus low malignancy fibromyxoid sarcoma. Distinct entities with similar names but different clinical course]. *Pathologe* 17: 116-121.

1418. Mentzel T, Mazzoleni G, Dei Tos AP, Fletcher CD (1997). Kaposiform hemangioendothelioma in adults. Clinicopathologic and immunohistochemical analysis of three cases. *Am J Clin Pathol* 108: 450-455.

1419. Mentzel T, Stengel B, Katenkamp D (1997). [Retiform hemangioendothelioma. Clinico-pathologic case report and discussion of the group of low malignancy vascular tumors]. *Pathologe* 18: 390-394.

1420. Merchant NB, Lewis JJ, Woodruff JM, Leung DH, Brennan MF (1999). Extremity and trunk desmoid tumors: a multifactorial analysis of outcome. *Cancer* 86: 2045-2052.

1421. Merchant W, Calonje E, Fletcher CD (1995). Inflammatory leiomyosarcoma: a morphological subgroup within the heterogeneous family of so-called inflammatory malignant fibrous histiocytoma. *Histopathology* 27: 525-532.

1422. Merck C, Angervall L, Kindblom LG, Oden A (1983). Myxofibrosarcoma. A malignant soft tissue tumor of fibroblastic-histiocytic origin. A clinicopathologic and prognostic study of 110 cases using multivariate analysis. *Acta Pathol Microbiol Immunol Scand Suppl* 282: 1-40.

1423. Merino S, Arrazola J, Saiz A, Blanco JA, Ortega L (1999). Post-Paget telangiectatic osteosarcoma of the skull. *Skeletal Radiol* 28: 470-472.

1424. Merkel H (1906). On a pseudolipoma of the breast (peculiar fat tumor). *Beitr Pathol Anat* 39: 152-157.

1425. Mertens F, Fletcher CD, Dal Cin P, de Wever I, Mandahl N, Mitelman F, Rosai J, Rydholm A, Sciot R, Tallini G, van den Berghe H, Vanni R, Willén H (1998). Cytogenetic analysis of 46 pleomorphic soft tissue sarcomas and correlation with morphologic and clinical features: a report of the CHAMP study group. *Genes Chromosomes Cancer* 22: 16-25.

1426. Mertens F, Jonsson K, Willén H, Rydholm A, Kreicbergs A, Eriksson L, Olsson-Sandin G, Mitelman F, Mandahl N (1996). Chromosome rearrangements in synovial chondromatous lesions. *Br J Cancer* 74: 251-254.

1427. Mertens F, Larramendy M, Gustavsson A, Gisselsson D, Rydholm A, Brosjö O, Mitelman F, Knuutila S, Mandahl N (2000). Radiation-associated sarcomas are characterized by complex karyotypes with frequent rearrangements of chromosome arm 3p. *Cancer Genet Cytogenet* 116: 89-96.

1428. Mertens F, Mandahl N, Örndal C, Baldetorp B, Bauer HC, Rydholm A, Wiebe T, Willén H, Åkerman M, Heim S, Mitelman F (1993). Cytogenetic findings in 33 osteosarcomas. *Int J Cancer* 55: 44-50.

1429. Mertens F, Pålsson E, Lindstrand A, Toksvig-Larsen S, Knuutila S, Larramendy ML, el Rifai W, Limon J, Mitelman F, Mandahl N (1996). Evidence of somatic mutations in osteoarthritis. *Hum Genet* 98: 651-656.

1430. Mertens F, Rydholm A, Kreicbergs A, Willén H, Jonsson K, Heim S, Mitelman F, Mandahl N (1994). Loss of chromosome band 8q24 in sporadic osteocartilaginous exostoses. *Genes Chromosomes Cancer* 9: 8-12.

1431. Mertens F, Willén H, Rydholm A, Brosjö O, Carlen B, Mitelman F, Mandahl N (1995). Trisomy 20 is a primary chromosome aberration in desmoid tumors. *Int J Cancer* 63: 527-529.

1432. Mervak TR, Unni KK, Pritchard DJ, McLeod RA (1991). Telangiectatic osteosarcoma. *Clin Orthop* 135-139.

1433. Mess D, Songer M (1986). Head and neck carcinoma metastases to the hand and foot. A case report of simultaneous involvement. *Orthopedics* 9: 975-977.

1434. Messineo A, Mognato G, d'Amore ES, Antoniello L, Guglielmi M, Cecchetto G (1998). Inflammatory pseudotumors of the lung in children: conservative or aggressive approach? *Med Pediatr Oncol* 31: 100-104.

1435. Meza-Zepeda LA, Forus A, Lygren B, Dahlberg AB, Godager LH, South A, Serra M, Nezetic D, Tarkkanen M, Knuutila S, Myklebost O (2002). Positional cloning identifies a novel cyclophilin as a candidate amplified oncogene in 1q21. *Oncogene* 21: 2261-2269.

1436. Mezzelani A, Sozzi G, Nessling M, Riva C, Della Torre G, Testi MA, Azzarelli A, Pierotti MA, Lichter P, Pilotti S (2000). Low grade fibromyxoid sarcoma. A further low-grade soft tissue malignancy characterized by a ring chromosome. *Cancer Genet Cytogenet* 122: 144-148.

1437. Michal M (1998). Inflammatory myxoid tumor of the soft parts with bizarre giant cells. *Pathol Res Pract* 194: 529-533.

1438. Michal M, Fetsch JF, Hes O, Miettinen M (1999). Nuchal-type fibroma: a clinicopathologic study of 52 cases. *Cancer* 85: 156-163.

1439. Michal M, Miettinen M (1999). Myoepitheliomas of the skin and soft tissues. Report of 12 cases. *Virchows Arch* 434: 393-400.

1440. Michal M, Mukensnabl P, Chlumska A, Kodet R (1992). Fibrous hamartoma of infancy. A study of eight cases with immunohistochemical and electron microscopical findings. *Pathol Res Pract* 188: 1049-1053.

1441. Michal M, Zamecnik M (2000). Hyalinized Uterine Mesenchymal Neoplasms with HMB-45-Positive Epithelioid Cells: Epithelioid Leiomyomas or Angiomyolipomas? Report of Four Cases. *Int J Surg Pathol* 8: 323-328.

1442. Michal M, Zamecnik M, Gogora M, Mukensnabl P, Neubauer L (1996). Pitfalls in the diagnosis of ectopic hamartomatous thymoma. *Histopathology* 29: 549-555.

1443. Miettinen M (1991). Keratin subsets in spindle cell sarcomas. Keratins are widespread but synovial sarcoma contains a distinctive keratin polypeptide pattern and desmoplakins. *Am J Pathol* 138: 505-513.

1444. Miettinen M (1991). Ossifying fibromyxoid tumor of soft parts. Additional observations of a distinctive soft tissue tumor. *Am J Clin Pathol* 95: 142-149.

1445. Miettinen M, Enzinger FM (1999). Epithelioid variant of pleomorphic liposarcoma: a study of 12 cases of a distinctive variant of high-grade liposarcoma. *Mod Pathol* 12: 722-728.

1446. Miettinen M, Fanburg-Smith JC, Virolainen M, Shmookler BM, Fetsch JF (1999). Epithelioid sarcoma: an immunohistochemical analysis of 112 classical and variant cases and a discussion of the differential diagnosis. *Hum Pathol* 30: 934-942.

1447. Miettinen M, Fetsch JF (1998). Collagenous fibroma (desmoplastic fibroblastoma): a clinicopathologic analysis of 63 cases of a distinctive soft tissue lesion with stellate-shaped fibroblasts. *Hum Pathol* 29: 676-682.

1448. Miettinen M, Hockerstedt K, Reitamo J, Totterman S (1985). Intramuscular myxoma – a clinicopathological study of twenty-three cases. *Am J Clin Pathol* 84: 265-272.

1449. Miettinen M, Lehto VP, Virtanen I (1983). Glomus tumor cells: evaluation of smooth muscle and endothelial cell properties. *Virchows Arch B Cell Pathol Incl Mol Pathol* 43: 139-149.

1450. Miettinen M, Rapola J (1989). Immunohistochemical spectrum of rhabdomyosarcoma and rhabdomyosarcoma-like tumors. Expression of cytokeratin and the 68-kD neurofilament protein. *Am J Surg Pathol* 13: 120-132.

1451. Miettinen M, Virtanen I (1984). Synovial sarcoma – a misnomer. *Am J Pathol* 117: 18-25.

1452. Miettinen MM, el Rifai W, Sarlomo-Rikala M, Andersson LC, Knuutila S (1997). Tumor size-related DNA copy number changes occur in solitary fibrous tumors but not in hemangiopericytomas. *Mod Pathol* 10: 1194-1200.

1453. Mii Y, Miyauchi Y, Hohnoki K, Maruyama H, Tsutsumi M, Dohmae K, Tamai S, Konishi Y, Yamanouchi T (1989). Neural crest origin of clear cell sarcoma of tendons and aponeuroses. Ultrastructural and enzyme cytochemical study of human and nude mouse-transplanted tumours. *Virchows Arch A Pathol Anat Histopathol* 415: 51-60.

1454. Mikami Y, Shimizu M, Hirokawa M, Manabe T (1997). Extraorbital giant cell angiofibromas. *Mod Pathol* 10: 1082-1087.

1455. Mikkelsen OA (1977). Dupuytren's disease – initial symptoms, age of onset and spontaneous course. *Hand* 9: 11-15.

1456. Milchgrub S, Ghandur-Mnaymneh L, Dorfman HD, Albores-Saavedra J (1993). Synovial sarcoma with extensive osteoid and bone formation. *Am J Surg Pathol* 17: 357-363.

1457. Milgram JW (1983). The origins of osteochondromas and enchondromas. A histopathologic study. *Clin Orthop* 264-284.

1458. Milgram JW (1988). Intraosseous lipomas. A clinicopathologic study of 66 cases. *Clin Orthop* 277-302.

1459. Miller CW, Aslo A, Tsay C, Slamon D, Ishizaki K, Toguchida J, Yamamuro T, Lampkin B, Koeffler HP (1990). Frequency and structure of p53 rearrangements in human osteosarcoma. *Cancer Res* 50: 7950-7954.

1460. Miller F, Whitehill R (1984). Carcinoma of the breast metastatic to the skeleton. *Clin Orthop* 121-127.

1461. Miller KK, Daly PA, Sentochnik D, Doweiko J, Samore M, Basgoz NO, Grinspoon SK (1998). Pseudo-Cushing's syndrome in human immunodeficiency virus-infected patients. *Clin Infect Dis* 27: 68-72.

1462. Miller MD, Ragsdale BD, Sweet DE (1992). Parosteal lipomas: a new perspective. *Pathology* 24: 132-139.

1463. Miller RL, Sheeler LR, Bauer TW, Bukowski RM (1986). Erdheim-Chester disease. Case report and review of the literature. *Am J Med* 80: 1230-1236.

1464. Mintzer CM, Klein JD, Kasser JR (1994). Osteochondroma formation after a Salter II fracture. *J Orthop Trauma* 8: 437-439.

1465. Miozzo M, Dalpra L, Riva P, Volonta M, Macciardi F, Pericotti S, Tibiletti MG, Cerati M, Rohde K, Larizza L, Fuhrman Conti AM (2000). A tumor suppressor locus in familial and sporadic chordoma maps to 1p36. *Int J Cancer* 87: 68-72.

1466. Miracco C, Laurini L, Santopietro R, De Santi MM, Sassi C, Neri E, Pepi F, Luzi P (1999). Intimal-type primary sarcoma of the aorta. Report of a case with evidence of rhabdomyosarcomatous differentiation. *Virchows Arch* 435: 62-66.

1467. Miralles GD, O'Fallon JR, Talley NJ (1992). Plasma-cell dyscrasia with polyneuropathy. The spectrum of POEMS syndrome. *N Engl J Med* 327: 1919-1923.

1468. Mirra JM (1989). *Bone Tumors. Clinical, Radiologic, and Pathologic Correlations*. Lea & Febiger: Philadelphia.

1469. Mirra JM (1989). Intramedullary cartilage- and chondroid-producing tumors. In: *Bone Tumors. Clinical, Radiologic, and Pathologic Correlations*. Lea & Febiger: Philadelphia.

1470. Mirra JM (1989). Metastases. In: *Bone Tumor: Clinical, Radiologic and Pathologic Correlations*. Lea & Febiger: Philadelphia, p. 1497.

1471. Mirra JM, Bullough PG, Marcove RC, Jacobs B, Huvos AG (1974). Malignant fibrous histiocytoma and osteosarcoma in association with bone infarcts; report of four cases, two in caisson workers. *J Bone Joint Surg Am* 56: 932-940.

1472. Mirra JM, Kameda N, Rosen G, Eckardt J (1988). Primary osteosarcoma of toe phalanx: first documented case. Review of osteosarcoma of short tubular bones. *Am J Surg Pathol* 12: 300-307.

1473. Mirra JM, Kessler S, Bhuta S, Eckardt J (1992). The fibroma-like variant of epithelioid sarcoma. A fibrohistiocytic/myoid cell lesion often confused with benign and malignant spindle cell tumors. *Cancer* 69: 1382-1395.

1474. Mirra JM, Wang S, Bhuta S (1984). Synovial sarcoma with squamous differentiation of its mesenchymal glandular elements. A case report with light-microscopic, ultramicroscopic, and immunologic correlation. *Am J Surg Pathol* 8: 791-796.

1475. Mirra M, Falconieri G, Zanconati F, Di Bonito L (1996). Inflammatory fibrosarcoma: another imitator of Hodgkin's disease? *Pathol Res Pract* 192: 474-478.

1476. Mitchell ML, di Sant'Agnese PA, Gerber JE (1982). Fibrous hamartoma of infancy. *Hum Pathol* 13: 586-588.

1477. *Mitelman Database of Chromosome Aberrations in Cancer* (2002). http://cgap nci nih gov/Chromosomes/Mitelman.

1478. Mitra A, Goldstein RY (1994). Dupuytren's contracture in the black population: a review. *Ann Plast Surg* 32: 619-622.

1479. Miyajima K, Oda Y, Oshiro Y, Tamiya S, Kinukawa N, Masuda K, Tsuneyoshi M (2002). Clinicopathological prognostic factors in soft tissue leiomyosarcoma: a multivariate analysis. *Histopathology* 40: 353-359.

1480. Miyake I, Tokumaru H, Sugino H, Tanno M, Yamamoto T (1995). Juvenile hyaline fibromatosis. Case report with five years' follow-up. *Am J Dermatopathol* 17: 584-590.

1481. Miyaki M, Konishi M, Kikuchi-Yanoshita R, Enomoto M, Tanaka K, Takahashi H, Muraoka M, Mori T, Konishi F, Iwama T (1993). Coexistence of somatic and germ-line mutations of APC gene in desmoid tumors from patients with familial adenomatous polyposis. *Cancer Res* 53: 5079-5082.

1482. Miyamoto Y, Satomura K, Rikimaru K, Hayashi Y (1995). Desmoplastic fibroma of the mandible associated with tuberous sclerosis. *J Oral Pathol Med* 24: 93-96.

1483. Miyoshi Y, Iwao K, Nawa G, Yoshikawa H, Ochi T, Nakamura Y (1998). Frequent mutations in the beta-catenin gene in desmoid tumors from patients without familial adenomatous polyposis. *Oncol Res* 10: 591-594.

1484. Mizukawa N, Nishijima Y, Nishijima K (1997). Metaphyseal fibrous defect (nonossifying fibroma) in the mandible. A case report. *Int J Oral Maxillofac Surg* 26: 129-130.

1485. Mohamed AN, Zalupski MM, Ryan JR, Koppitch F, Balcerzak S, Kempf R, Wolman SR (1997). Cytogenetic aberrations and DNA ploidy in soft tissue sarcoma. A Southwest Oncology Group Study. *Cancer Genet Cytogenet* 99: 45-53.

1486. Molenaar WM, DeJong B, Buist J, Idenburg VJ, Seruca R, Vos AM, Hoekstra HJ (1989). Chromosomal analysis and the classification of soft tissue sarcomas. *Lab Invest* 60: 266-274.

1487. Molenaar WM, DeJong B, Dam-Meiring A, Postma A, DeVries J, Hoekstra HJ (1989). Epithelioid sarcoma or malignant rhabdoid tumor of soft tissue? Epithelioid immunophenotype and rhabdoid karyotype. *Hum Pathol* 20: 347-351.

1488. Molenaar WM, van den Berg E, Dolfin AC, Zorgdrager H, Hoekstra HJ (1995). Cytogenetics of fine needle aspiration biopsies of sarcomas. *Cancer Genet Cytogenet* 84: 27-31.

1489. Molina A, Bangs CD, Donlon T (1989). Angiosarcoma of the scalp with complex hypotetraploid karyotype. *Cancer Genet Cytogenet* 41: 268.

1490. Momand J, Zambetti GP, Olson DC, George D, Levine AJ (1992). The mdm-2 oncogene product forms a complex with the p53 protein and inhibits p53-mediated transactivation. *Cell* 69: 1237-1245.

1491. Momeni P, Glockner G, Schmidt O, von Holtum D, Albrecht B, Gillessen-Kaesbach G, Hennekam R, Meinecke P, Zabel B, Rosenthal A, Horsthemke B, Lüdecke HJ (2000). Mutations in a new gene, encoding a zinc-finger protein, cause tricho-rhino-phalangeal syndrome type I. *Nat Genet* 24: 71-74.

1492. Monaghan H, Salter DM, Al Nafussi A (2001). Giant cell tumour of tendon sheath (localised nodular tenosynovitis): clinicopathological features of 71 cases. *J Clin Pathol* 54: 404-407.

1493. Monda L, Wick MR (1985). S-100 protein immunostaining in the differential diagnosis of chondroblastoma. *Hum Pathol* 16: 287-293.

1494. Monnat RJ, Jr. (2001). Cancer pathogenesis in the human RecQ helicase deficiency syndromes. In: *From Premature Gray Hair to Helicase: Werner Syndrome Implications for Aging and Cancer*, Goto M, Miller RW, eds. GANN Monograph on Cancer Research: 83-94.

1495. Montgomery E, Goldblum JR, Fisher C (2001). Myofibrosarcoma: a clinicopathologic study. *Am J Surg Pathol* 25: 219-228.

1496. Montgomery EA, Devaney KO, Giordano TJ, Weiss SW (1998). Inflammatory myxohyaline tumor of distal extremities with virocyte or Reed-Sternberg-like cells: a distinctive lesion with features simulating inflammatory conditions, Hodgkin's disease, and various sarcomas. *Mod Pathol* 11: 384-391.

1497. Montgomery EA, Meis JM (1991). Nodular fasciitis. Its morphologic spectrum and immunohistochemical profile. *Am J Surg Pathol* 15: 942-948.

1498. Montgomery EA, Meis JM, Mitchell MS, Enzinger FM (1992). Atypical decubital fibroplasia. A distinctive fibroblastic pseudotumor occurring in debilitated patients. *Am J Surg Pathol* 16: 708-715.

1499. Montgomery EA, Meis JM, Ramos AG, et al. (1993). Clear cell sarcoma of tendons and aponeuroses. A clinicopathologic study of 58 cases with analysis of prognostic factors. *Int J Surg Pathol* 1: 89-100.

1500. Montgomery H, Winkelmann RK (1959). Smooth-muscle tumors of the skin. *Arch Dermatol* 79: 32-41.

1501. Mooi WJ, Deenik W, Peterse JL, Hogendoorn PC (1995). Keratin immunoreactivity in melanoma of soft parts (clear cell sarcoma). *Histopathology* 27: 61-65.

1502. Moon NF (1994). Adamantinoma of the appendicular skeleton in children. *Int Orthop* 18: 379-388.

1503. Moon NF, Mori H (1986). Adamantinoma of the appendicular skeleton – updated. *Clin Orthop* 215-237.

1504. Moore JR, Weiland AJ, Curtis RM (1984). Localized nodular tenosynovitis: experience with 115 cases. *J Hand Surg [Am]* 9: 412-417.

1505. Moore PS, Chang Y (1995). Detection of herpesvirus-like DNA sequences in Kaposi's sarcoma in patients with and without HIV infection. *N Engl J Med* 332: 1181-1185.

1506. Morimitsu Y, Aoki T, Yokoyama K, Hashimoto H (2000). Sarcomatoid chordoma: chordoma with a massive malignant spindle-cell component. *Skeletal Radiol* 29: 721-725.

1507. Morris DM, House HC (1985). The significance of metastasis to the bones and soft tissues of the hand. *J Surg Oncol* 28: 146-150.

1508. Morris EJ, Dyson NJ (2001). Retinoblastoma protein partners. *Adv Cancer Res* 82: 1-54.

1509. Moser MJ, Bigbee WL, Grant SG, Emond MJ, Langlois RG, Jensen RH, Oshima J, Monnat RJ, Jr. (2000). Genetic instability and hematologic disease risk in Werner syndrome patients and heterozygotes. *Cancer Res* 60: 2492-2496.

1510. Moser MJ, Kamath-Loeb AS, Jacob JE, Bennett SE, Oshima J, Monnat RJ, Jr. (2000). WRN helicase expression in Werner syndrome cell lines. *Nucleic Acids Res* 28: 648-654.

1511. Moser MJ, Oshima J, Monnat RJ, Jr. (1999). WRN mutations in Werner syndrome. *Hum Mutat* 13: 271-279.

1512. Moses AM, Spencer H (1963). Hypercalcemia in patients with malignant lymphoma. *Ann Int Med* 59: 531-536.

1513. Motoyama T, Ogose A, Watanabe H (1996). Ossifying fibromyxoid tumor of the retroperitoneum. *Pathol Int* 46: 79-83.

1514. Muggia FM, Hansen HH (1972). Osteoblastic metastases in small-cell (oat-cell) carcinoma of the lung. *Cancer* 30: 801-805.

1515. Mukai M, Torikata C, Iri H, Hata J, Naito M, Shimoda T (1992). Immunohistochemical identification of aggregated actin filaments in formalin-fixed, paraffin-embedded sections. I. A study of infantile digital fibromatosis by a new pretreatment. *Am J Surg Pathol* 16: 110-115.

1516. Mukai M, Torikata C, Iri H, Hata J, Naito M, Shimoda T, Kageyama K (1986). Infantile digital fibromatosis. An electron microscopic and immunohistochemical study. *Acta Pathol Jpn* 36: 1605-1615.

1517. Mukai M, Torikata C, Iri H, Mikata A, Kawai T, Hanaoka H, Yakumaru K, Kageyama K (1984). Histogenesis of clear cell sarcoma of tendons and aponeuroses. An electron-microscopic, biochemical, enzyme histochemical, and immunohistochemical study. *Am J Pathol* 114: 264-272.

1518. Mulder JD, Schutte HE, Kroon HM, Taconis WK (1993). *Radiologic Atlas of Bone Tumors.* Elsevier: Amsterdam.

1519. Mulligan LM, Matlashewski GJ, Scrable HJ, Cavenee WK (1990). Mechanisms of p53 loss in human sarcomas. *Proc Natl Acad Sci U S A* 87: 5863-5867.

1520. Mundy GR (1988). Hypercalcemia of malignancy revisited. *J Clin Invest* 82: 1-6.

1521. Muroya K, Nishimura G, Douya H, Hasegawa T, Ogata T (2002). Diaphyseal medullary stenosis with malignant fibrous histiocytoma: further evidence for loss of heterozygosity involving 9p21-22 in tumor tissue. *Genes Chromosomes Cancer* 33: 326-328.

1522. Murphey MD, Gross TM, Rosenthal HG (1994). From the archives of the AFIP. Musculoskeletal malignant fibrous histiocytoma: radiologic-pathologic correlation. *Radiographics* 14: 807-826.

1523. Myers BW, Masi AT (1980). Pigmented villonodular synovitis and tenosynovitis: a clinical epidemiologic study of 166 cases and literature review. *Medicine (Baltimore)* 59: 223-238.

1524. Myhre-Jensen O (1981). A consecutive 7-year series of 1331 benign soft tissue tumours. Clinicopathologic data. Comparison with sarcomas. *Acta Orthop Scand* 52: 287-293.

1525. Myhre-Jensen O, Kaae S, Madsen EH, Sneppen O (1983). Histopathological grading in soft-tissue tumours. Relation to survival in 261 surgically treated patients. *Acta Pathol Microbiol Immunol Sand [A]* 91: 145-150.

1526. Nagamine N, Nohara Y, Ito E (1982). Elastofibroma in Okinawa. A clinicopathologic study of 170 cases. *Cancer* 50: 1794-1805.

1527. Naka N, Tomita Y, Nakanishi H, Araki N, Hongyo T, Ochi T, Aozasa K (1997). Mutations of p53 tumor-suppressor gene in angiosarcoma. *Int J Cancer* 71: 952-955.

1528. Naka T, Fukuda T, Shinohara N, Iwamoto Y, Sugioka Y, Tsuneyoshi M (1995). Osteosarcoma versus malignant fibrous histiocytoma of bone in patients older than 40 years. A clinicopathologic and immunohistochemical analysis with special reference to malignant fibrous histiocytoma-like osteosarcoma. *Cancer* 76: 972-984.

1529. Nakajima H, Sim FH, Bond JR, Unni KK (1997). Small cell osteosarcoma of bone. Review of 72 cases. *Cancer* 79: 2095-2106.

1530. Nakajima T, Watanabe S, Sato Y, Shimosato Y, Motoi M, Lennert K (1982). S-100 protein in Langerhans cells, interdigitating reticulum cells and histiocytosis X cells. *Gann* 73: 429-432.

1531. Nakamura Y, Okamoto K, Tanimura A, Kato M, Morimatsu M (1986). Elastase digestion and biochemical analysis of the elastin from an elastofibroma. *Cancer* 58: 1070-1075.

1532. Nakanishi H, Tomita Y, Myoui A, Yoshikawa H, Sakai K, Kato Y, Ochi T, Aozasa K (1998). Mutation of the p53 gene in postradiation sarcoma. *Lab Invest* 78: 727-733.

1533. Nakashima Y, Unni KK, Shives TC, Swee RG, Dahlin DC (1986). Mesenchymal chondrosarcoma of bone and soft tissue. A review of 111 cases. *Cancer* 57: 2444-2453.

1534. Nakashima Y, Yamamuro T, Fujiwara Y, Kotoura Y, Mori E, Hamashima Y (1983). Osteofibrous dysplasia (ossifying fibroma of long bones). A study of 12 cases. *Cancer* 52: 909-914.

1535. Nappi O, Ritter JH, Pettinato G, Wick MR (1995). Hemangiopericytoma: histopathological pattern or clinicopathologic entity? *Semin Diagn Pathol* 12: 221-232.

1536. Nascimento AG, Huvos AG, Marcove RC (1979). Primary malignant giant cell tumor of bone: a study of eight cases and review of the literature. *Cancer* 44: 1393-1402.

1537. Nascimento AG, Keeney GL, Sciot R, Fletcher CD (1997). Polymorphous hemangioendothelioma: a report of two cases, one affecting extranodal soft tissues, and review of the literature. *Am J Surg Pathol* 21: 1083-1089.

1538. Nascimento AG, Kurtin PJ, Guillou L, Fletcher CD (1998). Dedifferentiated liposarcoma: a report of nine cases with a peculiar neurallike whorling pattern associated with metaplastic bone formation. *Am J Surg Pathol* 22: 945-955.

1539. Nascimento AG, Ruiz R, Hornick JL, Fletcher CD (2002). Calcifying fibrous 'pseudotumour': clinicopathologic study of 15 cases and analysis of its relationship to inflammatory myofibroblastic tumour. *Int J Surg Pathol* (in press).

1540. Nascimento AG, Unii KK, Pritchard DJ, Cooper KL, Dahlin DC (1980). A clinicopathologic study of 20 cases of large-cell (atypical) Ewing's sarcoma of bone. *Am J Surg Pathol* 4: 29-36.

1541. Naumann M, Schalke B, Klopstock T, Reichmann H, Lange KW, Wiesbeck G, Toyka KV, Reiners K (1995). Neurological multisystem manifestation in multiple symmetric lipomatosis: a clinical and electrophysiological study. *Muscle Nerve* 18: 693-698.

1542. Naumann S, Krallman PA, Unni KK, Fidler ME, Neff JR, Bridge JA (2002). Translocation der(13;21)(q10;q10) in skeletal and extraskeletal mesenchymal chondrosarcoma. *Mod Pathol* 15: 572-576.

1543. Nayler SJ, Rubin BP, Calonje E, Chan JK, Fletcher CD (2000). Composite hemangioendothelioma: a complex, low-grade vascular lesion mimicking angiosarcoma. *Am J Surg Pathol* 24: 352-361.

1544. Naylor EW, Gardner EJ, Richards RC (1979). Desmoid tumors and mesenteric fibromatosis in Gardner's syndrome: report of kindred 109. *Arch Surg* 114: 1181-1185.

1545. Naylor MF, Nascimento AG, Sherrick AD, McLeod RA (1996). Elastofibroma dorsi: radiologic findings in 12 patients. *AJR Am J Roentgenol* 167: 683-687.

1546. Nellissery MJ, Padalecki SS, Brkanac Z, Singer FR, Roodman GD, Unni KK, Leach RJ, Hansen MF (1998). Evidence for a novel osteosarcoma tumor-suppressor gene in the chromosome 18 region genetically linked with Paget disease of bone. *Am J Hum Genet* 63: 817-824.

1547. Nemoto O, Moser RP, Jr., Van Dam BE, Aoki J, Gilkey FW (1990). Osteoblastoma of the spine. A review of 75 cases. *Spine* 15: 1272-1280.

1548. Newsham I, Daub D, Besnard-Guerin C, Cavenee W (1994). Molecular sublocalization and characterization of the 11;22 translocation breakpoint in a malignant rhabdoid tumor. *Genomics* 19: 433-440.

1549. Newton WA, Jr., Gehan EA, Webber BL, Marsden HB, van Unnik AJ, Hamoudi AB, Tsokos MG, Shimada H, Harms D, Schmidt D, . (1995). Classification of rhabdomyosarcomas and related sarcomas. Pathologic aspects and proposal for a new classification – an Intergroup Rhabdomyosarcoma Study. *Cancer* 76: 1073-1085.

1550. Newton WA, Jr., Soule EH, Hamoudi AB, Reiman HM, Shimada H, Beltangady M, Maurer H (1988). Histopathology of childhood sarcomas, Intergroup Rhabdomyosarcoma Studies I and II: clinicopathologic correlation. *J Clin Oncol* 6: 67-75.

1551. Ng SH, Ko SF, Wan YL, Tang LM, Ho YS (1998). Cervical ecchordosis physaliphora: CT and MR features. *Br J Radiol* 71: 329-331.

1552. Nichols GE, Cooper PH (1994). Low-grade fibromyxoid sarcoma: case report and immunohistochemical study. *J Cutan Pathol* 21: 356-362.

1553. Nicolaides A, Huang YQ, Li JJ, Zhang WG, Friedman-Kien AE (1994). Gene amplification and multiple mutations of the K-ras oncogene in Kaposi's sarcoma. *Anticancer Res* 14: 921-926.

1554. Niedt GW, Greco MA, Wieczorek R, Blanc WA, Knowles DM (1989). Hemangioma with Kaposi's sarcoma-like features: report of two cases. *Pediatr Pathol* 9: 567-575.

1555. Nielsen AL, Kiaer T (1989). Malignant giant cell tumor of synovium and locally destructive pigmented villonodular synovitis: ultrastructural and immunohistochemical study and review of the literature. *Hum Pathol* 20: 765-771.

1556. Nielsen GP, Dickersin GR, Provenzal JM, Rosenberg AE (1995). Lipomatous hemangiopericytoma. A histologic, ultrastructural and immunohistochemical study of a unique variant of hemangiopericytoma. *Am J Surg Pathol* 19: 748-756.

1557. Nielsen GP, Fletcher CD, Smith MA, Rybak L, Rosenberg AE (2002). Soft tissue aneurysmal bone cyst: a clinicopathologic study of five cases. *Am J Surg Pathol* 26: 64-69.

1558. Nielsen GP, Keel SB, Dickersin GR, Selig MK, Bhan AK, Rosenberg AE (1999). Chondromyxoid fibroma: a tumor showing myofibroblastic, myochondroblastic, and chondrocytic differentiation. *Mod Pathol* 12: 514-517.

1559. Nielsen GP, O'Connell JX, Dickersin GR, Rosenberg AE (1995). Chondroid lipoma, a tumor of white fat cells. A brief report of two cases with ultrastructural analysis. *Am J Surg Pathol* 19: 1272-1276.

1560. Nielsen GP, O'Connell JX, Dickersin GR, Rosenberg AE (1996). Collagenous fibroma (desmoplastic fibroblastoma): a report of seven cases. *Mod Pathol* 9: 781-785.

1561. Nielsen GP, O'Connell JX, Dickersin GR, Rosenberg AE (1997). Solitary fibrous tumor of soft tissue: a report of 15 cases, including 5 malignant examples with light microscopic, immunohistochemical, and ultrastructural data. *Mod Pathol* 10: 1028-1037.

1562. Nielsen GP, O'Connell JX, Rosenberg AE (1998). Intramuscular myxoma: a clinicopathologic study of 51 cases with emphasis on hypercellular and hypervascular variants. *Am J Surg Pathol* 22: 1222-1227.

1563. Nielsen GP, Oliva E, Young RH, Rosenberg AE, Dickersin GR, Scully RE (1995). Alveolar soft-part sarcoma of the female genital tract: a report of nine cases and review of the literature. *Int J Gynecol Pathol* 14: 283-292.

1564. Nielsen GP, Rosenberg AE, Young RH, Dickersin GR, Clement PB, Scully RE (1996). Angiomyofibroblastoma of the vulva and vagina. *Mod Pathol* 9: 284-291.

1565. Nielsen GP, Selig MK, O'Connell JX, Keel SB, Dickersin GR, Rosenberg AE (1999). Hyalinizing spindle cell tumor with giant rosettes: a report of three cases with ultrastructural analysis. *Am J Surg Pathol* 23: 1227-1232.

1566. Nielsen GP, Young RH, Dickersin GR, Rosenberg AE (1997). Angiomyofibroblastoma of the vulva with sarcomatous transformation ("angiomyofibrosarcoma"). *Am J Surg Pathol* 21: 1104-1108.

1567. Nilbert M, Mandahl N, Heim S, Rydholm A, Willén H, Mitelman F (1989). Cytogenetic abnormalities in an angioleiomyoma. *Cancer Genet Cytogenet* 37: 61-64.

1568. Nilbert M, Rydholm A, Willén H, Mitelman F, Mandahl N (1994). MDM2 gene amplification correlates with ring chromosome in soft tissue tumors. *Genes Chromosomes Cancer* 9: 261-265.

1569. Nilsson G, Skytting B, Xie Y, Brodin B, Perfekt R, Mandahl N, Lundeberg J, Uhlen M, Larsson O (1999). The SYT-SSX1 variant of synovial sarcoma is associated with a high rate of tumor cell proliferation and poor clinical outcome. *Cancer Res* 59: 3180-3184.

1570. Nilsson G, Wang M, Wejde J, Kanter L, Karlen J, Tani E, Kreicbergs A, Larsson O (1998). Reverse transcriptase polymerase chain reaction on fine needle aspirates for rapid detection of translocations in synovial sarcoma. *Acta Cytol* 42: 1317-1324.

1571. Nishida J, Sim FH, Wenger DE, Unni KK (1997). Malignant fibrous histiocytoma of bone. A clinicopathologic study of 81 patients. *Cancer* 79: 482-493.

1572. Nishida N, Yutani C, Ishibashi-Ueda H, Tsukamoto Y, Ikeda Y, Nakamura Y (2000). Histopathological characterization of aortic intimal sarcoma with multiple tumor emboli. *Pathol Int* 50: 923-927.

1573. Nistal M, Paniagua R, Picazo ML, Cermeno dG, Ramos Guerreira JL (1980). Granular changes in vascular leiomyosarcoma. *Virchows Arch A Pathol Anat Histol* 386: 239-248.

1574. Nixon HH, Scobie WG (1971). Congenital lipomatosis: a report of four cases. *J Pediatr Surg* 6: 742-745.

1575. Noer H, Krogdahl A (1991). Glomangiosarcoma of the lower extremity. *Histopathology* 18: 365-366.

1576. Nojima T, Yamashiro K, Fujita M, Isu K, Ubayama Y, Yamawaki S (1991). A case of osteosarcoma arising in a solitary osteochondroma. *Acta Orthop Scand* 62: 290-292.

1577. Nonomura A, Kurumaya H, Kono N, Nakanuma Y, Ohta G, Terahata S, Matsubara F, Matsuda T, Asaka T, Nishino T (1988). Primary pulmonary artery sarcoma. Report of two autopsy cases studied by immunohistochemistry and electron microscopy, and review of 110 cases reported in the literature. *Acta Pathol Jpn* 38: 883-896.

1578. Nora FE, Unni KK, Pritchard DJ, Dahlin DC (1983). Osteosarcoma of extragnathic craniofacial bones. *Mayo Clin Proc* 58: 268-272.

1579. Norman A, Abdelwahab IF, Buyon J, Matzkin E (1986). Osteoid osteoma of the hip stimulating an early onset of osteoarthritis. *Radiology* 158: 417-420.

1580. Norman A, Dorfman HD (1970). Juxtacortical circumscribed myositis ossificans: evolution and radiographic features. *Radiology* 96: 301-306.

1581. Norman A, Ulin R (1969). A comparative study of periosteal new-bone response in metastatic bone tumors (solitary) and primary sarcomas. *Radiology* 92: 705-708.

1582. North PE, Waner M, Mizeracki A, Mihm MC, Jr. (2000). GLUT1: a newly discovered immunohistochemical marker for juvenile hemangiomas. *Hum Pathol* 31: 11-22.

1583. Norton KI, Wagreich JM, Granowetter L, Martignetti JA (1996). Diaphyseal medullary stenosis (sclerosis) with bone malignancy (malignant fibrous histiocytoma): Hardcastle syndrome. *Pediatr Radiol* 26: 675-677.

1584. Nucci MR, Fletcher CD (2000). Vulvovaginal soft tissue tumours: update and review. *Histopathology* 36: 97-108.

1585. Nucci MR, Granter SR, Fletcher CD (1997). Cellular angiofibroma: a benign neoplasm distinct from angiomyofibroblastoma and spindle cell lipoma. *Am J Surg Pathol* 21: 636-644.

1586. Nucci MR, Weremowicz S, Neskey DM, Sornberger K, Tallini G, Morton CC, Quade BJ (2001). Chromosomal translocation t(8;12) induces aberrant HMGIC expression in aggressive angiomyxoma of the vulva. *Genes Chromosomes Cancer* 32: 172-176.

1587. Nunnery EW, Kahn LB, Guilford WB (1979). Locally aggressive fibrous histiocytoma of bone. A case report. *S Afr Med J* 55: 763-767.

1588. Nuovo MA, Norman A, Chumas J, Ackerman LV (1992). Myositis ossificans with atypical clinical, radiographic, or pathologic findings: a review of 23 cases. *Skeletal Radiol* 21: 87-101.

1589. O'Brien JE, Stout AP (1964). Malignant fibrous xanthomas. *Cancer* 17: 1445.

1590. O'Connell JX, Fanburg JC, Rosenberg AE (1995). Giant cell tumor of tendon sheath and pigmented villonodular synovitis: immunophenotype suggests a synovial cell origin. *Hum Pathol* 26: 771-775.

1591. O'Connell JX, Wehrli BM, Nielsen GP, Rosenberg AE (2000). Giant cell tumors of soft tissue: a clinicopathologic study of 18 benign and malignant tumors. *Am J Surg Pathol* 24: 386-395.

1592. O'Malley DP, Opheim KE, Barry TS, Chapman DB, Emond MJ, Conrad EU, Norwood TH (2001). Chromosomal changes in a dedifferentiated chondrosarcoma: a case report and review of the literature. *Cancer Genet Cytogenet* 124: 105-111.

1593. Ockner DM, Sayadi H, Swanson PE, Ritter JH, Wick MR (1997). Genital angiomyofibroblastoma. Comparison with aggressive angiomyxoma and other myxoid neoplasms of skin and soft tissue. *Am J Clin Pathol* 107: 36-44.

1594. Oda Y, Miyajima K, Kawaguchi K, Tamiya S, Oshiro Y, Hachitanda Y, Oya M, Iwamoto Y, Tsuneyoshi M (2001). Pleomorphic leiomyosarcoma: clinicopathologic and immunohistochemical study with special emphasis on its distinction from ordinary leiomyosarcoma and malignant fibrous histiocytoma. *Am J Surg Pathol* 25: 1030-1038.

1595. Odink AE, van Asperen CJ, Vandenbroucke JP, Cleton-Jansen AM, Hogendoorn PC (2001). An association between cartilaginous tumours and breast cancer in the national pathology registration in The Netherlands points towards a possible genetic trait. *J Pathol* 193: 190-192.

1596. Ogunsalu C, Smith NJ, Lewis A (1998). Fibrous dysplasia of the jaw bone: a review of 15 new cases and two cases of recurrence in Jamaica together with a case report. *Aust Dent J* 43: 390-394.

1597. Ohjimi Y, Iwasaki H, Ishiguro M, Isayama T, Kaneko Y (1994). Trisomy 2 found in proliferative myositis cultured cell. *Cancer Genet Cytogenet* 76: 157.

1598. Ohno T, Rao VN, Reddy ES (1993). EWS/Fli-1 chimeric protein is a transcriptional activator. *Cancer Res* 53: 5859-5863.

1599. Okada K, Frassica FJ, Sim FH, Beabout JW, Bond JR, Unni KK (1994). Parosteal osteosarcoma. A clinicopathological study. *J Bone Joint Surg Am* 76: 366-378.

1600. Okada K, Unni KK, Swee RG, Sim FH (1999). High grade surface osteosarcoma: a clinicopathologic study of 46 cases. *Cancer* 85: 1044-1054.

1601. Okada K, Wold LE, Beabout JW, Shives TC (1993). Osteosarcoma of the hand. A clinicopathologic study of 12 cases. *Cancer* 72: 719-725.

1602. Okada O, Demitsu T, Manabe M, Yoneda K (1999). A case of multiple subungual glomus tumors associated with neurofibromatosis type 1. *J Dermatol* 26: 535-537.

1603. Okamoto S, Hisaoka M, Ishida T, Imamura T, Kanda H, Shimajiri S, Hashimoto H (2001). Extraskeletal myxoid chondrosarcoma: a clinicopathologic, immunohistochemical, and molecular analysis of 18 cases. *Hum Pathol* 32: 1116-1124.

1604. Okamoto S, Hisaoka M, Meis-Kindblom JM, Kindblom LG, Hashimoto H (2002). Juxta-articular myxoma and intramuscular myxoma are two distinct entities – Activating Gsa mutation at Arg201 codon does not occur in juxta-articular myxoma. *Virchows Arch* 440: 12-15.

1605. Okamoto S, Hisaoka M, Ushijima M, Nakahara S, Toyoshima S, Hashimoto H (2000). Activating Gs(alpha) mutation in intramuscular myxomas with and without fibrous dysplasia of bone. *Virchows Arch* 437: 133-137.

1606. Oldfield MC (1954). The association of familial polyposis of the colon with multiple sebaceous cysts. *Br J Surg* 41: 534-541.

1607. Oliner JD, Kinzler KW, Meltzer PS, George DL, Vogelstein B (1992). Amplification of a gene encoding a p53-associated protein in human sarcomas. *Nature* 358: 80-83.

1608. Oliveira AM, Dei Tos AP, Fletcher CD, Nascimento AG (2000). Primary giant cell tumor of soft tissues: a study of 22 cases. *Am J Surg Pathol* 24: 248-256.

1609. Oliveira AM, Nascimento AG (2001). Pleomorphic liposarcoma. *Semin Diagn Pathol* 18: 274-285.

1610. Oliveira AM, Nascimento AG, Lloyd RV (2001). Leptin and leptin receptor mRNA are widely expressed in tumors of adipocytic differentiation. *Mod Pathol* 14: 549-555.

1611. Oliveira AM, Sebo TJ, McGrory JE, Gaffey TA, Rock MG, Nascimento AG (2000). Extraskeletal myxoid chondrosarcoma: a clinicopathologic, immunochemical, and ploidy analysis of 23 cases. *Mod Pathol* 13: 900-908.

1612. Olsen TG, Helwig EB (1985). Angiolymphoid hyperplasia with eosinophilia. A clinicopathologic study of 116 patients. *J Am Acad Dermatol* 12: 781-796.

1613. Onda M, Matsuda S, Higaki S, Iijima T, Fukushima J, Yokokura A, Kojima T, Horiuchi H, Kurokawa T, Yamamoto T (1996). ErbB-2 expression is correlated with poor prognosis for patients with osteosarcoma. *Cancer* 77: 71-78.

1614. Onikul E, Fletcher BD, Parham DM, Chen G (1996). Accuracy of MR imaging for estimating intraosseous extent of osteosarcoma. *AJR Am J Roentgenol* 167: 1211-1215.

1615. Ono K, Oshiro M, Uemura K, Ota H, Matsushita Y, Ijima S, Iwase T, Uchida M, Katsuyama T (1996). Erdheim-Chester disease: a case report with immunohistochemical and biochemical examination. *Hum Pathol* 27: 91-95.

1616. Oosthuizen SF, Barnetson J (1947). Two cases of lipomatosis involving bone. *Br J Radiol* 20: 426.

1617. Ordonez NG (1999). Alveolar soft part sarcoma: a review and update. *Adv Anat Pathol* 6: 125-139.

1618. Ordonez NG, Mackay B (1998). Alveolar soft-part sarcoma: a review of the pathology and histogenesis. *Ultrastruct Pathol* 22: 275-292.

1619. Ordonez NG, Ro JY, Mackay B (1989). Alveolar soft part sarcoma. An ultrastructural and immunocytochemical investigation of its histogenesis. *Cancer* 63: 1721-1736.

1620. Osgood PJ, Damron TA, Rooney MT, Goldschmidt AM, Sullivan TJ (1998). Benign fetal rhabdomyoma of the upper extremity. A case report. *Clin Orthop* 200-204.

1621. Oshiro Y, Fukuda T, Tsuneyoshi M (1994). Fibrosarcoma versus fibromatoses and cellular nodular fasciitis. A comparative study of their proliferative activity using proliferating cell nuclear antigen, DNA flow cytometry, and p53. *Am J Surg Pathol* 18: 712-719.

1622. Oshiro Y, Shiratsuchi H, Tamiya S, Oda Y, Toyoshima S, Tsuneyoshi M (2000). Extraskeletal myxoid chondrosarcoma with rhabdoid features, with special reference to its aggressive behavior. *Int J Surg Pathol* 8: 145-152.

1623. Ostrowski ML, Inwards CY, Strickler JG, Witzig TE, Wenger DE, Unni KK (1999). Osseous Hodgkin disease. *Cancer* 85: 1166-1178.

1624. Ostrowski ML, Johnson ME, Truong LD, Hicks MJ, Smith FE, Spjut HJ (1999). Malignant chondroblastoma presenting as a recurrent pelvic tumor with DNA aneuploidy and p53 mutation as supportive evidence of malignancy. *Skeletal Radiol* 28: 644-650.

1625. Ostrowski ML, McEnery KW (2002). Cartilaginous lesions of the skeleton. *Am J Clin Pathol* (in press).

1626. Ostrowski ML, Unni KK, Banks PM, Shives TC, Evans RG, O'Connell MJ, Taylor WF (1986). Malignant lymphoma of bone. *Cancer* 58: 2646-2655.

1627. Otano-Joos M, Mechtersheimer G, Ohl S, Wilgenbus KK, Scheurlen W, Lehnert T, Willeke F, Otto HF, Lichter P, Joos S (2000). Detection of chromosomal imbalances in leiomyosarcoma by comparative genomic hybridization and interphase cytogenetics. *Cytogenet Cell Genet* 90: 86-92.

1628. Otero LJ, Aragon dlC (1977). [Radiotherapy of osseous angiomas. Critical study on its indication]. *Rev Clin Esp* 144: 367-373.

1629. Outwater EK, Marchetto BE, Wagner BJ, Siegelman ES (1999). Aggressive angiomyxoma: findings on CT and MR imaging. *AJR Am J Roentgenol* 172: 435-438.

1630. Ozaki T, Inoue H, Sugihara S, Sumii H (1992). Radiological long-term follow-up of grafted xenogeneic bone in patients with bone tumors. *Acta Med Okayama* 46: 87-92.

1631. Ozisik YY, Meloni AM, Peier A, Altungoz O, Spanier SS, Zalupski MM, Leong SP, Sandberg AA (1994). Cytogenetic findings in 19 malignant bone tumors. *Cancer* 74: 2268-2275.

1632. Ozzello L, Stout AP, Murray MR (1963). Cultural characteristic of malignant histiocytomas and fibrous xanthomas. *Cancer* 16: 331.

1633. Örndal C, Carlen B, Åkerman M, Willén H, Mandahl N, Heim S, Rydholm A, Mitelman F (1991). Chromosomal abnormality t(9;22)(q22;q12) in an extraskeletal myxoid chondrosarcoma characterized by fine needle aspiration cytology, electron micro-scopy, immunohistochemistry and DNA flow cytometry. *Cytopathology* 2: 261-270.

1634. Örndal C, Mandahl N, Rydholm A, Willén H, Brosjö O, Mitelman F (1993). Chromosome aberrations and cytogenetic intratumor heterogeneity in chondrosarcomas. *J Cancer Res Clin Oncol* 120: 51-56.

1635. Örndal C, Rydholm A, Willén H, Mitelman F, Mandahl N (1994). Cytogenetic intratumor heterogeneity in soft tissue tumors. *Cancer Genet Cytogenet* 78: 127-137.

1636. Paal E, Miettinen M (2001). Retroperitoneal leiomyomas: a clinicopathologic and immunohistochemical study of 56 cases with a comparison to retroperitoneal leiomyosarcomas. *Am J Surg Pathol* 25: 1355-1363.

1637. Pack SD, Kirschner LS, Pak E, Zhuang Z, Carney JA, Stratakis CA (2000). Genetic and histologic studies of somatomammotropic pituitary tumors in patients with the "complex of spotty skin pigmentation, myxomas, endocrine overactivity and schwannomas" (Carney complex). *J Clin Endocrinol Metab* 85: 3860-3865.

1638. Paller AS, Gonzalez-Crussi F, Sherman JO (1989). Fibrous hamartoma of infancy. Eight additional cases and a review of the literature. *Arch Dermatol* 125: 88-91.

1639. Palmieri AJ, Kovarik JL (1962). Nonsteogenic fibroma of the rib. *Am Surg* 28: 794-798.

1640. Palmirotta R, Curia MC, Esposito DL, Valanzano R, Messerini L, Ficari F, Brandi ML, Tonelli F, Mariani-Costantini R, Battista P, Cama A (1995). Novel mutations and inactivation of both alleles of the APC gene in desmoid tumors. *Hum Mol Genet* 4: 1979-1981.

1641. Panagopoulos I, Höglund M, Mertens F, Mandahl N, Mitelman F, Åman P (1996). Fusion of the EWS and CHOP genes in myxoid liposarcoma. *Oncogene* 12: 489-494.

1642. Panagopoulos I, Mandahl N, Ron D, Höglund M, Nilbert M, Mertens F, Mitelman F, Åman P (1994). Characterization of the CHOP breakpoints and fusion transcripts in myxoid liposarcomas with the 12;16 translocation. *Cancer Res* 54: 6500-6503.

1643. Panagopoulos I, Mencinger M, Dietrich CU, Bjerkehagen B, Saeter G, Mertens F, Mandahl N, Heim S (1999). Fusion of the RBP56 and CHN genes in extraskeletal myxoid chondrosarcomas with translocation t(9;17)(q22;q11). *Oncogene* 18: 7594-7598.

1644. Panagopoulos I, Mertens F, Domanski HA, Isaksson M, Brosjö O, Gustafson P, Mandahl N (2001). No EWS/FLI1 fusion transcripts in giant-cell tumors of bone. *Int J Cancer* 93: 769-772.

1645. Panoutsakopoulos G, Pandis N, Kyriazoglou I, Gustafson P, Mertens F, Mandahl N (1999). Recurrent t(16;17)(q22;p13) in aneurysmal bone cysts. *Genes Chromosomes Cancer* 26: 265-266.

1646. Papadimitriou JC, Drachenberg CB (1994). Ultrastructural features of the matrix of small cell osteosarcoma. *Hum Pathol* 25: 430-431.

1647. Papagelopoulos PJ, Galanis E, Frassica FJ, Sim FH, Larson DR, Wold LE (2000). Primary fibrosarcoma of bone. Outcome after primary surgical treatment. *Clin Orthop* 88-103.

1648. Papagelopoulos PJ, Galanis EC, Sim FH, Unni KK (2000). Clinicopathologic features, diagnosis, and treatment of malignant fibrous histiocytoma of bone. *Orthopedics* 23: 59-65.

1649. Papkoff J, Rubinfeld B, Schryver B, Polakis P (1996). Wnt-1 regulates free pools of catenins and stabilizes APC-catenin complexes. *Mol Cell Biol* 16: 2128-2134.

1650. Pardo-Mindan FJ, Ayala H, Joly M, Gimeno E, Vazquez JJ (1981). Primary liposarcoma of bone: light and electron microscopic study. *Cancer* 48: 274-280.

1651. Parente F, Grosgeorge J, Coindre JM, Terrier P, Vilain O, Turc-Carel C (1999). Comparative genomic hybridization reveals novel chromosome deletions in 90 primary soft tissue tumors. *Cancer Genet Cytogenet* 115: 89-95.

1652. Parham DM, Reynolds AB, Webber BL (1995). Use of monoclonal antibody 1H1, anticortactin, to distinguish normal and neoplastic smooth muscle cells: comparison with anti-alpha-smooth muscle actin and antimuscle-specific actin. *Hum Pathol* 26: 776-783.

1653. Parham DM, Webber B, Holt H, Williams WK, Maurer H (1991). Immunohistochemical study of childhood rhabdomyosarcomas and related neoplasms. Results of an Intergroup Rhabdomyosarcoma study project. *Cancer* 67: 3072-3080.

1654. Park CH, Kim KI, Lim YT, Chung SW, Lee CH (2000). Ruptured giant intrathoracic lipoblastoma in a 4-month-old infant: CT and MR findings. *Pediatr Radiol* 30: 38-40.

1655. Park IC, Lee SY, Jeon DG, Lee JS, Hwang CS, Hwang BG, Lee SH, Hong WS, Hong SI (1996). Enhanced expression of cathepsin L in metastatic bone tumors. *J Korean Med Sci* 11: 144-148.

1656. Park KJ, Shin KH, Ku JL, Cho TJ, Lee SH, Choi IH, Phillipe C, Monaco AP, Porter DE, Park JG (1999). Germline mutations in the EXT1 and EXT2 genes in Korean patients with hereditary multiple exostoses. *J Hum Genet* 44: 230-234.

1657. Park YK, Cho CH, Chi SG, Han CS, Ushigome S, Unni KK (2001). Low incidence of genetic alterations of the p16CDKN2a in clear cell chondrosarcoma. *Int J Oncol* 19: 749-753.

1658. Park YK, Joo M (2001). Multicentric telangiectatic osteosarcoma. *Pathol Int* 51: 200-203.

1659. Park YK, Park HR, Chi SG, Kim CJ, Sohn KR, Koh JS, Kim CW, Yang WI, Ro JY, Ahn KW, Joo M, Kim YW, Lee J, Yang MH, Unni KK (2000). Overexpression of p53 and rare genetic mutation in mesenchymal chondrosarcoma. *Oncol Rep* 7: 1041-1047.

1660. Park YK, Unni KK, Beabout JW, Hodgson SF (1994). Oncogenic osteomalacia: a clinicopathologic study of 17 bone lesions. *J Korean Med Sci* 9: 289-298.

1661. Park YK, Unni KK, Kim YW, Han CS, Yang MH, Wenger DE, Sim FH, Lucas DR, Ryan JR, Nadim YA, Nojima T, Fletcher CD (1999). Primary alveolar soft part sarcoma of bone. *Histopathology* 35: 411-417.

1662. Parker JB, Marcus PB, Martin JH (1980). Spinal melanotic clear-cell sarcoma: a light and electron microscopic study. *Cancer* 46: 718-724.

1663. Parker SL, Tong T, Bolden S, Wingo PA (1996). Cancer statistics, 1996. *CA Cancer J Clin* 46: 5-27.

1664. Parkin DM, Stiller CA, Draper GJ, Bieber CA (1988). The international incidence of childhood cancer. *Int J Cancer* 42: 511-520.

1665. Parkin DM, Whelan SL, Ferlay J, Raymond L, Young J (1997). *Cancer Incidence in Five Continents*. IARC Press: Lyon.

1666. Paschall HA, Paschall MM (1975). Electron microscopic observations of 20 human osteosarcomas. *Clin Orthop* 42-56.

1667. Paterson DC (1970). Myositis ossificans circumscripta. Report of four cases without history of injury. *J Bone Joint Surg Br* 52: 296-301.

1668. Patterson H, Gill S, Fisher C, Law MG, Jayatilake H, Fletcher CD, Thomas M, Grimer R, Gusterson BA, Cooper CS (1994). Abnormalities of the p53 MDM2 and DCC genes in human leiomyosarcomas. *Br J Cancer* 69: 1052-1058.

1669. Pauwels P, Dal Cin P, Roumen R, van den Berghe H, Sciot R (1999). Intramuscular mixed tumour with clonal chromosomal changes. *Virchows Arch* 434: 167-171.

1670. Pauwels P, Sciot R, Croiset F, Rutten H, van den Berghe H, Dal Cin P (2000). Myofibroblastoma of the breast: genetic link with spindle cell lipoma. *J Pathol* 191: 282-285.

1671. Pavelic K, Spaventi S, Gluncic V, Matejcic A, Pavicic D, Karapandza N, Kusic Z, Lukac J, Dohoczky C, Cabrijan T, Pavelic J (1999). The expression and role of insulin-like growth factor II in malignant hemangiopericytomas. *J Mol Med* 77: 865-869.

1672. Payne C, Dardick I, Mackay B (1994). Extraskeletal myxoid chondrosarcoma with intracisternal microtubules. *Ultrastruct Pathol* 18: 257-261.

1673. Pea M, Bonetti F, Martignoni G, Henske EP, Manfrin E, Colato C, Bernstein J (1998). Apparent renal cell carcinomas in tuberous sclerosis are heterogeneous: the identification of malignant epithelioid angiomyolipoma. *Am J Surg Pathol* 22: 180-187.

1674. Pea M, Bonetti F, Zamboni G, Martignoni G, Riva M, Colombari R, Mombello A, Bonzanini M, Scarpa A, Ghimenton C. (1991). Melanocyte-marker-HMB-45 is regularly expressed in angiomyolipoma of the kidney. *Pathology* 23: 185-188.

1675. Pea M, Martignoni G, Bonetti F, Zamboni G, Colombari C, Manfrin E, et al. (1977). Tumors characterized by the presence of HMB45-positive perivascular epithelioid cell (PEC)—A novel entity in surgical pathology. *Electron J Pathol Histol* 3: 28-40.

1676. Pea M, Martignoni G, Zamboni G, Bonetti F (1996). Perivascular epithelioid cell. *Am J Surg Pathol* 20: 1149-1153.

1677. Peabody TD, Gibbs CP, Jr., Simon MA (1998). Evaluation and staging of musculoskeletal neoplasms. *J Bone Joint Surg Am* 80: 1204-1218.

1678. Pedeutour F, Forus A, Coindre JM, Berner JM, Nicolo G, Michiels JF, Terrier P, Ranchere-Vince D, Collin F, Myklebost O, Turc-Carel C (1999). Structure of the supernumerary ring and giant rod chromosomes in adipose tissue tumors. *Genes Chromosomes Cancer* 24: 30-41.

1679. Pedeutour F, Quade BJ, Sornberger K, Tallini G, Ligon AH, Weremowicz S, Morton CC (2000). Dysregulation of HMGIC in a uterine lipoleiomyoma with a complex rearrangement including chromosomes 7, 12, and 14. *Genes Chromosomes Cancer* 27: 209-215.

1680. Pedeutour F, Suijkerbuijk RF, Forus A, Van Gaal J, van de Klundert W, Coindre JM, Nicolo G, Collin F, Van Haelst U, Huffermann K, Turc-Carel C (1994). Complex composition and co-amplification of SAS and MDM2 in ring and giant rod marker chromosomes in well-differentiated liposarcoma. *Genes Chromosomes Cancer* 10: 85-94.

1681. Peh WC, Shek TW, Davies AM, Wong JW, Chien EP (1999). Osteochondroma and secondary synovial osteochondromatosis. *Skeletal Radiol* 28: 169-174.

1682. Pellat-Deceunynck C, Barille S, Jego G, Puthier D, Robillard N, Pineau D, Rapp MJ, Harousseau JL, Amiot M, Bataille R (1998). The absence of CD56 (NCAM) on malignant plasma cells is a hallmark of plasma cell leukemia and of a special subset of multiple myeloma. *Leukemia* 12: 1977-1982.

1683. Penman HG, Ring PA (1984). Osteosarcoma in association with total hip replacement. *J Bone Joint Surg Br* 66: 632-634.

1684. Penn I (1979). Kaposi's sarcoma in organ transplant recipients: report of 20 cases. *Transplantation* 27: 8-11.

1685. Penna C, Tiret E, Parc R, Sfairi A, Kartheuser A, Hannoun L, Nordlinger B (1993). Operation and abdominal desmoid tumors in familial adenomatous polyposis. *Surg Gynecol Obstet* 177: 263-268.

1686. Perez-Atayde AR, Newbury R, Fletcher JA, Barnhill R, Gellis S (1994). Congenital "neurovascular hamartoma" of the skin. A possible marker of malignant rhabdoid tumor. *Am J Surg Pathol* 18: 1030-1038.

1687. Perez-Losada J, Pintado B, Gutierrez-Adan A, Flores T, Banares-Gonzalez B, del Campo JC, Martin-Martin JF, Battaner E, Sanchez-Garcia I (2000). The chimeric FUS/TLS-CHOP fusion protein specifically induces liposarcomas in transgenic mice. *Oncogene* 19: 2413-2422.

1688. Perkins P, Weiss SW (1996). Spindle cell hemangioendothelioma. An analysis of 78 cases with reassessment of its pathogenesis and biologic behavior. *Am J Surg Pathol* 20: 1196-1204.

1689. Perlman EJ, Ali SZ, Robinson R, Lindato R, Griffin CA (1998). Infantile extrarenal rhabdoid tumor. *Pediatr Dev Pathol* 1: 149-152.

1690. Perniciaro C (1995). Gardner's syndrome. *Dermatol Clin* 13: 51-56.

1691. Perosio PM, Weiss SW (1993). Ischemic fasciitis: a juxta-skeletal fibroblastic proliferation with a predilection for elderly patients. *Mod Pathol* 6: 69-72.

1692. Perrone T, Swanson PE, Twiggs L, Ulbright TM, Dehner LP (1989). Malignant rhabdoid tumor of the vulva: is distinction from epithelioid sarcoma possible? A pathologic and immunohistochemical study. *Am J Surg Pathol* 13: 848-858.

1693. Peter M, Couturier J, Pacquement H, Michon J, Thomas G, Magdelenat H, Delattre O (1997). A new member of the ETS family fused to EWS in Ewing tumors. *Oncogene* 14: 1159-1164.

1694. Peter M, Gilbert E, Delattre O (2001). A multiplex real-time pcr assay for the detection of gene fusions observed in solid tumors. *Lab Invest* 81: 905-912.

1695. Peterson HA (1989). Multiple hereditary osteochondromata. *Clin Orthop* 222-230.

1696. Petit MM, Mols R, Schoenmakers EF, Mandahl N, Van de Ven WJ (1996). LPP, the preferred fusion partner gene of HMGIC in lipomas, is a novel member of the LIM protein gene family. *Genomics* 36: 118-129.

1697. Petit MM, Schoenmakers EF, Huysmans C, Geurts JM, Mandahl N, Van de Ven WJ (1999). LHFP, a novel translocation partner gene of HMGIC in a lipoma, is a member of a new family of LHFP-like genes. *Genomics* 57: 438-441.

1698. Petit MM, Swarts S, Bridge JA, Van de Ven WJ (1998). Expression of reciprocal fusion transcripts of the HMGIC and LPP genes in parosteal lipoma. *Cancer Genet Cytogenet* 106: 18-23.

1699. Petrik PK, Findlay JM, Sherlock RA (1993). Aneurysmal cyst, bone type, primary in an artery. *Am J Surg Pathol* 17: 1062-1066.

1700. Pettinato G, Manivel JC, De Rosa G, Petrella G, Jaszcz W (1990). Angiomatoid malignant fibrous histiocytoma: cytologic, immunohistochemical, ultrastructural, and flow cytometric study of 20 cases. *Mod Pathol* 3: 479-487.

1701. Pettinato G, Manivel JC, De Rosa N, Dehner LP (1990). Inflammatory myofibroblastic tumor (plasma cell granuloma). Clinicopathologic study of 20 cases with immunohistochemical and ultrastructural observations. *Am J Clin Pathol* 94: 538-546.

1702. Pettinato G, Manivel JC, Gould EW, Albores-Saavedra J (1994). Inclusion body fibromatosis of the breast. Two cases with immunohistochemical and ultrastructural findings. *Am J Clin Pathol* 101: 714-718.

1703. Pettit CK, Zukerberg LR, Gray MH, Ferry JA, Rosenberg AE, Harmon DC, Harris NL (1990). Primary lymphoma of bone. A B-cell neoplasm with a high frequency of multilobated cells. *Am J Surg Pathol* 14: 329-334.

1704. Picci P, Bacci G, Campanacci M, Gasparini M, Pilotti S, Cerasoli S, Bertoni F, Guerra A, Capanna R, Albisinni U, . (1985). Histologic evaluation of necrosis in osteosarcoma induced by chemotherapy. Regional mapping of viable and nonviable tumor. *Cancer* 56: 1515-1521.

1705. Pierce ER (1970). Gardner's syndrome: formal genetics and statistical analysis of a large canadian kindred. *Clin Genet* 1: 65-80.

1706. Pilotti S, Della Torre G, Lavarino C, Di Palma S, Sozzi G, Minoletti F, Rao S, Pasquini G, Azzarelli A, Rilke F, Pierotti MA (1997). Distinct mdm2/p53 expression patterns in liposarcoma subgroups: implications for different pathogenetic mechanisms. *J Pathol* 181: 14-24.

1707. Pinkard NB, Wilson RW, Lawless N, Dodd LG, McAdams HP, Koss MN, Travis WD (1996). Calcifying fibrous pseudotumor of pleura. A report of three cases of a newly described entity involving the pleura. *Am J Clin Pathol* 105: 189-194.

1708. Pinto A, Dold OR, Mueller D, Gilbert-Barness E (1993). Pathological cases of the month. Infantile fibrosarcoma. *Am J Dis Child* 147: 691-692.

1709. Pinto A, Tallini G, Novak RW, Bowen T, Parham DM (1997). Undifferentiated rhabdomyosarcoma with lymphoid phenotype expression. *Med Pediatr Oncol* 28: 165-170.

1710. Pisciotto PT, Gray GF, Jr., Miller DR (1978). Abdominal plasma cell pseudotumor. *J Pediatr* 93: 628-630.

1711. Pisters PW, Leung DH, Woodruff J, Shi W, Brennan MF (1996). Analysis of prognostic factors in 1,041 patients with localized soft tissue sarcomas of the extremities. *J Clin Oncol* 14: 1679-1689.

1712. Pollock M, Nicholson GI, Nukada H, Cameron S, Frankish P (1988). Neuropathy in multiple symmetric lipomatosis. Madelung's disease. *Brain* 111 (Pt 5): 1157-1171.

1713. Pollono DG, Tomarchio S, Drut R, Zaritzky M, Otero L, Vazquez AJ, Ripoll MC (1999). Retroperitoneal and deep-seated lipoblastoma: diagnosis by CT scan and fine-needle aspiration biopsy. *Diagn Cytopathol* 20: 295-297.

1714. Pomplun S, Goldstraw P, Davies SE, Burke MM, Nicholson AG (2000). Calcifying fibrous pseudotumour arising within an inflammatory pseudotumour: evidence of progression from one lesion to the other? *Histopathology* 37: 380-382.

1715. Popescu NC, Zimonjic DB, Leventon-Kriss S, Bryant JL, Lunardi-Iskandar Y, Gallo RC (1996). Deletion and translocation involving chromosome 3 (p14) in two tumorigenic Kaposi's sarcoma cell lines. *J Natl Cancer Inst* 88: 450-455.

1716. Popper H, Thomas LB, Telles NC, Falk H, Selikoff IJ (1978). Development of hepatic angiosarcoma in man induced by vinyl chloride, thorotrast, and arsenic. Comparison with cases of unknown etiology. *Am J Pathol* 92: 349-369.

1717. Porter DE, Emerton ME, Villanueva-Lopez F, Simpson AH (2000). Clinical and radiographic analysis of osteochondromas and growth disturbance in hereditary multiple exostoses. *J Pediatr Orthop* 20: 246-250.

1718. Porter DE, Simpson AH (1999). The neoplastic pathogenesis of solitary and multiple osteochondromas. *J Pathol* 188: 119-125.

1719. Portera CA, Jr., Ho V, Patel SR, Hunt KK, Feig BW, Respondek PM, Yasko AW, Benjamin RS, Pollock RE, Pisters PW (2001). Alveolar soft part sarcoma: clinical course and patterns of metastasis in 70 patients treated at a single institution. *Cancer* 91: 585-591.

1720. Posey Y, Valdivia E, Persons DL, Ally S, Smith DL, Pantazis CG, Smith SD (1998). Lipoblastoma presenting as a mesenteric mass in an infant. *J Pediatr Hematol Oncol* 20: 580-582.

1720a. Potepan P, Luksch R, Sozzi G, Testi A, Laffranchi A, Danesini GM, Parafioriti A, Giardini R, Spagnoli I (1999). Multifocal osteosarcoma as second tumor after childhood retinoblastoma. *Skeletal Radiol* 28: 415-421.

1721. Potocki L, Shaffer LG (1996). Interstitial deletion of 11(p11.2p12): a newly described contiguous gene deletion syndrome involving the gene for hereditary multiple exostoses (EXT2). *Am J Med Genet* 62: 319-325.

1722. Povysil C, Matejovsky Z (1979). Ultrastructural evidence of myofibroblasts in pseudomalignant myositis ossificans. *Virchows Arch A Pathol Anat Histol* 381: 189-203.

1723. Prat J, Woodruff JM, Marcove RC (1978). Epithelioid sarcoma: an analysis of 22 cases indicating the prognostic significance of vascular invasion and regional lymph node metastasis. *Cancer* 41: 1472-1487.

1723a. Pratt CB, Michalkiewicz EN, Rao BN, Lipson M, Cain A, Kaste S (1999). Multifocal osteosarcoma following retinoblastoma. *Ophthalmic Genet* 20: 23-29.

1724. Present D, Bacchini P, Pignatti G, Picci P, Bertoni F, Campanacci M (1991). Clear cell chondrosarcoma of bone. A report of 8 cases. *Skeletal Radiol* 20: 187-191.

1725. Present D, Bertoni F, Enneking WF (1986). Osteosarcoma of the mandible arising in fibrous dysplasia. A case report. *Clin Orthop* 238-244.

1726. Price AJ, Compson JP, Calonje E (1995). Fibrolipomatous hamartoma of nerve arising in the brachial plexus. *J Hand Surg [Br]* 20: 16-18.

1727. Price EB, Silliphant WM, Shuman R (1961). Nodular fasciitis: a clinicopathologic analysis of 65 cases. *Am J Clin Pathol* 35: 122-136.

1728. Prince PR, Emond MJ, Monnat RJ, Jr. (2001). Loss of Werner syndrome protein function promotes aberrant mitotic recombination. *Genes Dev* 15: 933-938.

1729. Pritchard-Jones K, Fleming S (1991). Cell types expressing the Wilms' tumour gene (WT1) in Wilms' tumours: implications for tumour histogenesis. *Oncogene* 6: 2211-2220.

1730. Pritchard DJ, Sim FH, Ivins JC, Soule EH, Dahlin DC (1977). Fibrosarcoma of bone and soft tissues of the trunk and extremities. *Orthop Clin North Am* 8: 869-881.

1731. Pritchard DJ, Soule EH, Taylor WF, Ivins JC (1974). Fibrosarcoma - a clinicopathologic and statistical study of 199 tumors of the soft tissues of the extremities and trunk. *Cancer* 33: 888-897.

1732. Propeck T, Bullard MA, Lin J, Doi K, Martel W (2000). Radiologic-pathologic correlation of intraosseous lipomas. *AJR Am J Roentgenol* 175: 673-678.

1733. Proust F, Laquerriere A, Constantin B, Ruchoux MM, Vannier JP, Freger P (1999). Simultaneous presentation of atypical teratoid/rhabdoid tumor in siblings. *J Neurooncol* 43: 63-70.

1734. Przygodzki RM, Finkelstein SD, Keohavong P, Zhu D, Bakker A, Swalsky PA, Soini Y, Ishak KG, Bennett WP (1997). Sporadic and Thorotrast-induced angiosarcomas of the liver manifest frequent and multiple point mutations in K-ras-2. *Lab Invest* 76: 153-159.

1735. Pujol LA, Erickson RP, Heidenreich RA, Cunniff C (2000). Variable presentation of Rothmund-Thomson syndrome. *Am J Med Genet* 95: 204-207.

1736. Pulitzer DR, Martin PC, Reed RJ (1989). Fibroma of tendon sheath. A clinicopathologic study of 32 cases. *Am J Surg Pathol* 13: 472-479.

1737. Pulitzer DR, Martin PC, Reed RJ (1995). Epithelioid glomus tumor. *Hum Pathol* 26: 1022-1027.

1738. Purdy LJ, Colby TV (1984). Infantile digital fibromatosis occurring outside the digit. *Am J Surg Pathol* 8: 787-790.

1739. Qureshi AA, Shott S, Mallin BA, Gitelis S (2000). Current trends in the management of adamantinoma of long bones. An international study. *J Bone Joint Surg Am* 82-A: 1122-1131.

1740. Rab GT, Ivins JC, Childs DS, Jr., Cupps RE, Pritchard DJ (1976). Elective whole lung irradiation in the treatment of osteogenic sarcoma. *Cancer* 38: 939-942.

1741. Rabbitts TH, Forster A, Larson R, Nathan P (1993). Fusion of the dominant negative transcription regulator CHOP with a novel gene FUS by translocation t(12;16) in malignant liposarcoma. *Nat Genet* 4: 175-180.

1742. Radig K, Buhtz P, Roessner A (1998). Alveolar soft part sarcoma of the uterine corpus. Report of two cases and review of the literature. *Pathol Res Pract* 194: 59-63.

1743. Radig K, Schneider-Stock R, Mittler U, Neumann HW, Roessner A (1998). Genetic instability in osteoblastic tumors of the skeletal system. *Pathol Res Pract* 194: 669-677.

1744. Radin R, Ma Y (2001). Malignant epithelioid renal angiomyolipoma in a patient with tuberous sclerosis. *J Comput Assist Tomogr* 25: 873-875.

1745. Rafal RB, Nichols JN, Markisz JA (1995). Pulmonary artery sarcoma: diagnosis and postoperative follow-up with gadolinium-diethylenetriamine pentaacetic acid-enhanced magnetic resonance imaging. *Mayo Clin Proc* 70: 173-176.

1746. Ragab AH, Heyn R, Tefft M, Hays DN, Newton WA, Jr., Beltangady M (1986). Infants younger than 1 year of age with rhabdomyosarcoma. *Cancer* 58: 2606-2610.

1747. Ragazzini P, Gamberi G, Benassi MS, Orlando C, Sestini R, Ferrari C, Molendini L, Sollazzo MR, Merli M, Magagnoli G, Bertoni F, Böhling T, Pazzagli M, Picci P (1999). Analysis of SAS gene and CDK4 and MDM2 proteins in low-grade osteosarcoma. *Cancer Detect Prev* 23: 129-136.

1748. Rahimi A, Beabout JW, Ivins JC, Dahlin DC (1972). Chondromyxoid fibroma: a clinicopathologic study of 76 cases. *Cancer* 30: 726-736.

1749. Rajani B, Smith TA, Reith JD, Goldblum JR (1999). Retroperitoneal leiomyosarcomas unassociated with the gastrointestinal tract: a clinicopathologic analysis of 17 cases. *Mod Pathol* 12: 21-28.

1750. Ramachandra S, Hollowood K, Bisceglia M, Fletcher CD (1995). Inflammatory pseudotumour of soft tissues: a clinicopathological and immunohistochemical analysis of 18 cases. *Histopathology* 27: 313-323.

1751. Ramani P, Cowell JK (1996). The expression pattern of Wilms' tumour gene (WT1) product in normal tissues and paediatric renal tumours. *J Pathol* 179: 162-168.

1752. Ramos A, Castello J, Sartoris DJ, Greenway GD, Resnick D, Haghighi P (1985). Osseous lipoma: CT appearance. *Radiology* 157: 615-619.

1753. Ramos CV, Gillespie W, Narconis RJ (1978). Elastofibroma. A pseudotumor of myofibroblasts. *Arch Pathol Lab Med* 102: 538-540.

1754. Ranchod M, Kempson RL (1977). Smooth muscle tumors of the gastrointestinal tract and retroperitoneum: a pathologic analysis of 100 cases. *Cancer* 39: 255-262.

1755. Raney RB, Anderson JR, Barr FG, Donaldson SS, Pappo AS, Qualman SJ, Wiener ES, Maurer HM, Crist WM (2001). Rhabdomyosarcoma and Undifferentiated Sarcoma in the First Two Decades of Life: A Selective Review of Intergroup Rhabdomyosarcoma Study Group Experience and Rationale for Intergroup Rhabdomyosarcoma Study V. *Am J Pediatr Hematol Oncol* 23: 215-220.

1756. Raney RB, Jr., Tefft M, Maurer HM, Ragab AH, Hays DM, Soule EH, Foulkes MA, Gehan EA (1988). Disease patterns and survival rate in children with metastatic soft-tissue sarcoma. A report from the Intergroup Rhabdomyosarcoma Study (IRS)-I. *Cancer* 62: 1257-1266.

1757. Rao AS, Vigorita VJ (1984). Pigmented villonodular synovitis (giant-cell tumor of the tendon sheath and synovial membrane). A review of eighty-one cases. *J Bone Joint Surg Am* 66: 76-94.

1758. Rao VK, Weiss SW (1992). Angiomatosis of soft tissue. An analysis of the histologic features and clinical outcome in 51 cases. *Am J Surg Pathol* 16: 764-771.

1759. Rappaport ZH (1989). Aneurysmal bone cyst associated with fibrous dysplasia of the skull. *Neurochirurgia (Stuttg)* 32: 192-194.

1760. Raskind WH, Conrad EU, Chansky H, Matsushita M (1995). Loss of heterozygosity in chondrosarcomas for markers linked to hereditary multiple exostoses loci on chromosomes 8 and 11. *Am J Hum Genet* 56: 1132-1139.

1761. Raskind WH, Conrad EU, III, Matsushita M, Wijsman EM, Wells DE, Chapman N, Sandell LJ, Wagner M, Houck J (1998). Evaluation of locus heterogeneity and EXT1 mutations in 34 families with hereditary multiple exostoses. *Hum Mutat* 11: 231-239.

1762. Rasmussen IS, Kirkegaard J, Kaasbol M (1997). Intermittent airway obstruction in a child caused by a cervical lipoblastoma. *Acta Anaesthesiol Scand* 41: 945-946.

1763. Raymond AK, Ayala AG (1988). Specimen management after osteosarcoma chemotherapy. *Contemp Issues Surg Pathol* 11: 157-183.

1764. Raymond AK, Chawla SP, Carrasco CH, Ayala AG, Fanning CV, Grice B, Armen T, Plager C, Papadopoulos NE, Edeiken J, . (1987). Osteosarcoma chemotherapy effect: a prognostic factor. *Semin Diagn Pathol* 4: 212-236.

1765. Raymond AK, Murphy GF, Rosenthal DI (1987). Case report 425: Chondroblastic osteosarcoma: clear-cell variant of femur. *Skeletal Radiol* 16: 336-341.

1766. Reddick RL, Michelitch HJ, Levine AM, Triche TJ (1980). Osteogenic sarcoma: a study of the ultrastructure. *Cancer* 45: 64-71.

1767. Redlich GC, Montgomery KD, Allgood GA, Joste NE (1999). Plexiform fibrohistiocytic tumor with a clonal cytogenetic anomaly. *Cancer Genet Cytogenet* 108: 141-143.

1768. Redmond OM, Stack JP, Dervan PA, Hurson BJ, Carney DN, Ennis JT (1989). Osteosarcoma: use of MR imaging and MR spectroscopy in clinical decision making. *Radiology* 172: 811-815.

1769. Reed RJ, Terazakis N (1972). Subcutaneous angioblastic lymphoid hyperplasia with eosinophilia (Kimura's disease). *Cancer* 29: 489-497.

1770. Reeves BR, Fisher C, Smith S, Courtenay VD, Robertson D (1987). Ultrastructural, immunocytochemical, and cytogenetic characterization of a human epithelioid sarcoma cell line (RM-HS1). *J Natl Cancer Inst* 78: 7-18.

1771. Rehring TF, Deutchman A, Cross JS (1999). Polymorphous hemangioendothelioma. *Ann Thorac Surg* 68: 1396-1397.

1772. Reid AH, Tsai MM, Venzon DJ, Wright CF, Lack EE, O'Leary TJ (1996). MDM2 amplification, P53 mutation, and accumulation of the P53 gene product in malignant fibrous histiocytoma. *Diagn Mol Pathol* 5: 65-73.

1773. Reid R, Barrett A, Hamblen DL (1996). Sclerosing epithelioid fibrosarcoma. *Histopathology* 28: 451-455.

1774. Reilly KE, Stern PJ, Dale JA (1999). Recurrent giant cell tumors of the tendon sheath. *J Hand Surg [Am]* 24: 1298-1302.

1775. Reiman HM, Dahlin DC (1986). Cartilage- and bone-forming tumors of the soft tissues. *Semin Diagn Pathol* 3: 288-305.

1776. Reis-Filho JS, Paiva ME, Lopes JM (2002). Congenital composite hemangioendothelioma: case report and reappraisal of the hemangioendothelioma spectrum. *J Cutan Pathol* 29: 226-231.

1777. Reiseter T, Nordshus T, Borthne A, Roald B, Naess P, Schistad O (1999). Lipoblastoma: MRI appearances of a rare paediatric soft tissue tumour. *Pediatr Radiol* 29: 542-545.

1778. Reissmann PT, Simon MA, Lee WH, Slamon DJ (1989). Studies of the retinoblastoma gene in human sarcomas. *Oncogene* 4: 839-843.

1779. Reitamo JJ, Hayry P, Nykyri E, Saxen E (1982). The desmoid tumor. I. Incidence, sex-, age- and anatomical distribution in the Finnish population. *Am J Clin Pathol* 77: 665-673.

1780. Reith JD, Bauer TW, Joyce MJ (1997). Paraarticular osteochondroma of the knee: report of 2 cases and review of the literature. *Clin Orthop* 225-232.

1781. Remagen W, Nidecker A, Prein J (1986). Case report 359: gigantic benign fibrous histiocytoma (nonossifying fibroma). Skeletal Radiol 15: 251-253.

1782. Remstein ED, Arndt CA, Nascimento AG (1999). Plexiform fibrohistiocytic tumor: clinicopathologic analysis of 22 cases. Am J Surg Pathol 23: 662-670.

1783. Renshaw AA (1995). O13 (CD99) in spindle cell tumors. Reactivity with hemangiopericytoma, solitary fibrous tumor, synovial sarcoma, and meningioma but rarely with sarcomatoid mesothelioma. Appl Immunohistochem 3: 250-256.

1784. Renwick PJ, Reeves BR, Dal Cin P, Fletcher CD, Kempski H, Sciot R, Kazmierczak B, Jani K, Sonobe H, Knight JC (1995). Two categories of synovial sarcoma defined by divergent chromosome translocation breakpoints in Xp11.2, with implications for the histologic sub-classification of synovial sarcoma. Cytogenet Cell Genet 70: 58-63.

1785. Resnick D, Greenway G, Genant H, Brower A, Haghighi P, Emmett M (1982). Erdheim-Chester disease. Radiology 142: 289-295.

1786. Ribalta T, Lloreta J, Munne A, Serrano S, Cardesa A (2000). Malignant pigmented clear cell epithelioid tumor of the kidney: clear cell ("sugar") tumor versus malignant melanoma. Hum Pathol 31: 516-519.

1787. Richkind KE, Romansky SG, Finklestein JZ (1996). t(4;19)(q35;q13.1): a recurrent change in primitive mesenchymal tumors? Cancer Genet Cytogenet 87: 71-74.

1788. Riddell RJ, Louis CJ, Bromberger NA (1973). Pulmonary metastases from chondroblastoma of the tibia. Report of a case. J Bone Joint Surg Br 55: 848-853.

1789. Ries LAG, Kosary CL, Hankey BF, et al (1999). SEER Cancer Statistics Review, 1973-1996. National Cancer Institute: Bethesda, MD.

1790. Rieske P, Bartkowiak J, Szadowska A, Debiec-Rychter M (1999). Malignant fibrous histiocytomas and H-ras-1 oncogene point mutations. Mol Pathol 52: 64-67.

1791. Rimareix F, Bardot J, Andrac L, Vasse D, Galinier P, Magalon G (1997). Infantile digital fibroma – report on eleven cases. Eur J Pediatr Surg 7: 345-348.

1792. Ritts GD, Pritchard DJ, Unni KK, Beabout JW, Eckardt JJ (1987). Periosteal osteosarcoma. Clin Orthop 299-307.

1793. Roarty JD, McLean IW, Zimmerman LE (1988). Incidence of second neoplasms in patients with bilateral retinoblastoma. Ophthalmology 95: 1583-1587.

1794. Robbins LB, Hoffman S, Kahn S (1970). Fibrous hamartoma of infancy; case report. Plast Reconstr Surg 46: 197-200.

1795. Roberts PF, Taylor JG (1980). Multifocal benign chondroblastomas: report of a case. Hum Pathol 11: 296-298.

1796. Roberts WM, Douglass EC, Peiper SC, Houghton PJ, Look AT (1989). Amplification of the gli gene in childhood sarcomas. Cancer Res 49: 5407-5413.

1797. Robinson W, Crawford AH (1990). Infantile fibrosarcoma. Report of a case with long-term follow-up. J Bone Joint Surg Am 72: 291-294.

1798. Rodgers WB, Mankin HJ (1996). Metastatic malignant chondroblastoma. Am J Orthop 25: 846-849.

1799. Rodriguez-Bigas MA, Mahoney MC, Karakousis CP, Petrelli NJ (1994). Desmoid tumors in patients with familial adenomatous polyposis. Cancer 74: 1270-1274.

1800. Rodriguez-Peralto JL, Lopez-Barea F, Gonzalez-Lopez J, Lamas-Lorenzo M (1994). Case report 821: Parosteal ossifying lipoma of femur. Skeletal Radiol 23: 67-69.

1801. Rodriguez E, Sreekantaiah C, Gerald W, Reuter VE, Motzer RJ, Chaganti RS (1993). A recurring translocation, t(11;22)(p13;q11.2), characterizes intra-abdominal desmoplastic small round-cell tumors. Cancer Genet Cytogenet 69: 17-21.

1802. Roebuck DJ (1996). The role of imaging in renal and extra-renal rhabdoid tumours. Australas Radiol 40: 310-318.

1803. Rogalla P, Lemke I, Kazmierczak B, Bullerdiek J (2000). An identical HMGIC-LPP fusion transcript is consistently expressed in pulmonary chondroid hamartomas with t(3;12)(q27-28;q14-15). Genes Chromosomes Cancer 29: 363-366.

1804. Rong S, Jeffers M, Resau JH, Tsarfaty I, Oskarsson M, Vande Woude GF (1993). Met expression and sarcoma tumorigenicity. Cancer Res 53: 5355-5360.

1805. Rosai J (1982). Angiolymphoid hyperplasia with eosinophilia of the skin. Its nosological position in the spectrum of histiocytoid hemangioma. Am J Dermatopathol 4: 175-184.

1806. Rosai J, Limas C, Husband EM (1984). Ectopic hamartomatous thymoma. A distinctive benign lesion of lower neck. Am J Surg Pathol 8: 501-513.

1807. Rose NC, Coleman BG, Wallace D, Gaupman K, Ruchelli E (1996). Prenatal diagnosis of a chest wall hamartoma and sternal cleft. Ultrasound Obstet Gynecol 7: 453-455.

1808. Rosenberg HS, Stenback WA, Spjut HJ (1978). The fibromatoses of infancy and childhood. Perspect Pediatr Pathol 4: 269-348.

1809. Rosenthal NS, Abdul-Karim FW (1988). Childhood fibrous tumor with psammoma bodies. Clinicopathologic features in two cases. Arch Pathol Lab Med 112: 798-800.

1810. Ross HM, Lewis JJ, Woodruff JM, Brennan MF (1997). Epithelioid sarcoma: clinical behavior and prognostic factors of survival. Ann Surg Oncol 4: 491-495.

1811. Ross JS, Del Rosario A, Bui HX, Sonbati H, Solis O (1992). Primary hepatic leiomyosarcoma in a child with the acquired immunodeficiency syndrome. Hum Pathol 23: 69-72.

1812. Rougraff BT, Kneisl JS, Simon MA (1993). Skeletal metastases of unknown origin. A prospective study of a diagnostic strategy. J Bone Joint Surg Am 75: 1276-1281.

1813. Rousseau-Merck MF, Versteege I, Legrand I, Couturier J, Mairal A, Delattre O, Aurias A (1999). hSNF5/INI1 inactivation is mainly associated with homozygous deletions and mitotic recombinations in rhabdoid tumors. Cancer Res 59: 3152-3156.

1814. Roux S, Amazit L, Meduri G, Guiochon-Mantel A, Milgrom E, Mariette X (2002). RANK (receptor activator of nuclear factor kappa B) and RANK ligand are expressed in giant cell tumors of bone. Am J Clin Pathol 117: 210-216.

1815. Rozmaryn LM, Sadler AH, Dorfman HD (1987). Intraosseous glomus tumor in the ulna. A case report. Clin Orthop 126-129.

1816. Rubin BP, Chen CJ, Morgan TW, Xiao S, Grier HE, Kozakewich HP, Perez-Atayde AR, Fletcher JA (1998). Congenital mesoblastic nephroma t(12;15) is associated with ETV6-NTRK3 gene fusion: cytogenetic and molecular relationship to congenital (infantile) fibrosarcoma. Am J Pathol 153: 1451-1458.

1817. Rubin BP, Fletcher JA, Renshaw AA (1999). Clear cell sarcoma of soft parts: report of a case primary in the kidney with cytogenetic confirmation. Am J Surg Pathol 23: 589-594.

1818. Rubin BP, Hasserjian RP, Singer S, Janecka I, Fletcher JA, Fletcher CD (1998). Spindle cell rhabdomyosarcoma (so-called) in adults: report of two cases with emphasis on differential diagnosis. Am J Surg Pathol 22: 459-464.

1819. Rubinfeld B, Albert I, Porfiri E, Fiol C, Munemitsu S, Polakis P (1996). Binding of GSK3beta to the APC-beta-catenin complex and regulation of complex assembly. Science 272: 1023-1026.

1820. Rubinfeld B, Souza B, Albert I, Muller O, Chamberlain SH, Masiarz FR, Munemitsu S, Polakis P (1993). Association of the APC gene product with beta-catenin. Science 262: 1731-1734.

1821. Ruco LP, Pilozzi E, Wedard BM, Marzullo A, D'Andrea V, De Antoni E, Silvestrini G, Bonetti F (1998). Epithelioid lymphangioleiomyomatosis-like tumour of the uterus in a patient without tuberous sclerosis: a lesion mimicking epithelioid leiomyosarcoma. Histopathology 33: 91-93.

1822. Ruggieri P, Sim FH, Bond JR, Unni KK (1994). Malignancies in fibrous dysplasia. Cancer 73: 1411-1424.

1823. Ruggieri P, Sim FH, Bond JR, Unni KK (1995). Osteosarcoma in a patient with polyostotic fibrous dysplasia and Albright's syndrome. Orthopedics 18: 71-75.

1824. Rushing EJ, Armonda RA, Ansari Q, Mena H (1996). Mesenchymal chondrosarcoma: a clinicopathologic and flow cytometric study of 13 cases presenting in the central nervous system. Cancer 77: 1884-1891.

1825. Rusin LJ, Harrell ER (1976). Arteriovenous fistula. Cutaneous manifestations. Arch Dermatol 112: 1135-1138.

1826. Russell WO, Cohen J, Enzinger F, Hajdu SI, Heise H, Martin RG, Meissner W, Miller WT, Schmitz RL, Suit HD (1977). A clinical and pathological staging system for soft tissue sarcomas. Cancer 40: 1562-1570.

1827. Ruszczak Z, Mayer-da-Silva A, Orfanos CE (1987). Angioproliferative changes in clinically noninvolved, perilesional skin in AIDS-associated Kaposi's sarcoma. Dermatologica 175: 270-279.

1828. Rutigliano MJ, Pollack IF, Ahdab-Barmada M, Pang D, Albright AL (1994). Intracranial infantile myofibromatosis. J Neurosurg 81: 539-543.

1829. Ruymann FB (1987). Rhabdomyosarcoma in children and adolescents. A review. Hematol Oncol Clin North Am 1: 621-654.

1830. Rydholm A (1983). Management of patients with soft-tissue tumors. Strategy developed at a regional oncology center. Acta Orthop Scand Suppl 203: 13-77.

1831. Rydholm A (1998). Improving the management of soft tissue sarcoma. Diagnosis and treatment should be given in specialist centres. BMJ 317: 93-94.

1832. Rydholm A, Gustafson P, Rööser B, Willén H, Åkerman M, Herrlin K, Alvegard T (1991). Limb-sparing surgery without radiotherapy based on anatomic location of soft tissue sarcoma. J Clin Oncol 9: 1757-1765.

1833. Saddegh MK, Lindholm J, Lundberg A, Nilsonne U, Kreicbergs A (1992). Staging of soft-tissue sarcomas. Prognostic analysis of clinical and pathological features. J Bone Joint Surg Br 74: 495-500.

1834. Saeed IT, Fletcher CD (1990). Ectopic hamartomatous thymoma containing myoid cells. Histopathology 17: 572-574.

1835. Saeter G, Elomaa I, Wahlqvist Y, Alvegard TA, Wiebe T, Monge O, Forrestier E, Solheim OP (1997). Prognostic factors in bone sarcomas. Acta Orthop Scand Suppl 273: 156-160.

1836. Safar A, Nelson M, Neff JR, Maale GE, Bayani J, Squire J, Bridge JA (2000). Recurrent anomalies of 6q25 in chondromyxoid fibroma. Hum Pathol 31: 306-311.

1837. Sagerman RH, Cassady JR, Tretter P, Ellsworth RM (1969). Radiation induced neoplasia following external beam therapy for children with retinoblastoma. Am J Roentgenol Radium Ther Nucl Med 105: 529-535.

1838. Saikevych IA, Mayer M, White RL, Ho RC (1988). Cytogenetic study of Kaposi's sarcoma associated with acquired immunodeficiency syndrome. Arch Pathol Lab Med 112: 825-828.

1839. Saint Aubain SN, Fletcher CD (1999). Leiomyosarcoma of soft tissue in children: clinicopathologic analysis of 20 cases. Am J Surg Pathol 23: 755-763.

1840. Saito R, Caines MJ (1977). Atypical fibrous histiocytoma of the humerus: a light and electron microscopic study. *Am J Clin Pathol* 68: 409-415.

1841. Saito T, Oda Y, Tanaka K, Matsuda S, Tamiya S, Iwamoto Y, Tsuneyoshi M (2001). beta-catenin nuclear expression correlates with cyclin D1 overexpression in sporadic desmoid tumours. *J Pathol* 195: 222-228.

1842. Sakabe T, Shinomiya T, Mori T, Ariyama T, Fukuda Y, Fujiwara T, Nakamura Y, Inazawa J (1999). Identifi-cation of a novel gene, MASL1, within an amplicon at 8p23.1 detected in malignant fibrous histiocytomas by comparative genomic hybridization. *Cancer Res* 59: 511-515.

1843. Sakakibara N, Seki T, Maru A, Koyanagi T (1989). Benign fibrous histiocytoma of the kidney. *J Urol* 142: 1558-1559.

1844. Sakamoto A, Oda Y, Iwamoto Y, Tsuneyoshi M (1999). Expression of membrane type 1 matrix metalloproteinase, matrix metalloproteinase 2 and tissue inhibitor of metalloproteinase 2 in human cartilaginous tumors with special emphasis on mesenchymal and dedifferentiated chondrosarcoma. *J Cancer Res Clin Oncol* 125: 541-548.

1845. Sakamoto A, Oda Y, Iwamoto Y, Tsuneyoshi M (2000). A comparative study of fibrous dysplasia and osteofibrous dysplasia with regard to Gsalpha mutation at the Arg201 codon: polymerase chain reaction-restriction fragment length polymorphism analysis of paraffin-embedded tissues. *J Mol Diagn* 2: 67-72.

1846. Salamah MM, Hammoudi SM, Sadi AR (1988). Infantile myofibromatosis. *J Pediatr Surg* 23: 975-977.

1847. Saleh G, Evans HL, Ro JY, Ayala AG (1992). Extraskeletal myxoid chondrosarcoma. A clinicopathologic study of ten patients with long-term follow-up. *Cancer* 70: 2827-2830.

1848. Salloum E, Caillaud JM, Flamant F, Landman J, Lemerle J (1990). Poor prognosis infantile fibrosarcoma with pathologic features of malignant fibrous histiocytoma after local recurrence. *Med Pediatr Oncol* 18: 295-298.

1849. Salm R, Sissons HA (1972). Giant-cell tumours of soft tissues. *J Pathol* 107: 27-39.

1850. Salmon SE, Cassady JR (1988). Plasma cell neoplasms. In: *Cancer, Principles and Practice of Oncology*, DeVita VT, Hellman S, Rosenberg S, eds. J.B.Lippincott: Philadelphia, p. 1854.

1851. Salmon SE, Seligmann M (1974). B-cell neoplasia in man. *Lancet* 2: 1230-1233.

1852. Salvati M, Ciappetta P, Raco A (1993). Osteosarcomas of the skull. Clinical remarks on 19 cases. *Cancer* 71: 2210-2216.

1853. Samaniego F, Markham PD, Gendelman R, Watanabe Y, Kao V, Kowalski K, Sonnabend JA, Pintus A, Gallo RC, Ensoli B (1998). Vascular endothelial growth factor and basic fibroblast growth factor present in Kaposi's sarcoma (KS) are induced by inflammatory cytokines and synergize to promote vascular permeability and KS lesion development. *Am J Pathol* 152: 1433-1443.

1854. Sandberg AA, Bridge JA (1994). *The Cytogenetics of Bone and Soft Tissue Tumors*. RG Landers Company: Austin, Texas.

1855. Sandberg AA, Bridge JA (2002). Updates on the cytogenetics and molecular genetics of bone and soft tissue tumors. Synovial sarcoma. *Cancer Genet Cytogenet* 133: 1-23.

1856. Sanders BM, Draper GJ, Kingston JE (1988). Retinoblastoma in Great Britain 1969-80: incidence, treatment, and survival. *Br J Ophthalmol* 72: 576-583.

1857. Sanerkin NG (1980). Definitions of osteosarcoma, chondrosarcoma, and fibrosarcoma of bone. *Cancer* 46: 178-185.

1858. Sanerkin NG (1980). The diagnosis and grading of chondrosarcoma of bone: a combined cytologic and histologic approach. *Cancer* 45: 582-594.

1859. Sanerkin NG, Mott MG, Roylance J (1983). An unusual intraosseous lesion with fibroblastic, osteoclastic, osteoblastic, aneurysmal and fibromyxoid elements. "Solid" variant of aneurysmal bone cyst. *Cancer* 51: 2278-2286.

1860. Sang DN, Albert DM (1982). Retinoblastoma: clinical and histopathologic features. *Hum Pathol* 13: 133-147.

1861. Santonja C, Martin-Hita AM, Dotor A, Costa-Subias J (2001). Intimal angiosarcoma of the aorta with tumour embolisation causing mesenteric ischaemia. Report of a case diagnosed using CD31 immunohistochemistry in an intestinal resection specimen. *Virchows Arch* 438: 404-407.

1862. Sara AS, Evans HL, Benjamin RS (1990). Malignant melanoma of soft parts (clear cell sarcoma). A study of 17 cases, with emphasis on prognostic factors. *Cancer* 65: 367-374.

1863. Sartoris DJ, Mochizuki RM, Parker BR (1983). Lytic clavicular lesions in fibromatosis colli. *Skeletal Radiol* 10: 34-36.

1864. Sato K, Kubota T, Yoshida K, Murata H (1993). Intracranial extraskeletal myxoid chondrosarcoma with special reference to lamellar inclusions in the rough endoplasmic reticulum. *Acta Neuropathol* (Berl) 86: 525-528.

1865. Satoh H, Nishiyama T, Horiguchi A, Nakashima J, Saito S, Murai M (2000). [A case of Collet-Sicard syndrome caused by skull base metastasis of prostate carcinoma]. *Nippon Hinyokika Gakkai Zasshi* 91: 562-564.

1866. Saw D, Tse CH, Chan J, Watt CY, Ng CS, Poon YF (1986). Clear cell sarcoma of the penis. *Hum Pathol* 17: 423-425.

1867. Sawada S, Honda M, Kamide R, Niimura M (1995). Three cases of subungual glomus tumors with von Recklinghausen neurofibromatosis. *J Am Acad Dermatol* 32: 277-278.

1868. Sawyer JR, Binz RL, Gilliland JC, Nicholas RW, Thomas JR (2001). A novel reciprocal (10;17)(p11.2;q23) in myxoid fibrosarcoma. *Cancer Genet Cytogenet* 124: 144-146.

1869. Sawyer JR, Sammartino G, Baker GF, Bell JM (1994). Clonal chromosome aberrations in a case of nodular fasciitis. *Cancer Genet Cytogenet* 76: 154-156.

1870. Sawyer JR, Swanson CM, Lukacs JL, Nicholas RW, North PE, Thomas JR (1998). Evidence of an association between 6q13-21 chromosome aberrations and locally aggressive behavior in patients with cartilage tumors. *Cancer* 82: 474-483.

1871. Sawyer JR, Tryka AF, Lewis JM (1992). A novel reciprocal chromosome translocation t(11;22)(p13;q12) in an intraabdominal desmoplastic small round-cell tumor. *Am J Surg Pathol* 16: 411-416.

1872. Schaberg J, Gainor BJ (1985). A profile of metastatic carcinoma of the spine. *Spine* 10: 19-20.

1873. Schaffler G, Raith J, Ranner G, Weybora W, Jeserschek R (1997). Radiographic appearance of an ossifying fibromyxoid tumor of soft parts. *Skeletal Radiol* 26: 615-618.

1874. Schajowicz F (1994). Cartilage-forming tumors. In: *Tumors and Tumor-like Lesions of Bone*. Springer: Berlin-Heidelberg-New York.

1875. Schajowicz F (1994). *Tumors and Tumor-like Lesions of Bone*. Springer: Berlin-Heidelberg-New York.

1876. Schajowicz F, Ackerman LV, Sissons HA (1972). *Histologic typing of bone tumours. International Histological Classification of Tumours*. World Health Orgnaization: Geneva, Switzerland.

1877. Schajowicz F, de Prospero JD, Cosentino E (1990). Case report 641: Chondroblastoma-like osteosarcoma. *Skeletal Radiol* 19: 603-606.

1878. Schajowicz F, Gallardo H (1970). Epiphysial chondroblastoma of bone. A clinico-pathological study of sixty-nine cases. *J Bone Joint Surg Br* 52: 205-226.

1879. Schajowicz F, Santini AE, Berenstein M (1983). Sarcoma complicating Paget's disease of bone. A clinicopathological study of 62 cases. *J Bone Joint Surg Br* 65: 299-307.

1880. Scheil S, Bruderlein S, Liehr T, Starke H, Herms J, Schulte M, Moller P (2001). Genome-wide analysis of sixteen chordomas by comparative genomic hybridization and cytogenetics of the first human chordoma cell line, U-CH1. *Genes Chromosomes Cancer* 32: 203-211.

1881. Scheithauer BW, Rubinstein LJ (1978). Meningeal mesenchymal chondrosarcoma: report of 8 cases with review of the literature. *Cancer* 42: 2744-2752.

1882. Scheithauer BW, Woodruff JM, Erlandson RE (1997). *Tumors of the Peripheral Nerve System*. Armed Forces Institute of Pathology: Washington.

1883. Schellenberg GD, Miki T, Yu CE, Nakura J (2001). Werner syndrome. In: *The Metabolic & Molecular Basis of Inherited Disease*, Scriver CR, Beaudet AL, Sly WS, Valle D, eds. McGraw-Hill: New York, pp. 785-797.

1884. Schepel JA, Wille J, Seldenrijk CA, van Ramshorst B (1998). Elastofibroma: a familial occurrence. *Eur J Surg* 164: 557-558.

1885. Schipani E, Kruse K, Juppner H (1995). A constitutively active mutant PTH-PTHrP receptor in Jansen-type metaphyseal chondrodysplasia. *Science* 268: 98-100.

1886. Schlesinger AE, Smith MB, Genez BM, McMahon DP, Swaney JJ (1989). Chest wall mesenchymoma (hamartoma) in infancy. CT and MR findings. *Pediatr Radiol* 19: 212-213.

1887. Schmale GA, Conrad EU, III, Raskind WH (1994). The natural history of hereditary multiple exostoses. *J Bone Joint Surg Am* 76: 986-992.

1888. Schmidt D, Harms D (1987). Epithelioid sarcoma in children and adolescents. An immunohistochemical study. *Virchows Arch A Pathol Anat Histopathol* 410: 423-431.

1889. Schneider-Stock R, Walter H, Radig K, Rys J, Bosse A, Kuhnen C, Hoang-Vu C, Roessner A (1998). MDM2 amplification and loss of heterozygosity at Rb and p53 genes: no simultaneous alterations in the oncogenesis of liposarcomas. *J Cancer Res Clin Oncol* 124: 532-540.

1890. Schoenmakers EF, Wanschura S, Mols R, Bullerdiek J, van den Berghe H, Van de Ven WJ (1995). Recurrent rearrangements in the high mobility group protein gene, HMGI-C, in benign mesenchymal tumours. *Nat Genet* 10: 436-444.

1891. Schofield DE, Conrad EU, Liddell RM, Yunis EJ (1995). An unusual round cell tumor of the tibia with granular cells. *Am J Surg Pathol* 19: 596-603.

1892. Schofield DE, Fletcher JA, Grier HE, Yunis EJ (1994). Fibrosarcoma in infants and children. Application of new techniques. *Am J Surg Pathol* 18: 14-24.

1893. Schofield DE, Yunis EJ, Fletcher JA (1993). Chromosome aberrations in mesoblastic nephroma. *Am J Pathol* 143: 714-724.

1894. Schofield JB, Krausz T, Stamp GW, Fletcher CD, Fisher C, Azzopardi JG (1993). Ossifying fibromyxoid tumour of soft parts: immunohistochemical and ultrastructural analysis. *Histopathology* 22: 101-112.

1895. Schreiber H, Barry FM, Russell WC, Macon WL, Ponsky JL, Pories WJ (1979). Stewart-Treves syndrome. A lethal complication of postmastectomy lymphedema and regional immune deficiency. *Arch Surg* 114: 82-85.

1896. Schuborg C, Mertens F, Rydholm A, Brosjö O, Dictor M, Mitelman F, Mandahl N (1998). Cytogenetic analysis of four angiosarcomas from deep and superficial soft tissue. *Cancer Genet Cytogenet* 100: 52-56.

1897. Schurch W, Begin LR, Seemayer TA, Lagace R, Boivin JC, Lamoureux C, Bluteau P, Piche J, Gabbiani G (1996). Pleomorphic soft tissue myogenic sarcomas of adulthood. A reappraisal in the mid-1990s. *Am J Surg Pathol* 20: 131-147.

1898. Schwartz HS, Dahir GA, Butler MG (1993). Telomere reduction in giant cell tumor of bone and with aging. *Cancer Genet Cytogenet* 71: 132-138.

1899. Schwartz HS, Unni KK, Pritchard DJ (1989). Pigmented villonodular synovitis. A retrospective review of affected large joints. *Clin Orthop* 243-255.

1900. Schwartz HS, Walker R (1997). Recognizable magnetic resonance imaging characteristics of intramuscular myxoma. *Orthopedics* 20: 431-435.

1901. Schwartz HS, Zimmerman NB, Simon MA, Wroble RR, Millar EA, Bonfiglio M (1987). The malignant potential of enchondromatosis. *J Bone Joint Surg Am* 69: 269-274.

1902. Schweitzer G, Pirie D (1971). Osteosarcoma arising in a solitary osteochondroma. *S Afr Med J* 45: 810-811.

1903. Schwindinger WF, Francomano CA, Levine MA (1992). Identification of a mutation in the gene encoding the alpha subunit of the stimulatory G protein of adenylyl cyclase in McCune-Albright syndrome. *Proc Natl Acad Sci U S A* 89: 5152-5156.

1904. Scinicariello F, Dolan MJ, Nedelcu I, Tyring SK, Hilliard JK (1994). Occurrence of human papillomavirus and p53 gene mutations in Kaposi's sarcoma. *Virology* 203: 153-157.

1905. Sciot R, Åkerman M, Dal Cin P, de Wever I, Fletcher CD, Mandahl N, Mertens F, Mitelman F, Rosai J, Rydholm A, Tallini G, van den Berghe H, Vanni R, Willén H (1997). Cytogenetic analysis of subcutaneous angiolipoma: further evidence supporting its difference from ordinary pure lipomas: a report of the CHAMP study group. *Am J Surg Pathol* 21: 441-444.

1906. Sciot R, Dal Cin P, Bellemans J, Samson I, Van den Berghe H., Van Damme B (1998). Synovial chondromatosis: clonal chromosome changes provide further evidence for a neoplastic disorder. *Virchows Arch* 433: 189-191.

1907. Sciot R, Dal Cin P, De Vos R, Van Damme B, de Wever I, van den Berghe H, Desmet VJ (1993). Alveolar soft-part sarcoma: evidence for its myogenic origin and for the involvement of 17q25. *Histopathology* 23: 439-444.

1908. Sciot R, Dal Cin P, Samson I, van den Berghe H, Van Damme B (1999). Clonal chromosomal changes in juxta-articular myxoma. *Virchows Arch* 434: 177-180.

1909. Sciot R, Dorfman H, Brys P, Dal Cin P, de Wever I, Fletcher CD, Jonson K, Mandahl N, Mertens F, Mitelman F, Rosai J, Rydholm A, Samson I, Tallini G, van den Berghe H, Vanni R, Willén H (2000). Cytogenetic-morphologic correlations in aneurysmal bone cyst, giant cell tumor of bone and combined lesions. A report from the CHAMP study group. *Mod Pathol* 13: 1206-1210.

1910. Sciot R, Rosai J, Dal Cin P, de Wever I, Fletcher CD, Mandahl N, Mertens F, Mitelman F, Rydholm A, Tallini G, van den Berghe H, Vanni R, Willén H (1999). Analysis of 35 cases of localized and diffuse tenosynovial giant cell tumor: a report from the chromosomes and morphology (CHAMP) study group. *Mod Pathol* 12: 576-579.

1911. Sciot R, Samson I, van den Berghe H, Van Damme B, Dal Cin P (1999). Collagenous fibroma (desmoplastic fibroblastoma): genetic link with fibroma of tendon sheath? *Mod Pathol* 12: 565-568.

1912. Scott L, Blair G, Taylor G, Dimmick J, Fraser G (1988). Inflammatory pseudotumors in children. *J Pediatr Surg* 23: 755-758.

1913. Scott RJ, Froggatt NJ, Trembath RC, Evans DG, Hodgson SV, Maher ER (1996). Familial infiltrative fibromatosis (desmoid tumours) (MIM135290) caused by a recurrent 3' APC gene mutation. *Hum Mol Genet* 5: 1921-1924.

1914. Scott SM, Reiman HM, Pritchard DJ, Ilstrup DM (1989). Soft tissue fibrosarcoma. A clinicopathologic study of 132 cases. *Cancer* 64: 925-931.

1915. Scrable HJ, Witte DP, Lampkin BC, Cavenee WK (1987). Chromosomal localization of the human rhabdomyosarcoma locus by mitotic recombination mapping. *Nature* 329: 645-647.

1916. Seelig MH, Klingler PJ, Oldenburg WA, Blackshear JL (1998). Angiosarcoma of the aorta: report of a case and review of the literature. *J Vasc Surg* 28: 732-737.

1917. Seki H, Kubota T, Ikegawa S, Haga N, Fujioka F, Ohzeki S, Wakui K, Yoshikawa H, Takaoka K, Fukushima Y (2001). Mutation frequencies of EXT1 and EXT2 in 43 Japanese families with hereditary multiple exostoses. *Am J Med Genet* 99: 59-62.

1918. Semmelink HJ, Pruszczynski M, Wiersma-van Tilburg A, Smedts F, Ramaekers FC (1990). Cytokeratin expression in chondroblastomas. *Histopathology* 16: 257-263.

1919. Sen-Gupta S, Van der Luijt RB, Bowles LV, Meera Khan P, Delhanty JD (1993). Somatic mutation of APC gene in desmoid tumour in familial adenomatous polyposis. *Lancet* 342: 552-553.

1920. Senzaki H, Kiyozuka Y, Uemura Y, Shikata N, Ueda S, Tsubura A (1998). Juvenile hyaline fibromatosis: a report of two unrelated adult sibling cases and a literature review. *Pathol Int* 48: 230-236.

1921. Sevenet N, Lellouch-Tubiana A, Schofield D, Hoang-Xuan K, Gessler M, Birnbaum D, Jeanpierre C, Jouvet A, Delattre O (1999). Spectrum of hSNF5/INI1 somatic mutations in human cancer and genotype-phenotype correlations. *Hum Mol Genet* 8: 2359-2368.

1922. Sevenet N, Sheridan E, Amram D, Schneider P, Handgretinger R, Delattre O (1999). Constitutional mutations of the hSNF5/INI1 gene predispose to a variety of cancers. *Am J Hum Genet* 65: 1342-1348.

1923. Shankman S, Desai P, Beltran J (1997). Subperiosteal osteoid osteoma: radiographic and pathologic manifestations. *Skeletal Radiol* 26: 457-462.

1924. Shankwiler RA, Athey PA, Lamki N (1989). Aggressive infantile fibromatosis. Pulmonary metastases documented by plain film and computed tomography. *Clin Imaging* 13: 127-129.

1925. Shannon FJ, Antonescu CR, Athanasian EA (2000). Metastatic thymic carcinoma in a digit: a case report. *J Hand Surg [Am]* 25: 1169-1172.

1926. Shannon P, Bedard Y, Bell R, Kandel R (1997). Aneurysmal cyst of soft tissue: report of a case with serial magnetic resonance imaging and biopsy. *Hum Pathol* 28: 255-257.

1927. Shapeero LG, Vanel D, Couanet D, Contesso G, Ackerman LV (1993). Extraskeletal mesenchymal chondrosarcoma. *Radiology* 186: 819-826.

1928. Shapiro DN, Parham DM, Douglass EC, Ashmun R, Webber BL, Newton WA, Jr., Hancock ML, Maurer HM, Look AT (1991). Relationship of tumor-cell ploidy to histologic subtype and treatment outcome in children and adolescents with unresectable rhabdomyosarcoma. *J Clin Oncol* 9: 159-166.

1929. Shapiro F, Simon S, Glimcher MJ (1979). Hereditary multiple exostoses. Anthropometric, roentgenographic, and clinical aspects. *J Bone Joint Surg Am* 61: 815-824.

1930. Shek TW, Peh WC, Leung G (1999). Chondromyxoid fibroma of skull base: a tumour prone to local recurrence. *J Laryngol Otol* 113: 380-385.

1931. Shen JC, Loeb LA (2000). The Werner syndrome gene: the molecular basis of RecQ helicase-deficiency diseases. *Trends Genet* 16: 213-220.

1932. Shen SH, Steinbach LS, Wang SF, Chen WY, Chen WM, Chang CY (2001). Primary leiomyosarcoma of bone. *Skeletal Radiol* 30: 600-603.

1933. Sheng WQ, Hisaoka M, Okamoto S, Tanaka A, Meis-Kindblom JM, Kindblom LG, Ishida T, Nojima T, Hashimoto H (2001). Congenital-infantile fibrosarcoma. A clinicopathologic study of 10 cases and molecular detection of the ETV6-NTRK3 fusion transcripts using paraffin-embedded tissues. *Am J Clin Pathol* 115: 348-355.

1934. Shenker A (1996). Activating mutations in G protein-coupled signaling pathways as a cause of endocrine disease. *Growth Genet Horm* 12: 33-37.

1935. Shenker A, Chanson P, Weinstein LS, Chi P, Spiegel AM, Lomri A, Marie PJ (1995). Osteoblastic cells derived from isolated lesions of fibrous dysplasia contain activating somatic mutations of the Gs alpha gene. *Hum Mol Genet* 4: 1675-1676.

1936. Shenker A, Weinstein LS, Moran A, Pescovitz OH, Charest NJ, Boney CM, Van Wyk JJ, Merino MJ, Feuillan PP, Spiegel AM (1993). Severe endocrine and nonendocrine manifestations of the McCune-Albright syndrome associated with activating mutations of stimulatory G protein GS. *J Pediatr* 123: 509-518.

1937. Shenker A, Weinstein LS, Sweet DE, Spiegel AM (1994). An activating Gs alpha mutation is present in fibrous dysplasia of bone in the McCune-Albright syndrome. *J Clin Endocrinol Metab* 79: 750-755.

1938. Shetty AK, Yu LC, Gardner RV, Warrier RP (1999). Role of chemotherapy in the treatment of infantile fibrosarcoma. *Med Pediatr Oncol* 33: 425-427.

1939. Shidham VB, Ayala GE, Lahaniatis JE, Garcia FU (1999). Low-grade fibromyxoid sarcoma: clinicopathologic case report with review of the literature. *Am J Clin Oncol* 22: 150-155.

1940. Shimizu S, Hashimoto H, Enjoji M (1984). Nodular fasciitis: an analysis of 250 patients. *Pathology* 16: 161-166.

1941. Shinjo K, Miyake N, Takahashi Y (1993). Malignant giant cell tumor of the tendon sheath: an autopsy report and review of the literature. *Jpn J Clin Oncol* 23: 317-324.

1942. Shipley J, Crew J, Birdsall S, Gill S, Clark J, Fisher C, Kelsey A, Nojima T, Sonobe H, Cooper C, Gusterson B (1996). Interphase fluorescence in situ hybridization and reverse transcription polymerase chain reaction as a diagnostic aid for synovial sarcoma. *Am J Pathol* 148: 559-567.

1943. Shives TC, Dahlin DC, Sim FH, Pritchard DJ, Earle JD (1986). Osteosarcoma of the spine. *J Bone Joint Surg Am* 68: 660-668.

1944. Shmookler BM, Enzinger FM (1981). Pleomorphic lipoma: a benign tumor simulating liposarcoma. A clinicopathologic analysis of 48 cases. *Cancer* 47: 126-133.

1945. Shmookler BM, Lauer DH (1983). Retroperitoneal leiomyosarcoma. A clinicopathologic analysis of 36 cases. *Am J Surg Pathol* 7: 269-280.

1946. Shugart RR, Soule EH, Johnson EW (1963). Glomus tumor. *Surg Gynecol Obstet* 117: 334.

1947. Siebenrock KA, Unni KK, Rock MG (1998). Giant-cell tumour of bone metastasising to the lungs. A long-term follow-up. *J Bone Joint Surg Br* 80: 43-47.

1948. Siegal GP (1998). Primary tumors of bone. In: *Pathology of Solid Tumors in Children*, Stocker JT, Askin FB, eds. Chapman& Hall Medical: London, pp. 183-212.

1949. Siegel MJ (2001). Magnetic resonance imaging of musculoskeletal soft tissue masses. *Radiol Clin North Am* 39: 701-720.

1950. Sigel JE, Fisher C, Vogt D, Goldblum JR (2000). Giant cell angiofibroma of the inguinal region. *Ann Diagn Pathol* 4: 240-244.

1951. Sigel JE, Smith TA, Reith JD, Goldblum JR (2001). Immunohistochemical analysis of anaplastic lymphoma kinase expression in deep soft tissue calcifying fibrous pseudotumor: evidence of a late sclerosing stage of inflammatory myofibroblastic tumor? *Ann Diagn Pathol* 5: 10-14.

1952. Silverman TA, Enzinger FM (1985). Fibrolipomatous hamartoma of nerve. A clinicopathologic analysis of 26 cases. *Am J Surg Pathol* 9: 7-14.

1953. Sim FH, Unni KK, Beabout JW, Dahlin DC (1979). Osteosarcoma with small cells simulating Ewing's tumor. *J Bone Joint Surg Am* 61: 207-215.

1954. Simmons AD, Musy MM, Lopes CS, Hwang LY, Yang YP, Lovett M (1999). A direct interaction between EXT proteins and glycosyltransferases is defective in hereditary multiple exostoses. *Hum Mol Genet* 8: 2155-2164.

1955. Simon MA, Aschliman MA, Thomas N, Mankin HJ (1986). Limb-salvage treatment versus amputation for osteosarcoma of the distal end of the femur. *J Bone Joint Surg Am* 68: 1331-1337.

1956. Simon RG, Irwin RB (1996). An unusual presentation of telangiectatic osteosarcoma. *Am J Orthop* 25: 375-379.

1957. Simons A, Schepens M, Jeuken J, Sprenger S, van de Zande G, Bjerkehagen B, Forus A, Weibolt V, Molenaar I, van den Berg E, Myklebost O, Bridge J, van Kessel AG, Suijkerbuijk R (2000). Frequent loss of 9p21 (p16INK4A) and other genomic imbalances in human malignant fibrous histiocytoma. *Cancer Genet Cytogenet* 118: 89-98.

1958. Singer S, Baldini EH, Demetri GD, Fletcher JA, Corson JM (1996). Synovial sarcoma: prognostic significance of tumor size, margin of resection, and mitotic activity for survival. *J Clin Oncol* 14: 1201-1208.

1959. Singer S, Corson JM, Demetri GD, Healey EA, Marcus K, Eberlein TJ (1995). Prognostic factors predictive of survival for truncal and retroperitoneal soft-tissue sarcoma. *Ann Surg* 221: 185-195.

1960. Singer S, Demetri GD, Baldini EH, Fletcher CD (2000). Management of soft tissue sarcomas: an overview and update. *Lancet Oncol* 1: 75-85.

1961. Sinovic JF, Bridge JA, Neff JR (1992). Ring chromosome in parosteal osteosarcoma. Clinical and diagnostic significance. *Cancer Genet Cytogenet* 62: 50-52.

1962. Sirvent N, Forus A, Lescaut W, Burel F, Benzaken S, Chazal M, Bourgeon A, Vermeesch JR, Myklebost O, Turc-Carel C, Ayraud N, Coindre JM, Pedeutour F (2000). Characterization of centromere alterations in liposarcomas. *Genes Chromosomes Cancer* 29: 117-129.

1963. Sjögren H, Meis-Kindblom J, Kindblom LG, Åman P, Stenman G (1999). Fusion of the EWS-related gene TAF2N to TEC in extraskeletal myxoid chondrosarcoma. *Cancer Res* 59: 5064-5067.

1964. Sjögren H, Wedell B, Kindblom JM, Kindblom LG, Stenman G (2000). Fusion of the NH2-terminal domain of the basic helix-loop-helix protein TCF12 to TEC in extraskeletal myxoid chondrosarcoma with translocation t(9;15)(q22;q21). *Cancer Res* 60: 6832-6835.

1965. Skalova A, Michal M, Husek K, Zamecnik M, Leivo I (1993). Aggressive angiomyxoma of the pelvioperineal region. Immunohistological and ultrastructural study of seven cases. *Am J Dermatopathol* 15: 446-451.

1966. Skytting B, Nilsson G, Brodin B, Xie Y, Lundeberg J, Uhlen M, Larsson O (1999). A novel fusion gene, SYT-SSX4, in synovial sarcoma. *J Natl Cancer Inst* 91: 974-975.

1967. Slater DN, Cotton DW, Azzopardi JG (1987). Oncocytic glomus tumour: a new variant. *Histopathology* 11: 523-531.

1968. Slullitel JA, Schajowicz F, Slullitel J (1971). [Solitary osteochondroma with malignant degeneration into osteogenic sarcoma]. *Rev Chir Orthop Reparatrice Appar Mot* 57: 471-478.

1969. Smith DM, Mahmoud HH, Jenkins JJ, III, Rao B, Hopkins KP, Parham DM (1995). Myofibrosarcoma of the head and neck in children. *Pediatr Pathol Lab Med* 15: 403-418.

1970. Smith KJ, Skelton HG, Barrett TL, Lupton GP, Graham JH (1989). Cutaneous myofibroma. *Mod Pathol* 2: 603-609.

1971. Smith ME, Costa MJ, Weiss SW (1991). Evaluation of CD68 and other histiocytic antigens in angiomatoid malignant fibrous histiocytoma. *Am J Surg Pathol* 15: 757-763.

1972. Smith ME, Fisher C, Weiss SW (1996). Pleomorphic hyalinizing angiectatic tumor of soft parts. A low-grade neoplasm resembling neurilemoma. *Am J Surg Pathol* 20: 21-29.

1973. Smith NM, Davies JB, Shrimankar JS, Malcolm AJ (1990). Deep fibrous histiocytoma with giant cells and bone metaplasia. *Histopathology* 17: 365-367.

1974. Smith S, Fletcher CD, Smith MA, Gusterson BA (1990). Cytogenetic analysis of a plexiform fibrohistiocytic tumor. *Cancer Genet Cytogenet* 48: 31-34.

1975. Smith SH, Weiss SW, Jankowski SA, Coccia MA, Meltzer PS (1992). SAS amplification in soft tissue sarcomas. *Cancer Res* 52: 3746-3749.

1976. Smith TA, Easley KA, Goldblum JR (1996). Myxoid/round cell liposarcoma of the extremities. A clinicopathologic study of 29 cases with particular attention to extent of round cell liposarcoma. *Am J Surg Pathol* 20: 171-180.

1977. Smith TA, Machen SK, Fisher C, Goldblum JR (1999). Usefulness of cytokeratin subsets for distinguishing monophasic synovial sarcoma from malignant peripheral nerve sheath tumor. *Am J Clin Pathol* 112: 641-648.

1978. Smythe JF, Dyck JD, Smallhorn JF, Freedom RM (1990). Natural history of cardiac rhabdomyoma in infancy and childhood. *Am J Cardiol* 66: 1247-1249.

1979. Sobin LH, Wittekind C (2002). *UICC TNM Classification of Malignant Tumours.* 6th ed. Wiley: New York.

1980. Soder S, Inwards C, Muller S, Kirchner T, Aigner T (2001). Cell biology and matrix biochemistry of chondromyxoid fibroma. *Am J Clin Pathol* 116: 271-277.

1981. Soini Y, Welsh JA, Ishak KG, Bennett WP (1995). p53 mutations in primary hepatic angiosarcomas not associated with vinyl chloride exposure. *Carcinogenesis* 16: 2879-2881.

1982. Sola JB, Wright RW (1998). Arthroscopic treatment for lipoma arborescens of the knee: a case report. *J Bone Joint Surg Am* 80: 99-103.

1983. Soler JM, Piza G, Aliaga F (1997). Special characteristics of osteoid osteoma in the proximal phalanx. *J Hand Surg [Br]* 22: 793-797.

1984. Somerhausen NS, Fletcher CD (2000). Diffuse-type giant cell tumor: clinicopathologic and immunohistochemical analysis of 50 cases with extraarticular disease. *Am J Surg Pathol* 24: 479-492.

1985. Somers GR, Tesoriero AA, Hartland E, Robertson CF, Robinson PJ, Venter DJ, Chow CW (1998). Multiple leiomyosarcomas of both donor and recipient origin arising in a heart-lung transplant patient. *Am J Surg Pathol* 22: 1423-1428.

1986. Somers KD, Winters BA, Dawson DM, Leffell MS, Wright GL, Jr., Devine CJ, Jr., Gilbert DA, Horton CE (1987). Chromosome abnormalities in Peyronie's disease. *J Urol* 137: 672-675.

1987. Sonobe H, Furihata M, Iwata J, Oka T, Ohtsuki Y, Hamasato S, Fujimoto S (1993). Morphological characterization of a new human epithelioid sarcoma cell line, ES020488, in vitro and in vivo. *Virchows Arch B Cell Pathol Incl Mol Pathol* 63: 219-225.

1988. Sonobe H, Iwata J, Komatsu T, Fukushima A, Hayashi N, Moriki T, Shimizu K, Ohtsuki Y (2000). A giant cell angiofibroma involving 6q. *Cancer Genet Cytogenet* 116: 47-49.

1989. Sonobe H, Ohtsuki Y, Mizobuchi H, Toda M, Shimizu K (1996). An angiomyoma with t(X;10)(q22;q23.2). *Cancer Genet Cytogenet* 90: 54-56.

1990. Sonobe H, Ohtsuki Y, Sugimoto T, Shimizu K (1997). Involvement of 8q, 22q, and monosomy 21 in an epithelioid sarcoma. *Cancer Genet Cytogenet* 96: 178-180.

1991. Sonobe H, Ro JY, Ordonez NG, Ayala AG (1994). Alveolar soft part sarcoma of the lung. *Int J Surg Pathol* 2: 57-62.

1992. Soper JR, De Silva M (1993). Infantile myofibromatosis: a radiological review. *Pediatr Radiol* 23: 189-194.

1993. Soravia C, Berk T, McLeod RS, Cohen Z (2000). Desmoid disease in patients with familial adenomatous polyposis. *Dis Colon Rectum* 43: 363-369.

1994. Sordillo PP, Hajdu SI, Magill GB, Golbey RB (1983). Extraosseous osteogenic sarcoma. A review of 48 patients. *Cancer* 51: 727-734.

1995. Sorensen PH, Lessnick SL, Lopez-Terrada D, Liu XF, Triche TJ, Denny CT (1994). A second Ewing's sarcoma translocation, t(21;22), fuses the EWS gene to another ETS-family transcription factor, ERG. *Nat Genet* 6: 146-151.

1996. Sorensen PH, Liu XF, Delattre O, Rowland JM, Biggs CA, Thomas G, Triche TJ (1993). Reverse transcriptase PCR amplification of EWS/FLI-1 fusion transcripts as a diagnostic test for peripheral primitive neuroectodermal tumors of childhood. *Diagn Mol Pathol* 2: 147-157.

1997. Sorensen SA, Mulvihill JJ, Nielsen A (1981). Long-term follow-up of von Recklinghausen neurofibromatosis. *N Engl J Med* 305: 1617.

1998. Sotelo-Avila C, Bale PM (1994). Subdermal fibrous hamartoma of infancy: pathology of 40 cases and differential diagnosis. *Pediatr Pathol* 14: 39-52.

1999. Souid AK, Ziemba MC, Dubansky AS, Mazur M, Oliphant M, Thomas FD, Ratner M, Sadowitz PD (1993). Inflammatory myofibroblastic tumor in children. *Cancer* 72: 2042-2048.

2000. Soule EH (1962). Proliferative (nodular) fasciitis. *Arch Pathol* 73: 437-444.

2001. Soule EH, Pritchard DJ (1977). Fibrosarcoma in infants and children: a review of 110 cases. *Cancer* 40: 1711-1721.

2002. Southwick GJ, Karamoskos P (1990). Fibroma of tendon sheath with bone involvement. *J Hand Surg [Br]* 15: 373-375.

2003. Sovani V, Velagaleti GV, Filipowicz E, Gatalica Z, Knisely AS (2001). Ossifying fibromyxoid tumor of soft parts: report of a case with novel cytogenetic findings. *Cancer Genet Cytogenet* 127: 1-6.

2004. Sozzi G, Miozzo M, Di Palma S, Minelli A, Calderone C, Danesino C, Pastorino U, Pierotti MA, Della Porta G (1990). Involvement of the region 13q14 in a patient with adamantinoma of the long bones. *Hum Genet* 85: 513-515.

2005. Spanta R, Lawrence WD (1995). Soft tissue chondroma of the fallopian tube. Differential diagnosis and histogenetic considerations. *Pathol Res Pract* 191: 174-176.

2006. Sparkes RS, Sparkes MC, Wilson MG, Towner JW, Benedict W, Murphree AL, Yunis JJ (1980). Regional assignment of genes for human esterase D and retinoblastoma to chromosome band 13q14. *Science* 208: 1042-1044.

2007. Speleman F, Colpaert C, Goovaerts G, Leroy JG, Van Marck E (1992). Malignant melanoma of soft parts. Further cytogenetic characterization. *Cancer Genet Cytogenet* 60: 176-179.

2008. Spencer H (1984). The pulmonary plasma cell/histiocytoma complex. *Histopathology* 8: 903-916.

2009. Spicer RD (1992). Neonatal soft tissue tumours. *Br J Cancer Suppl* 18: S80-S83.

2010. Spillane AJ, A'Hern R, Judson IR, Fisher C, Thomas JM (2000). Synovial sarcoma: a clinicopathologic, staging, and prognostic assessment. *J Clin Oncol* 18: 3794-3803.

2011. Spirio L, Olschwang S, Groden J, Robertson M, Samowitz W, Joslyn G, Gelbert L, Thliveris A, Carlson M, Otterud B (1993). Alleles of the APC gene: an attenuated form of familial polyposis. *Cell* 75: 951-957.

2012. Spitsbergen JM, Tsai HW, Reddy A, Miller T, Arbogast D, Hendricks JD, Bailey GS (2000). Neoplasia in zebrafish (Danio rerio) treated with N-methyl-N'-nitro-N-nitrosoguanidine by three exposure routes at different developmental stages. *Toxicol Pathol* 28: 716-725.

2013. Spjut HJ, Ayala AG, deSantos LA, et al (1977). *Proceedings of the Annual Clinical Conference on Cancer. Sponsored by The University of Texas System Cancer Center.* Year Book Medical Publishers: Chicago.

2014. Spouge AR, Thain LM (2000). Osteoid osteoma: MR imaging revisited. *Clin Imaging* 24: 19-27.

2015. Springfield DS, Capanna R, Gherlinzoni F, Picci P, Campanacci M (1985). Chondroblastoma. A review of seventy cases. *J Bone Joint Surg Am* 67: 748-755.

2016. Springfield DS, Rosenberg AE, Mankin HJ, Mindell ER (1994). Relationship between osteofibrous dysplasia and adamantinoma. *Clin Orthop* 234-244.

2017. Squire J, Gallie BL, Phillips RA (1985). A detailed analysis of chromosomal changes in heritable and non-heritable retinoblastoma. *Hum Genet* 70: 291-301.

2018. Sreekantaiah C, Karakousis CP, Leong SP, Sandberg AA (1992). Cytogenetic findings in liposarcoma correlate with histopathologic subtypes. *Cancer* 69: 2484-2495.

2019. Sreekantaiah C, Leong SP, Davis JR, Sandberg AA (1991). Cytogenetic and flow cytometric analysis of a clear cell chondrosarcoma. *Cancer Genet Cytogenet* 52: 193-199.

2020. Sreekantaiah C, Leong SP, Karakousis CP, McGee DL, Rappaport WD, Villar HV, Neal D, Fleming S, Wankel A, Herrington PN, Carmona R, Sandberg AA (1991). Cytogenetic profile of 109 lipomas. *Cancer* 51: 422-433.

2021. Staehelin F, Bissig H, Hosli I, Betts DR, Schafer BW, Scholl FA, Holzgreve W, Kuhne T (2000). Inv(11)(p13p15) and myf-3(MyoD1) in a malignant extrarenal rhabdoid tumor of a premature newborn. *Pediatr Res* 48: 463-467.

2022. Stanton RP, Abdel-Mota'al MM (1998). Growth arrest resulting from unicameral bone cyst. *J Pediatr Orthop* 18: 198-201.

2023. Steenman M, Westerveld A, Mannens M (2000). Genetics of Beckwith-Wiedemann syndrome-associated tumors: common genetic pathways. *Genes Chromosomes Cancer* 28: 1-13.

2024. Steeper TA, Rosai J (1983). Aggressive angiomyxoma of the female pelvis and perineum. Report of nine cases of a distinctive type of gynecologic soft-tissue neoplasm. *Am J Surg Pathol* 7: 463-475.

2025. Steiner GC (1979). Ultrastructure of benign cartilaginous tumors of intraosseous origin. *Hum Pathol* 10: 71-86.

2026. Steiner GC, Mirra JM, Bullough PG (1973). Mesenchymal chondrosarcoma. A study of the ultrastructure. *Cancer* 32: 926-939.

2027. Stener B, Gunterberg B (1978). High amputation of the sacrum for extirpation of tumors. Principles and technique. *Spine* 3: 351-366.

2028. Stenman G, Andersson H, Mandahl N, Meis-Kindblom JM, Kindblom LG (1995). Translocation t(9;22)(q22;q12) is a primary cytogenetic abnormality in extraskeletal myxoid chondrosarcoma. *Int J Cancer* 62: 398-402.

2029. Stenman G, Kindblom LG, Willems J, Angervall L (1990). A cell culture, chromosomal and quantitative DNA analysis of a metastatic epithelioid sarcoma. Deletion 1p, a possible primary chromosomal abnormality in epithelioid sarcoma. *Cancer* 65: 2006-2013.

2030. Stickens D, Brown D, Evans GA (2000). EXT genes are differentially expressed in bone and cartilage during mouse embryogenesis. *Dev Dyn* 218: 452-464.

2031. Stickens D, Clines G, Burbee D, Ramos P, Thomas S, Hogue D, Hecht JT, Lovett M, Evans GA (1996). The EXT2 multiple exostoses gene defines a family of putative tumour suppressor genes. *Nat Genet* 14: 25-32.

2032. Stickens D, Evans GA (1997). Isolation and characterization of the murine homolog of the human EXT2 multiple exostoses gene. *Biochem Mol Med* 61: 16-21.

2033. Stock C, Kager L, Fink FM, Gadner H, Ambros PF (2000). Chromosomal regions involved in the pathogenesis of osteosarcomas. *Genes Chromosomes Cancer* 28: 329-336.

2034. Stone CH, Lee MW, Amin MB, Yaziji H, Gown AM, Ro JY, Tetu B, Paraf F, Zarbo RJ (2001). Renal angiomyolipoma: further immunophenotypic characterization of an expanding morphologic spectrum. *Arch Pathol Lab Med* 125: 751-758.

2035. Stout AP (1948). Fibrosarcoma. The malignant tumor of fibroblasts. *Cancer* 1: 30-63.

2036. Stout AP (1949). Hemangiopericytoma. A study of twenty five new cases. *Cancer* 2: 1027-1035.

2037. Stout AP (1954). Juvenile fibromatosis. *Cancer* 7: 953.

2038. Stout AP (1962). Fibrosarcoma in infants and children. *Cancer* 15: 1028-1040.

2039. Stout AP, Hill WT (1964). Leiomyosarcoma of the superficial soft tissue. *Cancer* 11: 844-854.

2040. Stout AP, Murray MR (1942). Hemangiopericytoma: a vascular tumor featuring Zimmerman's pericytes. *Ann Surg* 116: 26-33.

2041. Stratton MR, Fisher C, Gusterson BA, Cooper CS (1989). Detection of point mutations in N-ras and K-ras genes of human embryonal rhabdomyosarcomas using oligonucleotide probes and the polymerase chain reaction. *Cancer Res* 49: 6324-6327.

2042. Stratton MR, Moss S, Warren W, Patterson H, Clark J, Fisher C, Fletcher CD, Ball A, Thomas M, Gusterson BA, Cooper CS (1990). Mutation of the p53 gene in human soft tissue sarcomas: association with abnormalities of the RB1 gene. *Oncogene* 5: 1297-1301.

2043. Stringer MD, Ramani P, Yeung CK, Capps SN, Kiely EM, Spitz L (1992). Abdominal inflammatory myofibroblastic tumours in children. *Br J Surg* 79: 1357-1360.

2044. Strong LC, Riccardi VM, Ferrell RE, Sparkes RS (1981). Familial retinoblastoma and chromosome 13 deletion transmitted via an insertional translocation. *Science* 213: 1501-1503.

2045. Strouse PJ, Ellis BI, Shifrin LZ, Shah AR (1992). Case report 710: Symmetrical eosinophilic granuloma of the lower extremities (proven) and Erdheim-Chester disease (probable). *Skeletal Radiol* 21: 64-67.

2046. Strutton G, Weedon D (1987). Acro-angiodermatitis. A simulant of Kaposi's sarcoma. *Am J Dermatopathol* 9: 85-89.

2047. Su LD, Atayde-Perez A, Sheldon S, Fletcher JA, Weiss SW (1998). Inflammatory myofibroblastic tumor: cytogenetic evidence supporting clonal origin. *Mod Pathol* 11: 364-368.

2048. Su W, Ko A, O'Connell T, Applebaum H (2000). Treatment of pseudotumors with nonsteroidal antiinflammatory drugs. *J Pediatr Surg* 35: 1635-1637.

2049. Suarez VD, Gimenez PA, Rio SM (1990). Vaginal rhabdomyoma and adenosis. *Histopathology* 16: 393-394.

2050. Sudo T, Kuramoto T, Komiya S, Inoue A, Itoh K (1997). Expression of MAGE genes in osteosarcoma. *J Orthop Res* 15: 128-132.

2051. Suh CH, Ordonez NG, Mackay B (2000). Malignant fibrous histiocytoma: an ultrastructural perspective. *Ultrastruct Pathol* 24: 243-250.

2052. Suh JS, Cho J, Lee SH, Shin KH, Yang WI, Lee JH, Cho JH, Suh KJ, Lee YJ, Ryu KN (2000). Alveolar soft part sarcoma: MR and angiographic findings. *Skeletal Radiol* 29: 680-689.

2053. Suijkerbuijk RF, Olde Weghuis DE, van den Berg M, Pedeutour F, Forus A, Myklebost O, Glier C, Turc-Carel C, van Kessel AG (1994). Comparative genomic hybridization as a tool to define two distinct chromosome 12-derived amplification units in well-differentiated liposarcomas. *Genes Chromosomes Cancer* 9: 292-295.

2054. Sumiyoshi K, Tsuneyoshi M, Enjoji M (1985). Myositis ossificans. A clinicopathologic study of 21 cases. *Acta Pathol Jpn* 35: 1109-1122.

2055. Sun TC, Swee RG, Shives TC, Unni KK (1985). Chondrosarcoma in Maffucci's syndrome. *J Bone Joint Surg Am* 67: 1214-1219.

2056. Sundaram M, Akduman I, White LM, McDonald DJ, Kandel R, Janney C (1999). Primary leiomyosarcoma of bone. *AJR Am J Roentgenol* 172: 771-776.

2057. Sundaram M, Herbold DR, McGuire MH (1986). Case report 370: Low grade (well-differentiated) intramedullary osteosarcoma. *Skeletal Radiol* 15: 338-342.

2058. Sundaresan N, Galicich JH, Chu FC, Huvos AG (1979). Spinal chordomas. *J Neurosurg* 50: 312-319.

2059. Suster S, Fisher C (1997). Immunoreactivity for the human hematopoietic progenitor cell antigen (CD34) in lipomatous tumors. *Am J Surg Pathol* 21: 195-200.

2060. Suster S, Fisher C, Moran CA (1998). Expression of bcl-2 oncoprotein in benign and malignant spindle cell tumors of soft tissue, skin, serosal surfaces, and gastrointestinal tract. *Am J Surg Pathol* 22: 863-872.

2061. Suster S, Moran CA (1997). Malignant cartilaginous tumors of the mediastinum: clinicopathological study of six cases presenting as extraskeletal soft tissue masses. *Hum Pathol* 28: 588-594.

2062. Suster S, Nascimento AG, Miettinen M, Sickel JZ, Moran CA (1995). Solitary fibrous tumors of soft tissue. A clinicopathologic and immunohistochemical study of 12 cases. *Am J Surg Pathol* 19: 1257-1266.

2063. Suster S, Wong TY, Moran CA (1993). Sarcomas with combined features of liposarcoma and leiomyosarcoma. Study of two cases of an unusual soft-tissue tumor showing dual lineage differentiation. *Am J Surg Pathol* 17: 905-911.

2064. Swanson PE, Lillemoe TJ, Manivel JC, Wick MR (1990). Mesenchymal chondrosarcoma. An immunohistochemical study. *Arch Pathol Lab Med* 114: 943-948.

2065. Swanson PE, Wick MR (1989). Clear cell sarcoma. An immunohistochemical analysis of six cases and comparison with other epithelioid neoplasms of soft tissue. *Arch Pathol Lab Med* 113: 55-60.

2066. Swanson PE, Wick MR, Dehner LP (1991). Leiomyosarcoma of somatic soft tissues in childhood: an immunohistochemical analysis of six cases with ultrastructural correlation. *Hum Pathol* 22: 569-577.

2067. Swarts SJ, Neff JR, Johansson SL, Bridge JA (1996). Cytogenetic analysis of dedifferentiated chondrosarcoma. *Cancer Genet Cytogenet* 89: 49-51.

2068. Swarts SJ, Neff JR, Johansson SL, Nelson M, Bridge JA (1998). Significance of abnormalities of chromosomes 5 and 8 in chondroblastoma. *Clin Orthop* 189-193.

2069. Sweet DE, Vinh TN, Devaney K (1992). Cortical osteofibrous dysplasia of long bone and its relationship to adamantinoma. A clinicopathologic study of 30 cases. *Am J Surg Pathol* 16: 282-290.

2070. Sybert V (1997). *Genetic Skin Disorders.* 1st ed. Oxford University Press: New York.

2071. Szymanska J, Mandahl N, Mertens F, Tarkkanen M, Karaharju E, Knuutila S (1996). Ring chromosomes in parosteal osteosarcoma contain sequences from 12q13-15: a combined cytogenetic and comparative genomic hybridization study. *Genes Chromosomes Cancer* 16: 31-34.

2072. Szymanska J, Tarkkanen M, Wiklund T, Virolainen M, Blomqvist C, Asko-Seljavaara S, Tukiainen E, Elomaa I, Knuutila S (1996). Gains and losses of DNA sequences in liposarcomas evaluated by comparative genomic hybridization. *Genes Chromosomes Cancer* 15: 89-94.

2073. Taccagni G, Sambade C, Nesland J, Terreni MR, Sobrinho-Simoes M (1993). Solitary fibrous tumour of the thyroid: clinicopathological, immunohistochemical and ultrastructural study of three cases. *Virchows Arch A Pathol Anat Histopathol* 422: 491-497.

2074. Taconis WK (1988). Osteosarcoma in fibrous dysplasia. *Skeletal Radiol* 17: 163-170.

2075. Taconis WK, Mulder JD (1984). Fibrosarcoma and malignant fibrous histiocytoma of long bones: radiographic features and grading. *Skeletal Radiol* 11: 237-245.

2076. Takahashi K, Kimura Y, Naito M, Yoshimura T, Uchida H, Araki S (1989). Inflammatory fibrous histiocytoma presenting leukemoid reaction. *Pathol Res Pract* 184: 498-506.

2077. Takanami I, Takeuchi K, Naruke M (1999). Low-grade fibromyxoid sarcoma arising in the mediastinum. *J Thorac Cardiovasc Surg* 118: 970-971.

2078. Takaoka K, Yoshikawa H, Masuhara K, Sugano N, Ono K (1994). Ectopic ossification associated with osteoid osteoma in the acetabulum. A case report. *Clin Orthop* 209-211.

2079. Takata H, Ikuta Y, Ishida O, Kimori K (2001). Treatment of subungual glomus tumour. *Hand Surg* 6: 25-27.

2080. Takeuchi T, Takenoshita Y, Kubo K, Iida M (1993). Natural course of jaw lesions in patients with familial adenomatosis coli (Gardner's syndrome). *Int J Oral Maxillofac Surg* 22: 226-230.

2081. Takigawa K (1971). Chondroma of the bones of the hand. A review of 110 cases. *J Bone Joint Surg Am* 53: 1591-1600.

2082. Tallini G, Dorfman H, Brys P, Dal Cin P, de Wever I, Fletcher CD, Jonson K, Mandahl N, Mertens F, Mitelman F, Rosai J, Rydholm A, Samson I, Sciot R, van den Berghe H, Vanni R, Willén H (2002). Correlation between clinicopathological features and karyotype in 100 cartilaginous and chordoid tumours. A report from the chromosomes and morphology (CHAMP) collaborative study group. *J Pathol* 196: 194-203.

2083. Tallini G, Vanni R, Manfioletti G, Kazmierczak B, Faa G, Pauwels P, Bullerdiek J, Giancotti V, van den Berghe H, Dal Cin P (2000). HMGI-C and HMGI(Y) immunoreactivity correlates with cytogenetic abnormalities in lipomas, pulmonary chondroid hamartomas, endometrial polyps, and uterine leiomyomas and is compatible with rearrangement of the HMGI-C and HMGI(Y) genes. *Lab Invest* 80: 359-369.

2084. Tanaka Y, Ijiri R, Kato K, Kato Y, Misugi K, Nakatani Y, Hara M (2000). HMB-45/melan-A and smooth muscle actin-positive clear-cell epithelioid tumor arising in the ligamentum teres hepatis: additional example of clear cell 'sugar' tumors. *Am J Surg Pathol* 24: 1295-1299.

2085. Tanda F, Rocca PC, Bosincu L, Massarelli G, Cossu A, Manca A (1997). Rhabdomyoma of the tunica vaginalis of the testis: a histologic, immunohistochemical, and ultrastructural study. *Mod Pathol* 10: 608-611.

2086. Tang TT, Segura AD, Oechler HW, Harb JM, Adair SE, Gregg DC, Camitta BM, Franciosi RA (1990). Inflammatory myofibrohistiocytic proliferation simulating sarcoma in children. *Cancer* 65: 1626-1634.

2087. Tarkkanen M, Aaltonen LA, Böhling T, Kivioja A, Karaharju E, Elomaa I, Knuutila S (1996). No evidence of microsatellite instability in bone tumours. *Br J Cancer* 74: 453-455.

2088. Tarkkanen M, Böhling T, Gamberi G, Ragazzini P, Benassi MS, Kivioja A, Kallio P, Elomaa I, Picci P, Knuutila S (1998). Comparative genomic hybridization of low-grade central osteosarcoma. *Mod Pathol* 11: 421-426.

2089. Tarkkanen M, Elomaa I, Blomqvist C, Kivioja AH, Kellokumpu-Lehtinen P, Böhling T, Valle J, Knuutila S (1999). DNA sequence copy number increase at 8q: a potential new prognostic marker in high-grade osteosarcoma. *Int J Cancer* 84: 114-121.

2090. Tarkkanen M, Kaipainen A, Karaharju E, Böhling T, Szymanska J, Helio H, Kivioja A, Elomaa I, Knuutila S (1993). Cytogenetic study of 249 consecutive patients examined for a bone tumor. *Cancer Genet Cytogenet* 68: 1-21.

2091. Tarkkanen M, Karhu R, Kallioniemi A, Elomaa I, Kivioja AH, Nevalainen J, Böhling T, Karaharju E, Hyytinen E, Knuutila S, Kalioniemi OP (1995). Gains and losses of DNA sequences in osteosarcomas by comparative genomic hybridization. *Cancer Res* 55: 1334-1338.

2092. Tarkkanen M, Nordling S, Böhling T, Kivioja A, Karaharju E Szymanska, Elomaa I, Knuutila S (1996). Comparison of cytogenetics, interphase cytogenetics, and DNA flow cytometry in bone tumors. *Cytometry* 26: 185-191.

2093. Tarkkanen M, Wiklund T, Virolainen M, Elomaa I, Knuutila S (1994). Dedifferentiated chondrosarcoma with t(9;22)(q34;q11-12). *Genes Chromosomes Cancer* 9: 136-140.

2094. Tarkkanen M, Wiklund TA, Virolainen MJ, Larramendy M, Mandahl N, Mertens F, Blomqvist C, Tukiainen E, Miettinen M, Elomaa I, Knuutila S (2001). Comparative genomic hybridization of postirradiation sarcomas. *Cancer* 92: 1992-1998.

2095. Tarkkanen M, Wolf M, Knuutila S (2002). *Genomic imbalances, their putative target genes and clinical significance in sarcomas and benign mesenchymal tumors* (in press).

2096. Taubert H, Berger D, Hinze R, Meye A, Wurl P, Hogendoorn PC, Holzhausen HJ, Schmidt H, Rath FW (1998). How is the mutational status for tumor suppressors p53 and p16INK4A in MFH of the bone? *Cancer Lett* 123: 147-151.

2097. Taubert H, Wurl P, Meye A, Berger D, Thamm B, Neumann K, Hinze R, Schmidt H, Rath FW (1995). Molecular and immunohistochemical p53 status in liposarcoma and malignant fibrous histiocytoma: identification of seven new mutations for soft tissue sarcomas. *Cancer* 76: 1187-1196.

2098. Taylor WF, Ivins JC, Dahlin DC, Edmonson JH, Pritchard DJ (1978). Trends and variability in survival from osteosarcoma. *Mayo Clin Proc* 53: 695-700.

2099. Taylor WF, Ivins JC, Unni KK, Beabout JW, Golenzer HJ, Black LE (1989). Prognostic variables in osteosarcoma: a multi-institutional study. *J Natl Cancer Inst* 81: 21-30.

2100. Tazelaar HD, Batts KP, Srigley JR (2001). Primary extrapulmonary sugar tumor (PEST): a report of four cases. *Mod Pathol* 14: 615-622.

2101. Tejpar S, Nollet F, Li C, Wunder JS, Michils G, Dal Cin P, Van Cutsem E, Bapat B, van Roy F, Cassiman JJ, Alman BA (1999). Predominance of beta-catenin mutations and beta-catenin dysregulation in sporadic aggressive fibromatosis (desmoid tumor). *Oncogene* 18: 6615-6620.

2102. Templeton SF, Solomon AR, Jr. (1996). Spindle cell lipoma is strongly CD34 positive. An immunohistochemical study. *J Cutan Pathol* 23: 546-550.

2103. Terzis JK, Daniel RK, Williams HB, Spencer PS (1978). Benign fatty tumors of the peripheral nerves. *Ann Plast Surg* 1: 193-216.

2104. Tetsu O, McCormick F (1999). Beta-catenin regulates expression of cyclin D1 in colon carcinoma cells. *Nature* 398: 422-426.

2105. Teyssier JR, Ferre D (1989). Frequent clonal chromosomal changes in human non-malignant tumors. *Int J Cancer* 44: 828-832.

2106. Thaete C, Brett D, Monaghan P, Whitehouse S, Rennie G, Rayner E, Cooper CS, Goodwin G (1999). Functional domains of the SYT and SYT-SSX synovial sarcoma translocation proteins and co-localization with the SNF protein BRM in the nucleus. *Hum Mol Genet* 8: 585-591.

2107. The I, Bellaiche Y, Perrimon N (1999). Hedgehog movement is regulated through tout velu-dependent synthesis of a heparan sulfate proteoglycan. *Mol Cell* 4: 633-639.

2108. Thomachot B, Daumen-Legre V, Pham T, Acquaviva PC, Lafforgue P (1999). Fibrous dysplasia with intramuscular myxoma (Mazabraud's syndrome). Report of a case and review of the literature. *Rev Rhum Engl Ed* 66: 180-183.

2109. Thomas R, Banerjee SS, Eyden BP, Shanks JH, Bisset DL, Hunt R, Byers RJ, Oogarah P, Harris M (2001). A study of four cases of extra-orbital giant cell angiofibroma with documentation of some unusual features. *Histopathology* 39: 390-396.

2110. Thompson AD, Braun BS, Arvand A, Stewart SD, May WA, Chen E, Korenberg J, Denny CT (1996). EAT-2 is a novel SH2 domain containing protein that is up regulated by Ewing's sarcoma EWS/FLI1 fusion gene. *Oncogene* 13: 2649-2658.

2111. Thompson J, Castillo M, Reddick RL, Smith JK, Shockley W (1995). Nasopharyngeal nonossifying variant of ossifying fibromyxoid tumor: CT and MR findings. *AJNR Am J Neuroradiol* 16: 1132-1134.

2112. Thurer RL, Thorsen A, Parker JA, Karp DD (2000). FDG imaging of a pulmonary artery sarcoma. *Ann Thorac Surg* 70: 1414-1415.

2113. Tigani D, Pignatti G, Picci P, Savini R, Campanacci M (1988). Vertebral osteosarcoma. *Ital J Orthop Traumatol* 14: 5-13.

2114. Tihy F, Scott P, Russo P, Champagne M, Tabet JC, Lemieux N (1998). Cytogenetic analysis of a parachordoma. *Cancer Genet Cytogenet* 105: 14-19.

2115. Tillotson C, Rosenberg A, Gebhardt M, Rosenthal DI (1988). Postradiation multicentric osteosarcoma. *Cancer* 62: 67-71.

2116. Toguchida J, Ishizaki K, Sasaki MS, Ikenaga M, Sugimoto M, Kotoura Y, Yamamuro T (1988). Chromosomal reorganization for the expression of recessive mutation of retinoblastoma susceptibility gene in the development of osteosarcoma. *Cancer Res* 48: 3939-3943.

2117. Toguchida J, Yamaguchi T, Ritchie B, Beauchamp RL, Dayton SH, Herrera GE, Yamamuro T, Kotoura Y, Sasaki MS, Little JB, . (1992). Mutation spectrum of the p53 gene in bone and soft tissue sarcomas. *Cancer Res* 52: 6194-6199.

2118. Tokano H, Sugimoto T, Noguchi Y, Kitamura K (2001). Sequential computed tomography images demonstrating characteristic changes in fibrous dysplasia. *J Laryngol Otol* 115: 757-759.

2119. Tomares SM, Jabra AA, Conrad CK, Beauchamp N, Phoon CK, Carroll JL (1994). Hemothorax in a child as a result of costal exostosis. *Pediatrics* 93: 523-525.

2120. Tongaonkar HB, Kulkarni JN, Kamat MR (1992). Solitary metastases from renal cell carcinoma: a review. *J Surg Oncol* 49: 45-48.

2121. Torok G, Meller Y, Maor E (1983). Primary liposarcoma of bone. Case report and review of the literature. *Bull Hosp Jt Dis Orthop Inst* 43: 28-37.

2122. Torres FX, Kyriakos M (1992). Bone infarct-associated osteosarcoma. *Cancer* 70: 2418-2430.

2123. Tosi P, Cintorino M, Toti P, Ninfo V, Montesco MC, Frezzotti R, Hadjistilianou T, Acquaviva A, Barbini P (1989). Histopathological evaluation for the prognosis of retinoblastoma. *Ophthalmic Paediatr Genet* 10: 173-177.

2124. Toth B, Patil K, Erickson J, Gannett P (1998). Carcinogenesis by benzenediazonium sulfate in mice. *In Vivo* 12: 379-382.

2125. Touriol C, Greenland C, Lamant L, Pulford K, Bernard F, Rousset T, Mason DY, Delsol G (2000). Further demonstration of the diversity of chromosomal changes involving 2p23 in ALK-positive lymphoma: 2 cases expressing ALK kinase fused to CLTCL (clathrin chain polypeptide-like). *Blood* 95: 3204-3207.

2126. Toyoda H, Kinoshita-Toyoda A, Selleck SB (2000). Structural analysis of glycosaminoglycans in Drosophila and Caenorhabditis elegans and demonstration that tout-velu, a Drosophila gene related to EXT tumor suppressors, affects heparan sulfate in vivo. *J Biol Chem* 275: 2269-2275.

2127. Trattner A, Hodak E, David M, Sandbank M (1993). The appearance of Kaposi sarcoma during corticosteroid therapy. *Cancer* 72: 1779-1783.

2128. Travis JA, Bridge JA (1992). Significance of both numerical and structural chromosomal abnormalities in clear cell sarcoma. *Cancer Genet Cytogenet* 64: 104-106.

2129. Trivers GE, Cawley HL, DeBenedetti VM, Hollstein M, Marion MJ, Bennett WP, Hoover ML, Prives CC, Tamburro CC, Harris CC (1995). Anti-p53 antibodies in sera of workers occupationally exposed to vinyl chloride. *J Natl Cancer Inst* 87: 1400-1407.

2130. Trojan A, Stallmach T, Kollias S, Pestalozzi BC (2001). Inflammatory myofibroblastic tumor with CNS involvement. *Onkologie* 24: 368-372.

2131. Trojani M, Contesso G, Coindre JM, Rouesse J, Bui NB, de Mascarel A, Goussot JF, David M, Bonichon F, Lagarde C (1984). Soft-tissue sarcomas of adults; study of pathological prognostic variables and definition of a histopathological grading system. *Int J Cancer* 33: 37-42.

2132. Troum S, Dalton ML, Donner RS, Besser AS (1996). Multifocal mesenchymal hamartoma of the chest wall in infancy. *J Pediatr Surg* 31: 713-715.

2133. Troup JB, Dahlin DC, Coventry MB (1960). The significance of giant cells in osteosarcoma: do they indicate a relationship between osteogenic sarcoma and giant cell tumor of bone? *Proc Staff Meet Mayo Clin* 35: 179-186.

2134. Tsai H, Whitney K, Kogan SJ (1997). Perineal lipoblastoma in a neonate. *J Urol* 158: 2272-2273.

2135. Tsang WY, Chan JK (1991). Kaposi-like infantile hemangioendothelioma. A distinctive vascular neoplasm of the retroperitoneum. *Am J Surg Pathol* 15: 982-989.

2136. Tsang WY, Chan JK, Lee KC, Fisher C, Fletcher CD (1992). Aggressive angiomyxoma. A report of four cases occurring in men. *Am J Surg Pathol* 16: 1059-1065.

2137. Tsokos M, Kouraklis G, Chandra RS, Bhagavan BS, Triche TJ (1989). Malignant rhabdoid tumor of the kidney and soft tissues. Evidence for a diverse morphological and immunocytochemical phenotype. *Arch Pathol Lab Med* 113: 115-120.

2138. Tsokos M, Webber BL, Parham DM, Wesley RA, Miser A, Miser JS, Etcubanas E, Kinsella T, Grayson J, Glatstein E, . (1992). Rhabdomyosarcoma. A new classification scheme related to prognosis. *Arch Pathol Lab Med* 116: 847-855.

2139. Tsuchiya H, Morikawa S, Tomita K (1990). Osteosarcoma arising from a multiple exostoses lesion: case report. *Jpn J Clin Oncol* 20: 296-298.

2140. Tsuchiya T, Sekine K, Hinohara S, Namiki T, Nobori T, Kaneko Y (2000). Analysis of the p16INK4, p14ARF, p15, TP53, and MDM2 genes and their prognostic implications in osteosarcoma and Ewing sarcoma. *Cancer Genet Cytogenet* 120: 91-98.

2141. Tsuneyoshi M, Daimaru Y, Hashimoto H, Enjoji M (1985). Malignant soft tissue neoplasms with the histologic features of renal rhabdoid tumors: an ultrastructural and immunohistochemical study. *Hum Pathol* 16: 1235-1242.

2142. Tsuneyoshi M, Dorfman HD, Bauer TW (1986). Epithelioid hemangioendothelioma of bone. A clinicopathologic, ultrastructural, and immunohistochemical study. *Am J Surg Pathol* 10: 754-764.

2143. Tsuneyoshi M, Enjoji M, Iwasaki H, Shinohara N (1981). Extraskeletal myxoid chondrosarcoma – a clinicopathologic and electron microscopic study. *Acta Pathol Jpn* 31: 439-447.

2144. Turc-Carel C, Dal Cin P, Rao U, Karakousis C, Sandberg AA (1988). Recurrent breakpoints at 9q31 and 22q12.2 in extraskeletal myxoid chondrosarcoma. *Cancer Genet Cytogenet* 30: 145-150.

2145. Turc-Carel C, Limon J, Dal Cin P, Rao U, Karakousis C, Sandberg AA (1986). Cytogenetic studies of adipose tissue tumors. II. Recurrent reciprocal translocation t(12;16)(q13;p11) in myxoid liposarcomas. *Cancer Genet Cytogenet* 23: 291-299.

2146. Turc-Carel C, Philip I, Berger MP, Philip T, Lenoir GM (1983). Chromosomal translocations in Ewing's sarcoma. *N Engl J Med* 309: 497-498.

2147. Turcotte RE, Kurt AM, Sim FH, Unni KK, McLeod RA (1993). Chondroblastoma. *Hum Pathol* 24: 944-949.

2148. Turgut M (1999). Spinal angiolipomas: report of a case and review of the cases published since the discovery of the tumour in 1890. *Br J Neurosurg* 13: 30-40.

2149. Turner DT, Shah SM, Jones R (1998). Intrascrotal lipoblastoma. *Br J Urol* 81: 166-167.

2150. Ugai K, Kizaki T, Morimoto K, Sashikata T (1994). A case of low-grade fibromyxoid sarcoma of the thigh. *Pathol Int* 44: 793-799.

2151. Umiker WO, Iverson L (1954). Postinflammatory "tumors" of the lung. Report of four cases simulating xanthoma, fibroma, or plasma cell tumor. *J Thorac Cardiovasc Surg* 28: 55-63.

2152. Unger EC, Gilula LA, Kyriakos M (1987). Case report 430: Ischemic necrosis of osteochondroma of tibia. *Skeletal Radiol* 16: 416-421.

2153. Unni KK (1996). Benign vascular tumors. In: *Dahlin's Bone Tumors : General Aspects and Data on 11,087 Cases*. 5th ed. Lippincott-Raven: Philadelphia, pp. 307-316.

2154. Unni KK (1996). Conditions that commonly simulate primary neoplasms of bone. In: *Dahlin's Bone Tumors : General Aspects and Data on 11,087 Cases*. 5th ed. Lippincott-Raven: Philadelphia, p. 369.

2155. Unni KK (1996). *Dahlin's Bone Tumors General Aspects and Data on 11,087 Cases*. 5th ed. Lippincott-Raven: Philadelphia.

2156. Unni KK, Dahlin DC, Beabout JW (1976). Periosteal osteogenic sarcoma. *Cancer* 37: 2476-2485.

2157. Unni KK, Dahlin DC, Beabout JW, Ivins JC (1974). Adamantinomas of long bones. *Cancer* 34: 1796-1805.

2158. Unni KK, Dahlin DC, McLeod RA, Pritchard DJ (1977). Intraosseous well-differentiated osteosarcoma. *Cancer* 40: 1337-1347.

2159. Urano F, Umezawa A, Hong W, Kikuchi H, Hata J (1996). A novel chimera gene between EWS and E1A-F, encoding the adenovirus E1A enhancer-binding protein, in extraosseous Ewing's sarcoma. *Biochem Biophys Res Commun* 219: 608-612.

2160. Uriburu IJ, Levy VD (1998). Intraosseous growth of giant cell tumors of the tendon sheath (localized nodular tenosynovitis) of the digits: report of 15 cases. *J Hand Surg [Am]* 23: 732-736.

2161. Ushigome S, Shimoda T, Nikaido T, Nakamori K, Miyazawa Y, Shishikura A, Takakuwa T, Ubayama Y, Spjut HJ (1992). Primitive neuroectodermal tumors of bone and soft tissue. With reference to histologic differentiation in primary or metastatic foci. *Acta Pathol Jpn* 42: 483-493.

2162. Ushigome S, Takakuwa T, Shinagawa T, Kishida H, Yamazaki M (1982). Chondromyxoid fibroma of bone. An electron microscopic observation. *Acta Pathol Jpn* 32: 113-122.

2163. Ushijima M, Hashimoto H, Tsuneyoshi M, Enjoji M (1986). Giant cell tumor of the tendon sheath (nodular tenosynovitis). A study of 207 cases to compare the large joint group with the common digit group. *Cancer* 57: 875-884.

2164. Ushijima M, Hashimoto H, Tsuneyoshi M, Enjoji M, Miyamoto Y, Okue A (1985). Malignant giant cell tumor of tendon sheath. Report of a case. *Acta Pathol Jpn* 35: 699-709.

2165. Uzoaru I, Chou P, Reyes-Mugica M, Shen-Schwartz S, Gonzalez-Crussi F (1993). Inflammatory myofibroblastic tumor of the pancreas. *Surg Pathol* 5: 181-188.

2166. Vaillo-Vinagre A, Ballestin-Carcavilla C, Madero-Garcia S, Pastor GS, Checa GA, Martinez-Tello FJ (2000). Primary angioleiomyoma of the iliac bone: clinical pathological study of one case with flow cytometric DNA content and S-phase fraction analysis. *Skeletal Radiol* 29: 181-185.

2167. Vallat-Decouvelaere AV, Dry SM, Fletcher CD (1998). Atypical and malignant solitary fibrous tumors in extrathoracic locations: evidence of their comparability to intra-thoracic tumors. *Am J Surg Pathol* 22: 1501-1511.

2168. Valmaggia C, Neuweiler J, Fretz C, Gottlob I (1997). A case of Erdheim-Chester disease with orbital involvement. *Arch Ophthalmol* 115: 1467-1468.

2169. Van Camp B, Durie BG, Spier C, De Waele M, van Riet I, Vela E, Frutiger Y, Richter L, Grogan TM (1990). Plasma cells in multiple myeloma express a natural killer cell-associated antigen: CD56 (NKH-1; Leu-19). *Blood* 76: 377-382.

2170. van de Rijn M, Barr FG, Xiong QB, Hedges M, Shipley J, Fisher C (1999). Poorly differentiated synovial sarcoma: an analysis of clinical, pathologic, and molecular genetic features. *Am J Surg Pathol* 23: 106-112.

2171. van de Rijn M, Barr FG, Xiong QB, Salhany KE, Fraker DL, Fisher C (1997). Radiation-associated synovial sarcoma. *Hum Pathol* 28: 1325-1328.

2172. van de Rijn M, Rouse RV (1994). CD34: a review. *Appl Immunohistochem* 2: 71-80.

2173. van den Berg E, Molenaar WM, Hoekstra HJ, Kamps WA, de Jong B (1992). DNA ploidy and karyotype in recurrent and metastatic soft tissue sarcomas. *Mod Pathol* 5: 505-514.

2174. van der Rest M, Garrone R (1991). Collagen family of proteins. *FASEB J* 5: 2814-2823.

2175. van der Woude HJ, Bloem JL, Holscher HC, Nooy MA, Taminiau AH, Hermans J, Falke TH, Hogendoorn PC (1994). Monitoring the effect of chemotherapy in Ewing's sarcoma of bone with MR imaging. *Skeletal Radiol* 23: 493-500.

2176. Van Dorpe J, Ectors N, Geboes K, D'Hoore A, Sciot R (1999). Is calcifying fibrous pseudotumor a late sclerosing stage of inflammatory myofibroblastic tumor? *Am J Surg Pathol* 23: 329-335.

2177. Van Geertruyden J, Lorea P, Goldschmidt D, de Fontaine S, Schuind F, Kinnen L, Ledoux P, Moermans JP (1996). Glomus tumours of the hand. A retrospective study of 51 cases. *J Hand Surg [Br]* 21: 257-260.

2178. van Haelst UJ, de Haas van Dorsser AH (1975). A perplexing malignant bone tumor. Highly malignant so-called adamantinoma or non-typical Ewing's sarcoma. *Virchows Arch A Pathol Anat Histol* 365: 63-74.

2179. van Hoeven KH, Factor SM, Kress Y, Woodruff JM (1993). Visceral myogenic tumors. A manifestation of HIV infection in children. *Am J Surg Pathol* 17: 1176-1181.

2180. Van Hul W, Wuyts W, Hendrickx J, Speleman F, Wauters J, De Boulle K, Van Roy N, Bossuyt P, Willems PJ (1998). Identification of a third EXT-like gene (EXTL3) belonging to the EXT gene family. *Genomics* 47: 230-237.

2181. van Lerberghe E, Van Damme B, van Holsbeeck M, Burssens A, Hoogmartens M (1990). Case report 626: Osteosarcoma arising in a solitary osteochondroma of the femur. *Skeletal Radiol* 19: 594-597.

2182. van Roggen JF, McMenamin ME, Fletcher CD (2001). Cellular myxoma of soft tissue: a clinicopathological study of 38 cases confirming indolent clinical behaviour. *Histopathology* 39: 287-297.

2183. van Unnik JA, Coindre JM, Contesso C, Albus-Lutter CE, Schiodt T, Sylvester R, Thomas D, Bramwell V, Mouridsen HT (1993). Grading of soft tissue sarcomas: experience of the EORTC Soft Tissue and Bone Sarcoma Group. *Eur J Cancer* 29A: 2089-2093.

2184. van Zelderen-Bhola SL, Bovée JV, Wessels HW, Mollevanger P, Nijhuis JV, van Eendenburg JD, Taminiau AH, Hogendoorn PC (1998). Ring chromosome 4 as the sole cytogenetic anomaly in a chondroblastoma: a case report and review of the literature. *Cancer Genet Cytogenet* 105: 109-112.

2185. Vanel D, Henry-Amar M, Lumbroso J, Lemalet E, Couanet D, Piekarski JD, Masselot J, Boddaert A, Kalifa C, Le Chevalier T, . (1984). Pulmonary evaluation of patients with osteosarcoma: roles of standard radiography, tomography, CT, scintigraphy, and tomoscintigraphy. *AJR Am J Roentgenol* 143: 519-523.

2186. Vang R, Kempson RL (2002). Perivascular epithelioid cell tumor ('PEComa') of the uterus: a subset of HMB-45-positive epithelioid mesenchymal neoplasms with an uncertain relationship to pure smooth muscle tumors. *Am J Surg Pathol* 26: 1-13.

2187. Vanhoenacker FM, Van Hul W, Wuyts W, Willems PJ, De Schepper AM (2001). Hereditary multiple exostoses: from genetics to clinical syndrome and complications. *Eur J Radiol* 40: 208-217.

2188. Vanni R, Marras S, Faa G, Uccheddu A, Dal Cin P, Sciot R, Samson I, van den Berghe H (1999). Chromosome instability in elastofibroma. *Cancer Genet Cytogenet* 111: 182-183.

2189. Vaquero J, Carrillo R, Leunda G, Cabezudo JM (1979). Primary osteogenic sarcoma of the skull. *Acta Neurochir (Wien)* 51: 97-104.

2190. Varela-Duran J, Dehner LP (1980). Postirradiation osteosarcoma in childhood. A clinicopathologic study of three cases and review of the literature. *Am J Pediatr Hematol Oncol* 2: 263-271.

2191. Varela-Duran J, Enzinger FM (1982). Calcifying synovial sarcoma. *Cancer* 50: 345-352.

2192. Varela-Duran J, Oliva H, Rosai J (1979). Vascular leiomyosarcoma: the malignant counterpart of vascular leiomyoma. *Cancer* 44: 1684-1691.

2193. Vargas SO, Perez-Atayde AR, Gonzalez-Crussi F, Kozakewich HP (2001). Giant cell angioblastoma: three additional occurrences of a distinct pathologic entity. *Am J Surg Pathol* 25: 185-196.

2194. Variend S, Bax NM, van Gorp J (1995). Are infantile myofibromatosis, congenital fibrosarcoma and congenital haemangiopericytoma histogenetically related? *Histopathology* 26: 57-62.

2195. Vayego SA, De Conti OJ, Varella-Garcia M (1996). Complex cytogenetic rearrangement in a case of unicameral bone cyst. *Cancer Genet Cytogenet* 86: 46-49.

2196. Vellios F, Baez J, Shumacker HB (1958). Lipoblastomatosis: a tumor of fetal fat different from hibernoma. Report of a case, with observations on the embryogenesis of human adipose tissue. *Am J Pathol* 34: 1149-1159.

2197. Vencio EF, Reeve CM, Unni KK, Nascimento AG (1998). Mesenchymal chondrosarcoma of the jaw bones: clinicopathologic study of 19 cases. *Cancer* 82: 2350-2355.

2198. Vennos EM, Collins M, James WD (1992). Rothmund-Thomson syndrome: review of the world literature. *J Am Acad Dermatol* 27: 750-762.

2199. Vennos EM, James WD (1995). Rothmund-Thomson syndrome. *Dermatol Clin* 13: 143-150.

2200. Vergel De Dios AM, Bond JR, Shives TC, McLeod RA, Unni KK (1992). Aneurysmal bone cyst. A clinicopathologic study of 238 cases. *Cancer* 69: 2921-2931.

2201. Versteege I, Sevenet N, Lange J, Rousseau-Merck MF, Ambros P, Handgretinger R, Aurias A, Delattre O (1998). Truncating mutations of hSNF5/INI1 in aggressive paediatric cancer. *Nature* 394: 203-206.

2202. Verstraete KL, De Deene Y, Roels H, Dierick A, Uyttendaele D, Kunnen M (1994). Benign and malignant musculoskeletal lesions: dynamic contrast-enhanced MR imaging – parametric "first-pass" images depict tissue vascularization and perfusion. *Radiology* 192: 835-843.

2203. Veyssier-Belot C, Cacoub P, Caparros-Lefebvre D, Wechsler J, Brun B, Remy M, Wallaert B, Petit H, Grimaldi A, Wechsler B, Godeau P (1996). Erdheim-Chester disease. Clinical and radiologic characteristics of 59 cases. *Medicine (Baltimore)* 75: 157-169.

2204. Vin-Christian K, McCalmont TH, Frieden IJ (1997). Kaposiform hemangioendothelioma. An aggressive, locally invasive vascular tumor that can mimic hemangioma of infancy. *Arch Dermatol* 133: 1573-1578.

2205. von Hochstetter AR (1990). Spontaneous necrosis in osteosarcomas. *Virchows Arch A Pathol Anat Histopathol* 417: 5-8.

2206. Voutsinas S, Wynne-Davies R (1983). The infrequency of malignant disease in diaphyseal aclasis and neurofibromatosis. *J Med Genet* 20: 345-349.

2207. Vujanic GM, Milovanovic D, Aleksandrovic S (1992). Aggressive inflammatory pseudotumor of the abdomen 9 years after therapy for Wilms tumor. A complication, coincidence, or association? *Cancer* 70: 2362-2366.

2208. Wadayama B, Toguchida J, Shimizu T, Ishizaki K, Sasaki MS, Kotoura Y, Yamamuro T (1994). Mutation spectrum of the retinoblastoma gene in osteosarcomas. *Cancer Res* 54: 3042-3048.

2209. Walsh SV, Evangelista F, Khettry U (1998). Inflammatory myofibroblastic tumor of the pancreaticobiliary region: morphologic and immunocytochemical study of three cases. *Am J Surg Pathol* 22: 412-418.

2210. Wang-Wuu S, Soukup S, Ballard E, Gotwals B, Lampkin B (1988). Chromosomal analysis of sixteen human rhabdomyosarcomas. *Cancer Res* 48: 983-987.

2211. Wang DH, Guan XL, Xiao LF, Zhang XP, Chen MG, Sun KM (1998). Soft tissue chondroma of the parapharyngeal space: a case report. *J Laryngol Otol* 112: 294-295.

2212. Wang LL, Levy ML, Lewis RA, Chintagumpala MM, Lev D, Rogers M, Plon SE (2001). Clinical manifestations in a cohort of 41 Rothmund-Thomson syndrome patients. *Am J Med Genet* 102: 11-17.

2213. Wang NP, Bacchi CE, Jiang JJ, McNutt MA, Gown AM (1996). Does alveolar soft-part sarcoma exhibit skeletal muscle differentiation? An immunocytochemical and biochemical study of myogenic regulatory protein expression. *Mod Pathol* 9: 496-506.

2214. Wang NP, Marx J, McNutt MA, Rutledge JC, Gown AM (1995). Expression of myogenic regulatory proteins (myogenin and MyoD1) in small blue round cell tumors of childhood. *Am J Pathol* 147: 1799-1810.

2215. Wang R, Lu YJ, Fisher C, Bridge JA, Shipley J (2001). Characterization of chromosome aberrations associated with soft-tissue leiomyosarcomas by twenty-four-color karyotyping and comparative genomic hybridization analysis. *Genes Chromosomes Cancer* 31: 54-64.

2216. Wapner KL, Ververeli PA, Moore JH, Jr., Hecht PJ, Becker CE, Lackman RD (1995). Plantar fibromatosis: a review of primary and recurrent surgical treatment. *Foot Ankle Int* 16: 548-551.

2217. Wargotz ES, Weiss SW, Norris HJ (1987). Myofibroblastoma of the breast. Sixteen cases of a distinctive benign mesenchymal tumor. *Am J Surg Pathol* 11: 493-502.

2218. Warter A, Satge D, Roeslin N (1987). Angioinvasive plasma cell granulomas of the lung. *Cancer* 59: 435-443.

2219. Watanabe K, Hoshi N, Tsu-Ura Y, Suzuki T (1995). A case of glomangiosarcoma. *Fukushima J Med Sci* 41: 71-77.

2220. Watanabe K, Sugino T, Saito A, Kusakabe T, Suzuki T (1998). Glomangiosarcoma of the hip: report of a highly aggressive tumour with widespread distant metastases. *Br J Dermatol* 139: 1097-1101.

2221. Watanabe K, Tajino T, Sekiguchi M, Suzuki T (2000). Inflammatory myofibroblastic tumor (inflammatory fibrosarcoma) of the bone. *Arch Pathol Lab Med* 124: 1514-1517.

2222. Waters BL, Panagopoulos I, Allen EF (2000). Genetic characterization of angiomatoid fibrous histiocytoma identifies fusion of the FUS and ATF-1 genes induced by a chromosomal translocation involving bands 12q13 and 16p11. *Cancer Genet Cytogenet* 121: 109-116.

2223. Weber-Hall S, Anderson J, McManus A, Abe S, Nojima T, Pinkerton R, Pritchard-Jones K, Shipley J (1996). Gains, losses, and amplification of genomic material in rhabdomyosarcoma analyzed by comparative genomic hybridization. *Cancer Res* 56: 3220-3224.

2224. Weeks DA, Malott RL, Arnesen M, Zuppan C, Aitken D, Mierau G (1991). Hepatic angiomyolipoma with striated granules and positivity with melanoma – specific antibody (HMB-45): a report of two cases. *Ultrastruct Pathol* 15: 563-571.

2225. Wehner MS, Humphreys JL, Sharkey FE (2000). Epididymal rhabdomyoma: report of a case, including histologic and immunohistochemical findings. *Arch Pathol Lab Med* 124: 1518-1519.

2226. Wehrli BM, Weiss SW, Coffin CM (2001). Gardner syndrome. *Am J Surg Pathol* 25: 694-696.

2227. Wehrli BM, Weiss SW, Yandow S, Coffin CM (2001). Gardner-associated fibromas (GAF) in young patients: a distinct fibrous lesion that identifies unsuspected Gardner syndrome and risk for fibromatosis. *Am J Surg Pathol* 25: 645-651.

2228. Wei G, Antonescu CR, de Alava E, Leung D, Huvos AG, Meyers PA, Healey JH, Ladanyi M (2000). Prognostic impact of INK4A deletion in Ewing sarcoma. *Cancer* 89: 793-799.

2229. Weibolt VM, Buresh CJ, Roberts CA, Suijkerbuijk RF, Pickering DL, Neff JR, Bridge JA (1998). Involvement of 3q21 in nodular fasciitis. *Cancer Genet Cytogenet* 106: 177-179.

2230. Weinstein LS, Shenker A, Gejman PV, Merino MJ, Friedman E, Spiegel AM (1991). Activating mutations of the stimulatory G protein in the McCune-Albright syndrome. *N Engl J Med* 325: 1688-1695.

2231. Weiss LM, Warhol MJ (1984). Ultrastructural distinctions between adult pleomorphic rhabdomyosarcomas, pleomorphic liposarcomas, and pleomorphic malignant fibrous histiocytomas. *Hum Pathol* 15: 1025-1033.

2232. Weiss RA, Whitby D, Talbot S, Kellam P, Boshoff C (1998). Human herpesvirus type 8 and Kaposi's sarcoma. *J Natl Cancer Inst Monogr* 51-54.

2233. Weiss SW (1982). Malignant fibrous histiocytoma. A reaffirmation. *Am J Surg Pathol* 6: 773-784.

2234. Weiss SW (1994). *Histologic Typing of Soft Tissue Tumours. World Health Organization Histological Classification of Tumours*. Springer: Berlin.

2235. Weiss SW, Dorfman HD (1977). Adamantinoma of long bone. An analysis of nine new cases with emphasis on metastasizing lesions and fibrous dysplasia-like changes. *Hum Pathol* 8: 141-153.

2236. Weiss SW, Enzinger FM (1977). Myxoid variant of malignant fibrous histiocytoma. *Cancer* 39: 1672-1685.

2237. Weiss SW, Enzinger FM (1978). Malignant fibrous histiocytoma: an analysis of 200 cases. *Cancer* 41: 2250-2266.

2238. Weiss SW, Enzinger FM (1982). Epithelioid hemangioendothelioma: a vascular tumor often mistaken for a carcinoma. *Cancer* 50: 970-981.

2239. Weiss SW, Goldblum JR (2001). Benign tumors and tumor-like lesions of synovial tissue. In: *Enzinger and Weiss's Soft Tissue Tumours*. 4th ed. Mosby-Harcourt: Philadelphia, pp. 1037-1062.

2240. Weiss SW, Goldblum JR (2001). Benign tumours and tumour-like lesions of blood vessels. In: *Enzinger and Weiss's Soft Tissue Tumours*. 4th ed. Mosby-Harcourt: Philadelphia, pp. 873-875.

2241. Weiss SW, Goldblum JR (2001). Cartilaginous soft tissue tumors. In: *Enzinger and Weiss's Soft Tissue Tumours*. 4th ed. Mosby-Harcourt: Philadelphia, pp. 1361-1388.

2242. Weiss SW, Goldblum JR (2001). *Enzinger and Weiss's Soft Tissue Tumors*. 4th ed. Mosby: St.Louis.

2243. Weiss SW, Goldblum JR (2001). Malignant fibrous histiocytoma. In: *Enzinger and Weiss's Soft Tissue Tumors,*. 4th ed. Mosby-Harcourt: Philadelphia, pp. 539-569.

2244. Weiss SW, Goldblum JR (2001). Malignant vascular tumours. In: *Enzinger and Weiss's Soft Tissue Tumours*. 4th ed. Mosby-Harcourt: Philadelphia, pp. 917-954.

2245. Weiss SW, Ishak KG, Dail DH, Sweet DE, Enzinger FM (1986). Epithelioid hemangioendothelioma and related lesions. *Semin Diagn Pathol* 3: 259-287.

2246. Weiss SW, Rao VK (1992). Well-differentiated liposarcoma (atypical lipoma) of deep soft tissue of the extremities, retroperitoneum, and miscellaneous sites. A follow-up study of 92 cases with analysis of the incidence of "dedifferentiation". *Am J Surg Pathol* 16: 1051-1058.

2247. Welch P, Grossi C, Carroll A, Dunham W, Royal S, Wilson E, Crist W (1986). Granulocytic sarcoma with an indolent course and destructive skeletal disease. Tumor characterization with immunologic markers, electron microscopy, cytochemistry, and cytogenetic studies. *Cancer* 57: 1005-1010.

2248. Wells GC, Whimster IW (1969). Subcutaneous angiolymphoid hyperplasia with eosinophilia. *Br J Dermatol* 81: 1-14.

2249. Wenger DE, Wold LE (2000). Benign vascular lesions of bone: radiologic and pathologic features. *Skeletal Radiol* 29: 63-74.

2250. Wenig BM, Devaney K, Bisceglia M (1995). Inflammatory myofibroblastic tumor of the larynx. A clinicopathologic study of eight cases simulating a malignant spindle cell neoplasm. *Cancer* 76: 2217-2229.

2251. Wesche WA, Fletcher CD, Dias P, Houghton PJ, Parham DM (1995). Immunohistochemistry of MyoD1 in adult pleomorphic soft tissue sarcomas. *Am J Surg Pathol* 19: 261-269.

2252. West DC, Grier HE, Swallow MM, Demetri GD, Granowetter L, Sklar J (1997). Detection of circulating tumor cells in patients with Ewing's sarcoma and peripheral primitive neuroectodermal tumor. *J Clin Oncol* 15: 583-588.

2253. Wester SM, Beabout JW, Unni KK, Dahlin DC (1982). Langerhans' cell granulomatosis (histiocytosis X) of bone in adults. *Am J Surg Pathol* 6: 413-426.

2254. Westra WH, Grenko RT, Epstein J (2000). Solitary fibrous tumor of the lower urogenital tract: a report of five cases involving the seminal vesicles, urinary bladder, and prostate. *Hum Pathol* 31: 63-68.

2255. Wetherington RW, Lyle WG, Sangueza OP (1997). Malignant glomus tumor of the thumb: a case report. *J Hand Surg [Am]* 22: 1098-1102.

2256. Weynand B, Draguet AP, Bernard P, Marbaix E, Galant C (1999). Calcifying fibrous pseudotumour: first case report in the peritoneum with immunostaining for CD34. *Histopathology* 34: 86-87.

2257. Whang-Peng J, Triche TJ, Knutsen T, Miser J, Douglass EC, Israel MA (1984). Chromosome translocation in peripheral neuroepithelioma. *N Engl J Med* 311: 584-585.

2258. Whitby D, Howard MR, Tenant-Flowers M, Brink NS, Copas A, Boshoff C, Hatzioannou T, Suggett FE, Aldam DM, Denton AS, . (1995). Detection of Kaposi sarcoma associated herpesvirus in peripheral blood of HIV-infected individuals and progression to Kaposi's sarcoma. *Lancet* 346: 799-802.

2259. White FV, Dehner LP, Belchis DA, Conard K, Davis MM, Stocker JT, Zuppan CW, Biegel JA, Perlman EJ (1999). Congenital disseminated malignant rhabdoid tumor: a distinct clinicopathologic entity demonstrating abnormalities of chromosome 22q11. *Am J Surg Pathol* 23: 249-256.

2260. White J, Chan YF (1994). Aggressive angiomyxoma of the vulva in an 11-year-old girl. *Pediatr Pathol* 14: 27-37.

2261. Whitehead RE, Melhem ER, Kasznica J, Eustace S (1998). Telangiectatic osteosarcoma of the skull base. *AJNR Am J Neuroradiol* 19: 754-757.

2262. Whyte P, Buchkovich KJ, Horowitz JM, Friend SH, Raybuck M, Weinberg RA, Harlow E (1988). Association between an oncogene and an anti-oncogene: the adenovirus E1A proteins bind to the retinoblastoma gene product. *Nature* 334: 124-129.

2263. Wick MR, Siegal GP, Unni KK, McLeod RA, Greditzer HG, III (1981). Sarcomas of bone complicating osteitis deformans (Paget's disease): fifty years' experience. *Am J Surg Pathol* 5: 47-59.

2264. Wicking C, Shanley S, Smyth I, Gillies S, Negus K, Graham S, Suthers G, Haites N, Edwards M, Wainwright B, Chenevix-Trench G (1997). Most germ-line mutations in the nevoid basal cell carcinoma syndrome lead to a premature termination of the PATCHED protein, and no genotype-phenotype correlations are evident. *Am J Hum Genet* 60: 21-26.

2265. Wicklund CL, Pauli RM, Johnston D, Hecht JT (1995). Natural history study of hereditary multiple exostoses. *Am J Med Genet* 55: 43-46.

2266. Wiedemann H (1964). Complexe malformatif familial avec hernie ombilicale et macroglossie, un "syndrome nouveau". *J Genet Hum* 13: 223-232.

2267. Wiggs J, Nordenskjöld M, Yandell D, Rapaport J, Grondin V, Janson M, Werelius B, Petersen R, Craft A, Riedel K, Liberfarb R, Walton D, Wilson W, Dryja TP (1988). Prediction of the risk of hereditary retinoblastoma, using DNA polymorphisms within the retinoblastoma gene. *N Engl J Med* 318: 151-157.

2268. Wile AG, Evans HL, Romsdahl MM (1981). Leiomyosarcoma of soft tissue: a clinicopathologic study. *Cancer* 48: 1022-1032.

2269. Wilke W, Maillet M, Robinson R (1993). H-ras-1 point mutations in soft tissue sarcomas. *Mod Pathol* 6: 129-132.

2270. Wilken JJ, Meier FA, Kornstein MJ (2000). Kaposiform hemangioendothelioma of the thymus. *Arch Pathol Lab Med* 124: 1542-1544.

2271. Willén H, Åkerman M, Dal Cin P, de Wever I, Fletcher CD, Mandahl N, Mertens F, Mitelman F, Rosai J, Rydholm A, Sciot R, Tallini G, van den Berghe H, Vanni R (1998). Comparison of chromosomal patterns with clinical features in 165 lipomas: a report of the CHAMP study group. *Cancer Genet Cytogenet* 102: 46-49.

2272. Williams AH, Schwinn CP, Parker JW (1976). The ultrastructure of osteosarcoma. A review of twenty cases. *Cancer* 37: 1293-1301.

2273. Williams SB, Ellis GL, Meis JM, Heffner DK (1993). Ossifying fibromyxoid tumour (of soft parts) of the head and neck: a clinicopathological and immunohistochemical study of nine cases. *J Laryngol Otol* 107: 75-80.

2274. Willis J, Abdul-Karim FW, di Sant'Agnese PA (1994). Extracardiac rhabdomyomas. *Semin Diagn Pathol* 11: 15-25.

2275. Willman CL, Busque L, Griffith BB, Favara BE, McClain KL, Duncan MH, Gilliland DG (1994). Langerhans'-cell histiocytosis (histiocytosis X) – a clonal proliferative disease. *N Engl J Med* 331: 154-160.

2276. Willms R, Hartwig CH, Bohm P, Sell S (1997). Malignant transformation of a multiple cartilaginous exostosis – a case report. *Int Orthop* 21: 133-136.

2277. Wilson JD, Montague CJ, Salcuni P, Bordi C, Rosai J (1999). Heterotopic mesenteric ossification ('intraabdominal myositis ossificans'): report of five cases. *Am J Surg Pathol* 23: 1464-1470.

2278. Wilson MB, Stanley W, Sens D, Garvin AJ (1990). Infantile fibrosarcoma – a misnomer? *Pediatr Pathol* 10: 901-907.

2279. Winik BC, Boente MC, Asial R (1998). Juvenile hyaline fibromatosis: ultrastructural study. *Am J Dermatopathol* 20: 373-378.

2280. Winnepenninckx V, De Vos R, Debiec-Rychter M, Samson I, Brys P, Hagemeijer A, Sciot R (2001). Calcifying/ossifying synovial sarcoma shows t(X;18) with SSX2 involvement and mitochondrial calcifications. *Histopathology* 38: 141-145.

2281. Winnepenninckx V, Debiec-Rychter M, Jorissen M, Bogaerts S, Sciot R (2000). Aneurysmal bone cyst of the nose with 17p13 involvement. *Virchows Arch* 439: 636-639.

2282. Wirman JA, Crissman JD, Aron BF (1979). Metastatic chondroblastoma: report of an unusual case treated with radiotherapy. *Cancer* 44: 87-93.

2283. Wise CA, Clines GA, Massa H, Trask BJ, Lovett M (1997). Identification and localization of the gene for EXTL, a third member of the multiple exostoses gene family. *Genome Res* 7: 10-16.

2284. Wiswell TE, Davis J, Cunningham BE, Solenberger R, Thomas PJ (1988). Infantile myofibromatosis: the most common fibrous tumor of infancy. *J Pediatr Surg* 23: 315-318.

2285. Woertler K, Lindner N, Gosheger G, Brinkschmidt C, Heindel W (2000). Osteochondroma: MR imaging of tumor-related complications. *Eur Radiol* 10: 832-840.

2286. Wold LE (1998). Fibrohistiocytic tumors of bone. In: *Bone Tumors*, Unni KK, ed. Livingstone: New York, pp. 183-197.

2287. Wold LE, McLeod RA, Sim FH, Unni KK (1990). *Atlas of Othopedic Pathology.* Saunders: Philadelphia-London.

2288. Wold LE, Unni KK, Beabout JW, Ivins JC, Bruckman JE, Dahlin DC (1982). Hemangioendothelial sarcoma of bone. *Am J Surg Pathol* 6: 59-70.

2289. Wold LE, Unni KK, Beabout JW, Sim FH, Dahlin DC (1984). Dedifferentiated parosteal osteosarcoma. *J Bone Joint Surg Am* 66: 53-59.

2290. Wolf M, el Rifai W, Tarkkanen M, Kononen J, Serra M, Eriksen EF, Elomaa I, Kallioniemi A, Kallioniemi OP, Knuutila S (2000). Novel findings in gene expression detected in human osteosarcoma by cDNA microarray. *Cancer Genet Cytogenet* 123: 128-132.

2291. Wolf RE, Enneking WF (1996). The staging and surgery of musculoskeletal neoplasms. *Orthop Clin North Am* 27: 473-481.

2292. Wong FL, Boice JD, Jr., Abramson DH, Tarone RE, Kleinerman RA, Stovall M, Goldman MB, Seddon JM, Tarbell N, Fraumeni JF, Jr., Li FP (1997). Cancer incidence after retinoblastoma. Radiation dose and sarcoma risk. *JAMA* 278: 1262-1267.

2293. Wong KF, So CC, Wong N, Siu LL, Kwong YL, Chan JK (2001). Sinonasal angiosarcoma with marrow involvement at presentation mimicking malignant lymphoma: cytogenetic analysis using multiple techniques. *Cancer Genet Cytogenet* 129: 64-68.

2294. Wong L, Dellon AL (1992). Soft tissue chondroma presenting as a painful finger: diagnosis by magnetic resonance imaging. *Ann Plast Surg* 28: 304-306.

2295. Wood GS, Beckstead JH, Medeiros LJ, Kempson RL, Warnke RA (1988). The cells of giant cell tumor of tendon sheath resemble osteoclasts. *Am J Surg Pathol* 12: 444-452.

2296. Woodruff JM, Antonescu CR, Erlandson RA, Boland PJ (1999). Low-grade fibrosarcoma with palisaded granulomalike bodies (giant rosettes): report of a case that metastasized. *Am J Surg Pathol* 23: 1423-1428.

2297. Wreesmann V, van Eijck CH, Naus DC, van Velthuysen ML, Jeekel J, Mooi WJ (2001). Inflammatory pseudotumour (inflammatory myofibroblastic tumour) of the pancreas: a report of six cases associated with obliterative phlebitis. *Histopathology* 38: 105-110.

2298. Wright CJE (1953). Benign giant cell synovioma. *Br J Surg* 38: 257.

2299. Wright RA, Hermann RC, Parisi JE (1999). Neurological manifestations of Erdheim-Chester disease. *J Neurol Neurosurg Psychiatry* 66: 72-75.

2300. Wu CT, Inwards CY, O'Laughlin S, Rock MG, Beabout JW, Unni KK (1998). Chondromyxoid fibroma of bone: a clinico-pathologic review of 278 cases. *Hum Pathol* 29: 438-446.

2301. Wu JP, Yunis EJ, Fetterman G, Jaeschke WF, Gilbert EF (1973). Inflammatory pseudo-tumours of the abdomen: plasma cell granulomas. *J Clin Pathol* 26: 943-948.

2302. Wu JX, Carpenter PM, Gresens C, Keh R, Niman H, Morris JW, Mercola D (1990). The proto-oncogene c-fos is over-expressed in the majority of human osteosarcomas. *Oncogene* 5: 989-1000.

2303. Wu YQ, Badano JL, McCaskill C, Vogel H, Potocki L, Shaffer LG (2000). Haploinsufficiency of ALX4 as a potential cause of parietal foramina in the 11p11.2 contiguous gene-deletion syndrome. *Am J Hum Genet* 67: 1327-1332.

2304. Wunder JS, Czitrom AA, Kandel R, Andrulis IL (1991). Analysis of alterations in the retinoblastoma gene and tumor grade in bone and soft-tissue sarcomas. *J Natl Cancer Inst* 83: 194-200.

2305. Wunder JS, Eppert K, Burrow SR, Gokgoz N, Bell RS, Andrulis IL, Gogkoz N (1999). Co-amplification and overexpression of CDK4, SAS and MDM2 occurs frequently in human parosteal osteosarcomas. *Oncogene* 18: 783-788.

2306. Wuyts W, Van Hul W (2000). Molecular basis of multiple exostoses: mutations in the EXT1 and EXT2 genes. *Hum Mutat* 15: 220-227.

2307. Wuyts W, Van Hul W, Bartsch O, Wilkie AO, Meinecke P (2001). Burning down DEFECT11. *Am J Med Genet* 100: 331-335.

2308. Wuyts W, Van Hul W, De Boulle K, Hendrickx J, Bakker E, Vanhoenacker F, Mollica F, Lüdecke HJ, Sayli BS, Pazzaglia UE, Mortier G, Hamel B, Conrad EU, Matsushita M, Raskind WH, Willems PJ (1998). Mutations in the EXT1 and EXT2 genes in hereditary multiple exostoses. *Am J Hum Genet* 62: 346-354.

2309. Wuyts W, Van Hul W, Hendrickx J, Speleman F, Wauters J, De Boulle K, Van Roy N, Van Agtmael T, Bossuyt P, Willems PJ (1997). Identification and characterization of a novel member of the EXT gene family, EXTL2. *Eur J Hum Genet* 5: 382-389.

2310. Wuyts W, Van Hul W, Wauters J, Nemtsova M, Reyniers E, Van Hul EV, De Boulle K, de Vries BB, Hendrickx J, Herrygers I, Bossuyt P, Balemans W, Fransen E, Vits L, Coucke P, Nowak NJ, Shows TB, Mallet L, van den Ouweland AM, McGaughran J, Halley DJ, Willems PJ (1996). Positional cloning of a gene involved in hereditary multiple exostoses. *Hum Mol Genet* 5: 1547-1557.

2311. Wyatt-Ashmead J, Bao L, Eilert RE, Gibbs P, Glancy G, McGavran L (2001). Primary aneurysmal bone cysts: 16q22 and/or 17p13 chromosome abnormalities. *Pediatr Dev Pathol* 4: 418-419.

2312. Xipell JM, Rush J (1985). Case report 340: Well differentiated intraosseous osteosarcoma of the left femur. *Skeletal Radiol* 14: 312-316.

2313. Xu L, Xia J, Jiang H, Zhou J, Li H, Wang D, Pan Q, Long Z, Fan C, Deng HX (1999). Mutation analysis of hereditary multiple exostoses in the Chinese. *Hum Genet* 105: 45-50.

2314. Yamada T, Irisa T, Nakano S, Tokunaga O (1995). Extraskeletal chondroma with chondroblastic and granuloma-like elements. *Clin Orthop* 257-261.

2315. Yamaguchi T, Dorfman HD (1998). Radiographic and histologic patterns of calcification in chondromyxoid fibroma. *Skeletal Radiol* 27: 559-564.

2316. Yamaguchi T, Toguchida J, Yamamuro T, Kotoura Y, Takada N, Kawaguchi N, Kaneko Y, Nakamura Y, Sasaki MS, Ishizaki K (1992). Allelotype analysis in osteosarcomas: frequent allele loss on 3q, 13q, 17p, and 18q. *Cancer Res* 52: 2419-2423.

2317. Yamamoto T, Marui T, Akisue T, Hitora T, Nagira K, Ohta R, Yoshiya S, Kurosaka M (2002). Intracortical lipoma of the femur. *Am J Surg Pathol* 26: 804-808.

2318. Yandell DW, Campbell TA, Dayton SH, Petersen R, Walton D, Little JB, McConkie-Rosell A, Buckley EG, Dryja TP (1989). Oncogenic point mutations in the human retinoblastoma gene: their application to genetic counseling. *N Engl J Med* 321: 1689-1695.

2319. Yang P, Hirose T, Hasegawa T, Gao Z, Hizawa K (1994). Ossifying fibromyxoid tumor of soft parts: a morphological and immunohistochemical study. *Pathol Int* 44: 448-453.

2320. Yang YJ, Damron TA, Ambrose JL (2001). Diagnosis of chondroid lipoma by fine-needle aspiration biopsy. *Arch Pathol Lab Med* 125: 1224-1226.

2321. Yaziji H, Ranaldi R, Verdolini R, Morroni M, Haggitt R, Bearzi I (2000). Primary alveolar soft part sarcoma of the stomach: a case report and review. *Pathol Res Pract* 196: 519-525.

2322. Yi ES, Shmookler BM, Malawer MM, Sweet DE (1991). Well-differentiated extraskeletal osteosarcoma. A soft-tissue homologue of parosteal osteosarcoma. *Arch Pathol Lab Med* 115: 906-909.

2323. Yip SK, Sim CS, Tan BS (2001). Liver metastasis and local recurrence after radical nephrectomy for an atypical angiomyolipoma. *J Urol* 165: 898-899.

2324. Yokoyama R, Mukai K, Hirota T, Beppu Y, Fukuma H (1996). Primary malignant melanoma (clear cell sarcoma) of bone: report of a case arising in the ulna. *Cancer* 77: 2471-2475.

2325. Yokoyama R, Tsuneyoshi M, Enjoji M, Shinohara N, Masuda S (1993). Prognostic factors of malignant fibrous histiocytoma of bone. A clinical and histopathologic analysis of 34 cases. *Cancer* 72: 1902-1908.

2326. Yoo J, Lee HK, Kang CS, Park WS, Lee JY, Shim SI (1997). p53 gene mutations and p53 protein expression in human soft tissue sarcomas. *Arch Pathol Lab Med* 121: 395-399.

2327. Yoshida MA, Ikeuchi T, Iwama T, Miyaki M, Mori T, Ushijima T, Hara A, Miyakita M, Tonomura A (1991). Chromosome changes in desmoid tumors developed in patients with familial adenomatous polyposis. *Jpn J Cancer Res* 82: 916-921.

2328. Yoshimoto K, Iwahana H, Fukuda A, Sano T, Itakura M (1993). Rare mutations of the Gs alpha subunit gene in human endocrine tumors. Mutation detection by polymerase chain reaction-primer-introduced restriction analysis. *Cancer* 72: 1386-1393.

2329. Yotov WV, Hamel H, Rivard GE, Champagne MA, Russo PA, Leclerc JM, Bernstein ML, Levy E (1999). Amplifications of DNA primase 1 (PRIM1) in human osteosarcoma. *Genes Chromosomes Cancer* 26: 62-69.

2330. Yousem SA, Shaw H, Cieply K (2001). Involvement of 2p23 in pulmonary inflammatory pseudotumors. *Hum Pathol* 32: 428-433.

2331. Yu CE, Oshima J, Fu YH, Wijsman EM, Hisama F, Alisch R, Matthews S, Nakura J, Miki T, Ouais S, Martin GM, Mulligan J, Schellenberg GD (1996). Positional cloning of the Werner's syndrome gene. *Science* 272: 258-262.

2332. Zagars GK, Goswitz MS, Pollack A (1996). Liposarcoma: outcome and prognostic factors following conservation surgery and radiation therapy. *Int J Radiat Oncol Biol Phys* 36: 311-319.

2333. Zahm SH, Fraumeni JF, Jr. (1997). The epidemiology of soft tissue sarcoma. *Semin Oncol* 24: 504-514.

2334. Zalupski MM, Ensley JF, Ryan J, Selvaggi S, Baker LH, Wolman SR (1990). A common cytogenetic abnormality and DNA content alterations in dedifferentiated chondrosarcoma. *Cancer* 66: 1176-1182.

2335. Zamboni G, Pea M, Martignoni G, Zancanaro C, Faccioli G, Gilioli E, Pederzoli P, Bonetti F (1996). Clear cell "sugar" tumor of the pancreas. A novel member of the family of lesions characterized by the presence of perivascular epithelioid cells. *Am J Surg Pathol* 20: 722-730.

2336. Zamecnik M, Dorociak F, Vesely L (1997). Calcifying fibrous pseudotumor after trauma. *Pathol Int* 47: 812.

2337. Zamecnik M, Michal M (2001). Nuchal-type fibroma is positive for CD34 and CD99. *Am J Surg Pathol* 25: 970.

2338. Zamecnik M, Michal M, Patrikova J (1994). [Atypical decubital fibroplasia (ischemic fasciitis) – a new pseudosarcomatous entity]. *Cesk Patol* 30: 130-132.

2339. Zavala-Pompa A, Folpe AL, Jimenez RE, Lim SD, Cohen C, Eble JN, Amin MB (2001). Immunohistochemical study of microphthalmia transcription factor and tyrosinase in angiomyolipoma of the kidney, renal cell carcinoma, and renal and retroperitoneal sarcomas: comparative evaluation with traditional diagnostic markers. *Am J Surg Pathol* 25: 65-70.

2340. Zelger B, Weinlich G, Steiner H, Zelger BG, Egarter-Vigl E (1997). Dermal and subcutaneous variants of plexiform fibrohistiocytic tumor. *Am J Surg Pathol* 21: 235-241.

2341. Zhao C, Yamada T, Kuramochi S, Yamazaki K, Mukai M, Kameyama K, Hata J (2000). Two cases of ectopic hamartomatous thymoma. *Virchows Arch* 437: 643-647.

2342. Zheng MH, Robbins P, Xu J, Huang L, Wood DJ, Papadimitriou JM (2001). The histogenesis of giant cell tumour of bone: a model of interaction between neoplastic cells and osteoclasts. *Histol Histopathol* 16: 297-307.

2343. Zheng MH, Siu P, Papadimitriou JM, Wood DJ, Murch AR (1999). Telomeric fusion is a major cytogenetic aberration of giant cell tumors of bone. *Pathology* 31: 373-378.

2344. Zietz C, Rossle M, Haas C, Sendelhofert A, Hirschmann A, Sturzl M, Lohrs U (1998). MDM-2 oncoprotein over-expression, p53 gene mutation, and VEGF up-regulation in angiosarcomas. *Am J Pathol* 153: 1425-1433.

2345. Zillmer DA, Dorfman HD (1989). Chondromyxoid fibroma of bone: thirty-six cases with clinicopathologic correlation. *Hum Pathol* 20: 952-964.

2346. Zimmerman LE, Burns RP, Wankum G, Tully R, Esterly JA (1982). Trilateral retinoblastoma: ectopic intracranial retinoblastoma associated with bilateral retinoblastoma. *J Pediatr Ophthalmol Strabismus* 19: 320-325.

2347. Zlatkin MB, Lander PH, Begin LR, Hadjipavlou A (1985). Soft-tissue chondromas. *AJR Am J Roentgenol* 144: 1263-1267.

2348. Zoubek A, Ladenstein R, Windhager R, Amann G, Fischmeister G, Kager L, Jugovic D, Ambros PF, Gadner H, Kovar H (1998). Predictive potential of testing for bone marrow involvement in Ewing tumor patients by RT-PCR: a preliminary evaluation. *Int J Cancer* 79: 56-60.

2349. Zu Y, Perle MA, Yan Z, Liu J, Kumar A, Waisman J (2001). Chromosomal abnormalities and p53 gene mutation in a cardiac angiosarcoma. *Appl Immunohistochem Mol Morphol* 9: 24-28.

2350. Zucman J, Delattre O, Desmaze C, Epstein AL, Stenman G, Speleman F, Fletchers CD, Aurias A, Thomas G (1993). EWS and ATF-1 gene fusion induced by t(12;22) translocation in malignant melanoma of soft parts. *Nat Genet* 4: 341-345.

2351. Zucman J, Melot T, Desmaze C, Ghysdael J, Plougastel B, Peter M, Zucker JM, Triche TJ, Sheer D, Turc-Carel C, Ambros P, Combaret V, Lenoir GM, Aurias A, Thomas G, Delattre O (1993). Combinatorial generation of variable fusion proteins in the Ewing family of tumours. *EMBO J* 12: 4481-4487.

2352. Zukerberg LR, Nickoloff BJ, Weiss SW (1993). Kaposiform hemangioendothelioma of infancy and childhood. An aggressive neoplasm associated with Kasabach-Merritt syndrome and lymphangiomatosis. *Am J Surg Pathol* 17: 321-328.

2353. Zura RD, Minasi JS, Kahler DM (1999). Tumor-induced osteomalacia and symptomatic looser zones secondary to mesenchymal chondrosarcoma. *J Surg Oncol* 71: 58-62.

Subject index